PRAISE FOR
CARING FOR THE MIND

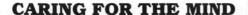

"The Haleses provide, in readable form, more information than most nonpsychiatric physicians have on these topics. . . . A treasure house . . . This title has no equal in breadth, depth, or timeliness."
—*Library Journal*

"This wonderful book will give people suffering from mental illnesses the knowledge that they need. It is packed with useful information about diagnosis, mechanisms, and treatment. Armed with this knowledge, they should be better empowered to cope with their symptoms, obtain quality treatment, and reduce misunderstanding and stigmatization."
—Nancy C. Andreasen, M.D., Ph.D.
Editor, *American Journal of Psychiatry*

"An informative and comprehensive book for everybody. Dianne and Robert Hales have met the thirst for knowledge in a clearly written, informative, and helpful guide. All who care about mental health and psychiatric illness will find it an invaluable resource."
—Herbert Pardes, M.D.
Dean and Chairman of Psychiatry, College of Physicians & Surgeons of Columbia University
Former Director, National Institute of Mental Health

"An absolute treasure house of invaluable information and practical guidance about every aspect of mental health. *Caring for the Mind* is the most valuable resource available today as a guide to the healing process."
—Joan Borysenko, Ph.D.
Author of *Minding the Body, Mending the Mind*

"The message Dianne and Robert Hales deliver is one of hope, engendered by giving readers the information and the tools they need to understand mental illness and to choose the most effective remedies available. This is a unique medical resource: clear enough to be accessible to the general public, authoritative enough to win the respect of professionals."
—H. Keith H. Brodie, M.D.
President Emeritus and James B. Duke Professor of Psychiatry, Duke University
Past President, American Psychiatric Association

Caring for the Mind

THE COMPREHENSIVE GUIDE TO MENTAL HEALTH

by Dianne Hales and Robert E. Hales, M.D.

Introduction by Allen Frances, M.D.

Bantam Books

NEW YORK • TORONTO • LONDON • SYDNEY • AUCKLAND

Readers are advised that the information in this book is not meant, and should not be used, to substitute for the advice and recommendations of a health professional. The authors believe that the more fully informed persons are about problems that may affect them or those close to them, the more they will be able to cope with such problems. Nonetheless, while accurate information and self-help strategies can play a significant part in living a satisfying and rewarding life, it is essential to remember that knowledge in this field is constantly evolving, and that mental disorders, like physical ones, are complex conditions that often require professional counseling and treatment.

The tables of diagnostic criteria for mental disorders have been adapted from American Psychiatric Association: *Diagnostic and Statistical Manual of Mental Disorders, Fourth Edition*, Washington, D.C., American Psychiatric Association, 1994, and are used with permission.

CARING FOR THE MIND:
The Comprehensive Guide to Mental Health
A Bantam Book
Bantam hardcover edition / May 1995
Bantam trade paperback edition / June 1996

Book produced by Current Medical Directions, Inc.
Library of Congress Card Number 92-40165

ISBN: 0-553-37511-3

Published simultaneously in the United States and Canada

Bantam Books are published by Bantam Books, a division of Bantam Doubleday Dell Publishing Group, Inc. Its trademark, consisting of the words "Bantam Books" and the portrayal of a rooster, is Registered in U.S. Patent and Trademark Office and in other countries. Marca Registrada. Bantam Books, 1540 Broadway, New York, New York 10036.

PRINTED IN THE UNITED STATES OF AMERICA
0 9 8 7 6 5 4 3 2 1

To Julia, our daughter and our delight, with love

Acknowledgments

Over the course of the five years that went into the making of *Caring for the Mind*, many people contributed in many different ways. We are grateful to them all, especially those who shared with us their personal stories and the mental health professionals and advocates who provided insight and inspiration as we developed this book.

The members of our editorial board—Charles Connor, M.D., Mary De May, M.D., Steven Dubovsky, M.D., Charles C. Engel, M.D., Allen Frances, M.D., Susan Friedland, M.D., T.B. Ghosh, M.D., Angela Lee, M.D., Hanna Levenson, Ph.D., John Morihisa, M.D., Thomas Neylan, M.D., Katharine A. Phillips, M.D., Jerilyn Ross, L.I.C.S.W., Chester Schmidt, M.D., David Spiegel, M.D., Michael Wise, M.D., and Stuart Yudofsky, M.D.—provided invaluable help and guidance. We are grateful for their time, effort, and expertise.

The leaders of many mental health advocacy and support groups have been extremely helpful. We offer special thanks to Laurie Flynn of the National Alliance for the Mentally Ill, Susan Dime-Meenan of the National Depressive and Manic-Depressive Association, Connie Lieber of the National Alliance for Research on Schizophrenia and Depression, and Jerilyn Ross of the Anxiety Disorders Association of America.

We are immensely thankful to our agent, Joy Harris, and our indefatigable editor, Ann Harris, whose commitment and highest standards of professionalism greatly enhanced the quality of *Caring for the Mind*. We also are grateful to Azrael Simone, Rhonda Anderson, Alexis Rubin, and Lynsey Rubin for their involvement in the research and preparation of this book. We owe a special debt to Jodie Corngold for her invaluable help when we needed her most.

Some interviews and other parts of this book have appeared in materials written by the authors for various publications, including *Parade, McCall's, Working Mother, Good Housekeeping, Woman's Day, American Health,* and *Invitation to Health.*

Contents

Introduction

Caring for the Mind is an important contribution to the mental health of patients and the peace of mind of their families. Perhaps the best way to combat mental illness is to become informed about its recognition, diagnosis, and treatment. As a psychiatrist, I have become convinced that education about mental disorders may be the single most important element in recovery. Again and again, I have found that patients improve a great deal simply by understanding what is happening to them and what treatments are available. Moreover, family members can provide much better help and support when they too understand what is happening.

This book provides just the right kind of education for consumers of mental health services and their families. It is extraordinarily comprehensive in its coverage of all the major mental disorders, of the special mental health needs and problems of children and the elderly, of the role of the family and of advocacy groups, and of the entire range of effective treatments.

This is an exciting time for the mental health field. We now have a much greater understanding of the various mental disorders and their causes. We have a more precise and scientific system for identifying these disorders, and we can draw on a host of new pharmacologic agents and psychotherapies to treat them. This book makes it possible for readers to understand the discoveries that have been made and to see how they or their loved ones may benefit from the remarkable progress that has occurred and the new advances that are on the horizon.

For the many millions of people whose lives are touched by mental disorders in themselves or in those close to them, *Caring for the Mind* offers help and hope. The writing style is clear, direct, and engaging. The symptom checklists featured in many chapters provide a practical tool for self-assessment. The diagnostic criteria drawn from the *Diagnostic and Statistical Manual of Mental Disorders, Fourth Edition (DSM-IV)*, ensure that readers have access to the very latest information about the major mental disorders. The descriptions of these disorders are fresh and incisive, and the case histories put a human face on mental illness.

Despite our progress, however, we who are mental health professionals and those whom we serve are faced with a new and very worrisome challenge. In an effort to lower costs and limit health care expenditures, mental health benefits have been greatly reduced. Many managed care plans have erected barriers to needed care rather than providing the means necessary to obtain it. As a result, many people are suffering needlessly, the costs in lost productivity are sizable and increasing, and the indirect costs to everyone in our society are great. Perhaps more than ever before, the public at large, as well as all of those involved in providing mental health services to those who need them, must remain aware that mental health is an integral, essential component of total health. They need to be able to recognize the signs of mental disorders, to know when to seek help, and to determine whether a treatment is appropriate and effective. *Caring for the Mind* can and will be of great assistance in achieving this.

I recommend this timely, authoritative, and insightful book as a reference you can use with confidence for problems that affect you and those close to you, and as a source of information and enlightenment now and for years to come.

ALLEN J. FRANCES, M.D.
Chairperson, Task Force on DSM-IV
Professor and Chairman, Department of Psychiatry
Duke University Medical Center

How to
Use this Book

This book represents the state of the art and the science of caring for the mind. Its purpose is to spread the good news about the advances that have been made in mental health care and to provide information readers can use to understand themselves better, to know when to seek help for themselves or loved ones, and to ensure that they receive the best and most appropriate care.

Caring for the Mind aims to inform, educate, illuminate, and reassure readers. While it cannot and should not take the place of a therapeutic relationship with a mental health professional, we hope that it will enrich such relationships by stimulating open and honest discussion. While it cannot take away the pain that mental illness may cause for individuals and their families, we hope that it will prevent the suffering bred of misunderstanding. And while it may not bring an end to the problems that affect so many, we hope that, at the least, it can serve as the beginning of the journey toward recovery and mental health. Among the ways in which this book may prove helpful are the following:

Recognizing problems. Each chapter in Part II begins with a straightforward checklist of symptoms. By reading through these lists, readers can get a sense of what may be wrong with them or someone close to them. In addition, Chapter 4, Is Something Wrong?, provides guidance on defining mental health and illness and dealing with problems of everyday living, as opposed to actual mental disorders.

Understanding specific disorders. Each chapter in Part II provides basic facts on specific disorders, including how common each one is and its types or stages. To convey the personal, human dimension of mental illness, we have included a subsection on how each disorder feels. We hope that this unique perspective will give readers a sense of the daily reality of living with a particular problem. The "personal voices" or case histories in the book should provide further insight.

In all instances, the names and identifying details for the individuals whose experiences are depicted throughout the book, which have been drawn from our clinical and journalistic experiences, have been changed to preserve their privacy.

Knowing when to seek help. Each chapter in Part II provides guidance on seeking help, including specific questions to ask yourself or a loved one. We also describe the risks and complications that can occur if a disorder is not treated. Chapter 4 offers advice on finding a therapist, while the Resource Directory at the back of the book list organizations, support groups, and other places to turn for more information and help.

Getting appropriate treatment. Each chapter provides descriptions of the various approaches that have proven effective in specific disorders, including the appropriate forms of psychotherapy and types of medication. Part IV, Healing the Mind, provides an in-depth look at talking therapies, psychiatric drugs, and self-help strategies.

Understanding those with a mental disorder. Mental disorders touch the lives, not only of those affected by them, but of their family, friends, and co-workers. Each chapter in Part II discusses the impact of specific disorders on relationships. In addition, Chapter 30, When Someone You Love Has a Mental Disorder, addresses the issues and concerns of partners, parents, children, and siblings.

Exploring special concerns and needs. Part III deals with key issues related to mental health, including its relationship to physical well-being, suicidal behavior, and violence. In addition, we have targeted chapters to two very special groups: children and the elderly. Both of these chapters provide guidance on recognizing problems, understanding their nature, and seeking effective treatment.

Caring for the Mind

THE COMPREHENSIVE GUIDE TO MENTAL HEALTH

PART I

A New Era in Mental Health

1

New Understanding, New Treatments, New Hope

A once-exuberant woman, drained of hope, wakes before dawn and tearfully waits for the sun. A teenager begins to hear voices that mock and criticize him. A lawyer finds herself gasping desperately for breath whenever she steps into an elevator. Every night a college student binges on chips and cookies and then forces herself to vomit. A businessman, so wired that he hardly sleeps, pours his company's cash reserves into a farfetched scheme that he's sure will make millions. A year after a brutal attack, a teacher is haunted by horrifying flashbacks. A doting grandfather bursts into sudden rages and curses at everyone around him.

These individuals are hardly unusual. More than one in every four Americans suffer from an emotional or behavioral problem so severe that it interferes with their ability to keep up with their daily routines, do their jobs, care for their families, or relate to others as they once did. No one, regardless of age, gender, education, or income, is immune. According to the National Institute of Mental Health's (NIMH) landmark Epidemiologic Catchment Area (ECA) survey, about 27 million adults and 7.5 million children in the United States have a diagnosable mental disorder—more than the combined total of individuals with cancer, heart disease, and lung disorders. In 1994 the National Comorbidity Survey found that mental illness is more common than had been thought. Almost half of those surveyed reported having at least one mental disorder over the course of their lifetimes; almost 30 percent had

3

been troubled by a disorder in the previous twelve months. According to some reports, the number of troubled children has increased to as many as 11 to 14 million youngsters.

The most surprising—and sad—fact is not that so many people are troubled but that so few get help. According to NIMH statistics, seven in every ten Americans with a mental disorder do not receive any treatment. These individuals may never realize why they are no longer able to function the way they once did or why their lives have become difficult and joyless. They may try to tell themselves that they are simply overworked or stressed out. Even when they suspect that something more serious is wrong, many hate to admit, even to themselves, that they have a problem. They blame themselves, as though becoming anxious or depressed or feeling out of control is somehow their fault in a way that diabetes or arthritis could never be. Often they fear that no matter where they might turn, no one will be able to help them. Nothing could be further from the truth.

During the last two decades the mental health field has undergone a quiet but profound revolution that has produced new forms of help and new reasons for hope. We now have a much better understanding of how the mind and the brain work, what can go wrong, and why. We know more about the complexity and variety of problems that can develop. We have identified patterns of vulnerability and the biological components of many mental illnesses. And we have an impressive collection of highly specific, carefully

HOW COMMON ARE MENTAL DISORDERS?

DISORDER	IN A GIVEN YEAR (% affected)	AT SOME POINT IN LIFE (% affected)
Anxiety disorders (panic disorder, agoraphobia, social phobia, specific phobia, generalized anxiety disorder)	17.2	24.9
Depressive disorders (major depression, manic depression, dysthymia)	11.3	19.3
Alcohol dependence or abuse	9.7	23.5
Drug dependence or abuse	3.6	11.9
Any mental disorder	29.5	48.0

Source: Kessler R., et al. Lifetime and 12-month prevalence of DSM-III-R psychiatric disorders in the United States. *Archives of General Psychiatry*, vol. 51, January, 1994.

tested, and scientifically proven therapies that can help most of those who seek treatment.

The new psychiatry

Thirty years ago a young girl in Michigan, whom we'll call Mary, developed some peculiar habits. Before going to bed at night she would arrange her shoes, teddy bears, dolls, and other toys with military precision in lines that had to be absolutely the same, absolutely perfect. During the day she would wash her hands ten or twelve times, often scrubbing so hard that they became raw and bloody. Although Mary was bright, perhaps even gifted, she did poorly at school because she would dot and redot every *i*, cross and recross every *t*, and check and recheck every word on every page to make sure it was aligned properly. Her rituals consumed so much time that she became isolated from other children and her own family.

Mary's worried parents brought her to the nearest university medical center, where doctors recommended hospitalization in a psychiatric institution. During her hospitalization she was allowed no contact with her family. She received no medication and was treated no differently from youngsters who were severely retarded or disturbed. When she returned home after two years, she discovered a strange and unwelcoming world. Her parents, who had been forced to pay all her bills out of pocket, had rented her room to a boarder. The other children in the neighborhood teased her mercilessly about having been "in the loony bin."

A few years ago, when Mary was a graduate student, the odd habits of her childhood returned and began to interfere with her work. She finally made the decision to see a psychiatrist, despite her fear that she would be once again locked up in a mental institution, cut off from everyone and everything she held dear.

But this time was different. In her childhood, psychiatry had no specific treatment for what had troubled Mary. In the decades since then, a "new" psychiatry, more research-based and more grounded in biology, had identified her problem as obsessive-compulsive disorder (OCD), which produces a particular form of often disabling anxiety and affects as many as 4 million Americans. Today, highly effective treatments enable most people with OCD to live essentially normal lives. Mary is now one of them.

As Mary's story illustrates, mental health care has entered a new and exciting era. During the last two decades, thanks to hundreds of rigorous studies, caring for the mind has become a science as well as an art. Through sophisticated psychotherapy, targeted pharmacotherapy (use of medications), or a combination of both, psychiatry has made enormous progress in overcoming disorders of the mind.

Because of large-scale epidemiological research, problems that were long unknown or overlooked, such as OCD, panic disorder, and social phobia (all forms of anxiety that cause different symptoms and respond to different treatments), have been recognized and studied. Because of a new symptom-based method for classifying serious disorders, diagnoses have become more precise and consistent. Because of a new consensus about what works and what doesn't, therapy is increasingly being tailored to meet each individual's problems and needs.

Treatments themselves have also changed. New psychiatric drugs have given the chance for a full and gratifying life back to many people suffering from anxiety disorders, depression, dementias, schizophrenia, and other problems. The talking therapies have been refined and streamlined to work effectively, not only with individuals but also with couples, families, and groups. Mental health professionals have recognized and addressed the special needs of children and of the elderly. And because of greater understanding about which treatments or combination of treatments work best for which problems, more people are not only getting better, they are staying well.

"The sun has shone in," observes Allen Frances, M.D., chairman of the Department of Psychiatry at Duke University. "We've been enlightened by the availability of new facts and insight. The bottom line is that we can help virtually everyone. It may take a series of treatments and a systematic and patient effort by both the individual and the clinician, but almost always those who seek treatment get better."

The last frontier

Traditionally, mental health professionals viewed the unconscious as the key to all mental illness. Yet Sigmund Freud, the pioneer explorer of the mind, predicted that some revelations might come only with greater understanding of the brain. "The deficiencies in our description [of the mind]," he wrote in 1920, "would probably vanish if we were already in a position to replace the psychological terms by physiological or chemical ones."

That is exactly what a new generation of brain explorers, called *neuropsychiatrists*, is doing. Because of discoveries made during the last ten years, they now can analyze behavior not only in psychological terms but also at the molecular level. Using dazzling new tools to study the brain at work, neuropsychiatrists have been able to correlate the symptoms of many mental disorders with specific changes in brain chemistry and activity. They are coming closer to identifying the genes that may transmit vulnerability to mental illnesses in which heritability may be a factor. Ultimately, they may be able to identify the biochemical defects associated with various mental disorders. With this knowledge, prevention or correction of these disorders may become possible.

Not even mental health professionals anticipated so much progress so quickly. "When the first report of CT [computed tomography] abnormalities in schizophrenia was published in 1976, most members of the psychiatric community predicted it would never be replicated," notes Nancy Andreasen, M.D., professor of psychiatry at the University of Iowa and a leader in brain research. "In fact, the finding of structural brain abnormalities in schizophrenia is now perhaps the most widely replicated finding in biological psychiatry."

New brain-imaging techniques offer even greater potential for understanding the mechanisms of mental illness. "We can see things that we simply could not see before," says Andreasen. "The contemporary psychiatrist is in a position much like that of an orthopedist or cardiologist at the time X-rays were invented. We now have the tools to explore, evaluate, and measure the functions and dysfunctions of the brain."

A common language

In 1840, in the first official attempt to gather information about mental illness in the United States, the Census Bureau recorded the frequency of a single category: idiocy/insanity. By the beginning of the twentieth century, early psychiatrists had identified more than a dozen mental illnesses. For decades, however, American psychiatry viewed mental illnesses, as psychiatrist Karl Menninger, M.D., put it, "as being essentially the same in quality, although differing quantitatively and in external appearance." This view has since given way to a search for greater specificity and precision in both diagnosis and treatment.

One of the major advances in this quest came in 1980, not in the form of a theory, technique, drug, or doctrine, but in a book: the third edition of the American Psychiatric Association's *Diagnostic and Statistical Manual of Mental Disorders*. The *DSM-III*, as it is commonly called, a revised edition published in 1987, and a completely overhauled fourth edition, the *DSM-IV*, published in 1994, spell out explicit characteristics, or diagnostic criteria, for almost three hundred disorders. Rather than focusing on the *why*s of mental illness, the *DSM* emphasizes the *what*s—the specific signs and symptoms that characterize various disorders.

As a result, even when mental health professionals disagree about, or do not know the possible causes of, a disorder, they can agree on how it manifests itself and can assess treatments most likely to bring about recovery.

The *DSM* has given mental health professions a common language. Psychology, psychiatry, and social work trainees, along with medical and nursing students, use the *DSM* as a textbook. Insurance companies base reimbursements on it. Research agencies and foundations fund investigations according to its criteria. Yet despite its acceptance as the clinical "bible" of these professions, the *DSM* remains controversial.

Some critics charge that the *DSM* transforms human foibles, such as excessive coffee consumption, into potential mental disorders (in this case, caffeine dependency). Others quibble with its arbitrary distinctions, such as requiring that an individual have no less than five of fourteen possible symptoms for a particular diagnosis to be made. Still others contend that the *DSM* is too specific, the ultimate triumph of "splitters," who prefer many categories based on small differences, over "lumpers," who group things together on the basis of loosely defined similarities.

Despite such criticisms, the *DSM* has had an enormous impact on mental health care. Because of its widespread use, clinicians today agree on diagnoses approximately 80 percent of the time, far more frequently than in the past. "There never will be a totally precise way of drawing the border between mental health and mental illness," says Allen Frances, M.D., head of the task force that created the *DSM-IV*. "But this is the most scientific, carefully tested system in the history of the field."

New options for treatment

The ancient Greeks pushed depressed individuals from the tops of cliffs into the sea to shock them out of their despair. In the Middle Ages, priests used exorcism to cast out the "demons" of madness. With the dawn of modern psychiatry, treatments were developed that were more humane but not necessarily more helpful. Only in recent years have mental health professionals been able to offer a wide range of therapies—more numerous, more varied, and more precisely targeted than ever before—that have proved effective against common and often crippling disorders.

New psychiatric medications are correcting chemical imbalances in the brain with far fewer side effects than older drugs. New psychotherapies are using cognitive, interpersonal, behavioral, and other techniques, to produce lasting benefits within weeks or months. The combination of biological and psychological treatments—an approach that, not very long ago, many doubted would ever work—has proved even more helpful for many individuals than either psychotherapy or medication alone.

Most importantly, there now is scientific proof that mental health care can and does help. According to the National Mental Health Advisory Council and the American Psychiatric Association, treatments for severe mental illnesses, such as major depression, bipolar (manic-depressive) illness, panic disorder, and schizophrenia, are as effective or more effective than those available in other branches of medicine, including surgery. Treatments tailored to the individual's particular condition and needs can help 80 to 90 percent of those who suffer from depression and bipolar disorder and 70 to 80 percent of those with panic disorder. More than 60 percent of those with schizophrenia can be relieved of acute symptoms with proper therapy, and advances in medication are pushing this percentage ever higher.

"The advances have been remarkable," observes former NIMH director Herbert Pardes, M.D., vice-president for Health Sciences, dean of Medicine, and chairman of the Department of Psychiatry at Columbia University. "We can now offer therapies that have a better chance of success than treatments in many other areas of medicine."

A new partnership

Just as scientific and therapeutic advances have revolutionized mental health care, changes in attitude have transformed the perspectives of those with mental disorders. "The discoveries about the biological nature of mental illness have lifted the oppressive weight of shame that so often has been part of the diagnosis of mental illness," says Laurie Flynn, executive director of the National Alliance for the Mentally Ill (NAMI), one of the oldest mental health advocacy groups. "They've given individuals a new lease on self-esteem and empowered them to accept illness and seek medical treatment because they now have a different way of looking at themselves and their possible futures."

Providers and consumers of mental health services have joined together to work toward common goals: unraveling the causes of mental disorders, improving treatments, and ultimately finding cures. "Science holds the key," says Flynn. "Even if we can't cure, as we learn more and translate research findings into more effective therapies, we can find ways to help more people overcome."

In 1986, several advocacy groups—NAMI, the National Mental Health Association, the National Depressive and Manic-Depressive

Association, and the Schizophrenia Research Foundation—formed the National Alliance for Research on Schizophrenia and Depression (NARSAD), which has contributed more than $20 million to psychiatric research. Most of this funding has come from families whose lives have been touched by mental illness.

"They are expressing their hope by supporting research," says Connie Lieber, NARSAD's president. "They believe there will be cures soon, there will be better medications soon. They know that progress has been made and that as more is done to find better treatments, more people can have productive lives."

The promise of prevention

The revolution that has brought so much excitement and hope to the mental health field is far from over. The coming years will undoubtedly yield new insights, advances, medications, therapies. However, the best hope lies in prevention. Both the federal government and advocacy groups, such as NAMI and the National Mental Health Association, are committed to promoting mental health and preventing mental disorders.

Mental health professionals are already taking steps toward these goals. They are teaching problem-solving skills to preschoolers whose backgrounds place them at risk for later behavioral problems. They are teaching coping skills to individuals who have recently lost their jobs, boosting their chances for re-employment. They are providing prenatal care and education about parenting skills to poor, pregnant, unmarried teenagers. They are helping children of divorcing parents adjust to the changes in their families. They are rushing to the scene of disasters to provide immediate intervention for the survivors. Such efforts are paying off in terms of reduced psychological distress, enhanced self-esteem, better social skills, and a reduced risk for long-term problems.

For individuals with mental disorders, the lines between prevention and treatment have blurred. In the past, those with manic-depressive illness typically spent one-half of their adult lives disabled, often in psychiatric hospitals. Thanks to medication that prevents debilitating mood swings, 75 to 80 percent now live essentially normal lives, saving the U.S. economy more than $40 billion since 1970. Preventing recurrences has also become increasingly important in major depression. As recent studies have shown, as many as 80 percent of those who become depressed experience a recurrence within ten years and face increased risk of job loss, marital breakups, and suicide. Maintenance treatment (described in Chapter 5) can prevent these terrible problems and keep individuals well.

The challenges that remain

Despite the progress that has been made, mental disorders continue to take an enormous toll on individuals, families, and society as a whole. If untreated—and, as noted, this is more often the case than not—they can forever alter a life course, destroy dreams, shatter relationships. Each year 29,000 Americans, most with treatable forms of mental illness, take their own lives. Moreover, the financial burden of mental disorders is staggering. The depressive disorders alone, both treated and untreated, cost the United States almost $44 billion a year, according to researchers from the Massachusetts Institute of Technology (MIT) and the Analysis Group of Boston. Direct costs, including medication and psychotherapy, come to about $12 billion, and indirect costs, such as decreased productivity and work absenteeism, total $23.8 billion annually. According to the National Foundation for Brain Research, about one in every seven dollars spent on health care goes toward treatment of disorders of the brain and nervous system, including psychiatric disorders. The mentally ill make up the largest single group of disabled persons in the nation and account for one-fourth of all recipients of federal disability funds.

It doesn't have to be this way. We now know, on the basis of solid scientific evidence, that treating mental disorders not only relieves suffering but pays huge dividends. Those who receive needed treatment use fewer health services, require shorter hospital stays for medical problems, and function more productively throughout their lives. Yet millions of Americans suffer needlessly simply because they do not seek help.

"Something is terribly wrong," the National Advisory Mental Health Council has reported to Congress. "The unfortunate truth is that most Americans do not yet understand that mental illness is a disease, and like heart disease or diabetes, it can be effectively treated." Moreover, many feel too ashamed to admit that they have a problem and to get help. In a nationwide poll of 2,503 men and women conducted for *Parade* magazine, more than two-thirds of the respondents said that there is a stigma attached to mental illness. One in ten said that the fear of what other people would say would keep them from seeking help if they had a mental or emotional problem.

Nevertheless, public attitudes are changing. "If you looked at epidemiological figures going back fifteen years, it used to be that one-third to two-thirds of people who realized that they had a problem wouldn't come for help," observes psychiatrist Pardes. "Now you're talking about a tenth. That's a big improvement."

The stigma surrounding mental illness should diminish even further as the good news about treatment successes spreads. There seems to be increasing openness about the subject. When a *Parade* magazine poll in 1993 invited readers to respond to several questions about mental illness and the mentally ill, more than 11,500 people phoned in their responses. Almost all (95 percent) said they believed that those with mental disorders can function normally with proper treatment, and more than seven out of ten (74 percent) said mental illnesses can be cured.

"There definitely is a growing sense of optimism about mental illness," says NAMI's Flynn, noting the *Parade* survey findings, "and I really believe that it is warranted. People are aware that mental illnesses are not hopeless diseases. We may not have cures yet, but for the vast majority of individuals, we have enormously effective treatments. And we have every reason to hope for even greater progress in the future."

2

The Final Frontier

It has been called the last and the greatest biological frontier, more complex and more challenging than anything else in the entire universe. The brain represents the sum of human knowledge, emotion, memory, and experience. It enables us to think and talk, to remember and anticipate, to work and play, to express our needs and control our desires. Some describe the spongy mass of gray and white matter within the skull as an enlightened machine that combines the analytic ability of a computer, the organizational skills of a filing system, and the communications network of a telephone switchboard. Yet no machine or invention, however sophisticated, can crack a joke, dream of daffodils, believe in a hereafter, or fall in love.

The brain has intrigued scientists for centuries, but only recently have its explorers made dramatic progress in unraveling its mysteries. Leaders in neuropsychiatry, the field that brings together the study of the brain and the mind, note that 95 percent of what is known about brain anatomy, chemistry, and physiology has been learned during the last decade. These discoveries have reshaped our understanding of the organ that is central to our identity and well-being, and have fostered great hope for more effective therapies for the more than one thousand disorders, psychiatric and neurological, that affect the brain and the nervous system.

There is so much scientific excitement centering on exploration of the brain that mental health professionals worry that the powers and potential of the mind will be neglected. In fact, the study of the brain is not only changing our understanding of mental illness but is challenging the conventional view that the mind and brain are completely distinct from each other. We are learning that these two aspects of consciousness work as one and that mental experiences affect brain processes, and vice versa. The more we discover about the molecular mysteries of the brain, about the energy that causes tiny clumps of cells to make an idea blossom or a feeling form, the more we may come to understand about how we think, learn, create, communicate—in essence, how the mind does all the things that make human beings unique.

Inside the brain

Each human brain contains hundreds of billions of nerve cells, or *neurons*, and support and scavenger cells, called *glia*. Most are present at birth, when the brain weighs less than a pound. The brain grows rapidly and over the first six years of life—the period during which we acquire more knowledge more rapidly than ever again—reaches its full weight of about three pounds. Thereafter, over the course of time, brain weight decreases gradually (about 10 percent in a normal lifetime) as neurons die.

The neurons are the basic working units of the brain. Like snowflakes, no two are exactly the same. Each consists of a cell body containing the nucleus; a long fiber called the *axon*, which can range from less than an inch to several feet in length; an axon terminal, or ending; and multiple branching fibers called *dendrites*. The glia assist in the growth of neurons, speed up the transmission of nerve impulses, and engulf and digest damaged neurons.

The brain is the master control center for the body, constantly receiving information from the senses and relaying messages to various parts of the body. Some of these messages travel through the spinal cord, which extends from the neck down about two-thirds of the length of the spine.

Historically, scientists have focused on the anatomy and structures of the brain in their attempts to understand how it functions and why it sometimes malfunctions. That emphasis has now changed, and modern neuropsychiatrists have shifted much of their attention to biochemical processes within the brain, particularly those involved in communication between neurons.

BASIC ANATOMY OF THE BRAIN

The three major parts of the brain are the *cerebrum*, the *cerebellum*, and the *brainstem*. The cerebrum, which accounts for about

85 percent of the weight of the brain, is divided into two halves or hemispheres by a large groove or fissure (see the figure on page 16). Although the two hemispheres of the brain appear almost identical, they process information in different ways. The left hemisphere regulates the right side of the body; the right hemisphere regulates the left side. Connecting the hemispheres is a bridging mini-highway of nerve fibers called the *corpus callosum.*

The outer layer of the cerebrum is a quarter-inch thick, deeply grooved cap of tissue called the *cerebral cortex.* The site of the brain's higher powers, it is divided into four regions, or lobes, where the activities we think of as the basic work of the brain— thought, perception, memory, language, communication—take place.

- The *frontal lobes*, behind the forehead, control movement, behavior, and memory. The prefrontal fibers, the most forward portion, regulate inhibitions (preventing us from blurting out an inappropriate comment or acting immediately on an impulse) and allow us to think, plan, and philosophize.

- The *temporal lobes*, at the sides and lower down, are involved in hearing, speech, and various aspects of emotion and memory.

- The *parietal lobes*, in the middle, play a role in interpreting sensations and positioning the body. When we stub a toe, the pain messages travel to these lobes, which tell us that it is a toe, not a finger, that has been hurt.

- The *occipital lobes*, at the back, control vision, visual images, and reading.

Deep within the cerebrum is the *limbic system*, a ring of structures that process the entire spectrum of human emotion. Below it, the *thalamus*, which processes all the senses other than smell, relays nerve impulses from various parts of the body to appropriate areas of the cerebral cortex. The *hypothalamus*, just below the thalamus, regulates many critical activities and physiological states, including body temperature and hunger.

The cerebellum, located below the rear of the cerebrum, has two hemispheres, joined by the finger-shaped vermis. It is made up of densely packed nerve cells. Although it accounts for only one-eighth of the weight of the brain, it plays the major role in coordinating movement, balance, and posture.

At the base of the brain is the brainstem, a stalk-like structure that connects the cerebrum to the spinal cord. It consists of the *midbrain*, the *pons*, and the *medulla*, which contain centers that control breathing, blood pressure, heart rate, and other "autonomic" physiological functions that occur without conscious awareness.

AREAS OF THE BRAIN

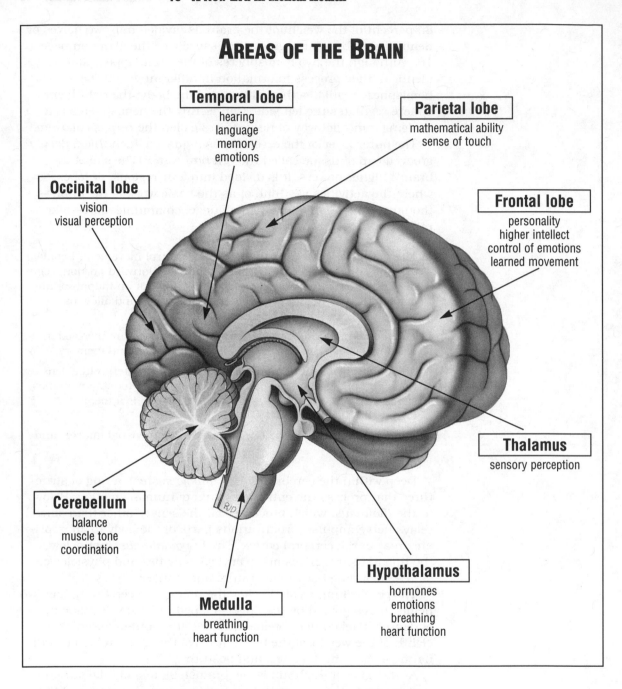

Temporal lobe
hearing
language
memory
emotions

Parietal lobe
mathematical ability
sense of touch

Occipital lobe
vision
visual perception

Frontal lobe
personality
higher intellect
control of emotions
learned movement

Thalamus
sensory perception

Cerebellum
balance
muscle tone
coordination

Hypothalamus
hormones
emotions
breathing
heart function

Medulla
breathing
heart function

COMMUNICATION WITHIN THE BRAIN

Neurons "talk" with each other by means of electrical and chemical processes. An electric charge or impulse travels along an axon to the terminal, where packets of chemicals called *neurotransmitters* are stored in *vesicles.* When released, these messenger molecules flow out of the axon terminal and cross the *synapse*, a specialized site at which the axon terminal of one neuron comes extremely close to a dendrite projecting from another neuron. On the surface of the dendrite are receptors, protein molecules designed to bind with specific neurotransmitters (see the figure on page 18). It takes only about a ten-thousandth of a second for a neurotransmitter and a receptor to come together, a union that noted neuropsychiatrist Richard Restak, M.D., author of *Receptors* and *The Brain*, has lyrically compared to an embrace between two lovers. Neurotransmitters that do not bind to receptors may remain in the synapse until they are broken down by enzymes or reabsorbed by the neuron that produced them—a process called *reuptake.*

Receptors relay a message—which can concern a wide variety of matters, from a physical signal to a thought, feeling, sensation, or behavior—from a neurotransmitter (the "first" messenger) to the rest of the neuron via chemical intermediaries known as *G-proteins* and *effectors.* A "second" messenger then triggers a cascade of chemical reactions to process the information.

A malfunction in the release of a neurotransmitter in its reuptake or elimination or in the receptors or second messengers may lead to abnormalities in thinking, feeling, or behavior. Some of the most promising research in neuropsychiatry is focusing on correcting such malfunctions. For example, the neurotransmitter *serotonin* and its receptors have been shown to affect mood, sleep, behavior, appetite, memory, learning, sexuality, and aggression, and to play a role in several mental disorders. The discovery of a possible link between low levels of serotonin and some cases of major depression has already led to the development of more precisely targeted antidepressant medications that boost serotonin to normal levels. During the next decade, neuropsychiatric research may yield a new generation of breakthrough medications for an ever-growing number of mental disorders. (Chapter 28 discusses psychiatric drugs and their effects on the brain.)

Windows on the brain

For centuries the brain remained the ultimate "black box," hidden within the skull and impossible to study in action. Just as medical scientists could not identify the mechanisms and molecules involved in infectious disease until the invention of the

NEURONAL SYNAPSE

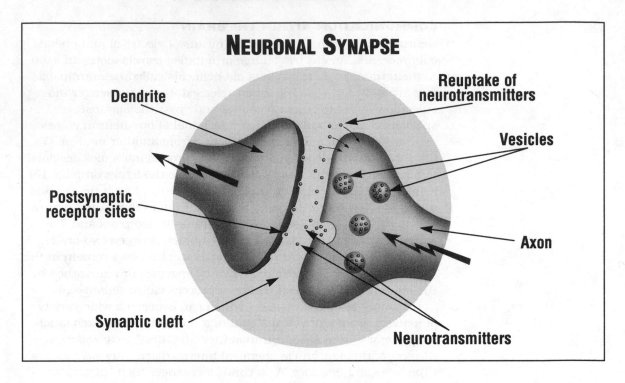

Dendrite

Reuptake of neurotransmitters

Vesicles

Postsynaptic receptor sites

Axon

Synaptic cleft

Neurotransmitters

microscope, neuropsychiatrists had to wait for tools to reveal the workings of the brain. The first was the electroencephalograph (EEG), which measures electrical signals in the brain by means of special sensors placed on the skull. For many decades, the EEG has been an invaluable tool in evaluating individuals with problems such as epilepsy and other seizure disorders.

The newest neuroimaging methods include structural techniques, which provide images of parts of the brain, and functional techniques, which study brain processes such as blood flow and glucose metabolism. In combination with powerful, high-speed computers for data processing, the neuroimaging techniques have revolutionized the study of the brain, enabling scientists to trace electrical currents and measure blood flow, study differences between the brains of people in good mental health and those with mental disorders, assess the effects of drugs on brain function, explore the interrelationship between mental activity and brain physiology, and monitor dynamic processes, such as brain development and aging.

Neuroimaging has also transformed our understanding of the biology of mental illness. In recent years, researchers have identified specific brain abnormalities in individuals with schizophrenia, Alzheimer's disease, autism and other developmental disorders, major depression, bipolar (manic-depressive) illness, panic disorder, obsessive-compulsive disorder (OCD), alcoholism, and eating disorders.

The primary structural imaging techniques are computed tomography (CT) and magnetic resonance imaging (MRI). In addition to research studies, psychiatrists may use these methods to assess patients with certain neuropsychiatric disorders, such as dementia (see Chapter 20), or patients with both neurological and psychiatric symptoms.

CT, the oldest of the newer imaging technologies, uses X-rays enhanced by computer processing to produce cross-sectional horizontal images of brain tissue and the surrounding cerebrospinal fluid (CSF). MRI, which uses magnetic forces rather than X-rays to generate images, is in many ways more powerful than CT and can produce clearer, more detailed images of smaller structures or those obscured by bone. With MRIs and computers, scientists can construct two- and three-dimensional images of portions of the brain and can distinguish structures as small as a millimeter.

Functional neuroimaging techniques, used primarily in neuropsychiatry research, study the brain at work by measuring cerebral blood flow. They trace small amounts of radioactive material, injected into the bloodstream, as it travels to a particular part of the brain. Regional cerebral blood flow (rCBF) is a reflection of the rate of glucose metabolism in various brain areas. Glucose is the brain's "fuel"; low levels of glucose utilization, visualized by means of these neuroimaging techniques, indicate low levels of brain activity. The most sophisticated method is positron emission tomography (PET), which monitors metabolic processes in the brain and produces clear, high-resolution, minute-to-minute images. Single-photon emission tomography (SPECT) is more widely used than PET, largely because it requires simpler imaging equipment that is available at most major medical centers.

On the horizon are faster, more sophisticated imaging techniques, such as echo-planar molecular MRI, which can capture changes in metabolism in the brain every 25 milliseconds, and SQUID (superconducting quantum interference device), which senses tiny changes in the magnetic fields produced by the electrical activity of neurons.

Genetics and mental illness

Mental health professionals have long noted that certain disorders, such as schizophrenia, alcoholism, major depression, and bipolar illness, appear to run in families. However, only in the last few years have advances in medical genetics—the study of inheritance—made it possible to start sorting out the influences of nature and nurture. Although the specific genes responsible for particular disorders remain elusive, epidemiological studies have shown that heredity plays a role in several common mental disorders.

The risk for an inherited susceptibility or predisposition to a mental disorder is highest in identical twins (who have the same genes), somewhat lower in fraternal twins (who have only half their genes in common), and lower still in first-degree relatives (such as siblings) of those with the disorder, although higher than for someone in the general population. (Genetic vulnerability to specific disorders is discussed in the chapters on these disorders in Part II of this book.)

Over the coming decades molecular biologists, who have been working to map the entire human complement of genes, called the *genome*, hope to trace vulnerability to particular mental disorders to specific strands of DNA. If they succeed in pinpointing the gene or genes responsible, tests can be developed to identify carriers of the genes. Genetic counseling could then provide these individuals with precise information about their risks for transmitting the disorder to their children and about the possibility of early intervention and correction—perhaps, someday, by altering or replacing the abnormal genes.

The promise of neuropsychiatry

The workings of the brain, neuroimaging techniques, and the genetics of mental illness are key aspects of neuropsychiatry, the medical subspecialty dedicated to the intricate relationships between the brain and the mind and between mental processes and physical functioning.

Neuropsychiatry first emerged as a discipline in the mid-1800s, a time when intense scientific interest focused on the brain. However, for much of the time thereafter, including most of this century, neuropsychiatry was eclipsed by psychoanalytic approaches to assessment and treatment of problems of the mind. The recent discoveries about the biology of mental illness have rekindled interest in neuropsychiatry and have made it one of the most exciting frontiers in all of medicine.

For those whose lives are touched by mental disorders, neuropsychiatry offers new hope for overcoming problems of the mind and brain. It also lifts the cruel burden of stigma and shame long attached to psychiatric disorders. For too many years, theorists blamed troubled individuals or their families for somehow causing mental illness, as when, for example, they contended that manipulative mothers—termed *schizophrenogenic*—were responsible for causing schizophrenia. Neuropsychiatry proved them wrong. Thanks to advances in neuroimaging and genetics, we now know beyond any doubt that schizophrenia is a biological disease characterized by abnormalities in brain structure and functioning.

"Neuropsychiatry places the focus where it belongs: on the prevention, early detection, and effective treatment of illnesses that can be disabling and deadly," says Stuart Yudofsky, M.D., chairman of the Department of Psychiatry at Baylor College of Medicine and editor of *The Journal of Neuropsychiatry.* "The millions of individuals with neuropsychiatric disorders deserve no less."

Silent No More

In August of 1982, at the age of twenty-seven, Susan Dime-Meenan of Chicago experienced the most important, defining moment of her life. "My husband committed me, his bride of two months, to a locked psychiatric ward. I have never fully thanked or forgiven him. And I've never forgotten how frightened I was as I watched the man I loved leave me, casting me off behind closed doors."

As horrible and horrifying as that experience was, it did provide Susan with something she had yearned for ever since she was a young child: a name for what was wrong with her. "I also have never fully thanked or forgiven the psychiatrist who came to the unit and told me I had bipolar illness [manic depression]. But I remember that, despite how scared I was, I was so relieved to think that at last someone might be able to help me."

Ever since she was a little girl growing up in Chicago, Susan had felt different, but no one could explain why she was plagued with crushing migraine headaches, uncontrollable nosebleeds, or bouts of deep sadness. By the time she was seventeen she had undergone seven exploratory operations.

"I was told that I might have neurological problems, gynecological problems, endocrine problems, a blood disease, a brain tumor," Susan recalls. "I saw every type of doctor except a psychiatrist. No one ever suspected that I might have a mental disorder. Yet I remember being a teenager and thinking that the desolation was never going to end, that I was never going to live to be older than forty, that the doctors eventually were going to find something terrible wrong with me. And somehow I felt that it had to be my fault, that I must be bad. I kept wondering, 'What did I do to cause this?'"

After high school, Susan went to court-reporting school and specialized in aviation litigation. At the age of twenty-three she opened her own court-reporting business, which became very successful. "On the surface, everything appeared wonderful," she recalls. "I lived in a beautiful high rise in Chicago. I had a new car. I vacationed any weekend I wanted anywhere I wanted. My closet was filled with clothes. I became engaged to an aviation attorney I'd met through my work."

Susan never realized that she was entering into the state of extreme emotional intensity called *mania*. "I started making irrational decisions. I'd travel and spend money outrageously. I hardly slept, which is one of the classic symptoms of mania, but that suited me fine. I'd transcribe notes from depositions until 2:00 or 4:00 A.M., sleep a few hours, and be back at work by 8:30 A.M. I looked in the mirror, and I was radiating energy."

Despite how seemingly fabulous life was, how invincible she felt, Susan knew something was not right. In the five months before her wedding, she charged $27,000 worth of clothes on her corporate credit card. "If I saw a sweater I liked, I'd buy it in nine different colors," she says. "I made thirty-two trips to Los Angeles to see friends in sixty days. I stopped eating. My wedding dress had to be sewn on my body because I'd lost so much weight you could practically see through me."

Two months after her wedding, Susan started to lose touch with reality. "I showed up for a deposition wearing blue jeans, gym shoes, a Chicago Cubs T-shirt, and no makeup. When a witness mentioned that his house had been bombed, I became paranoid about someone bombing my office." At the urging of her family and friends, she went to see her internist, who immediately called a psychiatrist.

"I was talking 285 words a minute and slurring my words—typical signs of mania," Susan remembers. "The psychiatrist told my husband and my parents that I had a classic case of manic depression and that I should be treated with antipsychotic medication and lithium [a mood-stabilizing drug]. Before I knew it, I was being escorted to the hospital's locked psychiatric unit."

Susan describes her involuntary commitment as "a moment of fear and humiliation, but also a breakthrough." Treatment with antipsychotic and mood-stabilizing drugs restored both her psychological and physical well-being, but left painful memories. "I was hospitalized for twenty-eight days, and it was demeaning and degrading. To have your rights taken away. To receive flowers from your friends and have them put in paper cartons because you're not allowed to have glass on a psych unit. To be threatened with being put in a quiet room in restraints. I don't think I'll ever get over that."

Two days after she got out of the hospital, Susan went to a meeting of the Depressive and Manic-Depressive Association (DMDA). "I was angry," she says. "I'd had classic symptoms of manic depression, yet the best doctors in Chicago hadn't recognized them. It felt wonderful to be among people who truly understood what I'd been through."

Susan credits such support, along with psychotherapy and medication, for helping her to stay well and for motivating her to help others: "I made the transformation from someone seeking support after hospitalization to an advocate within months. I couldn't do anything else. Soon after my diagnosis, someone handed me a newspaper article with the headline, 'Manic-Depressive Lawyer Kills Wife.' I called the writer and told him that the facts were incorrect. When he asked what made me such an expert, I explained that I have the illness. He wrote an article about me that was syndicated nationally."

Since then, Susan has appeared on almost all the top talk shows. "After I made my diagnosis public, I was asked to make more appearances, to speak to mental health groups, to talk to residents and interns at different hospitals. I became a full-time volunteer and advocate. Every time I turned a corner, there was another injustice, a new problem, a new need. I found myself investigating state hospitals, fighting insurance discrimination, lobbying for research funds."

In 1986, the DMDA became a national organization; it now has two hundred fifty chapters representing more than forty thousand people. Susan became its first executive director in 1989. "We are the only organization in health care run by patients," she says with pride. "Once when I was lobbying in a Senator's office, he said, 'You're not one of *them*, are you?' I said, 'Yes, I am.' He truly was surprised. I didn't know whether to take it as an insult or a compliment."

As the head of the National DMDA, Susan has addressed the American Psychiatric Association, lobbied on Capitol Hill, and traveled around the world to advocate improved recognition and treatment of mental disorders. She represents a new generation of individuals with mental disorders: informed, confident, competent, outspoken. "Advocacy is very fulfilling," she says. "But I don't see myself as a hero. What matters most to me are the people I've helped get treatment. It's wonderful to see how well they're doing."

Like other advocates, however, she realizes that a great deal remains to be done. "I am grateful to psychiatry for the life it has allowed me to take back for myself," she says. "If not for the medications I take and the therapy I've received, I would not be here. But current treatments can restore individuals with many mental disorders only to 60 or 80 percent of capacity. That's not good enough. We want and deserve 100 percent."

The age of advocacy

Millions of people like Susan Dime-Meenan, who once suffered silently, are speaking up for themselves, their families, and all of those whose lives have been touched by mental illness. "Consumers are demanding more information, more involvement in making decisions about their care, and more effective treatment," says Jerilyn Ross, head of the Anxiety Disorders Association of America (AADA).

This, in itself, represents a tremendous change. At one time, mental health professionals were viewed as all-knowing and all-powerful, and patients, as passive and helpless. Family members were shut out entirely or blamed for directly or indirectly causing the problem. "No one ever questioned a therapist or discussed a diagnosis," says Ross. "Patients and families were too mortified ever to ask for a second opinion. But things have changed. Individuals now see their problems as legitimate diseases that are not their fault." They also see themselves differently.

"When I was in a hospital, totally dependent on the care of others, I was a patient," comments a woman with a chronic mental disorder. "When I was discharged and relying on various services and therapists in the community, I was a client. When I recovered and was able to make choices for myself, I became a consumer."

Like savvy consumers in other areas, individuals who use mental health services and their families have banded together, forming dozens of nationwide groups. (See the Resource Directory at the back of the book for comprehensive listings.) "There has been a real coming of age of the consumer advocacy forces in the mental health field," says Laurie Flynn, executive director of the National Alliance for the Mentally Ill (NAMI), one of the oldest and largest organizations. "When NAMI started in 1980, it was viewed with hostility and suspicion. It was hard for psychiatrists to see anything positive in the anger that many members felt. But we have moved toward mutual respect and greater understanding of each other's roles."

NAMI and other consumer groups have emerged as powerful lobbyists for the rights of the mentally ill, adequate public funding for mental health programs, increased housing for the mentally disabled and homeless, and more basic and clinical research. To eliminate stigma and educate the public, they have prepared written and audiovisual materials and sponsored lectures and conferences. Many provide referral services to therapists, hospitals, and specialized programs around the country. Local chapters organize support and self-help groups and special programs for children, adolescents, and adults with mental disorders as well as for family members. Although they have accomplished much in many areas for millions of people, their greatest contribution has been in conveying a simple but vitally important message to those whose lives have been touched by mental illness: "You are not alone."

Although proud of their contributions to date, the leaders of advocacy groups feel their greatest challenges lie ahead. Research funding for psychiatry, which never has been high, is in jeopardy. Although schizophrenia is five times more common than multiple sclerosis and sixty times more common than muscular dystrophy, the government spends only $14 annually on research for each individual with schizophrenia, compared with $162 per person for multiple sclerosis and $1,000 for muscular dystrophy.

"What we need is an organization that is to the brain what the American Heart Association is to the heart and the American Cancer Society is to cancer," says Connie Lieber, president of the National Alliance for Research on Schizophrenia and Depression (NARSAD), a foundation that funds psychiatric research. "So many people have mental illnesses, and there is such a huge need for education and research. With the explosion in science and the explosion in technology, with the field progressing so fast, we need to keep the momentum up. What I want to see is NARSAD out of business, to hear the researchers say, 'We have the cures; we understand the diseases.' But that's the end of the rainbow, and it's a long way off."

A new openness

One major step forward in awareness and enlightenment has come with the growing realization that mental illnesses can strike anyone. Even national idols hailed as the best in their field can be totally demoralized by a problem of the mind. It happened to Earl Christian Campbell, the University of Texas football star who won a Heisman Trophy and became the National Football League's rookie of the year in 1978 and its most valuable player for three consecutive years. By the time he retired from professional football in 1989, Earl had become a football legend and the fourth official state hero of Texas, a distinction he shares with Stephen Austin, Davy Crockett, and Sam Houston.

Through it all, Earl kept his cool. "I worked at being calm. I became an athlete in the fifth grade, and I've been in the public eye ever since. I've always been the guy who said, 'Give me the baton. I'll get it done.'" All that changed on a Sunday afternoon in 1990, when Earl was singing along with a country tune on the radio and driving from Austin to Houston. At a stoplight, his heart began to pound. His chest muscles tightened. His hands shook. He could feel sweat breaking out all over his body. There didn't seem to be enough air to breathe. A horrible sense of doom came over him. Then thirty-six years old, Earl thought he was having a heart attack—just like his father, who had died of heart disease when Earl was only ten. Although the episode probably lasted no more than ten or fifteen minutes, it seemed like an eternity.

As the terror eased, Earl tried to figure out what had hit him. The sixth of eleven children, he had always been the quiet one, the one their mother described as different—"not so much shy as living in a slightly different world," as he puts it. In his years in the NFL, he faced off against some of the most physically intimidating athletes in America. As a public speaker and owner of a food products company in Austin, he handled his share of stressful situations. "I kept thinking, 'Why now? Why this?'"

The medical specialists in Houston who gave Earl a thorough examination were just as baffled. "All my life I'd avoided going to doctors. I was always healthy. When this happened, I went to eight different doctors, and they tested every part of me."

When the doctors proclaimed him healthy, Earl, who continued to have terrifying attacks, could scarcely believe they were telling him the truth. It took a while for his wife, Reuna, to convince him that the rigorous medical examinations truly had found nothing wrong. With each attack, Earl, the father of two boys, became more apprehensive. "I'd go to bed at night and just lie there because I knew that if I went to sleep, I'd have an attack," he recalls. As his anxiety intensified, he changed the way he lived. "I used to cherish being by myself, but for a while nothing terrified me more. I used to jog and work out all the time, but I stopped. I shut the world off and stayed at our home in Austin because I was afraid that I'd have an attack and no one would be around to help me."

His wife insisted that he keep searching for help. Finally, a physician neighbor suggested that Earl see the one type of doctor he'd never thought of consulting: a psychiatrist. "Where I grew up, we used to think that the only people who went to see psychiatrists were crazy. This guy—the ninth doctor I saw—listened to me and said, 'I think I know what's wrong. You're having panic attacks.' He gave me a pamphlet, and when I read it, I said, 'This is what's going on with me.' I'd never even heard of panic disorder."

As Earl discovered, panic disorder—repeated episodes of sudden, inexplicable, incapacitating dread—is both common and treatable, usually with a combination of medication and cognitive-behavioral techniques (see Chapter 7). "The important thing is that I went and got help," he says. "I learned what I needed to know. Now, it's just like in the country song, 'I'm back being me all over again.' And I want other people who have this problem to know that they can do the same."

Like Earl Campbell, more and more celebrities are speaking out about problems that they at one time would not have dared to admit. Patty Duke has chronicled her often-harrowing struggle with bipolar illness—manic depression—in autobiographies and television movies. Ally Sheedy, Jane Fonda, and other actresses have disclosed their problems with eating disorders. Communications mogul Ted Turner has openly discussed his bipolar illness. Writer William Styron and veteran newsman Mike Wallace have described the dark times they spent in major depression. Dick Cavett, the entertainer and talk show host, has told how his chronic depression convinced him that his brain was "broken," his intellect impaired, and his life hardly worth living. Treatment restored both his famed wit and his will to live.

Each celebrity voice, speaking out with honesty and dignity, has helped to shatter misleading myths and destructive stereotypes. "The mental health field is where cancer was twenty years ago," says Jerilyn Ross of the ADAA. "The celebrities who have come forward are doing what Betty Ford did for breast cancer and alcoholism. They are saying, 'Look at me. I had a problem. I got help, and now I feel better. You can too.'"

New reasons for hope

Just as dramatic as any celebrity's tale are the experiences of anonymous individuals who found their lives interrupted by mental disorders and who have slowly put the pieces of their dreams back together. Until her senior year, Shannon Flynn of Bethesda, Maryland, had been a "golden girl," the top-ranked student in her high school class. In the fall of 1984, her family noticed some differences in her behavior but dismissed them.

"Shannon seemed more anxious, but we thought it was because she was applying to colleges," her mother recalls. "She seemed more withdrawn, but we thought it was because she was sorting through scholarship offers. She did less socializing, but we thought she was working on her college application essays. Over eight weeks, we saw the breakdown coming, but we didn't realize what was happening. Finally she became suicidal and had to be hospitalized."

But the break wasn't as sudden as Shannon's parents thought. "I think I had depressive symptoms for years, but I'd been able to cope," Shannon recalls. "Then I couldn't handle it anymore. I had strong urges to cut myself, to punish myself. I was suicidal, paranoid. I thought people were reading my mind. I was afraid to look people in the eye. I was depressed, agitated. I paced the floor." Hospitalized at a private psychiatric hospital, Shannon, diagnosed as having schizophrenia, was almost catatonic for months.

"It was a radicalizing experience," Shannon's mother said. "We were treated like part of the problem, not allowed to talk to our daughter, expected to engage in intensive family therapy. At about the same time, my brother was in an automobile accident that left him in a coma and ultimately killed him. I would go to two hospitals every day. At my brother's, I was treated like a treasure, a partner in the process of trying to save his life. My daughter seemed no more or less likely to survive, but I wasn't allowed to touch her."

Shannon remembers little of her hospital stay or the limbo-like months she spent at home afterward. "When she was discharged, we got no information about what to expect," says her mother. "We were told she couldn't go back to school, but no one told us what she could do. We had to invent a program on our own. For a while, my husband and I took turns staying home with her. Then we took turns taking her to our offices. Eventually she got part-time work at a daycare center. But she felt terrible about making things hard on all of us."

Eventually Shannon took adult education classes and repeated her senior year, once again graduating at the top of her class. She chose to attend Georgetown University and lived at home during her first year. Gradually she spent more time on campus and ultimately moved into a dorm, where she educated her roommates about her problems. Several times she became so violently agitated that they had to take her to the emergency room. In 1991 her medications could no longer control her symptoms, and she was hospitalized again.

This time a remarkable antipsychotic drug called clozapine (Clozaril) restored Shannon's mental health. "It stopped the agitation, the paranoid feelings, and stopped making me want to hurt myself," she says. "My mind became a lot clearer." Thanks to this medication, Shannon has been able to work full-time as a psychologist, administering tests and monitoring patient records, at the National Institutes of Health in Bethesda, Maryland.

Success stories like hers are becoming increasingly common, and are fostering a sense of optimism about successes to come. "In all my years struggling with manic depression as a patient and being involved in the National DMDA as an advocate, I have never felt so hopeful," says Susan Dime-Meenan. "I truly believe that in my lifetime there will be more effective treatments. Those of us leading the fight in public for more research, more recognition, and more acceptance are not going to give up. A lot of days we wake up smiling. We know there's going to be a brighter tomorrow—for us and for millions of others." And this message is too important ever to keep silent again.

Individuals with a mental or emotional disorder may:

- ☐ **Feel depressed or sad for several weeks**
- ☐ **Lack energy or feel tired all the time**
- ☐ **Take no joy or pleasure in normally enjoyable activities**
- ☐ **Have problems falling or staying asleep or waking too early in the morning**
- ☐ **Think about suicide**
- ☐ **Experience extreme mood swings**
- ☐ **Feel helpless or hopeless**
- ☐ **Be nervous or restless**
- ☐ **Feel that life is out of control**
- ☐ **Be confused or find it difficult to concentrate and think clearly**
- ☐ **Have sudden feelings of panic or terror**
- ☐ **Become very suspicious or fear that people are out to get them**
- ☐ **Be extremely irritable, not get along well with people at home or work**
- ☐ **Drink excessively or use illegal drugs**
- ☐ **Be unable to control or stop destructive behavior, such as gambling or drinking**
- ☐ **Not be able to return to normal within a few months of a crisis or loss**
- ☐ **Lack interest in sex or have frequent sexual problems**
- ☐ **Develop troubling physical symptoms that have no known medical cause**
- ☐ **See, hear, or experience sensations that are imaginary**
- ☐ **Have fixed ideas that they believe despite proof that they are false**
- ☐ **Threaten violence or become aggressive and violent**

The more of these boxes that describe what you or someone close to you has been experiencing, the more reason you have to be concerned that something may be wrong. This chapter provides guidance on finding and evaluating a therapist and advice on coping with everyday problems.

PART II

Common Mental and Emotional Problems

4 Is Something Wrong?

We all live through bad days, sad times, crushing set-backs, heartbreaking losses. On occasion, any one of us might burst into tears, explode in anger, reach too often for a drink or a drug. Usually the bad patches in life give way to better times. Sometimes, though, a long night of anguished soul-searching turns into a string of dark and miser-able days. The jitters that cropped up once in a while don't go away. The urge to drink or use a drug becomes irresistible. The feeling of being out of control intensifies.

Is something wrong? Is it normal to feel this way? Could anyone help? With an aching knee or stomach pain, people often know, or can easily find out, what the problem is, what they can do about it, and whether they should see a doctor. Feelings and thoughts—invisible, untouchable, ephemeral, incapable of being X-rayed or biopsied—are harder to evaluate. If ignored, however, persistent emotional aches and pains can undermine an individual's ability to work, relate to others, and function normally.

Admitting that something is wrong does not mean that one has failed in any way or is "crazy." Just as the body can break down under the strain of day-to-day living, the mind, too, is vulnerable. No one is immune. As one psychiatrist puts it, "If a mind can function, it can malfunction." When that happens, it can often be repaired.

Defining mental health and illness

Mental health is not an absence of distress or conflict, but rather the capacity to think rationally and logically, and to cope with the transitions, stresses, traumas, and losses that occur in all lives, in ways that allow emotional stability and growth. In general, mentally healthy individuals value themselves, perceive reality as it is, accept its limitations and possibilities, respond to its challenges, carry out their responsibilities, establish and maintain close relationships, deal reasonably with others, pursue work that suits their talent and training, and feel a sense of fulfillment that makes the efforts of daily living worthwhile.

However, the borders between mental health and illness are not well marked. Where does eccentricity end and abnormality begin? When does sadness deepen into depression? When does stress intensify into endless anxiety? How does fantasy lose touch completely with reality? Where is the line between everyday ups and downs and serious problems that urgently need attention?

There are no clear answers. "Our view of mental illness is fuzzy," notes Laurie Flynn, executive director of the National Alliance of the Mentally Ill (NAMI). "On any given day almost everyone has a mental health problem—whether it's the stress of modern living, grief, or getting along with others. But these are not mental illnesses. They don't disable. They don't require medication. No one would identify themselves as mentally ill because of them. Someone who is stressed out and someone with schizophrenia may both need help, but one has a problem of everyday living and the other has a serious medical disease."

Although lay persons may speak of "nervous breakdowns" or "insanity," these are not scientific terms and have no official definitions. Mental health professionals prefer "mental disorder," which the *Diagnostic and Statistical Manual of Mental Disorders, Fourth Edition (DSM-IV)*, defines as "a clinically significant behavioral or psychological syndrome or pattern that occurs in an individual and that is associated with present distress (such as a painful symptom) or disability (such as impairment in one or more important areas of functioning) or with a significantly increased risk of suffering death, pain, disability, or an important loss of freedom." The U.S. government's official definition, as formulated in 1993, states that a serious mental illness is "a diagnosable mental, behavioral, or emotional disorder that interferes with one or more major activities in life, like dressing, eating, or working."

Who is troubled?

Individuals with mental and emotional problems often feel terribly alone, as though no one else experiences or understands the misery they feel. Yet, as epidemiological studies conducted in recent years have shown, mental disorders are common. As noted in Chapter 1, according to the National Comorbidity Study published in 1994, almost one in two Americans—48 percent of the population—has experienced a mental disorder at some point in life, and almost 30 percent suffer from one in any given year.

This study, based on interviews with 8,098 men and women from the ages of fifteen to fifty-four who were representative of the entire population of the United States, found that the most common disorders are major depression, alcohol dependence and abuse, drug dependence and abuse, social phobias, specific phobias, and dysthymia (a chronic form of mild depression). Although 25 percent report having had a single mental disorder, 14 percent have experienced three or more simultaneously.

Previous studies also documented a high rate of mental illness. The largest and most comprehensive of these, the National Institute of Mental Health's (NIMH) Epidemiologic Catchment Area (ECA) survey, referred to in Chapter 1, included initial interviews with twenty thousand men and women, with follow-up research on sixteen thousand of them. Published in 1993, this study found that 28 percent of the population—approximately 52 million Americans—suffer from a mental disorder during the course of a year. Nine million develop a new ailment, 8 million have a recurrent illness, 35 million suffer ongoing symptoms.

The actual number of people troubled by serious mental and emotional problems may be much higher. Epidemiological studies

THE MOST COMMON MENTAL DISORDERS

DISORDER	IN A GIVEN YEAR (% affected)	AT SOME POINT IN LIFE (% affected)
Major depression	10.3	17.1
Alcohol dependence or abuse	9.7	23.5
Specific phobias	8.8	11.3
Social phobias	7.9	13.3
Drug dependence or abuse	3.6	11.9
Dysthymia	2.5	6.4

Source: Kessler R., et al. Lifetime and 12-month prevalence of DSM-III-R psychiatric disorders in the United States. *Archives of General Psychiatry*, vol. 51, January, 1994.

usually include only persons who meet the official psychiatric criteria for mental disorders. Individuals who may be in considerable distress but are a symptom or two away from the diagnostic definition are not counted. However, as other studies have shown, they are at high risk for developing a full-blown mental disorder.

Problems of everyday living

No life is without problems—nor should it be. "Every problem brings the possibility of a widening of consciousness," Carl Jung once noted. As psychiatrist M. Scott Peck observed in *The Road Less Traveled*, the "whole process of meeting and solving problems" is what gives life meaning. "Problems," he writes, "are the cutting edge that distinguishes between success and failure. Problems call forth our courage and our wisdom. It is only because of problems that we grow mentally and spiritually."

The problems that most of us confront in daily life are not mental illnesses but difficulties that get in the way of happiness and fulfillment. Even though they are not as severe and incapacitating as major depression, anxiety, or the other disorders discussed in this book, they can affect daily life and personal relationships. The following are common reasons why people seek help.

TROUBLING FEELINGS

Although feelings are neither good nor bad in themselves, they can have powerful physical and psychological effects. Overwhelmed by emotion, we may cry in anguish, laugh in delight, sigh in sadness, grimace in anger. Sometimes we cut ourselves off from our feelings, if only because their intensity can frighten us. We can't always explain why we feel the way we do, nor may we want to admit, even to ourselves, that we are capable of negative feelings, such as anger or fear, as well as positive emotions, such as compassion and acceptance.

The feeling of depression is one of the most common and distressing emotions. Sooner or later everyone feels sad or discouraged. You want to pull the covers over your head and stay in bed all day. You can't imagine coping with one more thing. You pull away from others and lose interest in everything but your own misery. Under certain circumstances it's almost impossible not to feel this way: A flood or fire damages your home, the promotion you thought you deserved goes to a colleague, a back problem knocks you off your feet. Even a trauma that seems trivial to others, such as a fender-bending accident, can drag you into a funk.

Although it is perfectly normal to feel down occasionally, depression that lingers, not just for a few days but for weeks or months, is more than "the blues." If your spirits fail to lift, seek professional help. (Chapter 5 provides more information and advice.)

During the course of a week, a day, even an hour, feelings can change, with highs giving way to lows or tears dissolving into laughter. However, frequent mood swings can be deeply distressing. One of the best ways to monitor emotional changes is by keeping a record of your moods. In a small notebook or diary, record your mood at about the same time every day, from "0" for the worst you ever felt to "100" for the best you ever felt. This can help you get a better perspective on your moods. Chapter 6 describes the dramatic, often disabling mood changes that occur in bipolar illness (manic depression).

The symptoms of anxiety—a racing heart, a distracted mind, a general edginess—strike everyone occasionally. Life provides us with plenty of opportunities to become anxious: accidents, bankruptcies, layoffs, deadlines, sales quotas, shaky marriages, difficult children, crime, natural disasters. Sometimes talking with friends or family members, or setting aside a daily "worry period," can help. If you cannot dispel a vague but persisting sense of anxiety or find that your fears are intensifying, you may benefit from professional help. (Chapter 7 describes anxiety disorders.)

STRESS

People use the word *stress* in different ways: as an external force that causes a person to become tense or upset, as an internal state of arousal, and as the physical response of the body to various demands. Dr. Hans Selye, a pioneer in studying physiological responses to challenge, defined stress as "the nonspecific response of the body to any demand made upon it." In other words, the body reacts to all stressors—both the things that upset us and those that excite us—in the same way.

Stress isn't always negative. Some of life's happiest moments—births, reunions, weddings—are enormously stressful. While we may weep because of frustration or loss, we also shed tears of love and joy. Ideally, the level of stress in our lives should be just high enough to motivate us to satisfy our needs and not so high that it interferes with our ability to reach our fullest potential.

Stressors can be acute (such as an injury or a loved one's death), sequential (such as the series of events leading to a move or divorce), intermittent (such as project deadlines), or chronic (such as the daily challenges of coping with a serious illness). Our level of ongoing stress affects our ability to respond to a new day's stressors. Each of us has a breaking point for dealing with stress.

A series of too-intense pressures or too-rapid changes can push us closer and closer to that point.

Excessive, unmanaged stress can jeopardize physical well-being, psychological health, behavior, and performance at school or work. Watch for signals of stress overload, such as physical symptoms (fatigue, headaches, indigestion, diarrhea, sleep problems); frequent illness or worry about illness; problems in concentrating; feeling irritable, anxious, or apathetic; becoming accident-prone; breaking rules, such as speed limits on roadways; avoiding people; or self-destructive behavior, such as drinking too much. If these conditions increase or become more troubling, the best way of coping may be to seek professional help.

Sometimes even simple changes can help. In *Stress Without Distress*, Hans Selye provides these basic guidelines for coping when stress builds up:

- Admit that there is no perfection. But in each category of achievement, something is tops; be satisfied to strive for that.

- Do not underestimate the delight of real simplicity.

- Whatever situation you meet in life, consider first whether it is really worth fighting for.

- Try to keep your mind constantly on the pleasant aspects of life and on actions that improve your situation. Nothing paralyzes your efficiency more than frustration; nothing helps it more than success.

- Even after the greatest defeats, combat the depressing thought of being a failure by taking stock of all your past achievements, which no one can deny you.

- When faced with a task that is very painful yet indispensable to achieve your aim, don't procrastinate. Cut right into an abscess to eliminate the pain instead of prolonging it by gently rubbing the surface.

- Finally, do not forget that there is no ready-made success formula that will suit everybody.

WORK-RELATED PROBLEMS

Work is one of the most common sources of stress. The most troubled workers are those at the bottom of the job ladder: the bossed, rather than the bosses. They have far less control over their work situation than the powerful executives calling the shots from the top. People in "high-strain" jobs (such as assembly-line workers, waiters and waitresses, telephone operators) feel heavy pressure to perform but have little leeway in decision making and consistently have the highest rate of heart attacks, high blood pressure, and psychological problems. Those in "active" jobs (such as doctors, engineers, farmers, executives) work long hours but partly at their own discretion, and have opportunities to advance and learn new skills; they have the lowest rate of heart attacks.

Some people become so obsessed by their work and careers that they become workaholics, so caught up in racing toward the top that they forget what they are racing toward and why. One consequence is burnout, a state of physical, emotional, and mental exhaustion brought on by constant or repeated emotional pressure. This is particularly common in the helping professions, such as health care, in which men and women who have dedicated their lives to others may realize they have nothing left to give to themselves. The best way to avoid burnout is learning to cope well with smaller day-to-day stresses. Then tiny frustrations won't smolder into a blaze that may be impossible to put out. If burnout begins to undermine performance and happiness, professional help may be needed.

LIFE CHANGES AND CRISES

Every stage of life brings change and transitions. Past experiences, positive and negative, affect your attitude toward these changes and your resilience in handling them. Your general outlook on life can determine whether you expect the worst and feel stressed or anticipate a challenge and feel confident. An event such as a move to a new city becomes traumatic only when it is seen as an unwelcome upheaval rather than an exciting beginning of a new chapter in your life. (Chapter 12 discusses adjustment disorders.)

The number and frequency of changes in a person's life, along with the time and setting in which they occur, have a great impact on how the individual responds. Stress experts Thomas Holmes, M.D., and Richard Rahe, M.D., devised a scale to evaluate levels of stress and potential for coping, based on "life change units" that estimate the impact of each change. The death of a partner or parent ranks high on the list, but even changing apartments is considered a stressor. People who accumulate more than three hundred life change units in a year are more likely to suffer serious health problems.

If you develop troubling emotional or behavioral symptoms, take stock of the changes in your life. Have you had a child, changed jobs, relocated, retired, faced a milestone birthday? While many life transitions are difficult, most people make their way through them without therapy. The following suggestions can help:

- Seek accurate information about what is happening in your life. Knowledge—whether about the current job market or life after retirement—can bring vague fears down to earth.

- Share worries with someone you trust, love, or respect.

- Reframe an event by changing the way you look at it to emphasize the positive.

- Balance work and recreation. A set routine for relaxation will help.

- Avoid reliance on alcohol and other drugs to help you cope.

- Don't let yourself become obsessed with *you*. Doing something for others will take your mind off your concerns.

- Don't take yourself so seriously. You are a player in the human comedy—be able to laugh at yourself.

MARITAL PROBLEMS

Contemporary marriage has been described as an institution that everyone on the outside wants to enter and everyone on the inside wants to leave. All marriages change over time. According to one theory, most marriages go through four basic stages. In the first, the spouses are self-centered, interested in what the relationship can do for them. In the second stage, the couple starts negotiating, trading one service for another—for example, "I'll do the dishes if you take the car to the garage for a tune-up." During the third stage, the spouses begin to appreciate each other's individuality and to make accommodations for the good of the marriage. By the fourth stage, they have developed "rules of the relationship," by which they avoid or deal with problems.

Marital therapy (described in Chapter 27) may be useful to help spouses make it through rough times together. The benefits of saving or strengthening a marriage are many. As researchers have shown, marriage enhances happiness and health. Married people live longer than unmarried ones and, regardless of race or sex, are less likely to die of heart disease or other illnesses.

In one recent study, 23 percent of men aged forty-five to fifty-four years who lived without a spouse died within ten years, compared with 11 percent of men of similar ages who lived with their wives. The reason may be that single people may drink and smoke more, exercise less, and eat less nutritiously, whereas marriage may foster more stability and better living habits. Particularly for men, who often have few close friendships, marriage may also provide life-enhancing emotional support. In surveys that assess which adults are most happy and satisfied with their lives, the highest scores consistently come from married persons, especially husbands. For both spouses, marriage appears to serve as a protective barrier against life's stresses. Although it can't prevent economic and social upheavals, it buffers their impact so that married men and women are far less likely to be depressed or anxious than are divorced, separated, or single persons.

FAMILY PROBLEMS

No matter what form a family takes, one of its main roles is as a training ground for living. We use our experience in the family to learn how to behave in other groups and with other individuals. If parents behave lovingly and respectfully toward each other and their children, their youngsters may learn how to have loving and healthy relationships with others. If children are victims of abusive parents at home, they may become someone else's victim—or abuser—elsewhere.

A family is a system, a society in miniature, and our experience in this basic unit gives us a way of perceiving how we fit into the larger system. Like any complex creation, a family can develop all sorts of complications. Family dynamics are intricate, and although one person may be singled out as the source of a problem or conflict, everyone in the home is affected by it.

Although most families handle the majority of their problems without assistance, sometimes the difficulty is so upsetting or disruptive that parents seek professional help. As Chapter 27 explains, therapists skilled in working with families may meet with parents, children, or the entire family at different times and in different combinations over a period of several weeks. It may take "dysfunctional" families, those lacking in healthy and honest communication, even longer to work through their problems. (Chapter 26 focuses on children's issues.)

GRIEF

The death of a loved one may be the single most upsetting and feared event in a person's life. Obviously, a sudden death is more of a shock than one that follows a long illness. A suicide can be particularly devastating, because family members often wonder if they could have done anything to prevent it. Whether the death is anticipated or sudden, each loss in our lifetime can make us feel alone and vulnerable.

Grief is a psychological necessity, not self-indulgence. When parents die, their children, regardless of their age, mourn, not just for the father and mother who are gone but for their lost role of being someone's child. The loss of a mate has a profound impact. The death of a child is likely to be especially heartbreaking. Eventually some parents resolve their grief and accept the death as "God's will" or as "something that happens," but many continue to grieve for many years. Although the pain of their loss lessens with time, they describe an "emptiness" within themselves even when they have rich, meaningful, and happy lives.

Mental health professionals refer to grief as work, and it is— slow, tedious, and painful work. Yet it is only by working through grief that bereaved individuals can make their way back to the living world of hope and love. They may experience mood swings between sadness and anger, guilt and anxiety. They may feel physically sick, lose their appetites, sleep poorly, or fear they're going crazy because they keep "seeing" the deceased person in different places. Grief also produces physical changes in the respiratory, hormonal, and central nervous systems, and may affect the functioning of the heart, blood, and immune system.

All grieving people continue to need emotional support from family and friends for many months after their loss. The first anniversary of a death or the first holiday spent alone can be particularly difficult. Nevertheless, most do not need psychological counseling. The family members of a suicide victim are most likely to need and benefit from professional help in sorting out their feelings of failure, guilt, anger, and sorrow.

Sometimes a bereaved person halts in the middle of the process of normal grieving, becoming clinging and over-reliant on others, pining for the deceased, or showing signs of denial, avoidance, or anxiety. For individuals who remain intensely distressed or whose grief does not ease over time, therapy and medication can be enormously helpful and potentially life-saving. These grieving family members are at increased risk for serious physical and mental illness, suicide, and premature death.

Seeking help

According to the ECA survey, only 28 percent of individuals with mental disorders seek help: 43 percent of these turn to primary care physicians, 40 percent to mental health professionals, and 20 percent to members of the clergy or other counselors. Eighteen percent opt for self-care measures, such as joining a support group. The National Comorbidity Survey also found that less than half of those with diagnosable mental illnesses sought help from a mental health professional.

How do you know when you need help? A simple rule of thumb is to think about how intensely a problem is affecting you or a loved one and how long it has lasted. If the difficulty is causing great distress or interfering with work, relationships, or other aspects of life, it is wise to seek help. Symptoms that are not so severe or disturbing but continue not just for a few days but for weeks or months should also be evaluated. What distinguishes mental disorders from problems of daily living is their severity or persistence over time. But the sooner that individuals recognize they have a problem and get appropriate treatment, the sooner recovery can begin—and for disorders such as depression, early identification can improve the outcome.

If you are unsure about whether to seek help, the following questions may help you to make the decision:

- Are emotional problems getting in the way of your work, relationships, or other aspects of your personal life?

- Have you been feeling less happy, less confident, or less in control than usual for a period of several weeks or longer?

- Have you reached the point of being so unhappy that you want to do something about it?

- Have close, trusted friends or family members commented on changes in your behavior or personality?

- Have your own efforts to deal with a problem failed to resolve the situation?

- Is dealing with everyday problems more of a struggle than it used to be?

- Are you focusing less on external circumstances that cause stress and more on yourself and your inadequacies?

- Do you feel emotionally "stuck" and helpless to change your own behavior or circumstances?

The key question to ask yourself is not, "Am I mentally ill?" or "Do I have serious problems?" but "Could I use some help right now?" If the answer is "yes," do it. Therapy may turn out to be a tool for change or a source of support when you need it most. At the very least, the psychological equivalent of a checkup can assure you that a problem isn't more serious than you may have feared.

If your concern is about troubling changes in someone close to you, you may want to talk about it with other family members and friends. (Chapter 30 provides more information on what to do when someone you love has a mental disorder.) Anyone who feels that his or her own mental well-being is in jeopardy or who is worried about a relative or close friend should make an appointment for a consultation. A mental health professional may be able to help in deciding which steps to take next.

Cost can be a barrier to obtaining mental health care. Health insurance policies and health care programs and organizations may pay only part of a therapist's fee or may limit coverage to a preset number of therapy sessions or days of treatment in a hospital or residential facility. As mental health advocates contend and many financial analyses have shown, in the long run the costs of *not* getting needed care often are much higher than those of treatment—for individuals, for their families, and for society as a whole. Check your own health insurance or plan. If you do not have coverage, local and state agencies and advocacy groups may be able to direct you to publicly supported services or to suggest ways of handling the financial aspects of mental health care.

FINDING A THERAPIST

According to the nationwide poll conducted for *Parade* magazine in 1993 (described in Chapter 1), more than one in every five Americans—23 percent—have consulted a mental health professional at some time in their lives. Nevertheless, many people have no idea where to go for help. Asked if they would know where to turn if someone in their family showed signs of mental illness, 22 percent of those surveyed said no. Among those between ages eighteen and twenty-four, a time when many major mental disorders become evident, 35 percent did not know how to get help.

Yet, consumers today have more options than ever in terms of therapies and therapists. This book can help you begin sorting out these options. The descriptions of everyday problems in this chapter and the symptom checklists at the beginning of each chapter in this section of the book can provide some sense of what the problem might be. Depending on its nature and severity, treatment may involve psychotherapy (a general term for psychological or behavioral approaches that aim to change personality or behavior), medication, or a combination of both. (Chapter 27 describes the various forms of psychotherapy; Chapter 28 covers psychiatric medications.)

Many people refer to anyone in the mental health field as a "psychotherapist," but this is not an official designation. Furthermore, anyone, with or without formal training, can advertise as one. Therefore, before you select a therapist, be sure to check the person's background and credentials. Only trained professionals who have met state licensing requirements are certified as psychiatrists, psychologists, or social workers. Some individuals and groups try to take advantage of the vulnerability of those seeking mental health care. To protect yourself, the National Mental Health Association advises that you avoid any person or organization that does not answer questions clearly or satisfactorily, that promises financial rewards if you participate in a program, that pressures you through a third party, that offers or implies a guarantee of success, or that tries to involve you in a long-term financial commitment.

Many people turn to their family physicians or internists, who may be able to provide some counseling and who are authorized to prescribe psychiatric medications. Many such physicians are empathetic and caring and can draw on the trust that has developed through their ongoing relationship with their patients. However, there have been so many recent advances in the mental health sciences that not all physicians in primary care or other specialties are up to date about the latest options for treatment. As a result, they may not prescribe the most effective medications in the most appropriate doses, may not continue treatment for a long enough time, or may not offer newer forms of psychotherapy or combinations of treatment. A prescription for a psychiatric drug is only one step toward recovery. If this is chiefly what your primary care physician can offer you, ask for a referral to a psychiatrist or other mental health professional, if only for a consultation or a second opinion.

The most common types of mental health professionals are:

Psychiatrists, licensed medical doctors (M.D.s) who have completed medical school, a year-long internship that includes at least four months of internal medicine and usually two months of neurology, and a three-year residency program that provides training in various forms of psychotherapy (including couples, family, and group therapy), psychopharmacology (the study of drugs that affect the mind), and both outpatient and inpatient treatment of mental disorders. They can prescribe medications and make medical decisions. "Board-certified" psychiatrists have passed national oral and written examinations after completion of residency training. Child psychiatrists undergo additional academic and clinical training in working with children and adolescents; geriatric psychiatrists have special expertise in problems of the elderly.

Psychologists, who have completed a graduate program, which includes clinical training and internship, in human psychology but who have not studied medicine and cannot prescribe medication. Most states require that they be licensed in order to practice independently. An increasing number have a doctorate (either a Ph.D. or Psy.D.) plus postdoctoral training, and are trained in a variety of psychotherapeutic techniques rather than in one particular school or theory. Some have additional training in working with children and/or families.

Certified social workers (C.S.W.s) or licensed clinical social workers (L.C.S.W.s), who have usually completed a two-year graduate program and have specialized training in helping people with mental problems in addition to conventional social work. Some have doctoral degrees. Most states certify or license social workers and require two years of supervised postgraduate clinical work and a qualifying examination.

Psychiatric nurses, who have nursing degrees and have passed a state examination. They usually have special training and experience in mental health care, although no specialty licensing or certification is required.

Marriage and family therapists, licensed in some but not all states, who usually have a graduate degree, often in psychology, and at least two years of supervised clinical training in dealing with relationship problems. Psychiatrists, psychologists, and clinical social workers may also specialize in marriage and family counseling or may devote much of their practice to helping couples and families.

During the course of therapy, an individual may see several health professionals, each with a different type of expertise. Ideally, there should be close coordination of their efforts to ensure comprehensive care. A clinical social worker may refer a person to a psychiatrist to determine whether medications might help and to monitor the medical aspects of care. A primary care physician may recommend testing by a psychologist. A psychiatrist may suggest that an individual undergoing treatment for a mental disorder also participate in couples therapy with a marital counselor.

Other therapists include pastoral counselors, members of the clergy who offer psychological counseling; hypnotherapists, who use hypnosis for problems such as smoking and obesity; and stress management counselors, who teach relaxation methods. Anyone can use these terms as a professional description, and there are no licensing requirements.

In general, we recommend choosing *licensed* professionals. These individuals have received a certain amount of training and supervision, have demonstrated a basic level of competence, have passed state or national qualifying examinations, and must adhere to ethical standards and participate in continuing education programs in order to keep their licenses.

City or county health departments, neighborhood health centers, hospital clinics and services, and local branches of national service organizations, such as NAMI, may offer help or provide referrals. "Go to the best academic center, hospital, or clinic in your community and ask for the psychiatric program," advises former NIMH director Herbert Pardes, M.D., vice-president for Health Sciences, dean of Medicine, and chairman of the Department of Psychiatry in the College of Physicians & Surgeons of Columbia University.

Mental health clinics often use psychiatry residents or psychology trainees to provide care and usually charge lower fees, often based on a sliding scale according to income. They offer a wider range of services than any single therapist might. However, clinics may have waiting periods and limit the number of therapy sessions. In addition, therapists usually are assigned, rather than chosen by the consumer.

To obtain the names of several therapists, ask your physician, mental health professionals you know, or acquaintances who work with mental health care providers. If you belong to a health maintenance organization or another health care plan, it will provide you with a list of participating therapists, although you may have to request a referral from your primary care physician before seeing a therapist. The local chapters of support and advocacy groups usually provide names of specialists in certain disorders. (These groups are listed in the Resource Directory at the back of the book.) Hospitals will provide the names of affiliated psychiatrists who have met certain requirements in order to join the clinical staff. City or state psychiatric and psychological associations can provide information about a therapist's qualifications.

The usual way of making initial contact is by calling a therapist's office and arranging to talk by phone. Tell what is troubling you and who referred you, and say that you would like to find out more about the therapist's experience with and perspective on problems like yours. Increasingly, consumers are interviewing several mental health professionals to determine who might be most helpful. You should not hesitate to talk about fees, insurance coverage, payment plans, and other practical matters during this introductory call, or to state that you would like to work with someone who has experience in dealing with specific problems, such as eating disorders, or who has expertise in behavior therapy or in psychopharmacology (drug treatment for mental disorders).

If you have an explicit treatment in mind, such as a nicotine patch or hypnosis to help you quit smoking, say so. Therapists will let you know whether they have experience with or believe in the efficacy of an approach. They may suggest an alternative treatment or refer you to someone with the expertise you want.

Therapists will want to know the circumstances that led to your call, the nature of the current problem, whether there is a need for emergency evaluation or hospitalization, whether you are seeing or have seen a mental health professional or physician for it, and what you hope to gain by therapy. If you have a medical problem or are being referred by another mental health professional, the therapist may ask for permission to talk with your care providers to get more information. The initial phone conversation with a therapist sets the stage for building rapport in therapy. Ideally, you should feel that the therapist has listened to you and will work to understand you and your problem. If you decide that the therapist is likely to meet these criteria, the next step is to set up an appointment for a consultation. Be sure to inquire if there is a fee for this visit (usually there is) and, if so, what it will be.

WHAT TO EXPECT

During the initial consultation, you explain what is troubling you. The mental health professional listens and asks questions to get as clear an understanding of you and your problem as possible. This interview usually lasts for forty-five to ninety minutes. Therapists may begin by asking open-ended questions to encourage you to describe the current problem, as well as the feelings and reactions it has provoked. Typical questions include: What brings you here today? How have you been feeling? What do you think has caused your problem? Why do you think it started when it did? What do you think it does to you? How severe is it? What difficulties does it cause? What do you fear most about it?

The focus then shifts to you—your family history, significant relationships, occupation, education, leisure activities, values, religious and cultural background, medical history, developmental history, and sexual history. Depending on your responses, the therapist may explore topics that seem particularly sensitive or distressing. You may be asked to describe a typical day or to go into more detail about significant relationships.

Before the end of the session, the therapist will usually describe his or her impressions of what may be wrong, ask permission to obtain additional information (often from medical records or your primary care physician), suggest further testing if that seems warranted, and present an initial treatment plan and the reasons for these recommendations. You may be asked to schedule a medical examination with your primary care physician, because certain diseases, such as anemia (a deficiency of oxygen-carrying red blood cells) and hypothyroidism (a deficiency of thyroid hormone), may cause depression or other psychiatric symptoms.

Some therapists use standardized, structured diagnostic interviews based on the symptom descriptions in the *DSM-IV*. Many different types of assessments are available, including interactive software programs. Some of these are directed toward children and adolescents, and others are specifically designed for evaluating potential cases of depression, anxiety, alcoholism, schizophrenia, and other disorders. The "Structured Clinical Interview for the *DSM-IV*" (SCID), for example, systematically lists questions about the present problem, past episodes, and specific symptoms. There are different versions of the SCID, some involving self-assessments to complete before the interview and others designed for inpatients, outpatients, community members, individuals seeing their primary care physician, and family members.

DECIDING ON TREATMENT

Once you have met with one or more mental health professionals and discussed treatment options, you must make some basic decisions. In making your final choice of a therapist, here are some considerations and questions to keep in mind:

- Do you feel that you could work well together? Will the therapist treat you as a whole person, rather than an illness, and help you deal with the impact your problem may have on your personal development, your relationships, and your life?

- Do you feel that the therapist shows genuine concern, takes you seriously, treats you with respect, and shares or accepts your values? Regardless of qualifications or reputation, a therapist who is not understanding and caring probably is not the right choice.

- Is your therapist willing to explore all treatment options to find what works best for you? Will this include medication as well as specific psychotherapeutic techniques?

- If the therapist is not a physician and medication is necessary, who will prescribe and monitor your medication? Who will work with you to weigh the side effects of specific drugs against their benefits?

- If you may benefit from a specialized form of psychotherapy, such as behavior therapy, hypnosis, or couples or family therapy, will your therapist personally provide it? If you are referred to another professional, how will your care be coordinated? Who will be your primary therapist?

- Is your therapist ready to work with your partner or family? The choice of whether to include loved ones is yours. If you decide to include them, will your therapist help educate them about your problem and explain how they can help you manage it?

- Will your therapist be supportive if you want a second opinion about treatment? Will he or she work with you to evaluate others' recommendations?

Remember that you are choosing someone in whom you may confide your most intimate secrets and fears. Of course, you want a competent therapist with the right training, knowledge, skills, and experience, but competence is not the entire story. In making the choice, your instincts may be as helpful as your intelligence.

The chapters in this book that deal with specific disorders describe the treatments that most mental health professionals agree are effective for these conditions. If, after a few months, you don't feel that you are making progress, discuss this with your therapist. Almost always there are ways, such as combining therapies, to make treatment more effective.

There is a great deal that individuals can do to "supplement" their work with a therapist. Many people turn to self-help and support groups, either led by professionals or consisting solely of lay members. As described in Chapters 27 and 29, such groups can serve as invaluable resources providing information, insight, and the empathy that comes from sharing similar life experiences or problems. Groups offer support between therapy sessions as well as practical coping advice.

DIAGNOSING A MENTAL DISORDER

The mental health profession's gold standard for making a diagnosis—and the basis for reimbursement—is the pattern of symptoms, or diagnostic criteria, as defined for the almost three hundred disorders in the *DSM-IV*. This system, in a state of constant re-evaluation and refinement, makes certain distinctions for the sake of research purposes and consistency in the field. The fact that an individual has four rather than five symptoms of depression does not mean that he or she is not suffering or does not need help. These criteria establish a *threshold* for making a diagnosis; they do not indicate whether a person needs or could benefit from treatment. Whereas disorders can be classified and quantified, individuals cannot. For a skilled therapist, diagnosis is an art, based on clinical experience and knowledge, as well as a systematic scientific process.

It is possible to receive more than a single psychiatric diagnosis, such as panic disorder and agoraphobia (fear of being in places or situations from which it would be difficult to escape); this is called *comorbidity*. As many as half of those with mental disorders also have a substance abuse disorder, especially alcoholism; this is termed *dual diagnosis*. These individuals may turn to alcohol or drugs to ease the pain they feel, or an underlying vulnerability may precipitate both the mental illness and the substance abuse. In making a diagnosis, therapists also note any relevant general medical conditions and psychosocial and environmental problems that might affect that diagnosis, the treatment, or the prognosis, such as a recent divorce or the loss of a job. When appropriate, they may indicate any culturally related features and include an assessment of the individual's relationships.

As part of the *DSM-IV*'s approach to assessment, therapists also look for personality disorders, long-standing patterns of thinking and behaving that cause distress or interfere with normal functioning. Some individuals with personality disorders exaggerate their own guilt and innate badness; others blame everyone but themselves for what goes wrong in their lives. Some get involved in a series of intense all-or-nothing relationships; others remain completely aloof. Individuals with personality disorders are more likely to fall into a pattern of repeated crises in their lives and to develop other emotional and mental problems. (Chapter 21 discusses personality disorders.) In turn, mental disorders such as depression may influence personality and affect responses to stress.

Once you decide
to seek help

Obtaining help is not the end of a problem but rather the beginning of the quest for a solution. Individuals often wonder
whom, if anyone, they should tell about their decision to seek
mental health care. As with other illnesses, the only people who
need to know are you and the person or persons providing you
with care. The tendency to want to keep this confidential is understandable, but in fact it can be very helpful to inform close family
members and friends. They can provide support and understanding, work with you during difficult times, and offer encouragement
when needed. Moreover, when there is a possible or confirmed
genetic component to a disorder, family members may want to
learn more about their vulnerability to a similar problem.

No one can guarantee that any form of treatment will work.
The chances for success depend on the nature of the problem,
the therapies selected, the skills of the mental health professional
and, more than anything else, the commitment of the individual
who is seeking help. When people begin therapy with the attitude
that "nobody can really help me," recovery is all but doomed.
Within weeks, they typically declare, "I tried, but it didn't work."

For many disorders, medications can ease distressing symptoms, but they are no substitute for self-exploration. As they strive
to overcome a problem, individuals may have to face up to often
painful truths, acknowledge ways in which they have contributed
to their difficulties, and change some lifelong habits to break out
of a cycle of pain, blame, failure, and guilt. In this process, even
those who have endured overwhelming trauma or years of undiagnosed suffering often discover within themselves possibilities and
strengths they had never imagined. As they work toward recovery
they can learn more gratifying ways of living and behaving, rebuild
self-esteem and confidence, regain a sense of being in control, and
discover that they do have options and the ability to make competent choices. "Therapy opens doors of opportunity," says one mental health professional, "and makes individuals strong enough to
walk through them."

Is it depression?

Individuals with a depressive disorder may:

☐ **Feel chronically depressed, sad, empty, discouraged, tearful**

☐ **Lose interest or pleasure in once-enjoyable activities**

☐ **Eat more or less than usual and either gain or lose weight**

☐ **Have trouble sleeping or sleep much more than usual**

☐ **Feel slowed down or restless**

☐ **Be tired and listless and lack energy**

☐ **Feel helpless, hopeless, worthless**

☐ **Find it hard to concentrate or focus attention**

☐ **Become less effective or productive than in the past**

☐ **Have difficulty in thinking clearly or making decisions**

☐ **Be forgetful**

☐ **Have persistent thoughts of death or suicide**

☐ **Think poorly of themselves, put themselves down, feel inadequate**

☐ **Brood about the past**

☐ **Lack interest in sex or be less sexually active than usual**

☐ **Withdraw from others**

☐ **Develop physical symptoms (e.g., headaches, digestive problems, aches and pains)**

The more boxes that you or someone close to you checks, the more reason you have to be concerned about depressive disorders—especially if several symptoms have persisted for at least two weeks or if a feeling of depression has continued for a long time.

5

Depressive
Disorders

Ever since his girlfriend broke up with him, a college student has spent most of the time alone, brooding, not interested in any of the activities he used to enjoy. A young lawyer, convinced that she is not as smart and capable as others think, feels overwhelmed and inadequate. A research scientist snaps at his wife and children and criticizes everything his postdoctoral trainees do. Every winter a librarian finds herself craving rich, creamy foods and becoming so lethargic that she can hardly move. A somber bookkeeper describes herself as "living under a cloud."

Although feelings of depression, sadness, or discouragement occasionally tug at all of us, these individuals are experiencing something quite different: a state of psychological misery that does not go away. Like millions of others with depressive disorders, they have lost their joy in living. Food, friends, sex, and other forms of pleasure may no longer appeal to them. They may be unable to concentrate on their work or fulfill responsibilities. They may fight back tears throughout the day and toss and turn through long, empty nights. Gloom settles over their world like a thick, gray fog, creating an inescapable sense of deep sadness and utter hopelessness.

Unfortunately, fewer than one in every three depressed people ever seeks treatment. One reason is that many Americans still do not think of depression as a real illness that can and should be treated. In a poll by the National Mental Health Association,

43 percent of those surveyed said that they believed depression was a personal or emotional weakness rather than an illness, and blamed themselves, family members, friends, or circumstances for their symptoms. They are wrong.

Comparing everyday "blues" to *clinical depression* (a term commonly used to refer to any depressive disorder that requires treatment) is like comparing a cold to pneumonia. A manager laid off from his job may feel like a failure and not want to see anyone for a few days. A teacher whose mother is dying may have problems fighting back tears in class. Both *feel* depressed, but neither *is* depressed in the sense of having a mental disorder. However, if withdrawal or bouts of overwhelming sadness persist and intensify, clinical depression may develop.

This chapter provides information about "unipolar" depressive disorders, including major depression, seasonal affective disorder, depressions triggered by illness, medications, or childbirth, and dysthymia (chronic mild depression). Chapter 6 discusses "bipolar disorders," which involve emotional highs as well as lows. Chapter 12 describes adjustment disorders involving a depressed mood.

The depressive disorders are as real, as painful, and as disabling as any physical condition. A study of more than eleven thousand people in Los Angeles, Boston, and Chicago found that major depression impairs the ability to function at least as much as—if not more than—illnesses such as heart disease, back disorders, and diabetes. The annual costs to the economy, according to an analysis by researchers at the Massachusetts Institute of Technology, total almost $44 billion, including treatment and lost job productivity.

No one is too young or too old, too lucky or too likable, too successful or too secure to feel depression's downward tug. Kathy Cronkite, author of *On the Edge of Darkness*, describes it as "a great equalizer—the pain is the same, the floor is just as hard when you fall, and whether your window overlooks Malibu beach or a brick wall, all you see is gray."

Yet there is good news about depression: Treatment can and does work. The sooner a depressive disorder is diagnosed and treated, the sooner individuals can start feeling better and the brighter the long-term outlook. Thanks to an impressive array of well-researched treatments, as many as 80 percent of those suffering from depression improve significantly within a few months.

Major depression

Among the most common problems of the mind, major depression consists of a depressed mood or a loss of interest or pleasure in usual activities that persists for two weeks or longer.

In addition, individuals with this disorder typically develop other symptoms, including:

- *Changes in mood:* feeling sad, empty, hopeless, worried, irritable
- *Changes in thinking:* loss of interest or pleasure in usual activities, poor concentration, low self-esteem, indecisiveness, preoccupation with death, thoughts of suicide, guilt
- *Changes in behavior:* slowing down or increased restlessness, crying, social withdrawal, suicidal acts
- *Changes in physical condition:* increased or decreased appetite, disturbed sleep, decreased sexual drive, weight loss or gain, pain, digestive problems, fatigue.

Major depression can develop at any age or stage of life. (See Chapter 25 for a discussion of depression in the elderly, and Chapter 26 for information on depression in children and adolescents.) The incidence of this problem has soared over the last two decades, especially among young adults. Its symptoms can take many forms. Rather than feeling depressed, some people may become pessimistic, irritable, angry, or hostile. One person may chiefly be troubled by a loss of appetite, physical ailments, poor sleep, and lethargy. Another may be plagued by a sense of hopelessness, guilt, and feelings of worthlessness. Others may find that they cannot concentrate or think clearly, that it is hard to be around other people, and that thoughts of death or suicide keep pushing into their minds.

TYPES OF MAJOR DEPRESSION

Major depression can be mild, moderate, or severe. Mild cases involve a minimal number of symptoms (five are required for a diagnosis of major depressive disorder) and very little interference with normal functioning at work or in usual social activities and relationships. Individuals with moderate depression experience more symptoms and greater impairment in their daily lives. In severe depression, symptoms are increased in both number and severity, and take a much greater toll on the ability to function socially or professionally. In extreme cases, individuals are unable to work or even to feed or clothe themselves or to maintain basic hygiene.

Therapists identify three special forms of major depression as melancholic, atypical, and psychotic. Individuals with melancholic depression feel sad in a way they describe as different from other experiences of depression. They typically wake before dawn and cannot return to sleep; their depression is most intense in the morning. Many feel agitated or slowed down. They lose their appetite and weight loss often occurs. Their lack of pleasure in life's normal joys is complete and persistent. When something good happens they don't feel better, even briefly, and they may be haunted by excessive or unfounded guilt.

Individuals with atypical depression, in contrast, are capable of joy, however fleeting, and can feel temporarily happy in response to a pleasurable occurrence. Rather than losing their appetite or being unable to sleep, they may eat and sleep much more than usual. Some report a heavy, leaden feeling in their arms and legs. Often they have a chronic and extreme sensitivity to rejection that interferes with their ability to work and socialize.

In psychotic depression, which is uncommon, individuals lose touch with reality and may develop hallucinations, usually reflecting their sense of doom. They may think their insides are rotting out, for instance, or hear voices telling them to kill themselves. Treatment with antipsychotic medications is often essential. (Chapter 17 discusses the nature, symptoms, and treatment of psychotic disorders.)

▼

How common is major depression?

Young children, teenagers, men and women of every age and every social, racial, ethnic, and economic group can develop depression. According to epidemiological data from the National Institute on Mental Health (NIMH), 4.4 percent of Americans—about 9.4 million in all—develop major depression at some point in life. The National Comorbidity Survey found that major depression is the single most widespread mental disorder, affecting 10.3 percent of Americans in any given year.

At highest risk are those who have already experienced an episode of major depression, who have close relatives with severe depression, or who abuse alcohol or other drugs. Some researchers believe that many who abuse alcohol or drugs do so to ease or mask depression.

Women are two to three times more likely than men to develop major depression, dysthymia, seasonal affective disorder, or recurrent brief depression. According to the *Diagnostic and Statistical Manual of Mental Disorders, Fourth Edition (DSM-IV)*, a woman's lifetime risk for major depression ranges from 10 to 25 percent in community samples, compared with 5 to 12 percent for men. Rates for men and women are highest between the ages of twenty-five and forty-four years. The average age at onset is the mid-twenties.

In recent decades, major depression has been increasing and developing earlier in life. Epidemiological reports from China, Canada, France, Lebanon, New Zealand, and other countries indicate that the incidence of depression among individuals younger than age twenty-five is rising worldwide. Researchers have theorized that urbanization, a breakdown in family ties and traditional religion, and a rise in drug and alcohol abuse may be contributing factors.

An estimated 15 percent of adults over the age of sixty-five—and up to 25 percent of nursing home residents—have symptoms of major depression. In the elderly, physicians and family members often attribute many symptoms of depression to medical causes. A National Institutes of Health (NIH) panel of experts has warned that more than 60 percent of older Americans suffering from depression are not receiving appropriate therapy, often because both health care providers and individuals themselves misinterpret sad feelings as a normal response to the medical, social, and economic problems the elderly face. In other circumstances, what appears to be depression in the elderly may have physical roots, such as poor nutrition or anemia. (Chapter 25 discusses mental health in the elderly.)

▼

What causes major depression?

Depressed individuals may wonder, "Why did this happen?" or "Why do I feel this way?" Unfortunately, there are no definitive answers. Like many other illnesses, major depression can strike out of the blue without apparent reason. Various combinations of different factors—biological, genetic, chemical, psychological, social, developmental, and environmental—may lead to major depression. As with so many medical conditions, some individuals appear to have a biological vulnerability that makes them especially susceptible. Nevertheless, whatever its origins, depression is an illness characterized by neurochemical abnormalities that cause significant disability. It can be deadly, and it must be recognized and treated.

BIOLOGICAL FACTORS

Extensive research into the neurobiology of depression has shown that depression is a complex biological illness that affects the delicate balance of brain chemicals, the signaling system used for communication between neurons, the flow of blood through the brain, the hormones that regulate dozens of body processes, and the mechanisms involved in sleep and wakefulness.

Heredity The parents, siblings, and children of persons who have suffered major depression are more likely than others to become depressed themselves. In general, the rate of depression among close relatives is 1.5 to three times that of individuals with no family history of depression.

Studies of identical twins, who share identical genes, have suggested a genetic basis for depression. If one identical twin becomes

Women and depression: The sadder sex?

Women are two to three times more likely than men to develop a depressive disorder. According to data from the National Institute on Mental Health (NIMH), 2.6 to 3.9 percent of women in the United States suffer from depression during any one-month period, compared with 1.2 to 2.2 percent of men. Similar findings have emerged from more than forty studies in thirty different countries.

Why are women more vulnerable? According to the American Psychological Association's National Task Force on Women and Depression, there is no simple answer: "No one theory or set of theories fully explains gender differences in depression." However, some factors that may contribute to depression in women include:

☐ **Avoidant, passive, dependent behavior patterns and pessimistic, negative cognitive styles.** Women may become depressed more often and stay depressed longer because they may tend to react rather than act, rely too much on others as a source of their happiness, and dwell more on how tired or sad they feel. Men seem more likely to distract themselves, to seek out the company of others, and to focus on action and mastery strategies. In addition, women may have more difficulty than men in expressing anger, and may think that the price of emotional honesty is loss of love.

☐ **Physical and sexual victimization.** More than a third of all women are physically or sexually abused before the age of twenty-one; this may create a lifelong vulnerability to depression. Repeated abuse can instill a sense of helplessness that makes women feel out of control and incapable of change. In the recent National Comorbidity Survey, 12 percent of women reported that a traumatic experience, most often rape or sexual molestation, had resulted in a mental disorder.

☐ **Greater sensitivity to relationship problems.** In general, women base much of their self-esteem on relationships and suffer more when these are jeopardized or broken off. Women in unhappy marriages are three times more likely to become depressed than married men or single women. Women are more likely than men to become depressed after divorce; men may be more susceptible to depression after the death of a spouse.

☐ **The stress of female roles.** The gender differentials in depression occur at puberty, and some researchers believe that young girls become vulnerable to depression and eating disorders as they deal with ambivalence and anxiety about femininity, sexuality, and adulthood. Mothers of young children also are susceptible; their likelihood of depression increases with the number of children they must care for and with lack of support.

☐ **Social factors.** The relationship among women, work, and depression is complex, but non-employed depressed, the other faces a much greater chance of depression. In a study of more than a thousand pairs of female twins, the risk for an identical twin developing depression if her sister had the disease was 66 percent higher than the risk in the general population. Among fraternal twins, the risk was 27 percent higher. Children whose biological parents were depressed, and who were adopted at birth into families with no history of the disorder, are more likely to develop depression than the biological children of their adoptive parents. However, heredity is not the only determi-

women with high mental strain in their lives are most likely to become depressed. Women who are poor (women and children make up 75 percent of America's poor), non-white, lesbian, or chemically dependent are at increased risk.

Although it is impossible to separate biological and psychosocial factors, women do not seem *inherently* more susceptible to depression. As part of the preparation of the *DSM-IV*, a special task force reviewed all available data on women and depression and found no relation to levels of female hormones. Some women undergoing treatment for depression reported feeling worse before their periods, possibly because of premenstrual changes in the way they metabolize antidepressants. After five years of often heated debate, the *DSM-IV* task force distinguished premenstrual syndrome, which affects a great many women, from a newly designated form of depression, termed *premenstrual dysphoric disorder* (PMDD),

which is much less common. It occurs in an estimated 1 to 3 percent of all menstruating women, who experience symptoms of depression during the last week of their menstrual cycles and cannot function as usual at work, school, or home. They feel better a few days after menstruation begins.

PMDD remains controversial, primarily for political reasons. Some women's advocacy groups oppose labeling women with menstruation-linked symptoms as mentally ill. Others contend that a diagnosis of PMDD simply recognizes the distress some women experience and may make it easier for them to obtain help. "There is no way the diagnosis of PMDD should be used in a pejorative way against women," says psychiatrist Judith Gold, M.D., of Halifax, Canada, who chaired the *DSM-IV* task force, noting that PMDD does not mean a woman is "incompetent or psychotic."

In recent years, other long-standing theories about women and depression have been challenged.

The risk for becoming depressed after hysterectomy seems no greater than after any other major operation; indeed, women who had been depressed before surgery often feel better afterward. The notion of "menopausal depression" also may not hold up. Many therapists contend that women going through menopause are no more likely to suffer depression than women at other ages or than men, and that midlife depressions in women stem from psychological experiences or social circumstances rather than hormonal changes.

Most researchers feel that there never will be any simple or single explanation for why women have higher rates of depression. What we know now is that complex interactions among many variables appear to be responsible. As understanding grows, as social roles change, as we learn more about women's bodies and women's minds, we may find better answers to what makes anyone—male or female—vulnerable to depression.

nant. Individuals with no family history also can and do develop major depression.

Brain chemistry Depression alters the balance of certain crucial chemicals within the brain, including neurotransmitters, or messenger chemicals, such as serotonin and norepinephrine, that allow brain cells to communicate with each other. (Chapter 2 discusses the neurotransmitters and brain chemistry.)

In the past, scientists theorized that deficiency in either serotonin or norepinephrine or both may lead to depression. This hypothesis now seems simplistic. Other neurotransmitters may also be involved, or the underlying problem may stem from alterations in certain types of receptors, the specialized molecules that receive messages sent from neuron to neuron. In addition, some scientists studying depression are investigating the role of other brain chemicals, including the neuropeptides (short-chain amino acids that perform some of the same functions as the traditional neurotransmitters).

Hormonal systems   In addition to disrupting brain chemistry, depression may interfere with virtually every function of the endocrine system. It can cause subtle abnormalities in the production of hormones by the hypothalamus and the pituitary and adrenal glands. Many depressed persons have abnormal thyroid function. Sometimes psychiatrists give supplements of the thyroid hormone T_3 (not T_4, which is a treatment for hypothyroidism) to individuals who do not improve with antidepressants alone.

Sleep-wake controls   Depression has been linked with disruptions in the sleep-wake mechanisms within the brain. Depressed individuals often show characteristic changes in their sleep patterns, particularly a tendency to enter rapid eye movement (REM) or dream sleep much earlier in a night's sleep than usual. Researchers have been experimenting with sleep deprivation as a possible way of enhancing response to antidepressant drugs, speeding up their impact, preventing recurrences of the disorder, or predicting whether an individual will improve with treatment with a specific drug or electroconvulsive therapy (ECT).

PSYCHOLOGICAL FACTORS

Depression is an illness of the mind as well as the brain, and many theories about its psychological origins have emerged over the years. Freud traced adult depression back to childhood loss, a theory he later discounted. Many of his successors elaborated on this idea, arguing that loss, if not fully acknowledged and mourned, can result in sadness, anger, hopelessness, extreme sensitivity to rejection, and low self-esteem. Individuals who cannot express anger or assert their independence, often for fear of rejection or abandonment, may punish themselves for such "unacceptable" feelings by turning the anger inward and becoming depressed.

Therapists disagree as to whether some individuals have characteristic ways of behaving that put them at greater risk of depression. However, it has been observed that those who seek help for depression often share certain characteristics: Many are unable to fend off negative thoughts, have unrealistic expectations and standards for their own performance, or depend excessively on others. Having made a series of "safe" but unrewarding life choices, such people may end up in circumstances that provide little joy or satisfaction—with a dead-end job, an unloved mate, and overwhelming family responsibilities.

Cognitive and behavioral factors According to the creators of cognitive therapy, depression stems from a negative way of thinking about self, the environment, and the future. Automatically assuming that they, their world, or their future lacks something essential for happiness, individuals come to view themselves as inadequate or unworthy, their families as critical or unsupportive, and their prospects as bleak. Negative, distorted thoughts become more frequent as depression deepens.

Individuals who feel inadequate or unworthy may be particularly vulnerable to the sort of distorted thinking that can lead to depression. Their attitudes and reasoning processes lead them to faulty conclusions about the world and their own self-worth. They may also lack the social skills necessary to obtain positive feedback, such as praise for a job well done. Even when someone does compliment them, they may not believe they deserve the kind words.

Based on experiments with animals, psychologist Martin Seligman, Ph.D., developed the behavioral theory that past experiences of real helplessness (such as suffering from an accident or injury) can convince individuals that they will not be able to control current or future difficulties. As a result of such "learned helplessness" they become passive and resigned, accepting painful situations as inevitable and feeling overwhelmed and helpless.

Stress and life traumas Numerous or intensely stressful life events have often been linked with the development of depressive disorders, although they seem to have an impact primarily on initial episodes of major depression. Severe or unanticipated stress, major losses (such as the death of a loved one, a divorce, or the loss of a job), family or marital problems, financial problems, a move to a new town, a life transition (such as having a child), and chronic illness may trigger a first attack. But even among individuals facing similar amounts of stress, some seem inherently more vulnerable to depression than others.

Grief following the greatest possible life trauma—the death of a loved one—may lead to symptoms of depression (see Chapter 4 for a discussion of grief), and if it becomes particularly intense or prolonged it can develop into major depression. A bereaved person who has not begun to move on with life within six months, who becomes preoccupied with feelings of guilt or worthlessness, who develops hallucinations or delusions, or who contemplates suicide may have slipped into a major depression and needs treatment.

A lack of stable, close relationships may increase susceptibility to depression. Spouses (especially women) who describe their marriages as being in trouble are much more likely to be depressed than those in happy ones. As the box on women and depression notes, problems involving relationships may contribute to a woman's vulnerability. Men, who make up a third of depressed individuals, tend to get depressed for different reasons. Socialized to place great importance on being good providers and achievers, they are more likely to become depressed after the loss of a job, a promotion, or professional status. Paradoxically, success can have the same effect as failure for those who feel they don't deserve it or can't meet expectations. Some high achievers become depressed because they miss the challenge and stimulation of fighting their way to the top. For both men and women, ongoing tension or pressure, particularly in jobs that provide few rewards and little security, can set the stage for depression.

▼

How major depression feels

Developing a major depression is like falling into a bottomless pit. Although sufferers want to escape, they cannot muster the strength to move. They want to understand how they got there, yet they cannot concentrate or think clearly. Cut off by their depression from all they once cherished, they find that they simply don't care anymore. They feel themselves sliding into deeper, more terrifying depths, but they cannot help themselves or even hope that someone else might help them. They see no way out, and they may spend hours or days brooding about their past failures or future trials.

"What makes the condition intolerable is the foreknowledge that no remedy will come—not in a day, an hour, a month or a minute; it is hopelessness even more than pain that crushes the soul," writes author William Styron in *Darkness Visible*, his memoir of his struggle with what he calls "a howling tempest in the brain."

Others view depression as Winston Churchill did—as a "black dog" with a terrible bite. "It crouches in the corner of the room, waits for me to make a move. Or lies at the foot of the bed, like a shadow until I try to get up," writes Kathy Cronkite in *On the Edge of Darkness*. "I go nowhere alone; he is at my side."

Consumed by their own misery, depressed individuals pull away from others, isolating themselves within walls of apathy, indifferent to those around them. A loving mother no longer cuddles her children. An avid tennis player no longer picks up a racquet.

Even a long-awaited event, such as an exotic vacation, sparks no excitement. Life's pleasures are beyond reach, too remote to touch or even tempt. Very often individuals lose all interest in sex and pull away from any form of intimacy.

The face in the mirror turns into a despicable character with countless faults and no redeeming virtues. A straight-A student feels incapable of keeping up with schoolwork. A devoted spouse reproaches himself for every short-tempered remark. A hard-working manager accumulates evidence of her own incompetence. Guilt over current or past failings grows steadily. The most trivial incident, such as a forgotten errand, becomes further proof of inadequacy. When anything goes wrong, depressed individuals blame themselves. Even when they are clearly not responsible, they are guilty in their own eyes.

Often men react differently to depression than women. Denying the problem, men try to keep going and shake it off because they view it as a weakness. Far more than women, they mask their depression with irritability, since anger is an easier emotion than sadness for many men to express. They frequently self-medicate by drinking, but the depressant nature of alcohol only pulls them further down.

Yet both sexes suffer—and suffer deeply. "I am now the most miserable man living," Abraham Lincoln wrote during one of his depressions. "If what I feel were equally distributed to the whole human family, there would not be one cheerful face on earth." Baffled by what is happening within them, depressed individuals may wonder if they are losing their minds. Their families may share the same terrible fear.

Major depression distorts internal timing. A person may speak less or more slowly, pause longer before answering, speak in soft or monotonous tones, even stop talking at all. Some individuals move more slowly while others become incapable of sitting still. One woman recalls pacing back and forth day after day in her tiny apartment, wringing her hands as she walked.

Sleep patterns are shattered. Often a depressed person will sleep fitfully for a few hours and then wake long before dawn, unable to get more rest. Others will have the opposite response and sleep far more than usual, sometimes logging twelve or more unrefreshing hours in bed. Because depression saps vitality and stamina, getting out of bed in the morning seems a great burden. Routine tasks such as making dinner are exhausting. Any extra demand, such as getting an appliance or car repaired, may seem overwhelming.

The altered brain chemistry of depression can slow and cloud thought processes. Individuals often find it difficult to focus, remember, concentrate, make decisions, or think through an issue.

They may be easily distracted. Some people find it hard to absorb information or carry on a casual conversation. They read a newspaper without assimilating a single sentence or forget a question they have just been asked. Nothing lightens the load they feel.

Typically, depressed people lose their appetite and interest in food. Many shed ten pounds or more without any attempt at dieting. Conversely, some individuals, particularly women, crave sweets or other carbohydrates and eat more when they are depressed, often in binges. Those who put on a good deal of weight feel even worse about themselves.

Depressed individuals often have other psychological symptoms, including obsessive brooding, excessive concern about physical health, panic attacks, or phobias. Anxiety may be a symptom of depression or may develop at the same time. (See Chapter 7 for a discussion of mixed anxiety and depression.) This combination, which creates profound suffering at the core of one's being, can be lethal, since high levels of anxiety in depressed individuals may increase the risk for suicide.

But the pain of depression is never simply psychological. "Mysteriously, in ways difficult to accept by those who have never suffered it, depression comes to resemble physical anguish," William Styron writes. "Such anguish can become every bit as excruciating as the pain of a fractured limb, migraine, or heart attack."

As major depression deepens, thoughts of death may push ever more insistently into consciousness. Individuals may become preoccupied with death and wish they could succumb to a fatal illness or die in an accident. Some, assuming that their loved ones would be better off without them, contemplate what had once seemed unthinkable—ending their own lives.

▼

Seeking help Many depressed individuals do not realize that they are seriously ill. Some blame themselves and try to "tough it out"; others turn to alcohol or drugs. The inertia and despair bred by major depression keep many from obtaining help. Without treatment, they may suffer for months or even years. Often family members must take the initiative in seeking help because the depressed person may be too emotionally "stuck" to do so—or to recognize the need for it. Loved ones must reach through the isolation, show their concern, and encourage a depressed individual to go for help.

Major depression can develop over days or weeks or can occur suddenly, usually after a trauma. Some people experience mild symptoms or feelings of anxiety for several months before plunging into depression. Others experience relatively brief periods of depression that recur at least once a month.

The primary reason to suspect depression is a change from previous feeling and functioning that persists for most of the day, nearly every day, for two weeks or more. The most common symptom is feeling discouraged, sad, or hopeless—and not feeling better with some rest or relaxation, the passage of time, or good news. Major depression always affects the way a person works, copes with everyday tasks, and relates to others.

If you or someone close to you has not been able to function normally for two weeks or more, these are the questions that should be asked:

- Do you feel sad, anxious, tearful, irritable, or hopeless for most of the day, almost every day?

- Have you lost interest in eating, sex, socializing, or your favorite activities?

- Are you eating more or less than usual? Have you gained or lost weight?

- Are you sleeping more or less than usual?

- Do you feel as if you're talking or walking in slow motion? Do you fidget constantly or find yourself incapable of staying still?

- Are you always tired? Are you too weary to tackle even small chores?

- Do you feel worthless or guilty about something?

- Are you having problems in thinking, concentrating, or making decisions?

- Have you been thinking more and more about death? Do you ever think you'd be better off dead? Have you thought about killing yourself?

Many people will answer "yes" to at least one of these questions. If you are feeling down, you might respond "yes" to two or three, perhaps four. If you answer "yes" to more than four questions, you may need professional help. Keep in mind that depression is one of the most curable diseases of mind or body—but the key to getting better is getting help.

If you suspect that you or someone close to you is suffering from major depression, seek help from a mental health professional at once. If the urge to commit suicide is real, call 911 and ask for a paramedic team or police officer to come immediately. Another option is going to the nearest hospital emergency room (a friend or relative of the person should drive). Crisis intervention (see box) almost always reverses self-destructive urges and begins a process of understanding and recovery. Depressed individuals who develop psychotic symptoms, such as hearing voices or believing in delusions, are at especially high risk for suicide and should be taken to an emergency facility immediately.

Crisis intervention

This is the psychiatric equivalent of emergency medical care—an immediate response to a dangerous, even deadly situation, such as a person's intense wish to commit suicide. Special hotlines listed in the front of the telephone directory put callers in touch with trained personnel who can quickly determine what type of help they need most. Some hotlines focus on a specific problem, such as suicide or drug abuse. Others, staffed by local mental health centers, deal with any and all psychiatric problems, including almost uncontrollable feelings of rage or violence. Your local phone directory yellow or business pages will also carry listings of area mental health centers.

When calling during a crisis, keep these points in mind:

☐   If time is crucial—for instance, if someone is threatening to jump off a roof—call 911 rather than search through the phone book. The dispatcher will contact the appropriate agencies.

☐   If you call a mental health hotline, describe the primary problem, such as suicidal thoughts or uncontrollable anger, briefly and clearly. Allow the health workers to ask for details.

☐   Be patient. Your call may be transferred, or you may be referred to other numbers, before you finally reach the correct person or facility.

☐   If you cannot stay on the telephone, say where you are, give your phone number, and specify the kind of help you need. Be sure to state your location clearly.

☐   Always ask to be referred elsewhere if your initial contact cannot help you.

Because depression often develops insidiously and takes many different forms, it can be difficult to diagnose. According to the federal panel that prepared treatment guidelines for depression, primary care physicians fail to recognize depression in one in every three patients who have this disorder. A complete physical examination is important to rule out possible medical causes, such as thyroid disease, malnutrition, hormonal imbalances, vitamin deficiency, or drug abuse. Although researchers have developed several laboratory tests that detect biological changes in blood and urine, and have linked characteristic sleep patterns to depression, none provides definitive proof that a person is depressed.

▼

Risks and complications

Anyone experiencing a major depression is at risk for suicide. About 15 percent of those diagnosed as depressed kill themselves. Twice that number may attempt suicide. (See Chapter 22 on suicidal behavior.) Depressed individuals are at risk for suicide until they have fully recovered, and should see their physician or therapist regularly. This is especially important during the early phase of treatment, which usually restores them to a level of energy that may enable them to act on self-destructive impulses.

Substance abuse is a common complication of depression. Many individuals drink to blunt their sadness; others turn to alcohol to help them fall asleep (although in fact alcohol disrupts the usual rhythms of the brain during sleep and undermines deep, restorative sleep). Depressed individuals also may abuse or become dependent on drugs. Some try stimulants to lift their mood, but these drugs can produce a greater sense of depression when their effects wear off.

Depression complicates many physical conditions and can interfere with treatment and recovery from asthma, stroke, heart disease, cancer, epilepsy, multiple sclerosis, and Parkinson's disease. In a recent Canadian study, heart attack survivors who developed major depression had a three- to fourfold greater risk of dying within six months than those who were not depressed.

▼

Treating major depression

Both the federal Agency for Health Care Policy and Research and the American Psychiatric Association (APA) have issued practice guidelines for the treatment of adults with major depressive disorders. Years in the making and based on thousands of scientific studies, these guidelines represent the state of the science of therapy for depression. However, this does not mean that they spell out the best approach for a particular individual.

"For some people, finding the right treatment is as easy as taking aspirin for a headache. For others, the search involves trial and error, sometimes over an extended period of time," observes Kathy Cronkite, who spent twenty years in therapy before beginning on medications. For a long time she considered psychotherapy a failure in treating her depression and medication a success. But she has come to see her success story from a new angle—that without the therapy, "I would never have been able to flip that internal switch that illuminated my problems and allowed me to confront them. For many people, the medication is necessary to bring the disease under control before they are able to work consistently with a therapist. For me, much of that work was finished before medications were started."

Despite inevitable controversy, there is general agreement on certain key points about the treatment of depression:

- Most cases of major depression can be treated successfully, usually with psychotherapy, medication, or both.

- No single approach works for all depressed people, but individuals who do not improve with one form of therapy are highly likely to improve with a different one.

- Psychotherapy alone works in more than half of mild to moderate episodes of major depression. Two specific psychotherapies— cognitive-behavioral therapy and interpersonal therapy—have proven as helpful as antidepressant drugs in treating mild cases

Is it major depression?

According to the DSM-IV, a diagnosis of major depression should be based on these criteria:

■ **At least five of the following symptoms—one of which must be depressed mood or loss of interest or pleasure—that persist nearly every day for at least two weeks and represent a change from the way the individual felt or functioned in the past:**

1. **Depressed mood (feeling sad or empty or seeming sad or tearful)**
2. **Greatly diminished interest or pleasure in all or almost all activities**
3. **Significant weight gain or loss without dieting (e.g., more than 5 percent of body weight in a month) or increased or decreased appetite**
4. **Sleeping much less or much more than usual**
5. **Slowing down or speeding up of activity that is observable by others**
6. **Fatigue or loss of energy**
7. **Feelings of worthlessness or excessive or inappropriate guilt, not merely self-reproach about being sick**
8. **Diminished ability to think or concentrate, or indecisiveness**
9. **Recurrent thoughts of death (not just fear of dying), recurrent suicidal thoughts without a specific plan, or a suicide attempt or specific plan for committing suicide**

■ **Great distress or impairment in social, occupational, or other important areas of functioning**

■ **Symptoms are not due to the direct effects of a substance (e.g., drugs of abuse or medication) or a medical illness (e.g., hypothyroidism).**

■ **Symptoms persist for longer than two months after the loss of a loved one.**

Adapted from the Diagnostic and Statistical Manual of Mental Disorders, 4th Edition. *Used with permission.*

of depression, although they take longer than medication to achieve results.

- Antidepressant drugs work in more than half of those with moderate to severe depression and may be useful in treating mild depression in individuals who do not improve with psychotherapy alone. These medications usually take three or four weeks to produce significant benefits and may not achieve their full impact for up to eight weeks.

- Combined treatment with psychotherapy and medication benefits individuals with severe, chronic, or recurrent major depression and those who do not fully improve with medication or psychotherapy alone.

During the acute phase of depression, when symptoms are severe, the goal of treatment is to bring about improvement or remission (at least a brief period without any symptoms). Continuation treatment preserves the progress that has been made and prevents relapses. Maintenance treatment protects susceptible people from recurrences (new episodes of major depression).

Although some individuals suffering from major depression may receive only one form of therapy, most receive a combination of treatments, depending on their symptoms, medical and psychiatric history, life stressors, family and psychological make-up, social and cultural environment, and personal preferences. Mild depression may improve with therapy alone. When depression becomes severe or chronic, however, it usually requires biological treatment, most often with medication.

Electroconvulsive therapy (ECT) is recommended for individuals who do not improve after trying two different medications in succession for the recommended periods of time or who cannot tolerate the side effects of antidepressant drugs. Melancholic depression is particularly likely to improve with drug therapy or ECT. (ECT is discussed in detail in Chapter 28.)

A history of drug or alcohol abuse or dependence influences the choice of treatment and of medication for depression. Abstinence from alcohol or drugs is usually the first priority for depressed individuals who abuse these substances. Sometimes, simply not drinking or using drugs for six weeks or so reduces many of the depressive symptoms. In other cases, individuals who respond to treatment reduce their use of these substances. However, when depression and a substance abuse problem exist concurrently, it is always important that both be treated.

PSYCHOTHERAPY

Various forms of psychotherapy (all of which are more fully described in Chapter 27), often in combination with one another and with drug therapy, are used to treat depression. The individual's own preference, the stage and severity of the depression, and the nature of the person's symptoms and concerns all play a role in the choice of a particular type or types of psychotherapy. As noted above, two types—interpersonal and cognitive-behavioral therapy—have been proven effective in mild to moderate depression. Both approaches are brief therapies, usually requiring no more than twenty sessions.

During the acute phase of depression, the frequency of psychotherapy sessions can range from once a week or every other week to as often as several times a week. During continuation and maintenance treatment, therapists may see individuals one or more times a week to continue the work of psychotherapy or once every several weeks or months to provide ongoing support.

Supportive psychotherapy   A helpful, trusting relationship is the key to the supportive approach (also called *psychotherapeutic management*). Therapists educate individuals about their illness and symptoms, boost their morale and hopes for improvement, explore issues involving relationships, work, or health problems, recommend and discuss treatment options, set reasonable goals, encourage individuals to become more involved with others, and watch for destructive behaviors or impulses. This approach may be most useful during the initial phase of severe depression, when individuals may not have the emotional or cognitive resources for more probing forms of psychotherapy and may most need information about their illness and assistance in coping with its impact. It also provides encouragement during the period before antidepressant drugs begin to have a beneficial effect.

Interpersonal therapy   Interpersonal therapy (IPT) focuses on current relationships and social interactions and strategies for improving them so that a depressed person can relate to others more successfully. Techniques include clarifying and feeding back what the person says, encouraging individuals to recognize and accept painful feelings, and increasing effective communication. Unlike traditional psychodynamic therapy, which goes back to early development, interpersonal therapy focuses on the here and now. It may be most beneficial for depressed persons who are involved in troubled relationships or are having difficulty adjusting to a major life transition, such as divorce or retirement.

In the acute phase of depression, IPT alone has proven helpful in easing the distress of those with major depression that is not severe or melancholic. It is especially effective in dealing with social and occupational difficulties, and may also be useful during maintenance treatment to help individuals with their relationships, jobs, or handling social situations. The APA guidelines describe IPT as "an alternative maintenance treatment" for those who cannot take or are not helped by antidepressant medications.

Cognitive-behavioral therapy   Cognitive-behavioral therapy (CBT) focuses on identifying, testing, and changing irrational assumptions and distorted thought patterns and on changing behaviors that cause conflicts. Therapists may instruct individuals to record the events of the day and their reactions to them in order to identify errors in thinking. To alter behaviors, they may stress training in problem-solving and social skills. CBT has been reported effective in individuals with mild to moderately severe major depression, especially when combined with antidepressant medications.

Psychodynamic psychotherapy and psychoanalysis   These therapeutic approaches look beyond the loss, frustration, or rejection that may have precipitated a major depression to uncover its deeper meaning and to help individuals identify, confront, and master unconscious issues. There have been no controlled studies of long-term psychotherapy and psychoanalysis in the treatment of any phase of major depression, either alone or in combination with antidepressant medications. The APA guidelines note that these methods may "best help those with a chronic sense of emptiness; harsh self-expectations and self-underestimation; a history of childhood abuses, losses, or separations; chronic interpersonal conflicts," or co-existing personality disorders. Mild to moderately depressed individuals with a stable environment who are motivated and capable of psychological exploration and insight are most likely to benefit.

Marital and family therapy This approach helps depressed individuals, along with their family members or partners, to see the impact of their own behavior on others. Family relationships that are abusive, ambivalent, rejecting, or highly dependent may predispose individuals to depression. Family therapy can identify and correct such problems.

Marital and family therapy can reduce the symptoms of depression and the risk for relapse in those with troubled relationships, regardless of which developed first—the depression or the problem. It is not clear whether depressed individuals who do not have relationship difficulties also benefit from this approach.

Group therapy Although there have been no controlled studies of the usefulness of group therapy in depression, many therapists feel that it is helpful, especially for bereaved individuals or those dealing with a stressor such as a chronic disease. Groups enable individuals to learn from the experiences of others and, in time, to enhance their own self-esteem by serving as models and mentors for new members of the group. Groups also are useful for those receiving medications as maintenance therapy and for individuals and family members in search of a support network.

MEDICATION
The development of effective antidepressant medications, which first came into use in the 1950s, has had an enormous impact on the treatment of depression. Antidepressant drugs correct the neurotransmitter-receptor imbalances that tend to occur in depressed individuals. They are most likely to help individuals who:

- Cannot function normally because of depression or feel that they are unable to enjoy life as fully as they once did

- Have physical symptoms, such as loss of appetite and weight, sleep disturbances, and fatigue, that have persisted without interruption for two weeks or more

- Have a family history of depression

- Cannot identify any particular trigger for their depression.

Antidepressants are not stimulants or mood elevators that make individuals feel high. When those who are not depressed take these drugs, they feel no effect on their mood—although they do experience physiological side effects, such as the dry mouth or blurred vision caused by tricyclic antidepressants. Because antidepressants are not addictive, one cannot become "hooked" or dependent on these drugs.

The combination of antidepressants and psychotherapy is very effective in treating moderate to severe depression. Rather than medications and therapy interfering with each other—as some mental health professionals had feared—the two approaches complement each other. The medications improve mood, sleep, energy, and appetite, while therapy strengthens coping skills, deals with possible underlying issues, improves thought patterns and behavior, and consolidates the gains that medication may help to achieve.

In general, antidepressants alone help about 60 to 70 percent of those taking them. (Chapter 28 provides detailed information on psychiatric medications.) As noted above, these drugs do not have an immediate effect. Although a few individuals may experience some improvement by the end of the first week, most do not see significant benefits for three or four weeks, and it can sometimes take as long as eight weeks for a medication to achieve its full impact. It is critical that depressed individuals continue to take these drugs long enough for them to be beneficial. The exact mechanisms by which antidepressants work are not fully understood, but they appear to interfere with the chain of events that produce the abnormalities in brain chemistry characteristic of depression.

Recent years have brought the development of several generations of antidepressants. The first generation included tricyclic and heterocyclic antidepressants, such as amoxapine (Asendin) and maprotiline (Ludiomil), and the monoamine oxidase (MAO) inhibitors, such as phenelzine (Nardil) and tranylcypromine (Parnate). Trazodone (Desyrel), with a different chemical make-up, could be considered a second-generation antidepressant. The selective serotonin reuptake inhibitors (SSRIs), such as fluoxetine (Prozac), sertraline (Zoloft), paroxetine (Paxil), and fluvoxamine

(Luvox), and the atypical antidepressant bupropion (Wellbutrin), represent a third generation. The new "fourth generation" drugs include nefazodone (Serzone) and venlafaxine (Effexor).

In general, psychiatrists begin with a low dose of an antidepressant and gradually increase it for a period of several weeks. Both the initial dose and the "therapeutic" or effective dose vary from person to person. Younger adults typically need higher doses than older ones. For certain tricyclic antidepressants, monitoring of the level of a drug in the blood can help in optimizing its beneficial effects while keeping side effects to a minimum.

Better sleep often is the first positive effect of antidepressants, except for the SSRIs, which can cause sleep problems. Sleep usually improves within a week or so, followed by an easing of physical complaints. Gradually, the other symptoms of depression—lethargy, low self-esteem, depressed feelings, hopelessness, anxiety—improve, although family members or close friends rather than the individual may be the first to notice this.

Nevertheless, the road to recovery from depression is a rocky one. It is important not to become discouraged about feeling down occasionally. Most people have good days and bad days, but over time they find that they are consistently feeling better. One lingering side effect of major depression is a lack of energy. Even after they start to improve, depressed individuals may still have to struggle for months to keep up what once was their normal routine. The memory of past suffering—as well as the fear of its return—can also cloud recovery.

There is great variability in how individuals respond to antidepressant medications. Many people initially improve only partially and, when they realize this, may be at an increased risk for self-destructive behavior, including suicide. It is critically important that they and their therapists work very closely to deal with problems or setbacks. The therapist's personal experience in treating depression and using or combining different approaches can be crucial to an individual's recovery.

Side effects   Reading the list of all possible side effects of antidepressant medications may be more distressing than what individuals taking them actually experience. These effects don't all happen, don't always happen, and may be very mild if they do happen. Many abate after two or three weeks of use. Individuals and their psychiatrists have to balance possible side effects against potential benefits. For many people, medication makes a tremendous difference. "I can sleep again," says one depressed man after treatment with an antidepressant. "My indifference disappeared. I have more energy. I don't feel high or doped up. I just feel like myself again."

COMMON SIDE EFFECTS OF ANTIDEPRESSANTS

SIDE EFFECT	HOW TO COPE
Dry mouth	**Drink lots of water, chew sugarless gum or candy. Ask your doctor about using an oral rinse of 1 percent pilocarpine three or four times a day.**
Constipation	**Eat a high-fiber diet (bran cereals, prunes, fruit, vegetables); drink plenty of water.**
Bladder problems (trouble emptying bladder; weaker urine stream)	**Call your doctor if you experience pain while urinating.**
Blurred vision	**Check with your doctor about using pilocarpine eye drops.**
Dizziness	**Rise slowly from bed or chair.**
Drowsiness	**Do not operate machinery or drive. Check with your doctor about taking medication at bedtime rather than earlier in the day.**

Because individuals vary greatly in their response to different medications and because side effects vary in seriousness, it is very important to work closely with a psychiatrist in choosing and using an antidepressant. If the side effects of one drug are troublesome, it may be possible to choose another that causes fewer or more tolerable side effects.

Side effects indicate that an antidepressant is being absorbed into the bloodstream and brain, which is a positive sign. Because depressed persons are easily discouraged, family members may have to point this out to reassure them that, in time, they will indeed feel better. Most side effects begin to lessen within three weeks.

A common initial side effect with some drugs is drowsiness. Taking the medication before bedtime helps; the drowsiness often is considered a plus for people who have trouble sleeping. Another possible side effect, primarily with tricyclics and MAO inhibitors, is weight gain. To various degrees, tricyclics suppress mucous secretions in the body, causing dry mouth, difficulty focusing at close range, constipation, and problems in urinating. These may improve in time, and practical coping strategies can help.

Particularly at the beginning of treatment with tricyclic antidepressants, many people complain of feeling dizzy or "foggy." Mild dizziness usually goes away on its own in a few weeks. The psychiatrist should check out moderate to severe dizziness, which may be caused by low blood pressure; sometimes a change in medication is necessary to eliminate this problem. Fogginess can be the result of a drug's effects on the brain. If individuals become confused or forgetful, a psychiatrist can prescribe a different antidepressant less likely to produce these effects. Tricyclics can also cause light-headedness when sitting up or standing suddenly, a particular concern for the elderly because of the risk of injuries from a fall.

Because tricyclic antidepressants can affect the heart, physicians must carefully consider which medication might be best for people with cardiovascular problems, such as arrhythmias (irregular heartbeats). The SSRIs are often selected as alternatives. They are less sedating and do not affect heart rhythm, although they, too, can have side effects: nausea, headache, nervousness, anxiety, sleep disturbances, delayed orgasm in women, retarded ejaculation in men, diarrhea, and increased risk for seizures. Starting at a low dose minimizes such problems.

Individuals taking MAO inhibitors must conform to stringent dietary restrictions and avoid foods and beverages containing tyramine, an amino acid found in many common foods that normally causes no difficulty but, in combination with these medications, can lead to a sudden, extremely dangerous surge in blood pressure. Among the substances to be avoided are cheeses (except for cream, cottage, and ricotta cheese), chocolate (in large amounts), overripe or spoiled fruits, soy products, beer, chianti wine, and some common over-the-counter and prescription medications. (A complete guide to MAO inhibitor use appears in Chapter 28.)

HOSPITALIZATION

Hospitalization may be necessary for depressed individuals who cannot care for themselves or comply with outpatient treatment; are considered at high risk of suicide or harm to others; do not have a safe, supportive living environment; require detoxification from drugs or alcohol; have other complicating mental or medical problems that cannot be safely treated outside a hospital; or do not improve with outpatient drug therapy and psychotherapy. The length of the hospital stay—usually brief—depends on a number of factors, including the severity of the depression, the availability of supportive family members, and health insurance coverage.

CONTINUATION THERAPY

Stopping treatment as soon as the symptoms of depression lift can lead to relapse, especially during the first eight weeks after remission. To prevent this, practice guidelines recommend that persons who improve on antidepressant therapy continue to take the full therapeutic dose for at least sixteen to twenty weeks after they re-

Treading water

For three weeks after he lost his job, Matt, a marketing specialist in his thirties, got dressed every morning, picked up his briefcase, and kissed his wife Cheri good-bye. Cheri had no idea he'd been laid off until she opened a packet of medical insurance forms forwarded by his company. When she confronted Matt, tears filled his eyes. "I couldn't tell you," he said. "I didn't want you to know what a failure I am."

Although she reassured him that he was anything but a failure in her eyes, Cheri could tell that her words had little effect. Matt brooded constantly. If she woke early in the morning, she'd find him standing in front of the window and staring into the blackness outside. At first, Matt would put on a suit and tie and go out every day to check out job leads or touch base with former colleagues, but after a few weeks he hardly left the house. He'd go for days without shaving.

Once an enthusiastic athlete, Matt no longer jogged or worked out. Even when Cheri picked up his favorite desserts on her way home, he barely touched them. In the evenings, he chugged bottle after bottle of beer and slumped in a chair, flipping through the television channels with his remote control. When Cheri tried to snuggle next to him, he pulled away. She couldn't remember the last time they'd made love.

Cheri tried talking to Matt, reassuring him that they could get by for a while on her income, suggesting that they get away for a long weekend at a friend's country cabin. Invariably, whatever she said triggered an angry outburst. "Leave me alone!" Matt would bark. "Get off my back!" Wounded, Cheri pulled away and sought comfort and advice from her friends. One of them, a psychiatric social worker, speculated that Matt might be depressed. She gave Cheri the name of a psychiatrist she knew and advised her to make an appointment. "It sounds like he needs treatment," she said. "Do whatever you have to do to get him to go."

Despite Matt's protests, Cheri insisted he come with her to the psychiatrist. After a complete evaluation, the physician diagnosed Matt's problem as major depression and suggested two forms of therapy: an antidepressant medication and brief psychotherapy to correct his self-defeating thought processes. Matt, still mired in helplessness, heard the words with skepticism. But he did hear them. "I felt that I'd been treading water at sea for as long as I could remember and finally, in the distance, I'd caught a glimpse of a rescue ship. I wasn't sure I could reach it. I wasn't sure it would get to me in time. But at least there was some reason to hope."

Taking one of the new antidepressants that targets serotonin receptors, Matt experienced few side effects other than occasional nausea, a slight tremor, and transient nervousness. Within a few weeks Cheri noticed a difference in him—in the way he stopped dragging himself as if his body were a dead weight, in his energy level, in the welcome, almost forgotten sound of his laughter.

In his therapy sessions, Matt examined his highly critical views of himself and his pessimism about the future. When he made one of his typical comments, such as "I've screwed up everything in my life," the psychiatrist would point out that he was generalizing, tick off the evidence to the contrary, and teach him cognitive techniques such as thought-stopping.

Within three months Matt felt and looked like a changed man. He was consulting for several businesses and one of the finalists for a marketing director job at a good-sized company. He'd returned to the activities he'd loved and enjoyed spending time with Cheri. Matt continued to take antidepressants for about a year. A few months thereafter, he noticed a return of some of his earlier symptoms: irritability, sleep problems, a diminished sense of pleasure. "This time I didn't wait to feel worse," he says. "I got help immediately.

turn to normal functioning. When medication is gradually tapered off, they should be carefully monitored to ensure that symptoms do not return. Various forms of psychotherapy during the continuation phase may help them to deal with stresses and conflicts that might lead to a recurrence.

MAINTENANCE THERAPY

At least 50 percent of those who suffer an episode of major depression have a recurrence, often within two or three years. Continuing drug treatment with antidepressants or with lithium, a mood-stabilizing drug used in the treatment of bipolar disorder (see Chapters 6 and 28), can prevent such episodes; it may be advisable for some individuals to continue on medication indefinitely. Some psychiatrists believe that an episode of depression causes lasting alterations within the brain that increase the likelihood of future attacks. This may explain why stress or life traumas are most likely to play a role in an initial episode of major depression, whereas recurrences often strike out of the blue, without any link to an upsetting event.

The need for maintenance therapy depends on the frequency and severity of past depressions and the potential benefits and side effects of treatment. Recurrences are more likely when some symptoms of chronic mild depression (dysthymia) persist after recovery, when individuals have a concurrent mental or medical disorder, or when they have experienced previous depressive episodes. If such episodes involved suicide attempts or psychotic symptoms, such as hallucinations, or were extremely disabling, recurrences may be even more severe. Individuals with a family history of recurrent depression face a greater risk for recurrences and for not fully recovering between episodes.

Psychotherapy can be used along with drugs to prevent recurrences, depending on many factors, including any remaining difficulties that might make individuals more susceptible to another depression in the future. In one landmark study, the combination of medication and interpersonal psychotherapy proved most effective as a maintenance therapy.

ELECTROCONVULSIVE THERAPY

For persons with moderate or severe major depression who cannot take antidepressants because of medical problems or who do not improve with psychotherapy or drugs, electroconvulsive therapy (ECT) remains the safest and most effective treatment. (ECT is the administration, usually in the hospital, of a controlled electrical current through electrodes attached to the scalp.) About 50 percent of depressed individuals who do not get better with antidepressant medication and psychotherapy improve after ECT. It has proven especially useful for older people, who sometimes cannot tolerate the side effects of antidepressant drugs. (See Chapter 28 for further information on ECT.)

Although ECT remains politically controversial because of outdated misperceptions about its dangers, it has proven clinically very useful. Properly administered, ECT does not cause a shock; it induces a seizure. For those at high risk for suicide it can be life-saving. The technology involved has become increasingly sophisticated and far safer than was once the case. Treatment usually consists of six to twelve ECT sessions, each two or three days apart. Most individuals, although unable to remember the few hours before treatment, show no cognitive problems two or three weeks after treatment. About one in every two hundred reports memory problems that persist for six months.

Individuals treated with ECT may receive maintenance treatment thereafter with antidepressants and/or lithium (described at length in Chapters 6 and 28). However, if they cannot tolerate the medications or these are not effective, periodic ECT can be administered every three to six months. There has been only limited research on how well ECT works as a maintenance treatment or how long it should be continued.

SPECIAL ISSUES IN TREATMENT

Although depression is a highly treatable illness, finding the best therapy for a particular individual can be complicated. Mental health professionals sometimes talk about "treatment failures" or "poor responders." It is important to keep in mind that it is the *treatment*, not the person, that fails or does not improve.

When medication fails   Antidepressants initially fail to help about 20 to 30 percent of those with major depressive disorder. This can sometimes be the result of an incorrect diagnosis, inadequate doses, or failure to identify and treat another mental or medical problem; at other times the reason is unknown.

If a person does not return to normal functioning after eight weeks on a medication or feels only somewhat better, psychiatrists may increase the antidepressant dosage; initial doses are often too low to produce significant benefits. If there still is no improvement, they may switch to a different type of drug. If, after several weeks, this medication is also unsuccessful, they may use an additional drug to make the brain more receptive to the antidepressant. Among the agents used for "augmentation therapy" are:

- *Lithium*, a mood-stabilizing and antimania drug; it helps about half of those who fail to improve with antidepressants alone

- *T_3 thyroid hormone supplements* (not the T_4 supplements given for low thyroid function)
- *Anticonvulsants* (carbamazepine and valproic acid)
- *Stimulants,* such as methylphenidate (Ritalin).

In serious cases of depression in which other approaches have failed, psychiatrists may try a combination of antidepressants, such as an SSRI together with a tricyclic antidepressant. Such drug combinations must be carefully monitored by a psychiatrist or another physician experienced in the use of these medications because of the risk for potentially dangerous interactions.

Atypical depression This term refers to depression with unusual symptoms, such as extreme anxiety, increased appetite, weight, or sleep, intense moodiness, phobias, and severe fatigue that can cause a sense of heaviness in the arms and legs. Only 35 to 50 percent of individuals with this type of depression are helped by tricyclic antidepressants. MAO inhibitors are more effective, leading to improvement in as many as 75 percent of cases. For those who cannot take MAO inhibitors or comply with the necessary dietary restrictions, one of the SSRIs can also be very beneficial.

Depression and other mental disorders Many depressed individuals also suffer from other mental problems, including substance abuse, schizophrenia, anxiety disorders, panic, obsessive-compulsive disorder, dementia, and personality disorders (especially narcissistic personality disorder). No one knows as yet whether one problem causes or is caused by the other, whether both have a common cause, or whether they are separate entities.

Treatment of depressed individuals with another disorder can be more challenging than treating a single illness. Sometimes a single medication helps both problems. For instance, clomipramine (Anafranil) or an SSRI is effective in treating both depression and obsessive-compulsive disorder. In other cases, treating the depression eliminates symptoms of the other condition, such as the cognitive difficulties characteristic of pseudodementia (difficulty in thinking and processing information that can be mistaken for dementia). Antidepressant medications usually do not help individuals with personality disorders as much as others; however, psychodynamic psychotherapy or psychoanalysis—alone or in combination with medication—may be beneficial in treating both the depression and the personality disorder.

Medical problems An individual's general health or specific medical problems, including asthma, heart disease, hypertension, epilepsy, glaucoma, bladder obstruction, or Parkinson's disease, can affect and be affected by depression and its treatment. A psychiatrist or other physician with expertise in psychiatric drugs must carefully evaluate any medications the depressed person is taking before prescribing an antidepressant. In some cases, individuals with severe depression may not be able to use antidepressants because of potential side effects or interactions with the drugs they require for another medical problem; here, ECT is considered the best alternative.

▼

Self-help   For those who have sought treatment, self-care is an important complement to professional therapy. Many of the brief psychotherapies require "homework," such as monitoring daily activities and moods and providing incentives and rewards. Increasingly, therapists also add "prescriptions" for activity or enjoyment as well as for drugs or counseling. Among the most useful approaches are:

> **Exercise.** Since depression feeds on inactivity, regular physical workouts can help the mind as well as the body. Many studies of the psychological impact of exercise show that aerobic workouts, such as walking or jogging, significantly improve the mood of mildly depressed individuals. Even anaerobic exercise, such as weight-lifting, can boost spirits, improve sleep and appetite, reduce irritability and anger, and produce feelings of mastery and accomplishment. Exercise also can help lower the risk for recurrence of depression. In a major eighteen-year longitudinal study of almost seven thousand adults, researchers at the Human Population Laboratory in Alameda, California, found that inactive men and women faced two to three times the risk of becoming depressed again as those who exercised regularly.

> **Tuning into problems.** Analyzing recent events to identify possible sources of stress, either alone or with a close friend or loved one, can help a person to regain a better perspective. If life has been particularly tumultuous, a lazy Saturday at home or a weekend away can also make a difference.

> **Talking back.** All of us silently "talk" to ourselves and comment on how we look and act. People whose inner voice is constantly self-critical should try to make note of unrealistic or critical thoughts and focus instead on what they like about themselves or things that they do well. Those who fight off negative thoughts fare better than those who cave in in the face of unhappiness or who rely on others to make them feel better about themselves.

> **Self-help groups.** Many individuals who have suffered with depression have found that talking with people with similar problems is extremely useful. Hospitals and community mental health cen-

ters often sponsor informal support groups. Such groups, especially those associated with a specific problem linked to depression (such as alcoholism, loss of a loved one, or childhood sexual abuse), are also helpful in preventing recurrences.

Good nutrition. Depressed individuals may be at risk for nutritional deficiencies because they often eat less and lose weight. A well-balanced diet should be part of every treatment plan.

Courses. Some medical centers and psychiatric clinics offer self-help courses for coping with depression. Individuals attend sessions once or twice a week for eight weeks as a supplement to professional treatment. In these classes they listen to lectures, engage in role-playing and other structured exercises, and interact as a group. Follow-up studies have found definite improvement six months after "graduation" from these courses.

▼

Impact on relationships

By its very nature, depression makes it difficult, if not impossible, for people to relate normally to others. They often are too wrapped up in their own suffering to reach out to others; they also may feel they have nothing to offer or to give.

Family members should try to maintain as normal a relationship as possible, acknowledge the depressed person's pain, refrain from criticism, offer encouragement and kindness, and show that they continue to value and care for that person. (Chapter 30 deals with the issues that families face when a loved one has a mental disorder.)

Like other chronic illnesses, depression puts tremendous stress on a marriage, whether or not marital problems preceded the depression. Over time it can take a toll on every aspect of a couple's intimacy and interdependence. A loss of sexual desire is a symptom of depression, not a personal rejection, a fact that partners may need to remind themselves of often, since restoring sexual intimacy can take a long time, even after other symptoms improve.

Many well-intentioned spouses, trying to help, start "overfunctioning" around the house and doing more of the things their partner once did. This only makes the partner feel more helpless and inadequate. Depressed individuals should be given as much control and responsibility as possible and should be expected to contribute as partners and as parents. It is best for everyone in the family if they continue to do chores and help around the home rather than sit alone ruminating. Since depression tends to be immobilizing, any form of activity should be encouraged, from walking to weaving to working in the garden.

It is important that relatives and close friends not try to treat the depression themselves. If a husband is depressed, his wife may be tempted to jolly him out of his "blue funk." A husband may point out to his depressed wife that other people have much more serious problems. Such comments can make matters worse because they sound like a dismissal from a spouse who doesn't want to hear the truth about the other's condition or deal with the difficulty. Reassuring troubled spouses that they're competent or desirable doesn't help either; instead, it may make them feel they are being patronized. On the other hand, discussing troubling issues frankly can be useful. Encouraging a loved one to talk about an illness or a setback at work can help the person to realize that he or she is facing very real difficulties that may require some assistance to work through.

Depressed individuals can say and do hurtful things, and family members have to distinguish between the individual and the illness. A man who says that he hates everything in his life or a wife who claims she is miserable in the marriage is expressing inner desperation, not hidden truths. This doesn't mean that such statements do not sting or that the other partner may not come to question his or her own feelings. It is best to be honest and to acknowledge such negative emotions without retaliating with an equally cutting remark or concluding that the marriage is doomed.

Partners also have to protect themselves from "catching" depression—which happens to as many as a third of the spouses of depressed individuals. Talking to friends, getting away for a few hours, or attending a support group for the families of individuals with mental disorders can be very helpful.

A parent's depression is also likely to affect the children in a family. Focused on his or her own acute suffering, the parent may not be able to respond to youngsters' physical or psychological needs. Since children tend to assume that they are to blame when there is a serious family problem, an honest explanation that Mom or Dad has an illness that makes him or her feel bad can help. Youngsters also need reassurance that their parent will get better and is not unhappy with *them*. To the greatest extent possible, they should keep up their usual routines, including fun activities at school or in the neighborhood. This can help them to forget about the problems at home and to feel better about themselves.

Family members of any age may become impatient or resentful because they want the "old" John or Mary back. Feelings like this are natural. When they occur, it is important to keep in mind that depression is an illness, that illness is nobody's fault, and that people with this particular illness can and do get better.

▼

Outlook   If unrecognized and untreated, major depression typically lasts for six months or longer and recurs throughout a lifetime. The toll that untreated depression can take is great—not only in terms of personal happiness and fulfillment but in its impact on family, work, and physical health.

With treatment, about 75 to 80 percent of depressed patients improve dramatically within three to four months of starting psychotherapy and/or antidepressant medication; recovery may take longer for others. Signs of improvement should begin to be evident within eight weeks or so. If you or someone you know begins treatment for depression and does not show evidence of this, talk to the physician or therapist, or seek a second opinion. A change in therapy approach, medication, or dosage may make a difference.

Most of those who receive treatment recover from an episode of major depression. However, according to the *DSM-IV*, a significant number continue to have significant symptoms of depression a year after diagnosis and treatment. Five to 10 percent are still depressed two years after their symptoms first appeared. The reasons can vary. The person may have been taking too small a dose of medication for too short a time or may not have persisted with psychotherapy long enough. Sometimes the underlying problem is a chronic, low-grade depressive disorder called *dysthymia*, discussed later in this chapter. Continued use of alcohol can make recovery difficult if not impossible.

More than half of those who have become seriously depressed eventually do so again, especially if they have only partially recovered. Like many chronic illnesses, even when treated, episodes of major depression can and often do recur. The risk is highest during the first six months after recovery, and the chance of subsequent recurrence increases with each new episode. Some people experience a cluster of depressive episodes over a period of a few years, and others have increasingly frequent episodes as they grow older.

The treatment a person receives affects the risk for recurrence. According to some follow-up studies, individuals treated with drugs alone may be more likely to become depressed again than those who undergo psychotherapy, with or without medication. The talking therapies (discussed in Chapter 27) may help by dealing directly with underlying issues and by teaching people how to spot early signs of depression and how to pull themselves up before they plunge too deeply into an episode.

The dosage and duration of drug therapy also matter. In a University of Pittsburgh study, high daily doses of the drug imipramine, one of the oldest and most widely used antidepressants, greatly reduced recurrences over a three-year period in persons who had a history of developing deep depressions every 1.5 to two years. When the doses that helped them become well initially were sustained, they remained well; lower doses led to relapses. Continuing monthly interpersonal therapy sessions, in combination with the medication, reduced recurrences by about 50 percent.

The outlook for recovery is not as bright for those with psychotic depression, who usually have more frequent episodes, suffer greater impairment, require hospitalization more frequently, and may be at greater risk for suicide. Individuals with this uncommon form of major depression are less likely than others to improve with antidepressants or antipsychotic drugs alone, but they do respond when these medications are combined or are given along with or after ECT. (Chapter 17 provides more information on psychotic disorders.)

The best hope for recovery from depression comes with early detection and treatment. Getting help as soon as possible can help to avert complications and prevent more severe depression.

Seasonal affective disorder

Seasonal affective disorder (SAD) is marked by annual episodes of depression that develop at the same time each year. Some people experience only unipolar depression; others also suffer manic or hypomanic episodes. (These terms are explained in Chapter 6.) The onset of the depressive episode always occurs within characteristic times of the year, most often between the beginning of October and the end of November, as the days grow shorter, and it ends in March or April with the coming of spring. January and February, often cloudy and dark, are usually the worst months for persons with the disorder. (Summer seasonal depressions, which are much rarer, usually begin in the period between March and June and end in August or September.)

Although the gloomy, gray days of winter can dampen anyone's spirits, individuals with SAD feel more than the slight feelings of depression known as the "winter blues." In mild cases, however, individuals may experience a slump in energy but not become depressed. More commonly, the symptoms of SAD are similar to those of the atypical pattern of major depression described on page 79. People with SAD, like those with other forms of major depression, feel helpless, guilt-ridden, and hopeless, and have difficulty thinking and making decisions. They may feel such great distress that they cannot carry on normal social and work-related activities. But unlike those with major depression, rather than eating less and losing weight, they eat more and gain weight. Many crave rich carbohydrates. Rather than sleeping less, they spend many more hours asleep, yet feel chronically exhausted. In SAD, as with any severe depression, suicide can be a risk.

The NIMH estimates that about 10 million Americans have SAD. The incidence is higher in more northern latitudes; for instance, in New Hampshire 9.7 percent of residents develop SAD, compared with 1.4 percent in Florida. Most SAD sufferers are women who first developed seasonal depressions in their twenties.

SAD seems to be the result of alterations in brain chemistry, although researchers debate its exact cause. In the winter, northern cities get only about eight hours of daylight, compared to sixteen hours at the peak of summer, and some individuals may be especially sensitive to this change. Researchers had initially theorized that the loss of daylight in winter months might increase the brain's production of melatonin, a hormone produced by the pea-sized pineal gland in the center of the brain. However, melatonin itself is no longer believed to play a major role in SAD. Alterations in brain chemistry, including seasonal variations in the production of the neurotransmitter serotonin, are under investigation.

SAD often improves with a specialized treatment called *phototherapy* (exposure to bright light). Since the first reports on this approach in 1980, a number of studies have confirmed improvement in people with SAD who sit in front of a specially designed light box every day during winter months. There is still some debate over the best form, timing, and duration of phototherapy. Many individuals improve with only thirty minutes of light exposure, but longer exposure of up to two hours (which has proved just as effective as five or six hours) may produce more long-lasting benefits. Some researchers believe that morning is the best time for phototherapy; others feel that light exposure at other times of day can also be helpful. One team of researchers has found that persons exposed to very low levels of light—just bright enough to simulate dawn—while still asleep showed improvement in SAD symptoms.

The recommended light therapy system consists of a set of fluorescent bulbs, which do not produce harmful ultraviolet light, installed in a metal box with a plastic diffusing screen. Although the size of the box can vary, the level of light produced should match the intensity of outdoor light shortly after sunrise or before sunset. Most light boxes provide light with an intensity of 10,000 lux, ten to twenty times as bright as ordinary indoor light.

Light therapy should be monitored by a psychiatrist. With regular sessions, persons with SAD become happier and more energetic. Side effects are uncommon, although some individuals complain of irritability, eyestrain, headaches, or insomnia, usually when the lights are used in the late evening.

For severe forms of seasonal depression, therapists may combine phototherapy with antidepressant medications. This combination is also very beneficial for persons who improve only par-

PERSONAL VOICE

A season of sadness

For as long as she could remember, Claire, a teacher in Bangor, Maine, had bought winter clothes two sizes larger than her summer ones. As soon as the weather turned cold, she found herself craving rich, creamy foods and sweets. By Christmas, she was usually five pounds heavier than she'd been at Halloween. By the end of the holidays, she'd put on another five. "I just can't control my appetite," she told a friend. "Then I get so depressed about being fat that I feel miserable for months."

In fact, Claire not only looked different in the winter, she acted differently. In the summer she was full of pep, spending as much time as she could out in the sun. In the winter she holed up inside the house for entire weekends. Her husband once described her as "the original couch potato." It wasn't that she didn't want to get up and do things—she couldn't. She didn't have the energy. Her nerves also seemed more on edge. "Don't mind Mom," she heard her son tell a friend when she yelled for them to lower the volume on the TV. "She's just in one of her moods."

As she began her annual countdown to spring, she once told her husband, "I'd be better off hibernating." She couldn't wait for the first crocuses to push up through the earth. Whereas she usually didn't feel like fussing over Christmas, she celebrated Easter in grand style. And even though she cooked up a storm, she usually was able to curb her appetite and start losing weight. "Just getting ready for swimsuit time," she'd laugh.

One winter Claire's family decided to give themselves a special Christmas present: two weeks in Florida. "None of my clothes will fit," she wailed. But when she got into the sunshine, she started feeling so good she didn't care. As if it were as easy as taking off a heavy coat, Claire shed her winter gloom. The vacation was one of the happiest times of her life. But after returning to Maine, her spirits sank.

A few weeks later, Claire's seventeen-year-old son, working on a research paper, came across an article on a specific type of depression that strikes mainly in winter. "Read this, Mom," he said. "It sounds like you." As Claire read the article, she had to agree that the description of seasonal affective disorder fit her perfectly. The piece included an address for the National Institute of Mental Health, and Claire wrote away for more information on SAD. She also talked to the psychologist for her school district, who referred her to a psychiatrist in town. His recommendation: phototherapy, or daily exposure to bright light.

Claire purchased a specially designed light box, which she set up in her kitchen next to the table where she prepared her daily lesson plans in early morning. At school, she rearranged the classroom so that her seat was closer to the window. She took daily walks to get the benefit of whatever sunlight there was. Her food cravings diminished. She felt lighter, more energetic and upbeat. And although she still waited eagerly for the first flowers of spring, she felt relieved that winter had lost its terrible hold on her spirits.

tially with phototherapy. The medications most often used are the SSRIs and the atypical antidepressant bupropion (Wellbutrin).

Researchers understand less about the possible causes of summer SAD, but speculate that it may be caused by heat-induced changes in brain and body chemistry. The usual treatment is medication, based on the severity of the depression.

Depression caused by general medical conditions

Some illnesses and physical conditions can cause symptoms identical to those of major depression, such as depressed mood, weight loss, and fatigue. This is sometimes called "secondary" depression. Mental health professionals experienced in evaluating depression notice differences between those suffering from major depression and those whose depression stems from a medical condition. The latter are often bewildered by their change in mood, which seems imposed on them rather than welling up from within. Despite their feelings of depression, they still feel good about themselves, and they are more upset by the fact that their depression is interfering with their usual activities than by any imagined shortcomings or failures.

In some cases, a change in the drug being given for the medical condition can eliminate the problem. If this is not possible, secondary depression requires treatment, usually with antidepressants. These must be carefully selected and monitored by a psychiatrist experienced in treating individuals with medical problems, who consults with the physician treating the medical illness.

Thyroid problems are a particularly common source of secondary depression. Many physicians and psychiatrists routinely assess levels of thyroid hormones during their diagnostic work-up. Thyroid supplements can make up for a deficiency; treatments

SOME MEDICAL CONDITIONS THAT CAN CAUSE DEPRESSION

☐ **Cancer**

☐ **Cardiovascular illnesses (e.g., congestive heart failure or heart attack)**

☐ **Digestive disorders**

☐ **Hormonal disorders (e.g., Cushing's syndrome, adrenal and pituitary abnormalities, and thyroid disorders)**

☐ **Infectious illnesses, especially viral infections**

☐ **Collagen disorders, rheumatoid arthritis, systemic lupus erythematosus (SLE)**

☐ **Neurological conditions (e.g., Alzheimer's disease, brain tumors, Huntington's disease, multiple sclerosis, Parkinson's disease, stroke, and traumatic brain injury)**

☐ **Nutritional problems (e.g., malnutrition or vitamin deficiencies)**

that decrease thyroid hormone production can relieve problems caused by an excess of hormone.

Often depression is overlooked or else is regarded as inevitable in cases of serious illness, such as advanced cancer, AIDS, or Alzheimer's disease (each discussed in Chapter 24). However, treatment with psychotherapy, antidepressant medication, and/or both has proven effective in easing sadness and hopelessness in these individuals.

A number of other medical problems can cause secondary depression; for a fuller list, see the table on page 87. Chapter 24 discusses the impact that chronic illnesses and medical conditions can have on mental health—and vice versa.

Postpartum depression

Many new mothers experience temporary feelings of sadness or tearfulness during the first seven to ten days after childbirth. Such "baby blues" are not a mental disorder and do not require treatment. Postpartum depression, which *is* a mental disorder, develops after less than 1 percent of all births, usually within four weeks of delivery, although it can occur at any time in the baby's first year.

Common symptoms include sadness, decreased concentration, physical complaints, feelings of guilt and unworthiness, agitation, anxiety, lack of energy, loss of interest and pleasure, even in the newborn, and obsessive behaviors, such as constantly checking on the baby. "It was the most horrible time of my life," recalls one woman. "Everything loomed very large, and I'd get revved up turning things over in my head. I'd think about problems like homelessness and wonder how anyone could be happy. I was terrified of getting dizzy and dropping the baby. I thought I was going crazy. Neither my husband nor I had any idea of what was happening. The word depression never entered our vocabulary."

A very small percentage of women with postpartum depression develop psychotic symptoms, such as hallucinations and delusions; an example is thinking they are so worthless or horrible that they or their babies would be better off dead. Women who have a family history of a depressive disorder, have suffered major depression, or who stopped their treatment with antidepressants because of pregnancy are particularly vulnerable to postpartum depression. An episode of postpartum depression increases the risk for subsequent depression, not only after future births but at other times as well.

Postpartum depression is treated like other forms of major depression, except that women who are nursing are initially treated only with psychotherapy because antidepressants, which are secreted in breast milk, can have potentially harmful side effects on infants.

Substance-induced depression

Many substances, both licit and illicit, have been implicated in episodes of depression. The former include not only alcohol but a number of widely used medications, including birth control pills, steroids, diet pills, and antihypertensive drugs (used to lower high blood pressure). Among the latter are illegal drugs such as cocaine, heroin, and other narcotics. It is possible to determine whether a substance is the likely cause of a depressive episode by noting when the signs and symptoms of depression began and when they stopped. If they developed before the use of the substance and if they persist for more than a month after this use has been discontinued, the depression probably has other causes.

Any medication that slows down body systems, as many blood-pressure-lowering and cardiac drugs do, can cause depressive symptoms. Women tend to show more of the classic symptoms in a medication-induced depression, such as feeling sad or tearful, whereas men may not. Very often a man taking drugs for an irregular heart beat or angina (chest pain) will become cranky, have difficulty sleeping, work to excess, or become forgetful. When his wife tries to talk with him about it, he insists that she leave him alone. In such circumstances, she should call his doctor and say, "Look, I've noticed these changes in my husband. What's going on?" The physician needs to check out the situation and determine whether the behavior is a side effect of medication.

As many as 15 percent of women using oral contraceptives have reported mood changes, including depression. A switch to a different birth control pill or another form of contraception can help. Postmenopausal women who receive estrogen replacement therapy seem most likely to develop symptoms of depression *after* they stop taking it. Restarting estrogen at the lowest possible dose usually relieves the depressive symptoms.

Although switching to another medication often lifts a drug-induced depression, it is not always possible to do this, or even to lower the dose. One woman with multiple sclerosis became depressed while taking high doses of corticosteroids for a severe flare-up. Because the drug was essential for her treatment, her best option was antidepressant medication. Non-drug treatments, such as psychotherapy, are not useful when depression is caused

SOME SUBSTANCES THAT CAN CAUSE DEPRESSION

☐ **Alcohol**

☐ **Antihistamines, used for allergies and colds**

☐ **Anticancer drugs**

☐ **Anticonvulsant drugs for seizure disorders (e.g., Dilantin)**

☐ **Antihypertensive medications, including methyldopa (Aldomet), guanethidine (Ismelin), and clonidine (Catapres)**

☐ **Anti-inflammatory drugs for arthritis, including indomethacin (Indocin) and other nonsteroidal anti-inflammatory drugs**

☐ **Antiparkinsonian drugs (L-dopa)**

☐ **Benzodiazepines, such as diazepam (Valium)**

☐ **Cardiac drugs, including digitalis and beta-blockers (e.g., propranolol)**

☐ **Cocaine**

☐ **Corticosteroids used for asthma, certain autoimmune diseases, and cancer**

☐ **Estrogen in oral contraceptives; discontinuation of estrogen replacement therapy**

☐ **Heroin and other narcotics**

by a drug; but because depression can be a life-threatening illness, effective treatment is always of critical importance.

Alcohol is closely linked with depression. About 20 to 25 percent of alcoholic individuals are depressed before they start drinking, and if the condition is not treated they remain depressed even if they become sober. Increasingly, therapists are treating the combined problems of depression and substance abuse simultaneously. For example, depressed individuals may undergo regular psychotherapy, take antidepressants, and attend meetings of Alcoholics Anonymous or similar substance abuse groups. (Chapter 9 discusses substance abuse and Chapter 10 alcohol abuse.)

Dysthymia

Dysthymia, or chronic mild depression, is the clinical term for sadness that does not end. Although everyone feels discouraged, sad, or inadequate at times, people with dysthymia experience symptoms of depression most of the day, and more days than not, for a period of at least two years. They also may have low self-esteem, eat and sleep more or less than usual, lack energy, have problems concentrating or making decisions, and feel a sense of hopelessness. Their symptoms, however, are less intense than those of major depression.

Federal officials consider dysthymia to be a "very substantial public health problem that has been vastly overlooked and un-recognized." Mental health professionals, on the other hand, have long debated whether or not it is truly a separate entity from major depression. The answer remains unclear.

▼

How common is dysthymia?

In the past, it was estimated that about 3 percent of Americans develop chronic mild depression at some time in their lives. The National Comorbidity Survey showed a higher rate, with 6.4 per-cent developing this disorder at some point in life and 2.5 percent suffering from it within any twelve-month period. Dysthymia, which usually begins in childhood, adolescence, or early adult life, occurs equally in boys and girls, but in adults it is two to three times more common among women than men. Although it usually develops before the age of twenty-five, most affected individuals are not diagnosed until their thirties and forties. In the past, those who sought professional help were often treated for secondary symptoms, such as fatigue or low self-esteem, rather than for dys-thymia itself.

▼

What causes dysthymia?

Dysthymia may stem from the same complex causes as major de-pression. Individuals may inherit or develop a tendency towards imbalances in the levels of certain neurotransmitters. Many have experienced acute episodes of major depression and may never have fully recovered. (An estimated 5 percent of depressed persons remain sad two years after their initial diagnosis and despite treat-ment.) Whereas some adults with dysthymia can trace their sad feelings to a traumatic childhood experience, such as parental divorce or death, many recall becoming depressed as children for no clear reason. One woman, asked how long she had felt sad, told her therapist, "Since the sperm hit the egg."

Dysthymia often co-exists with other mental disorders. In the NIMH's epidemiological studies, 75 percent of individuals with dysthymia also had such concurrent disorders—most often epi-sodes of major depression, panic disorder, anxiety disorders, or substance abuse. Other studies have linked dysthymia with atten-tion deficit disorder, conduct disorder, and personality disorders.

▼

How dysthymia feels

People with dysthymia often describe themselves as having been down for so long they had forgotten what "up" felt like. They tend to be plagued by physical complaints, such as fatigue, aches, and pains, as well as emotional problems. If something good happens they think it's a fluke or a fraud; if something bad happens they blame themselves for it. In their mind's eye, they see themselves as lacking worth. They may bury themselves in work, typically at jobs that are not particularly fulfilling or interesting. Emotionally, they may find themselves mired in unsatisfying relationships from which they cannot pull out. Pessimism and poor self-esteem prevent them from ever developing their full potential. Their lives are bereft of spontaneity, fun, true intimacy, or satisfaction.

To those who know them, these individuals can seem like perennial wet blankets: moody, whiny, gloomy, sad, incapable of a spontaneous cry of delight or a quick hug straight from the heart. Unlike those with major depression, they do function—but joylessly.

▼

Seeking help   Many persons with dysthymia never seek help because they have no idea that their unhappiness is caused by a treatable disease. Because their symptoms are so enduring, they feel that their state of low-grade misery is normal, just "the way life is."

If you suspect that you or someone close to you may have dysthymia, these are the questions that should be asked:

- Have you been feeling depressed more often than not for at least two years?
- Have you been feeling inadequate or bad about yourself?
- Have you been feeling pessimistic or hopeless?
- Do you no longer feel a sense of joy or enjoy activities you once did?
- Have you pulled away from others and spent more time alone?
- Do you feel low in energy or chronically tired?
- Have you been brooding about the past or feeling guilty?
- Have you been irritable or excessively angry?
- Have you felt less effective or productive than you once were?
- Have you had problems concentrating and thinking?
- Have you found it hard to remember things or make decisions?
- During the two years or more that you have been feeling depressed, did good times or breaks in feeling bad always end in two months or less?

Several "yes" answers may indicate dysthymia or another depressive disorder. Whatever their source, these problems are a clear indication to seek help. Because it is more subtle and insidi-

Is it dysthymia?

According to the DSM-IV, a diagnosis of dysthymic disorder should be based on these criteria:

- Depressed mood, reported by the individual or observed by others, for most of the day, on more days than not, for at least two years

- At least two of the following symptoms while depressed:
  1. Poor appetite or overeating
  2. Sleeping less or more than usual
  3. Low energy or fatigue
  4. Low self-esteem
  5. Poor concentration or difficulty in making decisions
  6. Feelings of hopelessness

- During the two-year period (one year for children and teens), no symptom-free period lasting for more than two months

- No major depressive episode during the first two years of the disturbance (one year for children and teens)

- No manic or hypomanic episodes (described in Chapter 6)

- No other mental disorder (e.g., schizophrenia)

- No substance (drugs of abuse or medication) or general medical condition (e.g., hypothyroidism) is responsible for the symptoms.

- Significant distress or impairment in daily living

Adapted from the Diagnostic and Statistical Manual of Mental Disorders, 4th Edition. *Used with permission.*

ous, dysthymia can be even harder to identify than depression. The key factors in making the diagnosis are how long the depression has lasted and how severe the symptoms are.

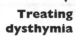

Risks and complications

Whereas major depression can destroy everything "normal" in a person's life, dysthymia's impact is more subtle. Although not as debilitating, it interferes with an individual's work and social life, if only because it continues for so long. The risks associated with dysthymia are similar to those linked with major depression: impaired performance at work or school, problems in relationships, substance abuse, self-destructive behavior, and suicide. Persons with dysthymia can also develop a major depression. If this happens, the resulting "double depression" can be extremely severe, and after recovery from this episode the dysthymia is likely to persist.

Treating dysthymia

As with other depressive disorders, dysthymia requires highly individualized treatment—a process that can take some time. There have been few careful, scientific studies to indicate which treat-

Shades of gray

"What's your favorite color?" Sylvia's niece asked her.

"Gray."

"Nobody's favorite color is gray," the girl replied.

"Your Aunt Sylvia's is," her mother interjected. "Suits her, don't you think?"

Everyone laughed as Sylvia struggled to smile. Ever since she'd been little, it had always been this way. Her sisters—rainbow girls who seemed to shimmer in the sun—giggled happily, while Sylvia, the quiet one, sat in the shadows. Even back then, Sylvia would marvel at how carefree her sisters and their friends seemed. Didn't they see how sad life could be? Didn't they worry about what could go wrong? But when Sylvia tried to explain how she felt, they called her a "Wendy Whiner." Even her mother would say that, for Sylvia, the glass was always half-empty, never half-full.

Sylvia didn't mean to rain on everyone's parade. She honestly couldn't help but see life the way she did—as trying and uncertain and filled with perils. Whenever she'd see her sisters run joyously into the surf, she'd long to join them but would hang back, thinking of how cold the water would feel or what a poor swimmer she was. As she got older, Sylvia watched her sisters charge on with their lives—one to study law, one to become a chef, one to try to make it as an actress.

Even though she'd always made good grades, Sylvia never thought of herself as being as bright or as talented. She went to a college in her hometown and lived at home. After graduation, she took a job as an administrative assistant at a local business. Six years later she was working for one of the vice-presidents. When this woman encouraged her to apply for positions that might put her on the management track, Sylvia declined. "I'm happy doing this," she said, not daring to admit that she feared being "found out" if she ever took on more responsibility. "They all think I'm so much smarter than I am," she'd tell herself when she earned a good performance report.

Sylvia never considered herself much of a "dater." "The moment a guy asks me out, I wonder how long it'll be till he dumps me," she once told a friend. "I wish I could skip the whole courtship thing and just get married." When she listened to her sisters gush about sweethearts and husbands and children, she'd think of how much energy it all seemed to take. Why put that much effort into other people's happiness?

But as she got older, Sylvia felt increasingly lonely. Her sisters and friends were wrapped up in their marriages and families. Her work seemed dull and repetitive. Her relationships with men never went anywhere. On the morning of her thirty-third birthday, Sylvia started crying and couldn't stop—not even when one of her sisters called to wish her a happy day. She was the one who urged Sylvia to see a therapist.

When the therapist used the term *dysthymia*, Sylvia had to ask what it was. She'd never heard the word before, although the symptoms—the feelings of inadequacy, the hopelessness, the lack of joy, the social withdrawal, the brooding and problems concentrating—were all too familiar. Asked how long she'd felt this way, she said she couldn't remember ever feeling any different. "All my life, I've felt that I was missing out on something—as if everyone else was tuned into music on the radio and all I could get was static."

The therapist recommended psychotherapy, including cognitive and interpersonal techniques to help Sylvia break out of her negative thought patterns and to enhance her social skills. She also recommended an antidepressant, although she explained that there was only a fifty-fifty chance that a drug would help—much lower than in major depression. After a few weeks of combined treatment, Sylvia hasn't magically been transformed. Yet she now has a new favorite color—bright yellow. And, as she tells her therapist, that's a start.

ments are best. Psychotherapy, antidepressant medications, or a combination of both may be effective. Aerobic exercise appears to be an especially helpful form of "adjunctive" or additional therapy.

Short-term psychotherapies help individuals with dysthymia to learn more healthful patterns of thinking, feeling, acting, and dealing with others. Cognitive therapy corrects typically negative and distorted thoughts, which can lead to self-destructive behavior. Interpersonal therapy strengthens social, coping, and communication skills. Behavioral therapy may combine aspects of other approaches and teach individuals practical skills, such as better time management and how to balance the ups and downs of daily living.

In the past, therapists often reserved antidepressant medications for major depressions, but research has shown that these drugs are effective in relieving dysthymia as well, although to a somewhat lesser extent; about 50 percent of those with this disorder improve with drug treatment. MAO inhibitors may be more effective than tricyclic antidepressants. The SSRIs and Wellbutrin may also help, although they have not been studied as extensively in dysthymia as in major depression. As in depression, antidepressants do not bring improvement for at least three to four weeks, and may take eight weeks for full benefit. Hospitalization is rarely required unless a person develops a major depression or is suicidal.

▼

Impact on relationships   Like other depressive disorders, dysthymia casts a gray shadow over everyone in the individual's life. At first, others may respond to the person's sadness with sympathy and support, but as it drags on, they may become irritated or pull away. Feeling rejected, the person may become even more isolated and despondent. With treatment, these relationship difficulties tend to diminish.

▼

Outlook   Without treatment, the sadness of dysthymia can continue for a lifetime. The prognosis for people who obtain help for the condition is good, and the vast majority improve significantly. In addition to a greater capacity for intimacy, they also do much better at work and attain significantly greater success than in the past. As with major depression, there is a risk for recurrence. If dysthymia does recur, many individuals opt to remain in treatment thereafter, usually with medication and maintenance psychotherapy, to prevent sliding back into dysthymia or depression.

Is it a bipolar disorder?

A bipolar disorder is characterized by mood swings that include episodes of depression and of mania or hypomania. The checklist at the beginning of Chapter 5 describes the most common symptoms of depression. In addition to such symptoms, individuals with bipolar illness may:

- ☐ **Feel unusual excitement, enthusiasm, energy, or irritability**

- ☐ **Experience an uncharacteristic change in mood or functioning**

- ☐ **Develop a sense of supreme self-confidence and inflated ability**

- ☐ **Have grandiose thoughts and plans**

- ☐ **Sleep very little and feel no need for more rest**

- ☐ **Talk more than usual and feel a sense of pressure to keep talking**

- ☐ **Think and talk rapidly, jumping from one idea to another**

- ☐ **Be easily distracted by irrelevant or unimportant comments or events**

- ☐ **Be physically and mentally restless**

- ☐ **Noticeably increase their usual social, sexual, or work-related activities**

- ☐ **Get involved in activities or pleasurable pursuits likely to lead to painful consequences (e.g., sexual indiscretions, poor business investments, buying sprees, potentially dangerous sports or adventures)**

The more boxes that you or someone close to you checks, the more reason you have to be concerned about bipolar illness. This chapter can provide insight and understanding about bipolar disorders, including guidance on seeking help.

Bipolar Disorders

Bipolar illness (manic depression) takes people to extremes. Individuals with bipolar disorders describe themselves as having "higher highs" and "lower lows" than others. When they are "up" they are on top of the world, absolutely euphoric, endlessly energetic, convinced that they can do anything they set out to do—whether that means skiing the expert run without ever having taken a lesson or dropping out of business school to become a screenwriter. People with bipolar disorders can and do go over the edge, often becoming self-destructive and sometimes losing touch with reality—and their plunge downward from the exhilarating highs of mania into the depths of depression can be so wrenching that life seems unbearably painful.

The various types of bipolar illness—bipolar I, bipolar II, and cyclothymia—account for about 20 percent of all depressive disorders. They are among the most treatable mental illnesses, *if* they are correctly diagnosed and treated. Unfortunately, affected individuals often are misdiagnosed or remain undiagnosed for years.

The cycles of despair and euphoria that are characteristic of bipolar illness can take various forms, but all involve episodes of hypomania (a mild form of mania) or mania, or mixed episodes (periods of at least one week of rapidly changing moods along with symptoms of mania and major depression). Hypomania usually imparts an intense sense of well-being, elation, and confidence and does not significantly impair functioning, although individuals may take dangerous risks or make impetuous decisions. Yet they also may become more productive, more passionate, or more charismatic than usual, all of which can be very appealing and enjoyable. In episodes of full-blown mania, impulsiveness and poor judgment become so extreme that they can destroy relationships, wreck careers, and wipe out personal finances. Some individuals develop psychotic symptoms, such as delusions and hallucinations, and require almost constant supervision to prevent physical harm. About 10 percent of people with a bipolar disorder experience only mania, without any depression. Mixed episodes seem to be more common among younger people and individuals with bipolar illness over the age of sixty.

Understanding bipolar disorders

First identified at the turn of the twentieth century, bipolar illness causes a wide range of symptoms, including the following signs of mania:

- *Changes in mood for a distinct period of time:* feeling happy, optimistic, euphoric, irritable

- *Changes in thinking:* thoughts speeding through one's brain; unrealistic self-confidence; difficulty concentrating; grandiose plans; delusions; hallucinations

- *Changes in behavior:* an increase in activity or socializing; immersion in plans and projects; talking very rapidly and much more than usual; excessive spending; impaired judgment; impulsive sexual involvement

- *Changes in physical condition:* less need for sleep; increased energy; fewer health complaints than usual.

The nine in ten people with bipolar illness who experience episodes of depression as well as mania or hypomania may develop the symptoms described in Chapter 5, including a depressed mood, loss of interest or pleasure in activities, feelings of worthlessness and hopelessness, lack of appetite, sleep difficulties, lack of energy, and thoughts of suicide.

CYCLES

The cycle of mood swings can vary greatly. Initially, in many instances, the period between episodes of depression, mania, or hypomania becomes shorter, with episodes occurring more and more frequently. In time, as part of its natural course, the condition may stabilize, with the interval between emotional extremes growing longer.

Although most people with bipolar disorders have some periods of normal moods, 5 to 15 percent of those seen in mood clinics (women more often than men) experience "rapid cycling"—four or more manic or major depressive episodes in a year, each lasting at least twenty-four hours and ending with a switch to the opposite psychological state, that is, from depression to mania or the reverse, or with a period of stability.

In ultra-rapid cycling, episodes of depression, mania, or hypomania may last only twenty-four hours. Some therapists have reported cases of ultra-ultra-rapid cycling, in which several or even many episodes occur daily. In continuous cycling, individuals swing from depression to mania or hypomania and back again without ever feeling normal for any sustained period of time.

Like unipolar depression, bipolar illnesses can follow a seasonal pattern, with individuals regularly sinking into depression at certain times of the year and then swinging into hypomania or mania a few months later. About half of those with bipolar disorder develop symptoms of psychosis (such as hallucinations and delusions), which may be consistent with their sense of power, knowledge, or inflated worth. More rarely, these symptoms involve completely different themes (such as a delusion of being controlled by others).

TYPES

Bipolar I disorder always includes at least one manic or mixed episode, often with one or more episodes of major depression. People in the depressive phase of bipolar I disorder feel worthless, helpless, and hopeless; derive no pleasure from life; cannot concentrate or remember clearly; eat and sleep more or less than usual; withdraw from friends and relatives; complain of insomnia, aches, pains, fatigue, and other physical problems; and may consider or attempt suicide.

Bipolar I disorder can begin with an episode of mania or of depression. In those who experience a depression first (which is more common in women), the interval from the first depression to the first manic episode is typically one to two years, although there have been instances in which mania did not develop for ten years or more. When individuals initially diagnosed as having major depression develop mania, their diagnosis changes to bipolar I disorder. More than 90 percent of persons who experience a single manic episode go on to have additional ones.

Bipolar II disorder, a new diagnosis added to the *Diagnostic and Statistical Manual of Mental Disorders, Fourth Edition (DSM-IV)*, consists of one or more major depressive episodes along with at least one episode of hypomania. Individuals with this type of bipolar disorder never develop full-blown mania; their "highs" are less extreme than those with bipolar I disorder. Because hypomania is more muted and lower-keyed than mania, bipolar II disorder can be more difficult to recognize. In people who have been depressed for a long time, a period of normal happiness may seem like hypomania or vice versa. An estimated 60 to 70 percent of hypomanic disorders occur immediately before or after a major depression.

▼

How common are bipolar disorders?

Nearly 2 million American adults suffer from a bipolar disorder. According to the National Institute of Mental Health (NIMH), about one in one hundred people will develop this illness. Bipolar disorders affect both sexes and all races equally, but are more common in upper socioeconomic and more highly educated groups.

Bipolar disorders usually begin in the late teens or early twenties. According to NIMH's epidemiological data, the median age for onset is eighteen years in men and twenty in women. In previous studies, the median age was somewhat older—in the mid-twenties—suggesting that, like major depression, bipolar illness is occurring earlier in life. If the illness is untreated, the average number of episodes of depression or mania over a ten-year period in bipolar I disorder is four; the number of episodes of depression and hypomania in bipolar II disorder tends to be higher.

Bipolar disorders have long been linked with creativity. The artist Vincent van Gogh, composers Robert Schumann and George Frederick Handel, poets Sylvia Plath and Robert Lowell, and writers Virginia Woolf and Ernest Hemingway suffered from what some have called this "brilliant madness." In her book, *Touched by Fire: Manic-Depressive Illness and the Artistic Temperament,* psychologist Kay Redfield Jamison, Ph.D., of Johns Hopkins University estimates that rates of bipolar illness are ten to forty times higher among artists than in the general public.

▼

What causes bipolar disorders?

Like major depression, bipolar disorders may stem from a complex combination of many factors: genetic, chemical, hormonal, psychological, social, and developmental. However, most mental health professionals now believe that bipolar illnesses are caused primarily by abnormal brain functioning.

Heredity plays an important role in susceptibility. Close relatives of people with bipolar illnesses are far more likely than others to develop either depression or a bipolar disorder themselves. The risks are highest if an individual's identical twin or both parents have bipolar disorder. (Some psychiatrists recommend preventive lithium therapy for a twin who has not yet developed symptoms.)

Researchers have theorized that bipolar illness stems from a defect in the brain's internal clock, or pacemaker, that controls daily and seasonal rhythms. Others feel that psychosocial stressors—a loved one's death, a serious accident, or other life traumas—may somehow sensitize the brain and make it more susceptible to mood swings. It is also possible that, as one researcher puts it, "episodes beget episodes"—in other words, that depression, mania, or hypomania alter brain chemistry in ways that create a predisposition to future episodes.

▼

How bipolar disorder feels

An episode of hypomania usually begins suddenly, with a pleasant sense of well-being or energy. In a letter to a friend, novelist Virginia Woolf wrote, "As an experience, madness is terrific, I can assure you, and not to be sniffed at." Sometimes this mild mania—hypomania—persists for a long period without becoming more severe. In other cases, it intensifies day by day. As the intensity increases, mania takes on an edge. The poet Robert Lowell described his mania as "pathological enthusiasm."

Bipolar disorders can cause great distress for affected individuals, who feel out of control of their emotions and behavior. Normally amiable people may become increasingly impulsive, emotional, irritable, angry. The euphoria of individuals in a manic state is so intense that not even a family tragedy or terrible disaster can dispel their high; yet if their plans are frustrated, their boisterous sense of well-being may turn to irritation that quickly shifts into uncontrollable fury. Some people typically become hostile rather than joyous; a few become paranoid and violent and may assault others, verbally or physically.

During a manic episode, individuals typically talk rapidly and incessantly, usually in loud voices. They answer questions at great length, continue talking when others speak, and sometimes talk when no one is listening. Their speech may be riddled with jokes, puns, word plays, or amusing but irrelevant witticisms. They may act in extremely theatrical ways, as if they were playing the part of a character in a play—dressing up in strange outfits, wearing garish make-up, offering money or advice to passing strangers.

Persons in a manic state may not be able to sit still or sleep. Some go for days with little more than two or three hours of rest, yet do not feel tired. In addition to being more physically active than usual, individuals in a manic state often become socially frenetic. They throw parties, go to bars, call friends up in the middle of the night. Throwing aside normal inhibitions, some become sexually hyperactive or promiscuous. They may initiate sex with

Higher highs, lower lows

Jack was a golden boy. He started reading when he was four, staged one-boy magic shows when he was six, skied the expert runs when he was eight. He captivated other youngsters with his daredevil exploits. As a teenager, he was a star athlete and an honor student, although he was always testing the limits, showing up late for practice or skipping classes. "Jack likes to live on the edge," his mother would say, with a mix of exasperation and indulgence. Over the years, she had seen a side of him few others ever did—sudden rages, bleak depressions, frenzied bursts of activity.

When he was in college, Jack set out to make his first million. As a design project, he developed a lightweight mesh backpack for hikers and bikers. Borrowing a girlfriend's sewing machine, he stayed up all night putting together a prototype. He hounded sporting goods manufacturers until they agreed to see him. His presentations were so persuasive that three companies bid on the manufacturing rights. By the time he turned twenty-one he had set up his own company, which he dubbed "Primo!"—the first.

Jack's schoolwork suffered as his business thrived. He would cut classes and buy others' notes to study for tests. During one finals week, he seemed to be running on sheer adrenaline. Night after night,

he stayed up writing papers or cramming for tests. Chugging coffee and chain-smoking, he'd talk non-stop to anyone who would listen, his mind flitting from one subject to the next. Even though he was sure he'd aced every course, Jack barely passed and was put on academic probation.

By the time grades were posted, Jack's spirits had plummeted. He retreated to his room, unable to get up, unwilling to talk with anyone. He felt that the faculty had finally discovered that he was a fast-talking fraud not nearly as smart as most people thought. Jack's worried friends called his parents, who packed his things and drove their subdued son home for the summer.

Jack didn't return to college for his final year. Instead he had a plan to develop an entire line of sporting accessories and market them by sponsoring adventure trips—white-water rafting, skydiving, skiing. Fired with enthusiasm, Jack rounded up backers. Primo's first line of sports gear, produced in eye-jolting neon colors, was a smash. But he had overestimated his production capabilities, and he couldn't keep up with retailers' demands. Some nights he'd go to the warehouse himself and package orders. Staff members coming to work in the morning would find him trying to pack six cartons at once, racing back and forth and babbling to himself.

When Jack's investors forced him to turn over the day-to-day management of Primo to experienced executives, he threw himself into plans for the adventure excursions. Borrowing against his company's assets, he spent a fortune on an elaborate launch, which included skydivers and a catered party for a thousand people. Jack was so wired that day that many thought he was high on cocaine. When he began rambling about the Star Trek crew beaming down to the party, his alarmed friends took him to the hospital. Tests revealed no drugs, but a consulting psychiatrist came up with the diagnosis: bipolar disorder (manic depression).

During his first week on a psychiatric ward, Jack remembers "the disease and the medications they gave me were fighting for control of my mind. I could feel myself slipping in and out of reality." By the time of his discharge four weeks later, Jack was definitely back in touch. "I had to survey the wreckage of my life and come to terms with the money I'd spent and the company I'd almost bankrupted," he says. With psychotherapy and ongoing treatment with drugs to control mood swings, Jack is building a new life, one he describes as "saner, with highs that are not quite so high and lows that aren't quite so low and a feeling, finally, of being in control."

their regular partner far more often than usual or enter into sexual liaisons with casual acquaintances or strangers.

Because mania impairs judgment, individuals sometimes make decisions with harmful long-term consequences—spending too much money, committing themselves to unrealistic deadlines, quarreling with family members who interfere with their plans. Others may announce that they are writing a book, marketing a brilliant invention, or starting a business. However, even when their plans are based in reality, these individuals are too easily distracted or are involved in too many projects to follow through.

In severe mania, thinking no longer is logical. The manic person speaks in an uncontrollable rush, flitting from subject to subject, sometimes becoming incoherent. Thoughts seem to take shape too quickly to be put into words. As in psychotic disorders, these individuals cannot distinguish between what is real and what is not. Some develop grandiose delusions and see themselves as invincible, all-powerful, or specially favored by God; some may even "hear" Jesus Christ explaining the need for a special crusade. Others become paranoid and so angry and frightened that they feel, as one person put it, trapped in "the bleakest caves of the mind caves you never knew were there." Some individuals with extremely severe mania may become catatonic, not speaking, barely moving, or assuming and maintaining weird postures.

▼

Seeking help   Bipolar disorders often strike people of great personal charm, creativity, and charisma. Initially it may be impossible for them—and difficult for those close to them—to understand or admit that anything is wrong. Often it is only when their behavior becomes outrageous, when they run up thousands of dollars on their credit

---

SOME DRUGS THAT CAN TRIGGER SYMPTOMS OF MANIA

☐ **Antidepressant medications**

☐ **Drugs of abuse (e.g., marijuana, LSD, cocaine, PCP, mescaline)**

☐ **Isoniazid (an antituberculosis medication)**

☐ **L-dopa, bromocriptine (for Parkinson's disease)**

☐ **Steroids (those medically prescribed as well as those used by body-builders and athletes)**

☐ **Stimulant medications prescribed for attention disorders (e.g., dextro-amphetamine, methylphenidate, pemoline)**

---

cards or get into a brawl, that friends or family members realize that something is seriously wrong.

If you suspect that you or someone close to you may be experiencing mania or hypomania, these are the questions to ask:

- Do you or does the other person feel or seem different—happier than usual, more talkative, more irritable? Has this change lasted for a week or more?

- Are ideas and plans unrealistic and grandiose?

- Has the need for sleep markedly diminished?

- Has speech become more rapid?

- Is there a tendency to jump from one idea to another?

- Is there increased distractibility?

- Is there a pattern of throwing oneself into work projects, social engagements, or other activities?

- Is there an increase in restlessness or agitation?

- Have there been imprudent actions, such as buying sprees or promiscuity?

- Has the usual level of performance at work or school fallen off?

- Has recent behavior affected relationships or social activities?

If the answer to most of these questions is "yes," you should seek help. If you see these telltale behaviors in a friend or loved one, insist that the person see a psychiatrist experienced in diagnosing and treating depressive disorders. If you or your loved one recall noting some of the characteristics of mania in the past but now feel depressed or have lost all interest or pleasure in most activities, see the "Seeking Help" section in Chapter 5 to ascertain whether the problem may be an episode of major depression.

As we have noted, mild forms of hypomania may be difficult for anyone, including many physicians and counselors, to recognize. Many people with bipolar illness are misdiagnosed as having other mental disorders, such as unipolar depression, schizophrenia, a personality disorder, or alcohol or drug dependence.

A recent survey by the National Depressive and Manic-Depressive Association found that it takes individuals with bipolar illness an average of seven to eight years to obtain a correct diagnosis and appropriate treatment; some of those surveyed did not seek or receive help for as long as ten years. During this time their lives were chaotic, and they reported financial difficulties, marital problems, drug use, aggression, crime, gambling, and personal injury. Yet, when finally treated, they were able to achieve greater stability and personal success.

A careful history of an individual's past mood changes can reveal a pattern of ups and downs. A detailed family history can identify persons who may have inherited a susceptibility to bipolar illness. In addition to a comprehensive psychiatric assessment, a thorough medical examination is essential because physical illnesses, such as epilepsy, multiple sclerosis, and hyperthyroidism, as well as certain drugs (see page 103), can mimic the symptoms of bipolar illness.

▼

Risks and complications

Mania can cause many personal and social complications: marital problems, divorce, business difficulties, lost jobs, bankruptcy, unsafe sexual encounters, illegal activities, accidents. Because bipolar disorders so often begin in youth or early adulthood, they can create one crisis after another. Unable to predict from one day to the next how they will feel, many individuals are always on edge. To relieve their anxiety, they may turn to drugs and alcohol, which is disturbingly common among those with bipolar illness. According to NIMH reports, 61 percent of those with bipolar illness (more than twice as many as those with major depression) develop a substance abuse or dependence disorder.

As many as 15 percent of those who receive no or inadequate

treatment for a bipolar disorder commit suicide. Mania can quickly lead to depression, and the risk for suicide is especially high when individuals become aware of their manic behavior and feel ashamed and remorseful because of what they did.

▼
Treating bipolar disorders
Professional therapy is essential in treating bipolar disorders. Medication is the cornerstone of treatment, although psychotherapy plays a critical role in helping individuals to understand their illness and to rebuild their lives.

MEDICATION

Lithium carbonate, a mood stabilizer, is used to treat both manic and depressive episodes and as maintenance therapy to prevent recurrences of mania. Other medications, primarily anticonvulsants, are also playing an increasingly important role in treatment of bipolar illness. (See Chapter 28 on psychiatric drugs.)

The treatment of episodes of major depression in bipolar disorder requires great care because of the possibility that certain biological therapies, including antidepressants and electroconvulsive therapy (ECT), can push bipolar individuals into a manic phase or speed up their cycling. To avoid this, psychiatrists usually prescribe lithium or another mood stabilizer before beginning an antidepressant. Sometimes the mood stabilizer alone proves to be adequate; if not, an antidepressant is added later.

Lithium No one knows precisely how lithium stabilizes the brain chemicals and neurons involved in mood swings. However, many studies have documented its effectiveness, showing that it successfully reduces both the number and the intensity of manic episodes for as many as 70 percent of those who take it. About 20 percent become completely free of symptoms. Those who respond best to lithium have a family history of mood disorders and periods of relatively normal mood between periods of mania and depression. Individuals who had experienced frequent episodes before they sought treatment tend to have a poorer response.

When taken early in a hypomanic episode, lithium can produce results in a few days. It usually takes seven to ten days to become effective in mania. However, if it is not given until full-blown mania develops, lithium alone may not be an adequate therapy, and individuals may need antipsychotic drugs and/or benzodiazepines—most often clonazepam (Klonopin) and lorazepam (Ativan)—to calm them during the period before the lithium takes effect. When used as a treatment for depression, lithium is usually combined with a tricyclic antidepressant or a monoamine oxidase (MAO) inhibitor.

Fairly common side effects of lithium include weight gain, ex-

Is it a hypomanic episode?

According to the DSM-IV, a diagnosis of a hypomanic episode should be based on these criteria:

■ A distinct period of sustained elevated, expansive, or irritable mood, lasting for four days or longer, which is clearly different from the individual's usual mood

■ During this period, at least three of the following symptoms (four if the only change in mood is increased irritability) are present to a significant degree:
   1. Inflated self-esteem or grandiosity
   2. Decreased need for sleep (e.g., feeling rested after three hours of sleep)
   3. More talkative than usual or pressure to keep talking
   4. Flight of ideas or feeling that one's thoughts are racing
   5. Distractibility
   6. Increase in goal-directed activity (socially, sexually, at work or school) or physical and mental restlessness or agitation
   7. Excessive involvement in pleasurable activities that are likely to lead to painful consequences, such as buying sprees or sexual indiscretions

■ An unequivocal change in functioning that is not characteristic of the individual

■ The changes in mood and functioning are observable by others.

■ The episode is not severe enough to cause significant impairment in the person's social or occupational functioning, does not necessitate hospitalization, and does not include any psychotic symptoms, such as delusions.

■ The episode is not due to the direct effects of a medication, an illicit drug, or a medical condition.

Adapted from the Diagnostic and Statistical Manual of Mental Disorders, 4th Edition. *Used with permission.*

cessive thirst and urination, digestive problems, hand tremors, and muscle weakness. Taking the medication on a full stomach can reduce nausea and other digestive symptoms. Some discomforts, such as extreme thirst, can be prevented by drinking eight to twelve glasses of water every day, restricting salt intake, and avoiding or limiting alcohol.

The gap between therapeutic and toxic levels of lithium is one of the narrowest of any drug routinely used in psychiatry. Excessive amounts can cause serious—although uncommon—problems, including hypothyroidism, kidney damage, confusion, delirium, seizures, coma, and even death. Because of its potential risks, lithium requires extremely conscientious monitoring by a psychiatrist or another physician experienced in the use of psychiatric drugs. Regular tests of the level of lithium in the blood and assessments of kidney and thyroid gland function are essential. It is also important to monitor for potential toxic effects, particularly those involving the central nervous system, such as slurred speech, dizziness, vertigo, incontinence, drowsiness, restlessness, confusion, stupor, and seizures.

Women should not become pregnant while taking lithium because use of the drug at the time of conception or during the first trimester of pregnancy has been linked to heart defects in the fetus. Those who wish to have a child are advised to wait until they have gone for at least two years without any episodes of mania or depression and then discontinue the medication. If treatment is needed early in pregnancy, ECT is a safer alternative. Lithium or certain antidepressants can be used later in pregnancy if a woman suffers a serious relapse but must be stopped two weeks before delivery. Women taking any of these medications should not breast-feed their babies.

Unfortunately, individuals with bipolar illness do not always follow their physicians' instructions about taking lithium. Some find the side effects too annoying or the weight gain too distressing. Others miss the confidence, drive, and energy of their hypomanic periods, although they admit that the consequences of their manic behavior are potentially too disastrous to risk. Some report that they feel "flat" or less creative, or have memory problems. Yet, in a survey of artists taking lithium, most found that their creativity had not diminished. For most people, the drug offers the opportunity for more "even" mood periods that can be devoted to work, family, or personal enjoyment.

To encourage compliance, physicians usually prescribe—through careful trial-and-error testing—the lowest possible dose that will prevent episodes of mania and depression. Group psychotherapy ("lithium groups") can help people cope with unavoidable side effects by sharing experiences and tips.

Anticonvulsant medications Anticonvulsant agents, primarily carbamazepine (Tegretol) and valproic acid (Depakene), have become increasingly important in the treatment of mania. It is thought that these may work by controlling "kindling"—changes in the pathways within the nervous system that transmit the impulses that produce manic behavior. Sometimes these are the only drugs used; sometimes they are prescribed along with lithium for individuals who do not improve on lithium alone. Anticonvulsants may be especially helpful for individuals who experience rapid cycling and who tend not to improve with lithium. Anticonvulsants should not be used during the first trimester of pregnancy.

Other medications Other drugs that have been used to treat mania are clonazepam (Klonopin), a benzodiazepine anticonvulsant; clonidine (Catapres), a medication primarily used for hypertension; and calcium-channel blockers such as verapamil (Isoptin or

Calan), which are more commonly used to treat irregular heartbeat and high blood pressure.

ELECTROCONVULSIVE THERAPY

Electroconvulsive therapy (ECT) is primarily recommended for treatment of severe mania in early pregnancy, when lithium and anticonvulsant medications should be avoided because of the risk of birth defects. It is said to be effective, although these reports are largely based on uncontrolled studies and anecdotal evidence.

MAINTENANCE THERAPY

Most individuals with bipolar disorders continue to take lithium indefinitely after remission of their symptoms. Some people dislike the idea of having to remain on medication, despite lithium's successful track record, even when they recognize that their need for it is similar to a diabetic's reliance on insulin. Those with such concerns should discuss them openly with their psychiatrists. They need to understand fully the nature of bipolar illness and the potential dangers of discontinuing lithium or trying to get by with doses too low to be effective.

Without maintenance therapy, the risk for recurrences after successful treatment is high: In one study, as many as half of the individuals developed new episodes of bipolar illness within five months after discontinuation of treatment. Recently, some psychiatrists have reported that, in people who suffered recurrences of bipolar disorders after discontinuing lithium, the drug no longer was as effective as it once had been. Small studies of the use of anticonvulsants alone for maintenance therapy have been promising but have not yet provided conclusive results. In clinical practice, the combination of lithium and an anticonvulsant appears helpful as a maintenance treatment for many people.

PSYCHOTHERAPY

Psychotherapy alone—whether behavioral, cognitive, or psychodynamic—has not proved effective in treating acute mania and does not affect the long-term course of bipolar disorders. However, therapy is useful in helping individuals to understand the stresses of both their illness and their everyday life, to restore their self-esteem, to adapt to a new range of emotions, and to work out ways to prevent relapses.

Psychotherapy can also help people learn how to establish healthy relationships with others and to recognize early signs of mood swings. By teaching practical coping strategies, it enables them to learn to manage the emotional roller coaster of the transition from a period of mania to a depression. No particular form of psychotherapy has proven significantly more useful than others, and therapists should be skilled and flexible enough to adapt their approach to the changing needs of each individual.

HOSPITALIZATION

Individuals with severe mania who develop psychotic symptoms may require hospitalization and continual supervision to prevent physical harm to themselves or others. Poor judgment can lead to personal danger; there have been rare cases in which persons with severe mania died as a result of physical exhaustion. Mania can be life-threatening in those who have heart disease. Treatment during hospitalization may consist of lithium, antipsychotic medication, or ECT, depending on the circumstances. Supportive psychotherapy, with a focus on education and reorientation to reality, can be beneficial during this acute phase.

Self-help   Although professional therapy is essential for persons with bipolar disorders, support groups, which meet in cities and towns across the country (many are affiliated with the National Depressive and Manic-Depressive Association or the National Alliance for the Mentally Ill), can make an invaluable contribution to recovery. Individuals can learn about their illness from experts who come to lecture at these meetings, and from people much like themselves who have similar problems. They can discuss variations in cycling or symptoms, tips for easing the side effects of medication, and ways of coping, such as keeping a "mood chart" to track fluctuations in mood and to spot early signs of mania or depression. Most important of all, they can reach out to others who understand, as no one else can, exactly how frightening and isolating bipolar illness can feel.

Impact on relationships   Bipolar illness can be especially hard for friends and family members, who are baffled and troubled by sudden transformations in their loved ones. During manic episodes, individuals with this disorder seem to be enjoying themselves while acting in alien and alienating ways. The consequences of their rash behavior often affect everyone around them. A husband and father may bankrupt the family by investing their savings in a wild scheme. A wife and mother may enter a series of dangerous sexual liaisons. A manic teenager high on drugs may crash into a car filled with young children.

When confronted with their destructive behavior, persons in a manic state typically deny being ill and resist getting help. Sometimes they explode in rage or into occasional violence. Often they insist they have never felt better in their lives. Then they may soon slide into a severe depression so disabling that they may not even

What is a mood chart?

One of the most important tools you and your doctor will use to design a treatment plan that is right for you is called a "mood chart" (like the one shown here). A mood chart is a chronological record tracking the feelings and behaviors associated with your condition. Its purpose is to let you and your doctor know the rhythms and cycles of your illness in order to design optimal treatment.

To use the mood chart shown here, you will need to begin by keeping a record of how you feel each day. Use a diary, for example, or a small notebook with dated pages. Each day rate your mood on a scale from 0 ("worst I've ever felt") to 100 ("best I've ever felt"). On the same page record other important information, including the medication you are taking and any key events that have taken place on that day. Because moods can vary with time of day, for accuracy and continuity try to record your mood at approximately the same time every day.

Then, each day, plot your mood on the chart at the lower right and connect each day's entry by a line. Over time the chart will provide you and your doctor a fairly objective history of the way you have been feeling and the effectiveness of your current treatments.

Blank mood chart page   DAY:_____

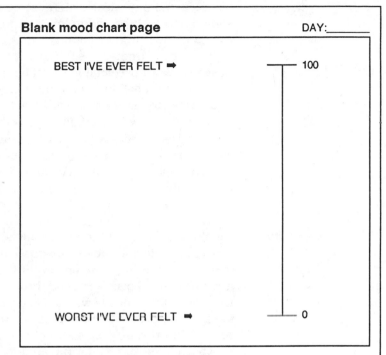

BEST I'VE EVER FELT ➡   ⊤— 100

WORST I'VE EVER FELT ➡   ⊥— 0

Completed diary page and mood scale

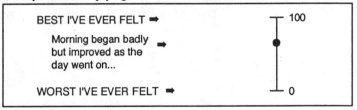

BEST I'VE EVER FELT ➡   ⊤ 100

Morning began badly ➡
but improved as the
day went on...

WORST I'VE EVER FELT ➡   ⊥ 0

Mood chart continuum after 14 days

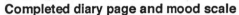

| 1 | 2 | 3 | 4 | 5 | 6 | 7 | 8 | 9 | 10 | 11 | 12 | 13 | 14 |

Blank continuum

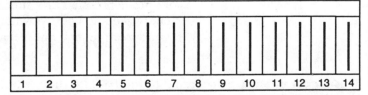

| 1 | 2 | 3 | 4 | 5 | 6 | 7 | 8 | 9 | 10 | 11 | 12 | 13 | 14 |

Source: National D.M.D.A. Used with permission.

be able to communicate. All these behaviors are threats to personal relationships and to family functioning. They also may affect the person's colleagues, supervisors, friends, or teachers.

Partners, parents, or siblings with milder forms of bipolar illness can be unpredictable—flipflopping from irritable to sad, affectionate to aloof, excited to indifferent—and relatives may never know what to expect or how to reach out to them. Because of the stress of living with an individual with bipolar illness, families benefit greatly from participating in support groups. Often family counseling helps to enhance understanding and develop effective ways of coping. (See Chapter 30 on coping when someone you love is mentally ill.)

▼
Outlook

Bipolar illnesses tend to be chronic and recurrent. Without treatment, a manic episode can last as long as three months, and a depressive episode even longer. With treatment, the prognosis for any particular episode is good, but many individuals continue to have persistent mood swings, particularly recurrent mild depressions. Even those receiving maintenance therapy with lithium may have "breakthrough" episodes of mania or depression, sometimes provoked by stress. Often the addition of an anticonvulsant proves more effective in preventing such problems than lithium alone. With treatment, these episodes usually occur less often.

Cyclothymic disorder

Cyclothymic disorder is a chronic bipolar illness that consists of swings from short periods of mild depression to short periods of hypomania. Mood swings can occur as often as every few days or weeks and persist for at least two years. Individuals with this disorder are never free of symptoms of hypomania or depression for more than two months at a time, yet they never develop a major depressive disorder.

Some individuals with cyclothymia experience more depressive than hypomanic episodes; others, more hypomanic ones. The persons most likely to seek help are those who alternate between periods of mild depression and times of intense irritability. Those who feel energized and creative when hypomanic and find their "lows" easy to tolerate may not feel a need for treatment.

▼
How common is cyclothymic disorder?

According to the *DSM-IV*, the lifetime prevalence of cyclothymia is 0.4 to 1 percent of the population. Most likely to begin in the late teens or early twenties, it is equally common in men and women.

▼
**What causes
cyclothymic
disorder?**

As with other bipolar disorders, there appears to be a genetic factor in cyclothymia. Many affected individuals have a family history of depression, bipolar illness, suicide, or drug dependence. Some researchers theorize that many relatives of people with cyclothymia, although not ill themselves, carry the gene for this illness and pass a predisposition on to their children.

▼
**How cyclothymia
feels**

Although it is not as severe as bipolar I and II disorders, cyclothymia can completely disrupt everyday life and create personal chaos. Zigzagging from euphoria to gloom, persons with this disorder never know how they will feel tomorrow or next week. Filled with enthusiasm, they may launch a project, only to abandon it a little while later. In personal relationships they are emotional yo-yos, alternately pulling close and pushing away. They may be cheerful, conscientious, considerate, charming, then become "blue" or turn mean. Their energy levels climb along with their spirits. Sleep disturbances are common, with individuals sleeping little during their high periods and barely pulling themselves out of bed during their lows. It is not uncommon for them to drink or take drugs to calm down.

Those whose cyclothymia is marked chiefly by periods of hypomania, during which they feel confident, creative, and energetic, may put these emotional surges to productive use and become leaders in industry, business, politics, or the arts. However, in most individuals, cyclothymia sabotages their chances for a stable life. They may repeatedly lose jobs. Their relationships tend to be volatile, and they may have a string of broken marriages. They may be impulsively promiscuous, dabble in different careers, or move from place to place.

Seeking help

If you suspect that mood swings may be interfering with your ability to function normally or may be affecting someone close to you, these are the questions that should be asked:

- Over the last two years, have you had many periods of feeling buoyantly energetic and optimistic?
- Have you also had many periods of feeling depressed or losing interest or pleasure in most activities? Do you sleep more when feeling down and less when feeling up?
- At times do you become much more talkative than usual?
- Does it sometimes seem that your thoughts are racing?
- Do you sometimes find yourself distracted by meaningless details?
- Do you sometimes feel restless or agitated and plunge from one type of activity to another?

Is it cyclothymic disorder?

According to the DSM-IV, a diagnosis of a cyclothymic disorder should be based on these criteria:

■ At least two years with many periods with hypomanic symptoms and many periods with depression or loss of interest or pleasure

■ No period of more than two months free of hypomanic or depressive symptoms

■ No major depressive, manic, or mixed episode during the first two years of the disturbance

■ Symptoms are not better accounted for by a schizophrenic or psychotic disorder.

■ Symptoms are not due to the direct effects of a medication, an illicit drug, or a medical condition.

■ Significant distress or impairment in daily living

Adapted from the Diagnostic and Statistical Manual of Mental Disorders, 4th Edition. *Used with permission.*

- Do you pursue pleasures without thinking of their consequences?

- Have your mood swings caused problems in your relationships, at work or school, or led to alcohol or drug abuse?

If the answer to many of these questions is "yes," you should consult a mental health professional. You may have cyclothymia or another bipolar disorder. A medical examination can rule out any physical problems that might cause mild mood swings, as well as the possibility that medications or alcohol or drug use are affecting your mood. A family history is important, as is the individual's recollection of fluctuations in mood over the preceding two years.

Risks and complications

Both relationships and work can suffer as a result of cyclothymia. During low periods, persons with this problem may alienate loved ones. At work, they may be less productive during times of depression and careless and disorganized during hypomanic periods. Substance abuse is common, as individuals turn to sedatives and alcohol during depressed periods or try stimulants and other drugs during hypomanic periods. Many are misdiagnosed with a borderline, antisocial, or histrionic personality disorder.

Treating cyclothymic disorder

There have not been rigorous scientific studies of treatments for cyclothymia. Individuals who feel productive during hypomanic states, whose behaviors are not destructive, and who can tolerate their mild depressions may prefer no treatment or supportive psychotherapy alone. In addition to individual psychotherapy, couples and family therapy may be especially helpful for dealing with problems in relationships.

Lithium, the primary medication used for bipolar illness, may help a substantial number of those with cyclothymia. It may take three or four months to have an effect and as long as a year for optimal results. After two years of successful maintenance, a psychiatrist may suggest stopping the drug, if only temporarily, to see how the individual might fare without it.

▼
Impact on relationships

Cyclothymia can baffle and frustrate even the most understanding family members. One day, their loved ones are thrilled to see them; the next, they're cold and indifferent. One night they're sexually charged; the next, they shy away from a kiss or touch. Sometimes spouses complain of never knowing what to expect.

Children may delight in parent's playful energy one day, only to be crushed when that parent loses interest or lacks the energy to follow through on plans or promises. Colleagues may feel that an affected individual is unreliable. Friends may be drawn to a person's exuberance, then hurt by seeming indifference.

With treatment, as the individual's moods become more stable, minor difficulties at work or in social relationships usually improve. Because cyclothymia can cause serious and lasting damage to intimate relationships, couples or family therapy is often recommended in addition to individual psychotherapy. In sessions with a therapist, partners can learn more about the illness and become skilled at spotting early clues of a mood shift and developing effective ways of responding.

▼
Outlook

If untreated, cyclothymia can continue for many years, with mood swings taking an ever-increasing toll on a person's relationships and happiness. Little is known about the long-term efficacy of psychotherapy or medication in treating cyclothymia, although clinical reports indicate that treatment helps individuals with this disorder achieve lasting balance and feel greater control over their lives.

Some individuals initially believed to suffer from cyclothymia eventually experience major depression, mania, and/or hypomania, and are diagnosed as having a bipolar I or II disorder. In one study, this occurred with more than one-third of those initially diagnosed with cyclothymia.

Is it an anxiety disorder?

Individuals with anxiety disorders may:

☐ **Experience episodes of overwhelming fear, rapid heartbeat, chest pain, profuse sweating, trembling, shaking, and other distressing symptoms**

☐ **Be afraid of losing control, going crazy, or dying during these attacks**

☐ **Worry about developing embarrassing symptoms or being in a place or situation that would be difficult to leave**

☐ **Avoid certain things, places, or situations because of anxiety**

☐ **Fear a particular object or situation, or the prospect of confronting that object or situation**

☐ **Worry about strangers' observations and criticisms**

☐ **Avoid or become extremely anxious in social situations**

☐ **Avoid or be extremely anxious about performing in front of others**

☐ **Have persistent feelings of anxiety, apprehension, restlessness, or irritability**

☐ **Worry about a variety of events or activities**

☐ **Find it hard to control their worrying**

☐ **Develop problems in concentrating**

☐ **Have physical symptoms, such as muscle tension**

☐ **Have problems in falling or staying asleep**

The more of these symptoms that describe what you or someone close to you has been experiencing recently, the more reason you have to be concerned about anxiety disorders, especially if they have persisted for six months or more or are interfering with routines, work, other activities, or relationships. This chapter provides information on the most common anxiety disorders, including guidance on getting help.

7 Anxiety Disorders

While taking an elevator to his office, a copywriter suddenly starts to tremble and sweat; unable to catch his breath, he thinks he is about to die. Certain that something dreadful might happen, a woman cannot leave her home unless her husband accompanies her. A model is so frightened of flying that she turns down out-of-town assignments. A biologist refuses a prestigious award because of the overwhelming anxiety he feels in any group. A popular singer becomes almost paralyzed with terror before every performance. A store owner feels "tied up in knots" by constant worries.

Although all of us feel vaguely uneasy, keyed up, nervous, or jumpy at times, the individuals described above live with something much more intense and disabling: anxiety disorders. The most common group of mental illnesses, they may involve episodes of sudden, inexplicable terror (panic attacks), inordinate fears of certain objects or situations (phobias), anxiety about social interactions or performances (social phobia), or chronic distress (generalized anxiety disorder, or GAD)—and they can trigger both physical and psychological symptoms.

Over a lifetime, according to the National Comorbidity Survey, as many as 25 percent—one in four—of the men and women in the United States may experience an anxiety disorder: either an acute or episodic one, such as a phobia, or a chronic or long-term one, such as GAD.

More than a third of all individuals who consult mental health professionals do so because of an anxiety disorder. In the past, their complaints were often misunderstood, misdiagnosed, or dismissed as primarily a psychological response to stress or conflict. These views have changed dramatically. As Jerilyn Ross, head of the Anxiety Disorders Association of America, says, "We have learned more about anxiety disorders in the past ten years than in the past one hundred."

Among the breakthroughs in understanding has been the discovery that some anxiety disorders, such as panic disorder, are primarily biological illnesses, associated with an underlying genetic vulnerability and alterations in brain chemistry. Stress and conflict can certainly make anxiety disorders worse, but they don't necessarily cause them. In most cases, an interplay of three major factors—biological, psychosocial (including stress), and behavioral—determines the nature and severity of the disorder.

Specific phobias are the most common anxiety disorder among the general population; panic disorder is the most common among those who seek psychiatric care. Other anxiety disorders include obsessive-compulsive disorder (OCD), discussed in Chapter 8, which involves distressing obsessions and senseless rituals, and posttraumatic stress disorder (PTSD) and other stress-related anxiety disorders, described in Chapter 12.

The new insights into the nature of anxiety disorders have led to major advances in treatment. For some problems, such as phobias, cognitive-behavioral therapy has proven highly effective. For others, such as panic disorders, medications, particularly in combination with cognitive-behavioral therapy, provide great relief. Self-help techniques, ranging from basics such as avoiding caffeine and exercising regularly to specialized strategies such as controlled breathing, can also be helpful.

Only one in every four persons with an anxiety disorder is correctly diagnosed and treated; many never seek help. Often individuals blame their distress on work, financial problems, or medical symptoms. Many hate to admit that they may be suffering from an anxiety disorder because they see it as a sign of weakness. Early recognition and treatment can prevent a great deal of suffering and help people to feel and function like themselves again. Most of those who do obtain help for these disorders, even those with severe and disabling problems, improve dramatically.

Panic attacks and panic disorder

Everyone has felt the abrupt stab of terror that comes, for example, with the sudden lurch of a plane in a storm or the sound of footsteps in a dark, empty parking garage. For those with panic disorder, however, there is often no impetus for the panic that overwhelms them; attacks typically strike during normal, everyday activities. A person may be washing dishes, driving to work, or shopping at a mall when an unexpected (or "uncued") panic attack hits. For others, attacks occur only when they confront or anticipate confronting a specific situation; these are called "situationally bound" or "cued" attacks. Panic attacks often lead to agoraphobia, fear and avoidance of places and situations in which individuals cannot readily escape or get help if needed. (Agoraphobia is discussed more fully later in this chapter.)

Most panic attacks reach peak intensity within ten minutes, a brief period that can feel like an eternity. During an attack, the person may hyperventilate (breathe very rapidly), tremble, shake, feel hot or cold, sweat profusely, become nauseated, experience heart palpitations or chest pain. Some people feel they are somehow outside of their bodies looking down at themselves, a phenomenon called *depersonalization*. Others experience the frightening sensation that their bodies feel unreal—*derealization*—or that they are somehow no longer themselves. Also common is an awful sense of impending doom, a fierce conviction that they are about to lose their minds, have a heart attack, or die. Each attack may bring greater apprehensiveness, called *anticipatory anxiety*, that can swell until it fills up the hours or days between attacks.

▼

How common are panic attacks and panic disorder?

About one-third of all young adults experience at least one panic attack between the ages of fifteen and thirty-five. According to data from the *Diagnostic and Statistical Manual of Mental Disorders, Fourth Edition (DSM-IV)*, 1.5 to 3.5 percent of people worldwide develop a full-blown panic disorder during their lifetimes.

Women are more than twice as likely as men to experience panic attacks, although no one knows precisely why. The parents, siblings, and children of individuals with panic disorders are more likely to develop them than others. Attacks typically begin between late adolescence and the mid-thirties. Panic disorder is most likely to develop in late adolescence; there is another, smaller peak in incidence in the thirties.

▼

What causes panic attacks and panic disorder?

The biological root of a panic attack appears to be a misfiring of the brain's alarm center, which normally triggers the classic fight-or-flight stress response. In a panic attack, the brain signals danger even though none exists.

There is a genetic risk factor, and close relatives of individuals with panic disorders may be born with a predisposition to panic attacks. One study found the risk to be about 25 percent among close relatives, compared with only 2 or 3 percent among others. In genetic studies of twins, panic disorder was more common among identical twins, who have an identical genetic make-up, than among fraternal twins, who have only half of their genes in common.

Researchers have identified distinctive differences in the autonomic nervous system (which controls mechanisms for breathing, blood pressure, heart rate, and sweating) and the breathing patterns of those with panic disorder. Certain medical conditions can cause anxiety or panic disorders. They include a usually benign heart problem called *mitral valve prolapse*; persons with this condition are much more likely than others to suffer panic attacks, although the association between these two problems remains unclear. Neither the differences in the autonomic nervous system nor mitral valve prolapse affect the treatment or prognosis of panic disorder.

Sometimes panic attacks begin after an illness, an accident, the break-up of a relationship, a separation from home (such as going away to college), or the birth of a child. Often, however, there is no obvious source of stress. Individuals with panic disorder do not appear to be more unstable or troubled than others; most, in fact, are in good psychological health.

Some people report that their first panic attacks occurred while they were using marijuana, LSD, cocaine, amphetamines, or other mind-altering drugs (including excessive amounts of caffeine). It is possible that their response to such substances is linked to an underlying susceptibility to panic; they continue to have attacks long after their drug use stops. Similarly, those who first suffered panic attacks when they developed a thyroid disorder may experience recurring attacks after this medical problem is treated.

Medical researchers have found that two-thirds of those who have had a panic attack and have not been treated for it will experience another if they are given an intravenous infusion of sodium lactate, a compound similar to the lactic acid produced in muscles during exercise. People who have not had attacks do not respond in this way to sodium lactate, nor do those who have been treated with antipanic medications. Those prone to panic attacks, unlike others, will also experience an attack if they inhale carbon dioxide. The fact that scientists can chemically induce a panic attack in certain people underscores the biological basis of this problem and confirms that medications can prevent attacks.

In seeking psychological roots for panic disorder, researchers have noted a variety of contributing factors, including an inborn susceptibility to fearfulness, frightening experiences in early childhood, discomfort with aggression, low self-esteem, and stressors that trigger frustration or resentment. Many individuals with panic

Is it a panic attack?

According to the DSM-IV, a panic attack is a period of intense fear or discomfort in which at least four of the following symptoms develop suddenly and reach a peak within ten minutes:

- Palpitations, pounding heart, or accelerated heart rate
- Sweating
- Trembling or shaking
- Sensations of shortness of breath or smothering
- Feeling of choking
- Chest pain or discomfort
- Nausea or abdominal distress
- Feeling dizzy, unsteady, light-headed, or faint
- Feelings of unreality or being detached from oneself (derealization)
- Fear of losing control or going crazy
- Fear of dying
- Numbness or tingling sensations (paresthesias)
- Chills or hot flushes

Adapted from the Diagnostic and Statistical Manual of Mental Disorders, 4th Edition. Used with permission.

disorder, especially those who also have agoraphobia, have a history of school phobia as children. Some researchers theorize that extreme separation anxiety in childhood—an enormous fear of being away from a parent—may increase the likelihood of developing panic attacks as an adult. In fact, attacks often do begin after a real or threatened loss.

How panic attacks and panic disorder feel

For most people, a panic attack is pure fear. Without reason or warning, they feel their hearts racing wildly. Some become light-headed or dizzy. Their throat muscles tighten. Their hands shake. Because they can't catch their breath, they may start to breathe rapidly and hyperventilate. Parts of their bodies, such as their lips, fingers, or toes, may tingle or feel numb. They may sweat profusely, flush, tremble, feel that they're choking, or become nauseated and vomit. Some report a surge of heat or an icy chill. Worst of all is a terrible, overwhelming sense that something horrible is about to happen. Individuals who have had panic attacks describe them as more profoundly frightening than anything else they have ever experienced. When an attack ends, they live in dread of having another one.

Panic disorder usually develops and worsens in stages. First, individuals experience a panic attack or a cluster of them. At least initially, the attacks are unexpected; later, they may occur immediately before or on confronting an anxiety-provoking object or situation. If, for example, a person has a spontaneous attack while driving a car or being in a crowded place, in time just the prospect of driving or going into a crowd may trigger attacks. As anticipatory anxiety—apprehension about having an attack—intensifies, many avoid the places or circumstances in which previous attacks occurred and develop agoraphobia, although often they do not realize that the panic attack is what they really fear and are avoiding. They may stop working, socializing, or going to school, may become increasingly dependent on a partner or parent, or may be unable to venture from their homes alone. Some try to relieve their dread with alcohol or drugs.

Panic attacks can recur several times a week or even within the same day, or only every few weeks or even months. In very rare instances there is an intense single attack. Some individuals may not have an attack for many years, then suddenly experience a new outburst. Most often the attacks come and go for years, varying in intensity and frequency, and can recur indefinitely if left untreated. Whatever the frequency of attacks, the anticipatory anxiety can be present all the time.

▼

Seeking help   Although panic disorder is among the most common and curable psychological problems, many with this problem never seek treatment, and those who do are often misdiagnosed. Many people think they are having a heart attack or stroke. If they rush to a nearby hospital or emergency room after the first attack, physicians find nothing physically wrong to explain their agonizing symptoms. If they have subsequent attacks and their doctors order more extensive medical tests, these will again show no signs of illness.

If you suspect that you or someone close to you may have panic disorder, these are the questions that should be asked:

- Are there times when you feel overwhelming fear, distress, or terror for no apparent reason?

- During these times, does your heart beat more quickly than usual? Does it seem to be pounding inside your chest? Do you feel pain in your chest?

- Do you break out in sweat?

- Do you tremble or shake?

- Do you feel as if there's not enough air to breathe or that you can't catch your breath?

- Do you think you're choking?

- Do you feel nauseated or have any other digestive symptoms?

- Do you feel dizzy, unsteady, light-headed, or faint?

- Do you ever have a sense of unreality or of being detached from yourself?

- Are you afraid of losing control or going crazy?

- Are you afraid that you might die?

- Do you experience numbness, tingling sensations, chills, or hot flushes?

- Do these episodes recur unexpectedly?

- Have your fears about having more attacks or your concern about their impact or implications lasted for a month or more?

- Have you changed your behavior because of the attacks or your anxiety about them?

If you or the person close to you answers "yes" to several of the questions, the problem may indeed be panic attacks. If they recur, cause great concern, or lead to a change in behavior, the problem may be panic disorder. In either case, it is advisable to seek professional help.

Individuals with panic disorder consult an average of ten physicians—cardiologists, neurologists, gastroenterologists, and others—before receiving an accurate diagnosis. The first step is to have a primary care physician perform a thorough physical examination and some basic laboratory tests to rule out physiological causes of panic, such as hypoglycemia, hyperthyroidism, excessive caffeine intake, overly rigorous exercise, or exposure to toxic chemicals, such as arsenic or mercury. Although there are experimental biological tests for panic disorder, such as the use of sodium lactate or carbon dioxide to trigger an attack, they are not usually done in a clinical evaluation.

If initial medical tests are negative, to prevent problems such as anticipatory anxiety and to avoid unnecessary medical work-ups and evaluation, it is advisable that individuals see a psychiatrist with expertise in anxiety disorders.

▼

Risks and complications   Initially, those who have panic attacks may be able to function normally or almost normally. If the attacks continue, however, or if the fear of them grows, they may progressively narrow the arena of their daily lives. By the time they seek treatment, many people with panic disorder have developed some symptoms of agoraphobia—anxiety about being in places in which they might not be able to get help or escape from if they were to have an attack. They either avoid such situations or endure them only with great anxiety or when a companion is present. They may have to sit on an aisle seat in a movie theater, may not be able to get on a bus or drive across a bridge, or may restrict their driving to particular "safety zones." In extreme cases they may not go out at all or may leave home only with a companion.

The longer the panic attacks persist, the more devastating their impact becomes. Many with panic disorder drink to relieve their anxiety; then, as the alcohol wears off, the anxiety and panic are likely to intensify. In time, both the panic disorder and the alcohol dependence become worse.

Overwhelmed by feelings of hopelessness, many people with panic disorder become depressed. About half of those with the disorder report an episode of major depression at some time in their lives. They often trace their depression to the demoralizing fear evoked by the attacks and to the severe restrictions they have made in their way of living.

There is an increased risk for suicide among affected individuals, but researchers disagree about the extent of this risk. In one study, about 20 percent of those with panic disorder had attempted suicide, but subsequent reports found a much lower risk.

▼

Treating panic attacks and panic disorder

The two primary treatments for panic disorder are medication and cognitive-behavioral techniques. No one knows yet which treatments work best for which people, but major studies are under way to compare medication, cognitive-behavioral therapy, and a combination of both.

Mental health professionals distinguish between panic disorder with and without agoraphobia. Agoraphobia, which involves fear and avoidance, is usually a direct consequence of untreated panic disorder. Once agoraphobia has developed, individuals usually require more extensive treatment.

COGNITIVE-BEHAVIORAL THERAPY

Cognitive-behavioral therapy changes the way people think about and respond to panic. First, they learn that what they are experiencing is a physiological response to danger and that, although it is frightening, it will not cause them harm. Therapists then desensitize individuals by recreating anxiety-provoking situations and

<table>
<tr><td>

Is it panic disorder?

According to the DSM-IV, a diagnosis of panic disorder should be based on these criteria:

</td><td>

■ **Both of the following:**

 1. **Recurrent, unexpected panic attacks**
 2. **At least one of the attacks is followed by a month or more of at least one of these:**
    a. **Persistent concern about having additional attacks**
    b. **Worry about the implications or consequences of an attack (e.g., losing control or having a heart attack)**
    c. **A significant change in behavior related to the attacks**

■ **The attacks are not due to the direct effects of a substance (e.g., drugs of abuse or a medication) or a medical condition (e.g., hyperthyroidism).**

■ **The attacks are not better accounted for by another mental disorder, such as obsessive-compulsive disorder, posttraumatic stress disorder, separation anxiety disorder, specific phobia, or social phobia.**

Panic disorder with agoraphobia also includes:

■ **Anxiety about being in places or situations from which escape might be difficult or embarrassing or in which help may not be available in the event of having a panic attack or panic symptoms (e.g., being on a bridge or traveling in a bus, train, or car)**

■ **Avoidance of such places or situations, enduring the experience with marked distress or anxiety about having a panic attack or symptoms, or requiring a companion's presence**

Adapted from the Diagnostic and Statistical Manual of Mental Disorders, 4th Edition. *Used with permission.*

</td></tr>
</table>

teaching relaxation and breathing techniques that take the punch out of an attack. A process called *cognitive restructuring* deals with the tendency of individuals with the disorder to "catastrophize" or assume the worst about their symptoms and provides rational, reassuring explanations for what they are feeling.

One of the most common symptoms of a panic attack is hyperventilation, or very rapid breathing. Hyperventilation affects the flow of oxygen and blood to the brain and can cause symptoms such as dizziness and confusion. Persons in therapy learn about the relationship between attacks and hyperventilation and how to breathe diaphragmatically. In one study, this technique greatly reduced the frequency of panic attacks within two weeks. Exposure therapy, discussed later in this chapter, is also helpful. Other behavioral approaches that play an adjunctive role in treatment include combinations of controlled breathing, relaxation training (involving the tensing and relaxing of various muscle groups), and biofeedback.

PSYCHOTHERAPY

Whereas cognitive-behavioral therapies teach specific strategies for coping with panic, psychodynamic psychotherapy explores possible unconscious meanings behind panic attacks. Although this approach may help some individuals, most therapists consider cognitive-behavioral therapy more effective.

MEDICATION

The primary medications used for panic disorder are antidepressants and anti-anxiety drugs. (Medications mentioned in this chapter are discussed in detail in Chapter 28.) Almost all antidepressants work well for panic because they "turn down" the danger response in the brain. For those with severe or persistent attacks, psychiatrists usually prescribe tricyclic antidepressants or monoamine oxidase (MAO) inhibitors, which block both the physical symptoms and the psychological aspects of a panic attack. These medications help the vast majority of affected individuals.

Imipramine (Tofranil) and desipramine (Norpramin, Pertofrane) are the tricyclic antidepressants most commonly used to treat panic disorder. It is possible that, in the future, selective serotonin reuptake inhibitors (SSRIs), such as the antidepressants fluoxetine (Prozac), sertraline (Zoloft), and paroxetine (Paxil), may become the preferred treatment. Although conclusive research has not yet been completed, they appear to be as effective as the tricyclic antidepressants and have fewer side effects.

Three anxiety-relieving benzodiazepines—alprazolam (Xanax), clonazepam (Klonopin), and lorazepam (Ativan)—have also proved helpful in panic disorder. Their advantage is that they work more rapidly than the antidepressants; their disadvantage is the potential for dependence. Although they are safe for most people, psychiatrists use them with caution, especially in those with personal or family histories of substance abuse. Sometimes low doses of benzodiazepines are prescribed for individuals who have severe anticipatory anxiety or whose symptoms intensify when they first begin to take an antidepressant drug. Once the antidepressant becomes effective at blocking the panic, the benzodiazepine can slowly be reduced. Medications for panic are usually taken for six months, then tapered slowly, and eventually discontinued. If the attacks recur, psychiatrists may recommend longer-term treatment with antidepressants to block the panic.

Many other psychiatric drugs—antipsychotic agents, barbiturates, other sedatives, and lithium—have been used to treat panic disorder, but they have not been proved safe or effective, and many have potentially hazardous side effects. None of these is recommended as a treatment for panic.

▼

Self-help Once individuals understand the nature of their problem, they can do a great deal to help themselves. By practicing diaphragmatic breathing or various cognitive-behavioral techniques, many learn to lessen the intensity of panic attacks or even to prevent them. Self-help groups provide support and understanding from others who share the same problem. (See the Resource Directory at the back of the book for information on the Anxiety Disorders Association of America and other groups.)

Individuals with panic disorder should limit their caffeine intake. Excessive amounts of caffeine can cause many symptoms associated with panic. Switching to herbal teas and decaffeinated coffee and cola beverages is advisable. Sensible nutrition, adequate rest, and regular exercise are also very helpful.

▼

Impact on relationships Panic disorder can change an individual's personality and family dynamics. People who had been outgoing, active, and independent may become extremely withdrawn, dependent, manipulative, and/or excessively agreeable or eager to please. Those close to them may be baffled and bothered by these changes. Although family members and friends often sympathize with the obvious distress that occurs during a panic attack, they may have difficulty understanding why individuals remain anxious between attacks or cannot bring themselves to go to places or do things they once enjoyed.

As the disorder leads to more and more avoidance, parents may be unable to visit their children's schools or games; spouses may refuse to accompany their partners to social or business events. Although individuals with panic disorder may long to be with those they love, their families and friends often feel disappointed, rejected, or resentful because of their behavior. If the affected person starts to drink heavily or to use drugs as a way of dealing with the disorder, relationship problems intensify.

Without treatment for the individual and counseling for couples and families, panic disorder can cause a great deal of emotional damage. Sometimes the strain of living with a spouse with panic disorder and agoraphobia is so great that a marriage breaks up.

▼

Outlook Panic disorder tends to wax and wane over time. As noted, less than one-quarter of those with panic disorder ever receive appropriate treatment. Most of those who do either improve significantly or recover completely. After receiving professional help, most persons feel better within six to eight weeks of treatment; those who do not improve over this time period should seek a re-evaluation. Individuals undergoing cognitive-behavioral therapy may need medication as well; those taking medication alone are likely to benefit from cognitive-behavioral therapy. Persons who receive both forms of treatment are less likely to suffer relapses than those who received only medication.

Phobic disorders

Most people have fears of some sort. They may be nervous about flying, feel awkward at large parties, or hate snakes, but they manage to travel, socialize, or walk in the woods despite their anxiety. Phobias—the most common anxiety disorder—are out-of-the-ordinary, irrational, intense, persistent fears of certain objects or situations. Over the course of a lifetime, an estimated 12.5 percent of adults develop such acute terror that they go to extremes to avoid whatever it is that they fear, even though they realize their feelings are excessive or unreasonable.

AGORAPHOBIA

The term *agoraphobia*, which comes from the Greek for "fear of the marketplace," refers to a condition in which individuals fear and avoid places or situations from which they perceive it would be difficult or embarrassing to escape. Although there is no real threat or danger, they fear having a panic attack and not being able to get to a safe place immediately. Large public places, such as shopping malls, theaters, stadiums, or parks, and crowds of any sort are most likely to trigger the dreaded fear. Many people with this problem cannot bring themselves to drive in rush-hour traffic or on busy expressways, to cross bridges, or to travel through tunnels because they feel trapped or cut off from help.

People with agoraphobia are often fearful of a panic attack or of specific symptoms, such as dizziness, loss of bladder or bowel control, vomiting, a racing heartbeat, or difficulty breathing. Their apprehension can be so overwhelming that they restrict their activities to avoid feared places; in extreme cases, they become virtual prisoners in their own homes.

Typically, agoraphobia develops after individuals have experienced the frightening symptoms of a panic attack or a series of attacks and associate them with specific places or situations. Occasionally they cannot articulate exactly what they fear will happen, only that they feel a vague sense of dread. Without treatment, they become increasingly fearful of future attacks.

▼

How common is agoraphobia?

According to epidemiological data from the National Institute of Mental Health (NIMH), an estimated 5.6 percent of adults develop agoraphobia at some point in their lives. Agoraphobia usually begins in the person's twenties or thirties and is diagnosed far more often in women than men. The rates of agoraphobia in college graduates are about half of those for non-graduates, and the disorder is more common among separated and divorced individuals than among those who are married.

▼

What causes agoraphobia?

Most psychiatric researchers believe that panic disorders and agoraphobia actually represent a single illness. Agoraphobia may share the same genetically based biological roots as panic disorder. Individuals who develop both panic disorder and agoraphobia sometimes report extreme separation anxiety in childhood. Very often, agoraphobia develops because individuals with panic disorder fear another attack occurring in a place in which they are trapped or will not be able to get help, or in circumstances that would be humiliating or dangerous. It is rare for a person to experience agoraphobia without panic attacks.

▼

How agoraphobia feels

Agoraphobia can range from mild, as in a feeling of distress when travelling alone, to severe, causing the person to become a complete shut-in. Individuals with agoraphobia are likely to have a fear of going outside their home, being alone, and being in a situation where they cannot quickly leave and help is not easily or readily available.

Most cases begin with panic attacks, often a cluster of uncued, spontaneous attacks. As these continue, affected individuals develop constant anticipatory anxiety about when and where the next attack might happen. In many cases the agoraphobia is linked to the particular settings in which the attacks occurred. For example, experiencing an attack while driving to work can lead to a fear of that specific freeway. If these persons experience an attack while boarding a bus, they begin to fear and avoid buses. If an attack develops while they are in a shopping mall, they may add malls to their list of feared places. The list can keep growing to include situations as well as places, such as simply being in a train or car or standing in line in the supermarket. In time, their fears may expand to include every setting and circumstance except being at home.

Some people with agoraphobia come to rely on a trusted companion and will travel or participate in normal activities only with

Fighting the fear

Emma's mom used to joke that she had to take her toddlers to the hospital so they could learn how to climb stairs. Most of the other buildings in their little town in west Texas were rambling, one-story structures. "You kids thought the stairwells at the hospital were the neatest thing you'd ever seen—until the time Emma took a header down an entire flight," she'd say.

Emma never thought much about her mother's story until decades later, when she took a job working for a petroleum firm on the twentieth floor of a Dallas high-rise. From her first day she felt uncomfortable riding the elevator. One day the elevator was extremely crowded, and she found it hard to catch her breath. When the doors opened on the fifteenth floor, Emma lunged through them and took the stairs the rest of the way up. From that day on, she would take the elevator to the fifteenth floor and walk up to her office.

Several weeks later Emma was supposed to meet her husband at his offices in another high-rise. She paced nervously around the downstairs lobby for ten minutes before getting on an elevator. As it ascended, Emma was sure she felt a lurch. Frantic, she punched all the floor numbers on the elevator panel until the doors opened. When she told her husband what had happened, he tried to reassure her with a detailed explanation of the safety mechanisms of modern elevators, yet all she could think of was, "What if it happened again?"

Emma started wearing a pair of running shoes to work and walking all twenty floors up to her offices. She didn't go out to lunch anymore because she couldn't face the climb.

Her life began to revolve around avoiding elevators. When friends invited her and her husband to brunch in their elegant penthouse apartment, she cancelled at the last minute. When she went on business trips she refused to accept hotel rooms any higher than the third floor. Sometimes merely thinking about elevators would fill her with dread. Irritated by the excuses she was constantly making to explain why she couldn't go somewhere, her husband said, "Why don't you just lock yourself inside the house and stay there for the rest of your life?"

"I must be crazy," Emma thought. "That actually sounds good to me." She had read stories about people who had become prisoners in their own homes, trapped by their fears. She didn't want that to happen to her. When a talk show featured the stories of people with fears like hers, she contacted the local branch of a national advocacy organization. One of the therapists she was referred to was starting a group for people with phobias, and Emma decided to join.

It was a relief just to talk openly about what she had been going through with people who truly understood. The therapist outlined the steps the group members could take to confront and overcome their fears. For Emma, this would mean doing what frightened her most: getting on an elevator. The first time she saw the elevator doors close in front of her, she had to fight not to pound on them, but with her therapist at her side she made it as far as two floors. The next time they went a little higher, then higher yet.

In the group, members shared a host of practical strategies that worked for them—everything from breathing techniques to wearing rubber bands around their wrists and snapping them to distract them from their particular fear. Emma experimented until she found some strategies that worked for her. She also kept forcing herself to ride up one floor higher on her office building elevator each day. When she finally made it to the twentieth floor, her smile was so bright that the receptionist asked if she'd just gotten some good news. "You could say that," Emma said with a wink.

this "phobic partner." Because they become so dependent, they may try overly hard to please and accommodate others.

▼ Seeking help

If you suspect that you or someone close to you may have agoraphobia, these are the questions that should be asked:

- Do you worry about what might happen if you suddenly feel anxious or panicky in a place or situation from which it would be difficult or embarrassing to leave?

- Do you worry about fainting, experiencing a sudden attack of diarrhea, or developing other embarrassing symptoms when you are in such settings?

- Do particular places, such as bridges or elevators, or certain situations, such as being in a shopping mall or attending a concert, make you anxious?

- Do you avoid certain places or certain things because they make you anxious?

- If you cannot avoid such places and situations, do you feel extremely anxious or upset while you're in them? Can you endure them only with someone you trust?

If you or the person close to you answers "yes" to several of these questions, the problem may be agoraphobia or another anxiety disorder, and professional help should be sought. The earlier that treatment begins, the less disabling agoraphobia is.

Many people with mental disorders do not leave their homes for a variety of reasons, and therapists must carefully distinguish agoraphobia from other problems. Individuals who are severely depressed, for example, may not go out because they have lost all interest in outside activities and assume that no one wants their company anyway. By comparison, those with agoraphobia may be eager to enjoy the world's pleasures but are held back by fear. Diagnosis is based on a comprehensive interview, the person's history and symptoms, and a complete medical examination to rule out other possible causes of anxiety and fear.

▼ Risks and complications

Some individuals with mild cases of agoraphobia can maintain a relatively normal lifestyle. They may travel alone when necessary, such as commuting to work, but they may need to take a certain route or to sit close to the bus door. Other than that, they may be able to go only to certain places or may avoid going out alone. Symptoms tend to worsen over time and, as they do, there is increased risk for depression and substance use.

According to the DSM-IV, a diagnosis of agoraphobia without a history of panic disorder should be based on these criteria:

■ Anxiety about being in places or situations from which escape might be difficult or embarrassing, or in which help may not be available in case of a panic attack or panic-like symptoms. Agoraphobic fears typically involve characteristic clusters of situations that include being outside the home alone, being in a crowd or standing in a line, being on a bridge, or traveling in a bus, train, or car.

■ Agoraphobic situations are avoided, endured with marked distress or anxiety about having a panic attack, or require a companion's presence.

■ The avoidance or anxiety is not better accounted for by another mental disorder, such as specific phobia, separation anxiety disorder, obsessive-compulsive disorder, posttraumatic stress disorder, or social phobia.

■ The disturbance is not due to the direct effects of a substance, such as drugs of abuse or a medication, or a medical condition.

■ When a medical condition is present, the anxiety is clearly much greater than that usually associated with the condition.

Adapted from the Diagnostic and Statistical Manual of Mental Disorders, 4th Edition. *Used with permission.*

▼
Treating agoraphobia

Because most persons with this problem also have panic disorder, the first step is treating the underlying panic, usually with cognitive-behavioral therapy (see Chapter 27) and antidepressants or anti-anxiety drugs. (Medical treatment of panic disorder is discussed on page 126.) In general, agoraphobia improves along with the panic disor-der. As the panic attacks disappear, individuals feel more confident about facing the situations they fear.

The goal of cognitive-behavioral therapy is to encourage individuals to confront or enter the place or situation they fear so they can prove to themselves that they will not undergo the anticipated reaction. Exposure to the actual place or situation, rather than simply imagining it, is the most effective way to accomplish this. The best techniques are graduated or graded exposure (beginning with the least frightening situation and gradually working up to those that are more strongly feared) and flooding (confronting people with their most intensely feared situation). Although both may work equally well, graduated exposure is much more widely used. Therapists can work with individuals one-on-one or in groups. Many find that two exposure sessions a week, each lasting for two hours, lead to greater success than less frequent exposure for a shorter time. (If the exposure is too brief, it can increase the anxiety because it fails to give affected individuals the confidence that they can ride it through.) Daily self-practice, reinforcing the techniques learned during therapy sessions, is critical.

Other psychotherapeutic treatments can also contribute to recovery. Cognitive therapy can help to reduce irrational beliefs about feared places. Assertiveness training helps affected persons learn to express their own needs and desires and to gain more confidence in dealing with the world. Biofeedback, hypnosis, meditation, and relaxation can be useful as adjunctive therapies, although they are not effective by themselves. Individuals who have become extremely dependent on a partner may benefit from couples counseling.

▼
Self-help

Once they understand what is wrong and develop cognitive-behavioral strategies for coping with their fears, many people benefit greatly from the understanding and support that self-help groups can provide. Groups can also offer encouragement in practical ways, as when members go together to shopping malls, restaurants, or other places that individual participants may fear.

▼
Impact on relationships

As noted, people with agoraphobia, terrified of some unknown threat to their well-being, may become extremely dependent on one individual, a "support person," and may not leave home without this companion. Some support persons help individuals to cope with the limitations imposed by their agoraphobia; others may consciously or unconsciously encourage the dependency by reinforcing the person's fears. Agoraphobia can place great stress on a marriage, and couples or marital therapy can help both partners to change their ways of relating to each other. Many couples report greater marital satisfaction once the partner with the disorder receives treatment.

Agoraphobia can also affect family members, friends, and colleagues. Although they may find the person's avoidance of various situations puzzling or frustrating, they often adapt to it. Individuals with agoraphobia may arrange to work at home or may regularly host parties in their houses to keep up social ties. Particularly if they rely on a support person, they may be able to keep their agoraphobia a secret to all but those closest to them. In time, however, the constant need to make excuses or to devise complex arrangements to deal with the routines of daily living is likely to take its toll both on the affected persons and those who care about them. Without supportive companions, individuals with agoraphobia can become increasingly isolated and lonely.

Outlook   Untreated agoraphobia typically lasts for many years and can be very disabling. With treatment for both panic disorder and the agoraphobia, most individuals are able to return to a normal life. About 75 percent of those treated by exposure therapy benefit from it, but as many as 10 to 20 percent who begin treatment drop out. Those who complete the therapy report less anxiety and avoidance, improved morale, a better quality of life and functioning at home and work, expanded interests and activities, and more gratifying relationships.

SPECIFIC PHOBIAS

Specific phobias (previously called *simple phobias*) are characterized by intense, unfounded, and persistent fear of a particular object, activity, or situation. Individuals with specific phobias typically develop anticipatory anxiety at the prospect of confronting whatever they fear and will do anything they can to avoid it. The most common types are animal phobia (most often involving dogs, snakes, insects, or mice); blood-injection-injury phobia (a fear of hypodermic needles or any bodily injury involving blood); situational phobia (being in closed spaces, such as elevators, or air travel); and natural environment phobia (fear of storms, heights, or water). In adults, situational phobias occur most frequently.

How common are specific phobias?   According to the National Comorbidity Survey and NIMH's epidemiological data, specific phobias are the most common anxiety disorders. As many as 11 percent of all men and women develop a specific phobia at some point in their lives. About 9 percent are affected within any six- to twelve-month period. These phobias occur more often in women than men. Some, especially those involving animals, begin in childhood, most of them before the age of seven. Blood and injury phobias typically develop in adolescence or early adulthood, and the onset of phobias involving heights, driving, closed spaces, and air travel peaks in childhood and again in the mid-twenties.

What causes specific phobias?   Specific phobias may stem from a combination of influences, including a genetic predisposition. Close relatives of individuals with specific phobias are at greater risk for developing such problems themselves. Specific phobias involving injury or blood have a particularly strong genetic component. Relatives of those with these phobias are much more likely than others to develop similar fears.
  Environmental and developmental factors, such as a traumatic

event in childhood, can play a significant role. At any age, for instance, someone who chokes or almost chokes may develop a phobia about choking. A classic example reported by Freud is the case of "Little Albert," who heard a loud, upsetting noise while playing with a white rat when he was two. Thereafter, he became extremely fearful of rats, which he unconsciously associated with the fear triggered by the loud noise. However, many phobias cannot be traced back to such a trauma.

▼

How specific phobias feel

People with intense fear—of dogs, for example—become extremely anxious, even panicky, if they approach a dog on the street. They sweat, have difficulty breathing, their hearts race, and they calm down only when they are no longer near the animal. Because the prospect of being around a dog provokes extreme anxiety, they do everything possible to stay away from dogs. As with other specific phobias, the dog itself is not what the person fears; rather, the fear is of some frightening consequence that might occur, such as being bitten. Moreover, although the reactions to the feared object are strong and although specific phobias are unquestionably upsetting, the anxieties associated with them are not as intense as those that occur in panic attacks.

▼

Seeking help

Individuals with specific phobias rarely seek help, probably because they perceive their fears as trivial and usually can live normally despite them. Many do not realize that treatment is relatively simple and highly successful. If you suspect that you or someone close to you may have a specific phobia, these are the questions that should be asked:

- Is there a particular object (such as a hypodermic needle) or a situation (such as being in an airplane) that terrifies you?
- Do you become extremely frightened almost every time you confront this object or situation?
- Do you become intensely anxious and fearful even before you actually confront it?
- Do you believe that your fear is much greater than normal or makes no sense?
- Do you avoid whatever makes you so fearful? If you cannot avoid it, do you feel extremely anxious and upset?
- Have you changed your normal routine because of your fear? Has it affected your ability to work or interfered with your family and social life?
- Are you very upset or concerned about this fear?

If you or the person close to you answers "yes" to many of these questions, the problem may be a specific phobia. It is best to seek professional help before it begins to have an even greater impact on your life.

Therapists diagnose specific phobias on the basis of an individual's history and symptoms and a clinical interview. In evaluating someone who might have a specific phobia, they check for other anxiety disorders, such as panic disorder, agoraphobia, generalized anxiety disorder, and obsessive-compulsive disorder. Some people appear to have a specific phobia that on closer evaluation proves to be a more pervasive panic disorder. Therapists also make sure the irrational fear is not really a symptom of a more severe mental disorder, such as schizophrenia or bipolar illness.

▼
Risks and complications

If the cause of a specific phobia—spiders, for example—is relatively easy to avoid, it may not interfere with the affected person's life to any great extent. If the feared object cannot be easily avoided, however—such as flying when work requires regular travel—a specific phobia can create daily stress and anxiety. In extreme cases, individuals may limit their social activities or change jobs just to avoid the thing they fear. They are also at higher risk for depression and substance abuse, both of which may be related to the impact of their fear on their lives.

▼
Treating specific phobias

Behavior therapy is the best approach. Although various medications have been tried, none is effective by itself in relieving phobias. Treatment usually consists of gradual, systematic exposure to the feared object, a process called *systematic desensitization*. Using graded exposure, therapists usually begin with the least stressful situation. Some use ungraded exposure, in which individuals confront the most stressful situations first.

As with agoraphobia, a number of studies have proven that exposure, especially "in vivo" or actual exposure in which individuals are exposed to the actual source of their fear rather than simply imagining it, is highly effective. Real-life experience greatly enhances a person's sense of self-efficacy (that is, of competence and capacity for change).

Although psychotherapy is not considered the first choice of treatment for specific phobias, therapists usually provide emotional support in addition to teaching behavioral techniques. Some individuals also benefit from gaining a better understanding of the impact their fear has had on their relationships and their lives.

Is it specific phobia?

According to the DSM-IV, a diagnosis of specific phobia should be based on these criteria:

■ Marked, persistent fear that is excessive or unreasonable and is triggered (cued) by the presence or anticipation of a specific object or situation, such as flying, heights, animals, getting an injection, or seeing blood

■ Exposure to the object or situation invariably provokes an immediate anxiety response, which may take the form of a panic attack (children may cry, cling, or throw tantrums).

■ Recognition by the person that his or her fear is excessive or unreasonable (except for children)

■ Avoidance of the feared object or situation or enduring it only with intense anxiety or distress

■ Avoidance, anxious anticipation, or distress in the feared situations interferes significantly with normal routine, work, academic performance, or social activities or relationships, or causes marked distress about having the phobia.

■ Duration of at least six months in those under eighteen years of age

■ Avoidance, anxiety, or panic attacks are not better accounted for by another mental disorder, such as obsessive-compulsive disorder, posttraumatic stress disorder, separation anxiety disorder, social phobia, panic disorder, or agoraphobia.

Adapted from the Diagnostic and Statistical Manual of Mental Disorders, 4th Edition. *Used with permission.*

Self-help   Because of the intense fear phobias trigger, most people—at least initially—may find it difficult to overcome this problem on their own. With the help of a trusted friend or partner, however, they can sometimes overcome mild phobias through a process of gradually exposing themselves to the thing or situation they fear. Support groups can be helpful because members benefit from one another's example and encouragement.

Impact on relationships   Mild phobias that do not cause great distress or interfere with a person's usual routine have little, if any, impact on relationships. However, if the phobia involves something important in a couple's or family's life, it can become a trigger for conflict and misunderstanding. A person's fear of flying, for example, may interfere with vacation plans, or a phobia about horses may become an issue if the other partner loves to ride.

▼

Outlook   Most phobias that develop in childhood disappear without treatment. As individuals mature, they may simply outgrow their fears. Specific phobias that persist into adulthood usually don't go away without treatment, although they tend not to be disabling. Behavioral treatment is highly effective in overcoming them.

SOCIAL PHOBIA

Social phobia (social anxiety disorder) centers on the fear of acting in a way that will be publicly humiliating. Individuals with this problem fear and try to avoid situations in which they must interact or perform a task in public, such as signing their names, eating, or using a public lavatory when others are present. In performance anxiety—a subtype of social phobia—the main fear is of speaking, dancing, singing, or playing a musical instrument in front of others.

Many people feel nervous about socializing or speaking in public. Professional entertainers almost always feel some tension prior to a performance. Those with social phobia experience greatly intensified anxiety in such situations. In addition to psychological symptoms, such as fear and tension, they develop physical symptoms similar to those that occur during a panic attack: shakiness, rapid heartbeat and breathing, sweating, dry mouth, nausea, tremors, heartburn, vomiting, and diarrhea, as well as others particular to their circumstances, such as not being able to swallow or freezing up. Usually their fear is general rather than specific; they are afraid of eating in any public place rather than of eating at a very formal dinner party. They may try to avoid all situations that make them anxious and may also develop a panic disorder or specific phobia.

▼

How common is   During the course of a lifetime, according to the National Comor-
social phobia?   bidity Survey, 13.3 percent of Americans may experience social phobia, with 7.9 percent affected during any twelve-month period. Other studies have found rates as low as 2 or 3 percent. Unlike many other anxiety disorders, men appear to be as vulnerable as women. Social phobia typically develops in the mid-teens. Most people who seek help for social phobia fear more than one type of situation.

▼

What causes   Early traumas, along with a lack of social skills, negative self-
social phobia?   evaluation, and hypersensitivity to rejection or criticism, may lead to a social phobia. Often the affected individuals can pinpoint a

particularly embarrassing event, such as forgetting their lines in a class play or tripping in front of a large crowd, or an instance in which they were humiliated by a public criticism or rebuke, as the trigger that initiated their anxiety. In others, social phobia may be a response to constant criticism by parents or partners at home. Some persons become anxious in public immediately after an incident that they experience as traumatic, although more often social phobia develops gradually over a period of months or years.

Social phobia appears to be more common among first-degree relatives of individuals with this disorder. Some traits associated with this problem, such as fear of strangers, shyness, social introversion, and fear of criticism, may be inherited. Persons vulnerable to social phobia may have greater-than-normal increases in adrenaline (epinephrine) during stress or may be more sensitive to its effects.

▼

How social phobia feels

Being in or anywhere near the limelight is a nightmare for those with social phobia. Whether they are answering a teacher's question in class, outlining a sales plan at work, or speaking at a community meeting, individuals with this anxiety disorder feel extremely self-conscious, shy, and embarrassed. They may blush and sweat profusely. Their mouths become dry. Their hands tremble. Their heart rate speeds up; they have difficulty breathing. They may become nauseated, vomit, or develop diarrhea. Before the event begins, they feel severe anticipatory anxiety, worrying that their words will sound foolish, that they'll "freeze," that they'll choke on their food, that their hand will tremble as they write, that they will make disgusting noises when they use a public restroom, that others will notice how nervous they are and think less of them.

Some individuals try to avoid social events entirely. Those who fear making presentations before others may hold themselves back professionally so that they can avoid such situations. If they force themselves to endure a public outing, they may suffer immense psychological distress during the entire time. If they try to perform, their symptoms may affect how well they do, creating even greater anxiety in the future.

▼

Seeking help

If fear of social settings or of performing before others is troubling you or someone close to you, these are the questions that should be asked:

- Do public gatherings almost always make you extraordinarily anxious?

- Does the prospect of performing in any way in front of others make you extremely fearful?

- Has your anxiety or avoidance of certain situations interfered with your normal routine?

- Has your fear of making a presentation or appearing before others affected your performance at school or work, your usual social activities, or your relationships with others?

- Do you worry about strangers observing and criticizing you when you meet them or do something in front of them?

- Do you ever suffer panic attacks at social gatherings?

- Do you worry that others will notice how anxious you are? Are you afraid of doing something embarrassing?

- Do you believe that your fear is irrational or much greater than the occasion warrants?

- Do you try to avoid social situations or public performances? If you must be in such situations, do you feel anxious or upset throughout the event?

If you or someone close to you answers "yes" to many of these questions, the problem may be a social phobia or another anxiety disorder, and a mental health professional should be consulted.

A diagnosis of social phobia is based on a thorough history and clinical interview, as well as a medical examination to make certain that no substance or general medical condition is directly responsible for the fear or avoidance of certain situations. Therapists must also ascertain that no other mental disorder might be causing the symptoms of social phobia, and that those individuals who do have physical or other mental disorders are truly suffering from social phobia, rather than embarrassment about noticeable symptoms or their appearance.

▼

Risks and complications

Social phobia has a wide range of intensity and may or may not be incapacitating. Some individuals have only mild symptoms and manage reasonably well except in specific—but important—circumstances, such as addressing a group of co-workers or being interviewed for a job. Those with more severe social phobia may become demoralized, withdraw from others, and be unable to lead a normal social life or achieve all that they might in their careers. In very severe cases, these affected persons may lose their jobs, suffer in academic and professional evaluations, and lose self-esteem. They may also turn to alcohol and drugs to relieve their anxious feelings. If their anxiety interferes with their social or work functioning, they face an increased risk of depression.

Is it social phobia?

According to the DSM-IV, a diagnosis of social phobia should be based on these criteria:

■ Marked and persistent fear of one or more social or performance situations in which the individual is exposed to unfamiliar people or possible scrutiny by others. The individual fears acting in a way or showing symptoms of anxiety that will be humiliating or embarrassing. (In the case of children, those capable of normal age-appropriate relationships must develop anxiety when with peers, not just with adults.)

■ Exposure to the feared social situation almost invariably provokes anxiety, which may take the form of a panic attack. (Children may cry, throw tantrums, freeze or shrink from social situations with unfamiliar people.)

■ Recognition that the fear is excessive or unreasonable (except in children)

■ The feared situation is avoided, or endured with intense anxiety or distress.

■ The avoidance, anxious anticipation, or distress in the feared situation interferes significantly with the person's normal routine, occupational or academic functioning, or with social activities or relationships with others, or there is marked distress about having the phobia.

■ Duration of at least six months in those under eighteen years of age

■ Fear or avoidance is not due to the direct effects of a substance (a drug of abuse or a medication) or medical condition and is not better accounted for by panic disorder, separation anxiety disorder, body dysmorphic disorder, pervasive developmental disorder, schizoid personality disorder, or other mental disorder.

■ In individuals with a physical or mental disorder, the fear is not related to it; for example, in Parkinson's disease the fear is not of stuttering or trembling.

Adapted from the Diagnostic and Statistical Manual of Mental Disorders, 4th Edition. *Used with permission.*

▼

Treating social phobia The primary treatment for social phobia is cognitive-behavioral therapy. By means of exposure techniques, individuals imagine or actually confront the situation they fear. Training in social skills, involving modeling, rehearsing, role-playing, and assigned practice, helps them to become more assertive and less anxious. Anxiety management, a form of cognitive restructuring, enables them to identify negative or self-defeating thoughts, to become aware of their tendency to blame themselves for what goes wrong and to credit luck for what goes right, and to rehearse alternative, more positive ways of thinking. These individuals improve most with a combination of these approaches, either in individual or in group sessions. Moreover, supportive psychotherapy can help people with a social phobia to rebuild their self-confidence and improve their self-esteem. In some cases, psychodynamic psychotherapy reveals a problem, such as hypersensitivity to even a hint of disapproval or criticism, that may be contributing to the social phobia.

Medication   Some individuals with social phobia may also require medication, usually with the antidepressant phenelzine (Nardil), an MAO inhibitor. Its chief drawback is the need for dietary restrictions for safe use (see Chapter 28). Some psychiatrists prescribe tricyclic antidepressants, but persons with social phobia tend to be very sensitive to their side effects and may develop irritability, insomnia, and nervousness, even at low doses.

The primary medications prescribed for performance anxiety are a group of drugs called *beta-blockers*, which are prescribed primarily for hypertension (high blood pressure). They block the beta receptors in the nervous system that are responsible for producing anxiety-like physical symptoms—racing heart, rapid breathing, dry mouth, and tingling in the hands—and can lessen the physical manifestations of stress, such as rapid heartbeat, sweating, or "butterflies" in the stomach.

Although the FDA has not yet approved any drug specifically for performance anxiety, more than twenty studies have assessed the effectiveness of beta-blockers in persons in a variety of stressful or competitive situations, such as giving speeches, taking examinations, and performing in public, and in the majority of cases the drugs relieved anxiety and improved performance.

Beta-blockers are powerful medications that have some potentially serious side effects, particularly for those with illnesses such as asthma, congestive heart failure, insulin-dependent diabetes, and hyperthyroidism. Beta-blockers can be taken safely by individuals who have these conditions, but they must be very carefully supervised by physicians experienced in their use. They also increase the risk for a depressive episode in persons with a prior history of major depression. Therefore, these medications should *never* be taken without a complete medical evaluation, and must be used only under the direct care of a psychiatrist with expertise in this area.

By far the most widely used beta-blocker for performance anxiety is propranolol (Inderal), which lowers blood pressure and heart rate and prevents constriction of blood vessels in the lungs. It is usually prescribed in a low dose to be taken an hour or two before a rehearsal or performance that normally causes mild anxiety. In cases of particularly severe performance anxiety, some psychiatrists suggest long-term preventive treatment with higher doses of propranolol. This requires frequent monitoring of blood pressure and heart rate to make certain that these parameters do not drop too low. Individuals should report any dizziness, loss of coordination, or wheezing.

It can take six to eight weeks to determine whether a beta-blocker is having an effect on performance anxiety. Persons who take these medications should never discontinue them suddenly; they must be gradually reduced to avoid possible complications, such as high blood pressure or a racing heartbeat.

▼

Self-help Self-help groups, classes in social skills, or assertiveness training can be very helpful for those with a social phobia. Some also find that working with a trusted partner who accompanies them to various social situations can help in overcoming apprehension.

▼

Impact on relationships Performance anxiety is less likely to affect personal relationships than the person's professional or academic life. However, social phobia can have a major impact, creating difficulties for couples when one partner refuses to accompany the other to parties or other public events. The other's understanding and sensitivity may be crucial in overcoming this problem. If a dysfunctional relationship is contributing to the social phobia, as when one spouse has become self-conscious with other people because the other spouse makes criticisms in public, marriage or family counseling is sometimes needed.

▼

Outlook Without treatment, social phobia may be lifelong, although it may remit or become less severe in adulthood. There are few long-term studies of current treatments. Symptoms tend to recur when medications are discontinued, unless individuals with this disorder also undergo cognitive-behavioral therapy.

Generalized anxiety disorder

The hallmark of a generalized anxiety disorder (GAD) is chronic unrealistic worry about several events or activities so intense that it produces physical symptoms as well as psychological distress and is so persistent that it lasts for six months or longer. This disorder involves certain characteristic types of symptoms:

- Constant apprehension, with individuals always expecting the worst and not being able to control their worry
- Physical tension, which leads to complaints of sore muscles, feeling shaky, being unable to relax, and being easily startled

- Physiological changes similar to those produced by fear, such as a rapid heart rate, sweating, clammy hands, increased blood pressure, dry mouth, lump in the throat, trouble swallowing, light-headedness, upset stomach, frequent urination, and diarrhea

- Increased arousal or hypervigilance, which may cause irritability, impatience, problems concentrating, and insomnia.

▼

How common is GAD?

According to the *DSM-IV*, 3 percent of the population experiences a generalized anxiety disorder in any one-year period; the lifetime prevalence rate is 5 percent. Symptoms often begin in childhood or young adulthood, and the disorder affects women somewhat more than men. Among the anxiety disorders, generalized anxiety is second only to phobias in frequency.

▼

What causes GAD?

GAD may have multiple causes. Genetic factors may create an inherent vulnerability that makes some people more likely to become anxious under certain conditions. One family study found a 19.5 percent risk for GAD in close relatives of those with this disorder, compared with only 3.5 percent in others. About half of individuals with GAD develop their symptoms after stressful life events. It may be that those with a predisposition to anxiety cannot bounce back from a trauma in the same way as others and therefore become anxious. However, there is less clear-cut evidence of a biological basis for GAD as compared with panic disorder. According to psychodynamic theories, "free-floating" anxiety stems from unconscious conflicts.

▼

How GAD feels

Individuals with this disorder live in a state of unending tension. They worry—not just some of the time, not just about the stresses and strains of ordinary life, but constantly and about almost everything: their health, families, finances, marriages, jobs, potential problems, and dangers. They often wake up feeling apprehensive that something bad will happen that day. A vague sense of unease hangs over them regardless of what they do. One person described himself as feeling as though he were taking a final exam with every task he performed at work.

Many of these anxious individuals become keyed up and irritable, often finding it hard to fall asleep at night or to concentrate during the day. They may snap at friends and co-workers. When asked a question, their minds may suddenly go blank. Although they realize that something is wrong, they cannot pinpoint the source of their unease.

Is it generalized anxiety disorder?

According to the DSM-IV, a diagnosis of generalized anxiety disorder should be based on these criteria:

- Excessive anxiety and worry (apprehensive expectation) about a number of events or activities (e.g., work or school performance), occurring more days than not for at least six months

- Difficulty controlling the worry

- At least three (one in children) of the following symptoms associated with the anxiety:
  1. Restlessness or feeling keyed up or on edge
  2. Being easily fatigued
  3. Difficulty concentrating or mind going blank
  4. Irritability
  5. Muscle tension
  6. Sleep disturbances (difficulty falling or staying asleep; restless, unsatisfying sleep)

- The focus of the worry and anxiety is not limited to the concerns associated with other mental disorders, such as the fear of having a panic attack associated with panic disorder or the fear of being contaminated that can occur in obsessive-compulsive disorder.

- Significant distress or impaired functioning socially, at work, or in other important ways because of the anxiety, worry, or physical symptoms

- This disorder is not due to the direct effects of a substance (a drug of abuse or a medication) or a general medical condition and does not occur only during a mood disorder, psychotic disorder, or pervasive developmental disorder.

Adapted from the Diagnostic and Statistical Manual of Mental Disorders, 4th Edition. *Used with permission.*

GAD produces physical as well as psychological symptoms. Most commonly, individuals complain that their heads ache or their muscles are tense. They may hyperventilate and feel they cannot get enough air. This may cause faintness or tingling in various parts of the body. They may experience dizziness, heart palpitations, excessive sweating, skin flushing, dry mouth, and frequent urination. Even though they are exhausted, they cannot sit still. Never truly comfortable, they always feel too cold or too hot, too restless or too weary. They cannot forget or put off their worries, and their excessive fretting about finances, children, work, or other aspects of their lives seems to breed still more worry and anxiety.

Seeking help   Usually no dramatic event or specific episode persuades those with a generalized anxiety disorder to seek help. In time, however, they may realize that their chronic worrying is not normal and that they should be able to feel better.

If generalized anxiety may be affecting you or someone close to you, the questions that should be asked are:

- Do you feel extremely anxious, worried, or apprehensive?
- Have you felt this way for at least six months?
- Do you feel this way more days than not?
- Do you worry about a variety of events or activities?
- Are you having a hard time controlling your worry?
- Do you usually feel restless, keyed up, or on edge?
- Do you tire easily?
- Are you having problems concentrating? Does your mind go blank?
- Have you been more irritable than usual?
- Do your muscles feel tense?
- Are you having problems falling or staying asleep? Are you restless during the night? Do you wake up feeling unrefreshed?
- Are you unable to work or relate to others the way you once did because of your anxiety, worry, or physical symptoms?

Because some degree of anxiety is part of the experience of living, many people will answer "yes" to a few of these questions. However, if you or someone close to you answers "yes" to most of them and cannot function as in the past, the problem may be an anxiety disorder and help should be sought.

A comprehensive physical examination is essential because many conditions, especially somatoform disorder (described in Chapter 19), can mimic generalized anxiety. To rule out anxiety produced by a medical condition (discussed later in this chapter), the examination should include a thorough assessment of physical complaints, vital signs, heart and blood pressure, skin and mucous membranes, neurological symptoms such as tics and tremors, abdominal pain, and breathing problems. In some cases, physicians may order laboratory tests, such as a complete blood count, thyroid function, liver and kidney function, electrolytes, and glucose tolerance. Individuals also may be asked to complete standardized screening tests to help identify an anxiety problem and gauge its seriousness.

▼
Risks and complications   At the very least, GAD diminishes the quality of life. Some people miss work, withdraw from contact with others, and cut back on

social activities. Others may become so hopeless and demoralized that they develop major depression or abuse alcohol or drugs. Those with GAD tend to worry excessively about illness; they often visit doctors repeatedly and undergo unnecessary tests and treatments.

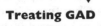

Treating GAD   Among the treatments for this disorder are cognitive-behavioral therapy, psychotherapy, and anti-anxiety drugs. At present there are no firm scientific data indicating which type of treatment is the most effective or which will work best for which patients.

COGNITIVE-BEHAVIORAL THERAPY

Various cognitive-behavioral approaches have proved helpful in treating GAD, especially when combined with relaxation techniques. One behavioral strategy, anxiety symptom management, consists of explaining the symptoms of the disorder, training individuals in ways to distract themselves from their constant worries, and practice in balancing anxious thoughts with reassuring ones. Cognitive restructuring targets distorted assumptions that lead to apprehension and worry. A combination of cognitive therapy, relaxation training (which helps to reduce tension and other physical symptoms), and systematic desensitization also has proved beneficial.

PSYCHODYNAMIC PSYCHOTHERAPY

Although psychodynamic psychotherapy alone is not the treatment of choice for GAD, it can play an important role in motivating those who feel overwhelmed and demoralized by their anxiety by helping them look beyond their symptoms to the roots of their feelings. It can also prove beneficial when unconscious conflict may be the cause for an individual's chronic anxiety disorder.

MEDICATION

Individuals with more severe or persistent symptoms of GAD may benefit from psychiatric medications. The most commonly prescribed drugs for this disorder are buspirone (BuSpar) and the benzodiazepines (see Chapter 28). The benzodiazepines take effect quickly but can impair memory and cause drowsiness, and they have the potential for dependence. Buspirone, which belongs to a drug family called the *azapirones*, is not sedating or habit-forming, and it does not impair driving or motor skills. Its side effects (dizziness, nausea, diarrhea, headache, nervousness) are usually mild and temporary. However, it can take from one to four weeks for buspirone to be effective. Buspirone can be used to treat patients with both generalized anxiety disorder and associated depressive symptoms.

Tricyclic antidepressants, such as imipramine (Tofranil), may be as, if not more, effective than benzodiazepines for GAD. A tricyclic may also be prescribed when individuals have symptoms of both anxiety and depression. As described in Chapters 5 and 28, tricyclics can initially cause side effects such as blurred vision and constipation, but these usually ease after the first weeks of treatment.

In treating GAD, physicians may prescribe medication for a six-month period, along with nondrug approaches, and then gradually reduce and discontinue the drug.

▼

Self-help

Learning about anxiety disorders can in itself lessen their impact. Many individuals are not aware that muscle tension can lead to aching, that hyperventilation can cause light-headedness, or that caffeine, nicotine, and alcohol can make them feel much worse.

Exercise is also an effective means of anxiety reduction. Regular workouts reduce tension and aggression, enhance the sense of well-being, and improve overall health. Recommended forms of exercise include walking, swimming, other aerobic activities, and working with exercise equipment. Individuals should build up gradually to thirty minutes of exercise three or four days a week. Other good health habits that are helpful include sensible nutrition and adequate rest.

Progressive relaxation exercises, yoga, transcendental meditation, or biofeedback can help to lessen the feeling of loss of control that many individuals experience with GAD. Playing a musical instrument or creative writing (including keeping a journal) can also serve as a form of psychological release. In time, individuals can learn to monitor themselves for anxiety symptoms and turn to their own coping strategies whenever the pressures on them increase. (See the Resource Directory at the back of the book for information on the Anxiety Disorders Association of America and other consumer groups.)

▼

Impact on relationships

Generalized anxiety disorder can undermine emotional stability and intimate relationships. The slightest incident—a glass of spilled milk at dinner, a traffic jam, a forgotten phone message— can trigger an outburst of anger. Unaware that increased irritability is a hallmark of the disorder, family members may take such tirades personally. Anxious individuals are often so involved in their own worries, aches, and pains that their loved ones may feel ignored or emotionally abandoned. Marital problems can intensify if the disorder leads to alcohol or drug use.

Learning about generalized anxiety disorder can help family members to understand the reasons underlying these behaviors. Marital stresses can be eased when partners become involved in treatment or participate in counseling that enables them to educate themselves, voice their concerns and feelings, and work with the anxious person in overcoming difficulties.

▼

Outlook   Without treatment, GAD may persist, unrecognized, for many years, worsening during times of stress. Although treatment may not eliminate all symptoms, it can reduce them significantly, freeing individuals of the burden of constant anxiety.

Mixed anxiety and depression

Individuals sometimes develop persistent mild symptoms common to both anxiety and depressive disorders: problems in sleeping, changes in appetite, difficulty in concentrating, irritability, fatigue. These symptoms may represent an early stage of either type of problem. "Mixed anxiety and depression" is not an official psychiatric diagnosis, and little research has been done on this combination. In clinical practice, mental health professionals sometimes do see depressed individuals with "anxiety-like" symptoms such as irritability and insomnia or panic attacks, phobias, obsessive-compulsive rituals, or generalized anxiety. In addition to psychotherapy (usually cognitive-behavioral and supportive therapy), psychiatrists may prescribe antidepressants that also ease anxiety or may recommend an anxiety-relieving medication in addition to an antidepressant.

Distinguishing between anxiety and depressive disorders can be challenging when symptoms of both are present, but there are some characteristic differences, including the following:

Mood. Individuals with anxiety disorders are predominantly fearful—of a panic attack, of an object or situation, or of vague dangers. Depressed people are typically sad and joyless. Even when they are anxious or tense, there is an underlying sense of despair.

Age at onset. Depression can develop at any age, although the average is the late twenties. Most anxiety disorders, such as panic and social phobia, begin during the teens and early twenties. Older individuals who become depressed and anxious are more likely to be suffering from a primary depression than an anxiety disorder.

Sleep patterns. Although both depressed and anxious individuals may have difficulty sleeping, those with an anxiety disorder tend to have more problems falling asleep, whereas depressed individuals typically fall asleep but wake up very early and cannot get back to sleep, or sleep much more than usual.

Slowing down. Depressed individuals often become much less active than usual, even speaking at a slower rate. Those with an anxiety disorder may be fidgety or may show no change in their activity level, but they rarely slow down.

Family history. Individuals with panic and other anxiety disorders are likely to report similar symptoms in their relatives. Depressed individuals are more likely to have a family history of depression.

Other symptoms. Both depressed and anxious people may have difficulty concentrating or making decisions and may develop physical symptoms. Chronic pain is more common in depression, however. Individuals with an anxiety disorder usually feel best on waking, but their symptoms worsen as the day goes on. Depressed individuals, on the other hand, feel worse in the morning than later in the day.

Response to exercise. Individuals with mild or moderate depression may feel temporarily better after exercising; those with severe depression may find it impossible to exercise.

Sexual interest. Persons with anxiety disorders often have normal sex lives, whereas depressed men and women tend to lose interest in sex and pull away from loved ones.

It is critical to determine the primary problem so that treatment can be targeted as precisely as possible. For individuals who appear to have both an anxiety and a depressive disorder, psychiatrists usually treat the depression, often with an antidepressant that also can ease anxiety, such as imipramine (Tofranil). In contrast, treatment of depressed persons for an anxiety disorder (whether by medication or by other approaches) usually does not relieve depression. If individuals with symptoms of depression and anxiety do not improve within eight weeks of treatment on antidepressants, they should be reassessed.

Anxiety caused by medical conditions or substances

Physical, or organic, problems (such as hyperthyroidism or the disorders listed in the table on the opposite page) and substances, including drugs of abuse and medication, can cause symp-

SOME MEDICAL CONDITIONS THAT CAN CAUSE ANXIETY OR PANIC

☐ **Cardiovascular disorders, such as arrhythmias, congestive heart failure, coronary artery disease, and mitral valve prolapse**

☐ **Respiratory diseases, such as asthma, chronic obstructive pulmonary disease, emphysema, hyperventilation, and hypoxia**

☐ **Hormonal imbalance disorders, such as Cushing's syndrome, hyper-thyroidism, hypoparathyroidism, menopause, and premenstrual syndrome**

☐ **Metabolic conditions, such as anemia, hypoglycemia (low blood sugar), hyponatremia (low blood levels of sodium), and hypokalemia (low blood levels of potassium)**

☐ **Neurological disorders, such as encephalopathy (degenerative disease of the brain), temporal lobe epilepsy, Huntington's disease, multiple sclerosis, delirium, dementia, and Wilson's disease**

toms of an anxiety disorder. Depending on the underlying cause and how rapidly it develops, a "secondary" anxiety disorder can range from mild to severe, may cause great distress, and may interfere with normal functioning. Unlike a true anxiety disorder, anxiety induced by illness or substances typically causes significant impairment in thinking and attentiveness. Individuals may experience panic attacks, anxiety symptoms, or obsessions or compulsions.

Diagnosis is based on a thorough assessment of physical complaints, vital signs, heart and blood pressure, skin and mucous membranes, neurological symptoms (such as tics and tremors), abdominal pain, and breathing problems. In some cases, doctors may order laboratory tests, such as a complete blood count, thyroid function, liver and kidney function, electrolytes, and glucose tolerance. Treatment of the underlying medical condition usually eases secondary anxiety, although some symptoms may linger and may require treatment with the same approaches used for specific anxiety disorders. If the underlying physical problem is not corrected, other mental syndromes may develop, including delirium, a state of disorganized thinking, and diminished ability to focus and shift attention (see Chapter 20).

DRUGS THAT CAN CAUSE ANXIETY

Many drugs, both medications and substances of abuse, can produce, worsen, or mimic the physical or psychological symptoms of

SOME SUBSTANCES THAT CAN CAUSE ANXIETY OR PANIC

☐ **Anticholinergic drugs, such as diphenhydramine hydrochloride (Benadryl)**

☐ **Antidepressants, including fluoxetine (Prozac), bupropion (Wellbutrin), and desipramine (Norpramin, Pertofrane)**

☐ **Aspirin (in persons with intolerance)**

☐ **Asthma medications (e.g., theophylline)**

☐ **Caffeine**

☐ **Cocaine**

☐ **Decongestants (e.g., pseudoephedrine)**

☐ **Hallucinogens, including PCP (phencyclidine)**

☐ **Steroids**

☐ **Thyroid supplements (in too high a dose)**

☐ **Withdrawal from certain drugs, such as benzodiazepines, alcohol, and narcotics**

anxiety, either while the person is taking them or afterwards. Because some of these drugs can cause withdrawal symptoms that mimic anxiety if they are discontinued suddenly, their use should be reduced gradually.

Drugs that stimulate or "speed up" the central nervous system can cause agitation and anxiety. These include over-the-counter cold and congestion remedies that contain pseudoephedrine, caffeine, and theophylline, a chemical relative of caffeine found in more than one hundred different prescription and over-the-counter drugs. All these substances act like mild amphetamines in the body, making people feel "hyper" and restless.

Ironically, long-term use of some medications that people initially take to help them relax or sleep—among them the familiar benzodiazepines Valium, Librium, and Halcion—makes them become anxious when they cut back or try to stop using these medications. These drugs should be taken in the lowest possible doses and only for a limited time because they can induce dependence. They should be tapered off, not discontinued abruptly, to avoid withdrawal problems.

Other types of anxiety

Many people experience brief periods of nervousness or worry about a specific circumstance, such as looking for a job, and may feel jittery for days or even several weeks. Self-help strategies, such as exercise, reassurance from others, or brief counseling, can ease such anxiety. Individuals are especially likely to become anxious after experiencing a stressful event or a significant life change. Such stress-related anxiety is discussed in Chapter 12. When symptoms of anxiety persist for more than a few weeks and affect relationships, social activities, or performance at work or school, it is advisable to see a mental health professional for a complete evaluation.

Is it an obsessive-compulsive disorder?

Individuals with an obsessive-compulsive disorder may:

☐ **Experience senseless, upsetting, or bizarre thoughts or images**

☐ **Repeatedly try but invariably fail to ignore or block troubling thoughts**

☐ **Worry excessively about dirt, germs, or contamination**

☐ **Be afraid of losing or giving away something that may be important**

☐ **Feel compelled to think certain thoughts or perform certain acts repeatedly**

☐ **Wash or clean excessively**

☐ **Check things repeatedly to make sure they are done**

☐ **Do the same thing over and over again**

☐ **Keep useless things because they think they may need them someday**

☐ **Spend more than an hour a day on odd thoughts or behaviors**

☐ **Feel upset or embarrassed because of these thoughts or behaviors**

☐ **Find it difficult to carry on normal daily routines because of intrusive thoughts or the need to perform certain acts repeatedly**

The more boxes that you or someone close to you checks, the more reason there is to be concerned about obsessive-compulsive disorder. This chapter describes this problem and provides guidance on seeking help in overcoming it.

Obsessive-Compulsive Disorder

A realtor returns home a half dozen times a day to make sure she has unplugged the iron. A software specialist washes his hands and genitals several times a day to prevent HIV infection, even though he knows that the virus is not spread by casual contact. A young mother spends hours scrubbing her bathroom and kitchen floors every day to protect her baby from germs. A bright college student is late for his morning classes because it takes him so long to go through a precise sequence of steps as he shaves, showers, and gets dressed. A dentist has a garage jammed with old magazines that she cannot bring herself to throw away.

These men and women have very different symptoms, but they all suffer from the obsessions and compulsions that are characteristic of obsessive-compulsive disorder (OCD). This malfunctioning of information-relaying mechanisms within the brain causes repetitive thoughts or ritualistic behaviors to spin out of control. As a result, the small rituals of daily living, such as washing hands, locking doors, turning off lights, checking to make sure nothing is forgotten—tasks so trivial that most people do them without thinking—take over the individual's life.

Although they realize there is no sense to what they do, individuals with OCD cannot block out disturbing thoughts or stop compulsive behavior. Unable to convince themselves that they actually did turn off the headlights or put out the trash, they may check again, and again, and yet again. Unsure that their hands are truly clean, they may scrub them not once but dozens of times a day, until the skin is raw and bleeding. Incapable of deciding that they no longer need old newspapers or worn-out clothes, they may hoard worthless items and live in a sea of clutter. Worried that something bad may happen if they don't count up to a certain number before leaving a room or crossing a street, they may spend hours on meaningless mental gymnastics.

The American Psychiatric Association's *Diagnostic and Statistical Manual of Mental Disorders, Fourth Edition (DSM-IV)*, classifies OCD as an anxiety disorder because obsessions and attempts to resist compulsions are often linked with anxiety, because performance of compulsive acts often relieves anxiety, and because other anxiety disorders, such as phobias, often occur along with OCD. This categorization is controversial. As some therapists argue, the fear and anxiety that individuals with OCD feel are of a different nature from those that occur in phobias or generalized anxiety disorder. Moreover, giving in to a compulsion does not necessarily ease anxiety.

However, the question of classifying OCD is primarily a concern for mental health professionals, not for individuals with OCD. As many as one in every fifty Americans suffers from this disorder, and for these persons the critical issues are recognizing its symptoms and getting appropriate therapy. The good news is that highly effective treatments can relieve potentially disabling symptoms for as many as 90 percent of those with OCD.

Obsessions and compulsions

More than 90 percent of those with OCD have both obsessions and compulsions, although some are troubled more by one than by the other. Obsessions are intrusive, irrational ideas that repeatedly well up in a person's mind. They can take different forms, ranging from thoughts such as "There are germs on my cup" or "I forgot to turn off the coffeemaker," to images of stealing something or shooting someone. Some people may see themselves doing something harmful, such as hurting a child, and the image—at once both repulsive and irresistible—will not leave them. They know that this obsession is irrational; they know that they will not act on it. Yet they cannot force it away, so they may try to suppress or neutralize it by counting, repeating a phrase, touching a wall, taking a specific number of steps. They are not only distressed by such images themselves, they feel horrible about "being a bad person" because they have thoughts like these—even though they are not to blame for them in any way.

Compulsions are repetitive rituals such as handwashing, checking, doing things in a certain order, or mental acts such as praying, counting, repeating words silently, that a person feels driven to perform. The aim of these behaviors or mental acts is to ease anxiety or prevent some dreaded event or situation. But the compulsions usually provide only momentary relief, if any, and they give no sense of satisfaction or completion.

By the broadest definition, obsessions and compulsions might include uncontrollable nail-biting or a fear of losing bowel control so intense that individuals frantically search for restrooms wherever they go. Certain activities—eating, sex, gambling, drinking—are commonly referred to as "compulsive" if engaged in excessively, but such behaviors do not conform to the definition of OCD. They provide fleeting pleasure or excitement, whereas true obsessions and compulsions (see the tables on pages 158 and 159) are joyless attempts to reduce anxiety and distress.

▼

How common is OCD?   Once thought to be relatively rare, obsessive-compulsive disorder is actually more common than many better-known psychiatric disorders, such as schizophrenia and anorexia nervosa. According to the National Institute of Mental Health (NIMH), in the course of a lifetime 2 to 3 percent of the population develop OCD. As many as 4 million Americans—equal numbers of men and women—may be affected. People with OCD are often bright and talented. If it were not for this disorder, they would be normal in every way and function well socially and professionally.

OCD may begin in childhood, adolescence, or early adulthood. About one-third of those with the disorder are children or teenagers. Boys are most likely to develop OCD between the ages of 6 and 15; women usually develop OCD between the ages of 20 and 29.

▼

What causes OCD?   OCD may be one of the most biologically based of all mental illnesses. Psychiatrist Judith Rapoport, M.D., an NIMH researcher and a leading expert on OCD, describes it as "a severe, chronic, biologically rooted syndrome . . . associated with abnormalities in the basal ganglia region of the brain." In very simple terms, this means that those with OCD may experience a "hiccup" in the brain that makes them mistrust their eyes, knowledge, or good judgment. Because they doubt what they see and know, they must check and recheck or repeat the same acts over and over. This constant questioning is the reason why the French have dubbed the disorder "the doubting disease."

Brain-imaging techniques have found distinctive differences in

COMMON OBSESSIONS

- ☐ **Extreme concern with dirt, germs, urine, feces, toxic chemicals, sticky substances**

- ☐ **Disgusting images of filth or human waste**

- ☐ **Extreme concern with contamination (either becoming ill oneself or making others ill)**

- ☐ **Perverse sexual images or impulses (e.g., molesting a child)**

- ☐ **Violent images (e.g., stabbing or beating someone)**

- ☐ **Fears of harming oneself or others, either deliberately or by not being cautious**

- ☐ **Fears of causing something bad to happen (e.g., an accident) or of committing a crime**

- ☐ **Fears of saying something obscene or offensive**

- ☐ **Extreme concern about religious issues, morality, or values**

- ☐ **Extreme concern for order, exactness, or symmetry (sometimes accompanied by the belief that something bad will happen if things are out of order)**

- ☐ **Persistent thoughts of colors, lucky and unlucky numbers, senseless sounds or words**

- ☐ **Superstitions**

glucose metabolism, neuroanatomy, and blood flow in certain regions of the brain in persons with OCD. Perhaps because of these abnormalities, something goes wrong with the way the senses register information and the way the body responds to it. The result, as Rapoport puts it, is "grooming behaviors gone wild."

An imbalance in neurotransmitters, such as serotonin, which may affect doubting and certainty, plays an important role. Some of the medicines that have proven highly effective in controlling OCD reduce serotonin levels in the brain. The role of dopamine, a neurotransmitter linked with thought and movement disorders, also is under investigation. In addition, researchers theorize that a stress-related neurotransmitter, norepinephrine, may contribute to the anxiety that individuals with OCD feel. OCD has also been linked with neurological illness and injury, including birth trauma and head injury.

Heredity may contribute to vulnerability to the disorder; as many as 25 percent of those affected have relatives with OCD. Sometimes they share the same obsessions and compulsions. One adopted child with OCD constantly checked the doors to make sure they

COMMON COMPULSIONS

- ☐ **Prolonged, repeated, or ritualized handwashing, bathing, etc.**

- ☐ **Prolonged, repeated, or ritualized cleaning of objects, furniture, floors, etc.**

- ☐ **Repeated checking of appliances, lights, door locks, etc.**

- ☐ **Repeated checking for possible damage to something or harm to someone (e.g., checking to see if a car has hit a child or animal)**

- ☐ **Repeated checking for mistakes**

- ☐ **Writing or reading the same material over and over again**

- ☐ **Counting the number of vowels or words in a paragraph before or after reading**

- ☐ **Repeating certain movements (e.g., sitting, standing, climbing stairs, turning) a set number of times**

- ☐ **Repeatedly drawing up lists**

- ☐ **Mental rituals**

- ☐ **Repeated need to say certain things or to ask for reassurance**

were locked—a behavior that was not seen in his adoptive family. Later, he discovered that his biological father was a compulsive door-checker. Studies of twins and first-degree relatives of persons with the disorder show a higher than normal incidence of OCD.

The family members of those with OCD also have a higher than normal incidence of major depression, bipolar illness, panic attacks, severe phobias, and neurological problems, such as uncontrollable tics, Tourette's syndrome, and epilepsy. Often individuals suffer from both OCD and major depression. Those with either disorder often exhibit similar abnormalities in sleep patterns and hormonal activity, and experience similar symptoms, such as guilt, indecisiveness, low self-esteem, anxiety, and exhaustion. Some psychiatrists theorize that depressed persons may try to use the rituals of OCD to keep from plunging deeper into depression.

OCD also often occurs together with other mental disorders, such as trichotillomania (compulsive hair-pulling) and personality disorders. OCD is sometimes confused with *obsessive-compulsive personality disorder*, a different condition that refers to an enduring personality type characterized by a preoccupation with perfectionism, control, and orderliness. Although some—but far from all—individuals with obsessive-compulsive personality disorder (discussed in Chapter 21) also develop OCD, OCD is a distinct biochemical disorder characterized by obsessions and rituals.

Is it obsessive-compulsive disorder?

According to the DSM-IV, a diagnosis of OCD should be based on these criteria:

- *Obsessions,* as defined by
  1. Recurrent and persistent thoughts, impulses, or images that are experienced, at some time during the disturbance, as intrusive and inappropriate, and cause marked anxiety or distress
  2. These thoughts, impulses, or images that are not simply excessive worries about real-life problems
  3. Attempts to ignore, suppress, or neutralize them with some other thought or action
  4. Recognition that the obsessional thoughts, impulses, or images are a product of the person's own mind, not imposed from without

  OR

- *Compulsions,* as defined by
  1. Repetitive behaviors (e.g., handwashing, ordering, checking) or mental acts (e.g., praying, counting, repeating words silently) that the person feels driven to perform in response to an obsession or according to rules that must be applied rigidly
  2. The behaviors or mental acts are aimed at preventing or reducing distress or preventing some dreaded event or situation, but are not connected in a realistic way with what they are designed to neutralize or prevent, or are clearly excessive.

- Recognition, at some point during the course of the disorder, that the obsessions or compulsions are excessive or unreasonable (except in children)

- The obsessions or compulsions cause marked distress, consume more than an hour a day, or significantly interfere with normal routine, occupational functioning, or usual social activities or relationships.

- The content of the obsessions and compulsions is not restricted to another mental disorder, such as a preoccupation with food in someone with an eating disorder or with drugs in someone with a substance abuse disorder.

- The obsessions and compulsions are not the direct effects of a substance, such as a drug of abuse or medication, or a general medical condition.

Adapted from the Diagnostic and Statistical Manual of Mental Disorders, 4th Edition. *Used with permission.*

▼

How OCD feels   Some people experience only mild symptoms of OCD. They may worry obsessively about thinking or saying something sinful, or they may not be able to go to bed at night until they have personally checked every door and window no more and no less than three times. Although they realize that their thoughts and actions make little sense, they shrug them off and are not upset by them.

The most common obsessions in OCD concern dirt and con-tamination, as was the case with famed billionaire Howard Hughes. Others may involve endless brooding over issues such as the fate of the planet, the existence of God, or fear of great harm to oneself or others. By definition, obsessions recur again and again, resisting all attempts the person may make to ignore or control them.

Compulsions can be equally tenacious. Compulsive hoarders cannot throw anything out because they fear they might someday need it. Compulsive cleaners scrub everything in sight. Compul-sive organizers meticulously arrange and rearrange objects on a table or desk. Those with numerical compulsions perform an act a certain number of times, for example, in threes or sevens, because of a superstitious association with that particular number. When individuals try to resist a compulsion, they feel a sense of mount-ing tension that can be relieved only by yielding to it. As the dis-order progresses, having so often failed in resisting, they may no longer try. Most of these people know, to variable degrees, that their acts are irrational, but they *must* perform them nevertheless. Others usually do not recognize that their obsessions or compul-sions are excessive or unreasonable.

Change is very upsetting for individuals with OCD, and in times of stress or change they may find themselves devoting more time to their compulsions or developing new obsessions. In serious cases of the disorder, odd behaviors take on greater and greater importance in a person's life and become disabling. "At first I'd walk up and down the stairs only three to four times," says one man who started this behavior when he was eight years old. "Later I had to run up and down sixty-three times in forty-five minutes. If I failed, I had to start all over again from the beginning." Eventu-ally he developed other compulsions, and they persisted for twenty years—until he sought treatment.

▼
Seeking help   People with OCD are very secretive about their problem. They think that they are crazy or the only ones with such weird thoughts or behaviors. Often they feel too embarrassed to seek help. On average most wait more than seven years before seeing a therapist, and then usually only because of another serious prob-lem, such as major depression, anxiety, or panic attacks. Even then, they may not bring up their symptoms unless the mental health professional specifically asks about them.

If you suspect that you or someone close to you may be suffer-ing from obsessions or compulsions, these are the questions that should be asked:

- Are you bothered by senseless or bizarre thoughts that repeatedly enter your mind and interfere with what you're thinking or doing? For example, are you extremely concerned about contamination, dirt, germs, human waste, or toxic chemicals? Do perverse sexual images or impulses, such as molesting a child, enter your mind?

- Do these thoughts make you anxious?

- Do they keep coming back?

- Do you try to get them out of your head by thinking of something else or performing a certain ritual?

- Do you ever feel compelled to think or do something over and over in precisely the same way? For example, do you repeatedly wash your hands, shower, clean, check lights or locks, check for possible damage or harm to someone, or read or write the same thing over and over again?

- Do you feel that doing this will make you feel less anxious or somehow prevent something bad from occurring?

- Do these thoughts or behaviors take up more than an hour a day?

- Do you think that they make no sense or occur too often?

- Do they upset or embarrass you?

- Can you carry on your day-to-day routine? Has your job, social life, or family been affected in any way?

If you or someone close to you answers "yes" to several of these questions, the problem may be OCD, and you should consider talking with a mental health professional. Ideally, you should seek help as soon as intrusive thoughts or compulsive behaviors begin to affect your life, even if they seem innocuous.

Although scientists have identified biological and neuropsychiatric markers associated with OCD, a comprehensive psychiatric examination and history, along with a complete medical history, remain the keys to diagnosis. OCD must be distinguished from obsessive-compulsive personality disorder, which is characterized by a preoccupation with details and rules, perfectionism, excessive devotion to work, inflexibility about matters of morality, rigidity, and stubbornness. (This problem is described in Chapter 21.)

▼

Risks and complications

As symptoms progress, OCD can be extremely disabling. Because individuals devote so much time to their compulsions, it can be virtually impossible for them to work or relate to others normally. Irrational fears and thoughts can lead to crippling anxiety or to phobias stemming from an obsession, such as avoiding public restrooms because of a fear of germs. Some people end up spending all their waking hours consumed by obsessions and compulsions.

Persons with OCD tend to be socially isolated, marry at an older age, and have fewer children than others, if any. Men, in particular, may not be sexually active. Individuals may try to relieve their symptoms by drinking or taking anti-anxiety drugs. Many OCD sufferers become anxious or depressed, sometimes to the point of considering suicide.

▼

Treating OCD

Behavioral therapy and medication have proved equally helpful in treating OCD. Symptoms disappear completely for some. In others they are substantially reduced, so that the person feels a significant difference in daily living. Some persons choose behavioral therapy because they want to avoid the side effects that may accompany medication. Others prefer medication because they do not have the time or energy for the demands of behavioral therapy, or begin with it because they want relief from their symptoms before they start behavioral treatment. The combination of the two is often the most effective treatment. Medication helps individuals to follow through with behavioral treatment; behavioral therapy helps to prevent relapses after medication is stopped.

BEHAVIORAL THERAPY

The goals of behavioral therapy are easing the anxiety associated with obsessions and decreasing the frequency of compulsive thoughts or behaviors. (The principles of behavioral therapy are explained in Chapter 27.) Among the techniques that have proved most helpful for OCD is *systematic desensitization*. First, individuals imagine themselves doing or not doing whatever they usually feel compelled to do or to avoid. Thus, a "checker" may imagine leaving the kitchen and not returning to make sure the refrigerator door is closed. Someone obsessed with contamination may picture himself picking up a used tissue. As part of their homework assignments, individuals may progressively have to limit the number of times they check on something or how often they wash their hands until these rituals consume less and less of their day. Therapists often use a treatment contract to implement this. The contract specifies limits on the compulsive behavior, such as showering for no more than ten minutes once a day or checking doors only once before going to bed. The therapist and the individual decide on some behavioral consequence if the contract is broken, such as donating time or money to an organization the person dislikes or opposes.

Another effective approach, exposure and "response prevention," involves exposure to a feared object or to a situation that triggers self-doubt and not responding to it with the obsessive

Making magic

After her parents died in a plane crash, eleven-year-old Annie went to live at her aunt's house, a noisy, cheerful place filled with the giggles of her three young cousins, Annie didn't think of it as home, except for her room. There she kept all the treasured mementos of her life with the parents she'd loved so much and lost so young. As she carefully dusted the frames of their family photos, arranged her mother's jewelry, and lined up her father's pens, she wondered if there were some sort of magic that could protect her or, at least, keep the bad feelings at bay. She made up some rituals—silly little things, she knew—like always counting to ten before leaving her room or kissing each doll two times in exactly the same sequence before going to bed at night. Maybe, just maybe, if she kept making her magic and taking very good care of everything that was precious to her, she would be safe.

Even in college, when she lived with the world's messiest roommate, Annie kept her things in meticulous order. An accounting major, Annie did well in her first jobs, but as she won promotions and took on greater responsibilities, she worried more and more about making mistakes. She would check and recheck her work—and often that of her staff members as well. Even though she ended up working later than anyone else in the office, she was convinced that she needed the extra time. However, her performance reviews began to note problems in meeting deadlines and an "over-attention to often meaningless details."

Obsessed with germs, Annie showered several times a day, carried a toothbrush with her and used it every time she went to a ladies' room, and scoured every inch of her apartment. At work she got in early to clean out the coffee pot and dust her office, even though the building staff had cleaned the night before. She also found herself resorting to her "magic"-counting, repeating things in a certain sequence, checking and rechecking everything she did. She realized that what she was doing didn't make any sense, but she couldn't stop.

When Annie was put in charge of a major project with the potential to make or break her career, she knew she couldn't go on the way she had been. She called the only doctor she knew, her gynecologist, who referred her to a psychiatrist. Annie was apprehensive before her first session, afraid that the doctor would tell her she was losing her mind. When she heard the words "obsessive-compulsive disorder" she wasn't sure what they meant. But the description of OCD's characteristic symptoms suited her to a T. The psychiatrist suggested Prozac, an antidepressant that has also proven effective in the treatment of OCD, along with behavioral therapy.

At first Annie found it hard to comply with some of her "homework" assignments, such as not scrubbing the sink for an entire day. But with continued practice and medication, she began to let go of the rituals that had been taking over her life. Within three months she reported a dramatic decrease in her compulsive behavior. The habits she had held onto for so long didn't go away completely, and they still tended to increase at times of stress, but Annie felt more productive and relaxed.

or compulsive behavior. Someone obsessed by dirt is told not to wash; a driver who backtracks again and again to make sure he hasn't run over a child or a pet, or a homeowner who keeps returning to make certain a door or window is closed, is directed not to check. Initially, individuals may simply delay giving in to the urge to wash or check, but gradually they work toward overcoming such behaviors entirely.

Regardless of whether medication is also being used, behavioral therapy requires active participation and intensive practice. Even after therapy ends, individuals with OCD must continue to apply what they have learned to prevent relapses and make further progress. If behavioral therapy alone does not help or is only partially effective, or if individuals drop out (as 25 percent do), medication is the best alternative.

MEDICATION

Antidepressant drugs that inhibit or block serotonin reuptake in the brain have revolutionized the treatment of OCD, bringing improvement to 60 to 70 percent of those who take them. In 1989, clomipramine (Anafranil), used to treat depression and OCD in Europe for more than twenty years, became the first medication to win FDA approval in the United States as a therapy for OCD. Fluoxetine (Prozac) has since been approved for this purpose, too, and fluvoxamine (Luvox) was approved for treating OCD in 1995. Other selective serotonin reuptake inhibitors (SSRIs) will probably prove useful as well. (All of the medications mentioned in this chapter are discussed in Chapter 28.)

The primary side effects of clomipramine are dry mouth, drowsiness, tremor, dizziness, nausea, and constipation. A small number of those taking this medication—about 1 percent—suffer seizures. The SSRIs tend to have fewer side effects, although individuals may complain of nausea, weight loss, and insomnia. In addition, the SSRIs may cause sexual dysfunction, particularly retarded ejaculation in men and delayed orgasm in women.

Medication should be taken consistently for ten to twelve weeks before a psychiatrist determines whether it is helping. In some cases it is continued for six months to a year or longer. Higher doses of antidepressants may be required in the treatment of OCD than would be used to treat depression (such as 60 to 80 mg of fluoxetine for OCD compared with 20 to 40 mg for depression).

Scientists do not know why medications that block serotonin reuptake are effective for many people with OCD but not for all. When clomipramine or an SSRI fails to help or causes troubling side effects, psychiatrists may augment these drugs with other medications, selecting a specific agent based on an individual's symptoms. For example, buspirone (BuSpar), an anti-anxiety medication, can be used for those troubled by associated anxiety; fenfluramine (Pondomin), for those with symptoms of depression; trazodone (Desyrel), for those with insomnia and depression; clonazepam (Klonopin), for those with panic attacks or anxiety; or lithium, for those with mood swings and other signs of bipolar illness. Although these combinations have proved clinically helpful, they have not been fully tested, and a psychiatrist experienced in their use should monitor them carefully.

PSYCHOTHERAPY

Psychodynamic psychotherapy alone usually does not bring relief from OCD, and many individuals with the disorder have failed to improve despite years of this therapy or analysis. However, supportive psychotherapy (see Chapter 27) is an important adjunct to other treatments. Because they doubt everything around and about them, persons with OCD usually require extra reassurance during the early stages of treatment. In addition, supportive psychotherapy can educate individuals and family members about OCD, boost morale and self-confidence, enhance optimism, and improve compliance with prescribed treatments.

FAMILY THERAPY

Individual family therapy, multifamily support groups, and educational meetings can help family members to learn more about OCD and what they can do to offer support. Often parents or partners, trying to help or to avoid arguments, go along with or even participate in the person's compulsions—for example, repeating the same phrase several times or following the sequence specified in performing a task, just as requested. Family therapy can help to break this pattern.

Seeking reassurance from family members may become a compulsion in itself for individuals with this disorder. They may ask again and again if they have spelled a word right or if they are spreading germs. Told that everything is fine, they can feel better for a while, but as their doubts return—as inevitably happens—they again seek reassurance. Torn between a sincere desire to put their loved one's doubts at ease and their own irritation, family members may not know what to do. The best response is withholding reassurance—not meanly or sarcastically, but with a straightforward refusal, perhaps coupled with the explanation that the demand for reassurance is part of the compulsion. Often therapists work with family members so that they can fully understand the dynamics of the situation, rehearse possible responses, and draw up contracts for handling sensitive issues.

▼

Self-help OCD can be a serious, extremely disruptive illness, and it requires professional help. However, learning as much as possible about the disorder, joining a support group or the OCD Foundation (see the Resource Directory at the back of the book), and talking about obsessions and compulsions with others who have this problem or with friends and family can make a difference in recovery and in preventing relapses.

▼

Impact on relationships

People with mild symptoms of OCD often have normal or nearly normal interactions and relationships with others. However, if they begin to spend more and more time on their obsessions or compulsions, usually trying desperately to keep them secret, their family members may not understand what is going on. When they find out about a ritual, they may be critical and demand that the person give up his or her "crazy" behavior. According to the OCD Foundation, family members tend to respond in three different ways: assisting with the rituals to keep peace, tolerating compulsive behavior but not participating in it, or refusing to acknowledge or allow compulsions in their presence. None of these responses is ideal. Family members benefit from learning more about OCD and about helpful responses, such as projecting a nonjudgmental attitude yet not tolerating the behavior, and not allowing one person's symptoms to disrupt the normal household routine.

Once individuals begin treatment, family members can help by offering encouragement and providing a strong, supportive home environment. It is important for everyone in the family to realize that individuals improve at different rates and that symptoms may recur or intensify at times.

▼

Outlook

OCD rarely improves on its own, although symptoms may come and go over the years, often flaring up during times of change or crisis. With either behavioral therapy or medication, about 70 percent of individuals with OCD show at least moderate improvement. A combination of these two approaches can help as many as 90 percent, with symptoms disappearing entirely for about a third of affected persons. Most of those treated with drugs alone relapse after they stop taking medication.

Is it substance dependence or abuse?

Individuals with a substance dependence or abuse disorder may:

☐ **Use more of an illegal drug or a prescription medication or use a drug for a longer period of time than they desire or intend**

☐ **Try repeatedly and unsuccessfully to cut down or control their drug use**

☐ **Spend a great deal of time getting drugs, taking them, or recovering from their use**

☐ **Be so "high" or feel so bad after drug use that they often cannot do their jobs or fulfill other responsibilities**

☐ **Give up or cut back on important social, work, or recreational activities because of drug use**

☐ **Continue to use drugs even though they realize that they are causing or worsening physical or mental problems**

☐ **Use more and more of a drug to achieve a "high" or desired effect, or feel fewer such effects than in the past**

☐ **Use drugs in dangerous ways or situations**

☐ **Experience repeated drug-related legal problems, such as arrests for possession**

☐ **Continue to use drugs even though they cause or worsen social or personal problems, such as arguments with a spouse**

☐ **Develop hand tremors or other withdrawal symptoms if they cut down or stop drug use**

☐ **Take drugs to relieve or avoid withdrawal symptoms**

The more boxes that you or someone close to you checks, the more reason there is to be concerned about drug use. This chapter provides information on drug dependence and abuse and specific drugs of abuse.

Substance Dependence and Abuse

A t the end of the day, a stressed-out executive downs a couple of scotches to relax. College students pass around a marijuana joint while listening to a concert. A bored teenager in an affluent suburb swallows a tab of LSD. At a party, a group of twenty-something singles snort lines of cocaine. A middle-aged woman, troubled by worries and unable to relax, starts taking more and more of the medications she's gotten from various doctors to relieve her anxiety symptoms.

These people may not fit the image of the desperate "junkie" that many conjure up when they think about drug users. Yet drugs are a fact of life for all of them, and all face a risk of developing a substance abuse disorder. They are far from unusual—in this or any other time.

Although drugs have been identified as a modern plague, they are not new. People have been using mind-altering, or *psychoactive*, chemicals for centuries. Citizens of ancient Mesopotamia and Egypt used opium. More than three thousand years ago Hindus included cannabis products in religious ceremonies. For centuries the Incas in South America chewed the leaves of the coca bush. Although drugs have long existed in most societies, their use was usually limited to small groups. Today, millions of Americans regularly turn to drugs to pick them up, bring them down, alter perceptions, or ease psychological pain. (Chapter 10 discusses alcohol use and abuse.)

The 1960s ushered in an explosive increase in drug use and in the number of drug users in our society. Marijuana use soared during the 1960s and 1970s, and cocaine during the 1980s. In 1986, crack—a cheap, smokable form of cocaine—hit the streets and cities of America, and the numbers of regular cocaine users soared. Since that time, government officials, describing drugs as the number-one public health threat in our society, have declared war against them. Yet the abuse of both legal and illegal drugs continues to be an enormous problem. An estimated 5 million Americans are in need of treatment for drug abuse and dependence. Millions more are struggling to live drug-free lives.

None of these millions ever set out to get hooked on drugs. Those who try them believe that they are smart enough, strong enough, or lucky enough to stay in control. But after continued use, a person's need for a drug can outweigh everything else in life, including the people, relationships, and values once held dearest. This chapter first discusses the general problems of substance dependence and abuse and then describes specific drugs of abuse.

Understanding substance dependence and abuse

Until the 1960s, many people imposed moral judgments on drug users, viewing them as weak, immoral, or criminal. Since then, we have come to regard chemical addiction as a lifelong chronic illness that affects mind, body, and spirit. The key characteristics of addiction are repeated drug use, loss of control over how much or how often a person takes a drug, and continued use despite harmful consequences. Because addiction is considered too broad and judgmental a term for scientific use, mental health professionals describe drug-related problems in terms of dependence and abuse.

When individuals feel a strong craving for a psychoactive substance because it produces pleasurable feelings or relieves stress or anxiety, they have developed *psychological dependence* on it. *Physical dependence* occurs when the body develops *tolerance* to the effects of a substance, so that the person needs larger and larger doses to achieve the desired effect—sometimes in amounts that would produce intoxication or an overdose in someone who was not a regular user. If these individuals reduce or stop drug use, they suffer *withdrawal*, a state of acute physical and psychological distress with symptoms that range in severity from mild to life-threatening. These persons are diagnosed as having a substance dependence disorder, which the *Diagnostic and Statistical*

Manual of Mental Disorders, Fourth Edition (DSM-IV), defines as a "maladaptive pattern of substance use, leading to clinically significant impairment or distress." (See the table, Is it substance dependence? on page 175.)

Intoxication is a major aspect of psychoactive substance disorders. The term refers to maladaptive behavioral, psychological, and physiological changes that occur as a result of substance use. (Intoxication and withdrawal from specific drugs are discussed later in this chapter.)

Individuals with substance dependence become intoxicated or high on a regular basis, every day, every weekend, or in several binges a year. They may repeatedly try but fail to discontinue their drug use, even though they realize that it is adversely affecting their health, family life, relationships, and work, and sometimes literally putting them in dangerous situations, as when they get behind the wheel of a car while high.

Some drug users do not develop the symptoms of tolerance and withdrawal that characterize physical dependence, yet they use drugs in ways that are clearly harmful. These individuals are diagnosed as having a psychoactive substance abuse disorder. The *DSM-IV* defines substance abuse as a "maladaptive pattern of substance use, leading to clinically significant impairment or distress." (See the table, Is it substance abuse? on page 177.) Like those with substance dependence, individuals with a substance abuse disorder continue to use drugs despite their awareness of the problems they are causing in every aspect of their lives.

The symptoms of dependence vary with the particular drug. Certain substances induce psychological but not physical dependence, so stopping does not cause withdrawal symptoms; among these are cannabis (marijuana), hallucinogens, and phencyclidine (PCP). The degree of dependence also varies. In mild cases, a person may function normally most of the time. In severe cases, the person's entire life may revolve around obtaining, using, and recuperating from the effects of a drug.

Increasingly, psychiatrists have recognized that there is a great deal of overlap between mental disorders and substance abuse disorders. "A little more than a third of those with a psychiatric disorder also have a chemical dependence problem, and a little more than a third of those with a chemical dependency problem have a psychiatric disorder," notes psychiatrist Richard Frances, M.D., the founding president of the American Association of Addiction Psychiatry. Individuals with such *dual diagnoses* require careful evaluation and appropriate treatment for the complete range of complex and chronic difficulties that they face.

▼
How common are drug dependence and abuse?

The National Academy of Science's Institute of Medicine in Washington, D.C., estimates that more than 5 million Americans use drugs to the extent of suffering physical and psychological distress if they stop. According to the National Comorbidity Survey, 11.6 percent of the population become dependent on or abuse drugs at some point in their lives; 3.6 percent do so during a given year.

Although recreational use of drugs by some segments of the population has dropped since the 1980s, heavy drug use and abuse have not diminished. Cocaine and crack use remains very high in inner cities, where prices are low and supplies plentiful. Marijuana continues to be the most common illegal drug on college campuses. LSD use is increasing among high school students, especially suburban youths. There are signs that even elementary school students are now experimenting with drugs.

▼
What causes drug dependence and abuse?

No one fully understands why some people develop drug dependence or abuse disorders whereas others, who may experiment briefly with drugs, do not. Inherited body chemistry, still-unknown genetic factors, and sensitivity to drugs may make some individuals more susceptible. Many complex causes play a part, including:

Biochemical factors. More than twenty years ago, scientists located specific opiate receptors in the brain to which opium, heroin, morphine, and other opioids attach. Subsequently, they identified natural opioids, called *endorphins*, which the body itself produces to relieve pain and stress. Since then, researchers have located receptor mechanisms for other psychoactive drugs as well, including LSD, nicotine, cocaine, and tetrahydrocannabinol (THC), the active ingredient in marijuana. These receptors are involved in drug highs and in dependence. When a person repeatedly uses a psychoactive drug, the number of these receptor sites in the brain is reduced and the drug loses some of its effectiveness. As a result, the user must take larger amounts to achieve the same effect as before. Researchers are also working to identify biological markers that may indicate increased genetic vulnerability to the neurochemical processes of tolerance and dependence.

Psychological factors. Although scientists do not believe that there is such a thing as an "addictive personality," certain individuals are at greater risk for drug dependence because of psychological risk factors, including difficulty in controlling impulses, a lack of the values that might prevent drug use (whether based in religion, family, or society), low self-esteem, feelings of powerlessness, and depression. The one psychological trait most often linked with drug use is denial. It is especially evident in young people, many of whom are absolutely convinced that they will never lose control or suffer in any way as a result of drug use.

Mental disorders. Many of those diagnosed with substance abuse or dependence disorders have at least one mental disorder, particularly depression or anxiety, and many people with psychiatric disorders abuse drugs. Individuals sometimes self-administer drugs to treat psychiatric symptoms—for example, they take sedating drugs to suppress panic attacks—and develop dependence on them.

Environment. Individuals who are isolated from friends and family, or who live in communities such as poor inner city areas in which drugs are widely used, have higher rates of drug abuse. Young people from lower socioeconomic backgrounds are more likely to use drugs than their more affluent peers, possibly because of economic disadvantage, family instability, a lack of opportunities, a dearth of positive role models, and a sense of hopelessness.

Peers and family. Individuals whose companions are substance abusers are far more likely to use drugs. Young people growing up in families in which parents or older siblings abuse drugs tend to develop drug problems themselves. The likelihood of drug abuse is also related to family instability, parental rejection, and divorce.

The nature of the drug. Substances such as crack cocaine that produce an intense, brief high lead to dependence more quickly than slower-acting agents such as cocaine powder. Drugs that cause distressing withdrawal symptoms, such as barbiturates, may lead to continued use by those trying to avoid such discomfort.

Conditioned learning. Drug use involves certain behaviors, situations, and settings that users may, over time, associate with getting high. Even after long periods of abstinence, former drug users sometimes find that they crave the drug when they return to a site of past drug use or meet people with whom they once used drugs. Former cocaine users report that the sight of white powder alone can serve as a cue that triggers a craving.

Drug experimentation. Most individuals who use drugs first try them as adolescents. Teens are likely to begin experimenting with tobacco, beer, wine, or hard liquor, then smoke marijuana or sniff inhalants. Some then go on to try sedative-hypnotics, stimulants (including cocaine), and hallucinogens, such as LSD. A much smaller percentage will try the opioids. Over time, some individuals give up certain drugs, such as hallucinogens, and return to old favorites such as alcohol and marijuana. A smaller number continue using several drugs, a pattern called *polysubstance abuse.* Mental health professionals have long debated whether experimentation with certain drugs, chiefly marijuana, serves as a gateway to other substances of abuse. Many now agree that positive experiences with any drug, including marijuana, can encourage experimentation with stronger, potentially less controllable substances.

▼

Seeking help   If you suspect that you or someone close to you has a problem with drugs, these are some questions that should be asked:

- Do you find yourself using more of a prescription medication or drug of abuse than you expected, or take the substance over a longer period of time than you intended?

- Have you wanted or tried to cut down or control your drug use, but failed?

- Do you spend a great deal of time doing whatever you have to in order to get drugs, use drugs, or recover from their effects?

- Have you given up or cut down on activities at work, at home, or socially because of your drug use?

- Have you continued to use drugs even though you realize that they are creating or worsening a physical or mental problem?

- Have you developed tolerance to a drug so that you have to use much more of it than in the past to feel the way you once did with a much smaller amount?

- If you cut down or stop drug use, do you develop physical or psychological withdrawal symptoms, such as anxiety, insomnia, restlessness, or nausea?

- Do you use drugs to relieve or avoid these withdrawal symptoms?

If you or someone close to you answers "yes" to several of these questions, the problem is probably substance dependence, and you should consult a mental health professional. Even if you feel these questions are not applicable to you, ask yourself the following:

- Are you often so intoxicated or high, or do you feel so bad after drug use, that you cannot do your job or fulfill your responsibilities at home or work?

- Do you use drugs in dangerous ways or situations, such as while driving or operating machinery?

- Have you had repeated drug-related legal problems, such as being arrested for possession of illegal drugs?

- Do you continue to use drugs even though they cause or worsen social or personal problems, such as arguments with relatives?

If you or someone close to you answers "yes" to any of these questions, the problem is probably substance abuse, and you should seek professional help.

The most difficult step for anyone with a substance use disorder is to admit to the problem. Sometimes a drug-related crisis, such as being arrested or fired, forces individuals to acknowledge

Is it substance dependence?

According to the DSM-IV, a diagnosis of drug dependence should be based on three or more of these criteria, occurring during any twelve-month period:

■ *Tolerance,* as defined by either
1. Need for markedly increased amounts of a drug to achieve intoxication or desired effect, or
2. Markedly diminished effect with continued use of the same amount

■ *Withdrawal,* as manifested by
1. Characteristic symptoms, including at least two of the following: sweating, rapid pulse, or other signs of autonomic hyperactivity; increased hand tremor; insomnia; nausea or vomiting; temporary hallucinations or illusions; physical agitation or restlessness; anxiety; or grand mal seizures; or
2. Drug use to avoid or relieve these symptoms

■ Consuming larger amounts of a drug or over a longer period than was intended

■ Persistent desire or unsuccessful efforts to cut down or control drug use

■ A great deal of time spent in activities necessary to obtain drugs, use them, or recover from their effects

■ Important social, occupational, or recreational activities given up or reduced because of drug use

■ Continued drug use despite knowledge that the drug is likely to cause or exacerbate a persistent or recurring physical or psychological problem

Adapted from the Diagnostic and Statistical Manual of Mental Disorders, 4th Edition. *Used with permission.*

the impact of their drug use. If not, those who care—family, friends, boss, physician—may have to confront them and insist that they do something about it. This confrontation, planned beforehand, is called an *intervention* (discussed more fully on page 180), and it can be the turning point for drug users and their families.

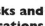

Risks and complications

Drugs affect a person's physical, mental, social, and spiritual health. These effects can be acute (resulting from a single dose or series of doses) or chronic (resulting from long-term use). Acute effects vary with different drugs: stimulants may trigger unpredictable rage; marijuana can produce intense anxiety; cocaine can affect blood pressure and heart rate, and may trigger arrhythmias or seizures; PCP can cause a psychotic episode; LSD can lead to irrational and sometimes fatal acts, such as jumping from a window.

Over time, chronic drug users may become physically, mentally, and spiritually debilitated. They may feel chronically fatigued or suffer from multiple symptoms, such as insomnia, poor concentration, memory impairment, malnutrition, and weight loss. They may develop mental disorders, such as depression or paranoia. They may experience blackouts (periods of memory lapse), flashbacks (vivid reliving of a previous experience), and episodes of impulsive or bizarre behavior, often triggered by escalating paranoia.

With continued drug use and ever-increasing doses, the risk for overdose rises steadily. Chronic users live in a state of continual fear and stress: fear of being arrested for possession, fear of losing a job if they test positive for drugs, preoccupation with getting enough money for the next supply, and the danger of associating with drug dealers. Life loses all sense of meaning or purpose, and the risk for suicide increases.

▼

Treating drug dependence and abuse

Once a person has made the decision to seek help for substance abuse, the first step is usually detoxification, the process of clearing the drug from the body. "Detoxing" can take place in an outpatient setting, a residential facility, or a hospital. A treatment plan thereafter may consist of individual psychotherapy, marital and family therapy, medication, and behavior therapy. Increasingly, treatment is being tailored to address co-existing, or dual, diagnoses.

Controlled and supervised withdrawal in a medical or psychiatric hospital may be recommended if an individual has not been able to stop using drugs as an outpatient or in a residential treatment program. Other reasons for inpatient treatment include the absence of a drug-free living environment, a lack of psychosocial support for maintaining abstinence, or a complicated drug history with addiction to multiple substances. Detoxification is likely to be most complicated when a person is a polysubstance abuser, and it may require close monitoring and the treatment of severe, potentially fatal withdrawal symptoms. Even when inpatient care is advisable, however, restrictions on insurance coverage may limit the number of days of such care. More and more often, persons continue treatment in residential programs or as outpatients as soon as they complete detoxification.

Medications are used in detoxification to alleviate withdrawal symptoms and to prevent medical and psychiatric complications. After withdrawal is complete, these medications are discontinued, so that the individual is in a drug-free state. However, those with mental disorders or symptoms (such as psychotic symptoms after

Is it substance abuse?

According to the DSM-IV, a diagnosis of drug abuse should be based on one or more of these criteria, occurring at any time during a twelve-month period:

- Recurrent drug abuse resulting in a failure to fulfill major role obligations at work, school, or home

- Recurrent drug abuse in situations in which it is physically hazardous

- Recurrent drug-related legal problems

- Continued drug use despite persistent or recurring social or interpersonal problems caused or exacerbated by drug use

- Has never had drug dependence, as defined in the *DSM-IV*

Adapted from the Diagnostic and Statistical Manual of Mental Disorders, 4th Edition. *Used with permission.*

PCP use) may require appropriate psychiatric medication to manage their symptoms and to reduce the risk for relapse. A person suffering from major depression or panic disorder, for instance, may require ongoing treatment with antidepressants.

The aim of chemical dependence treatment is to help individuals establish and maintain their recovery from drugs of abuse and alcohol (discussed in Chapter 10). Recovery is a dynamic process of personal growth and healing that takes place as the person makes the transition from a lifestyle of active substance use to the drug-free lifestyle of recovery.

Whatever their setting, chemical dependence treatment programs involve an initial period of intensive treatment, followed by one to two years of continuing aftercare. Most freestanding programs—those not affiliated with a hospital—follow what is known as the "Minnesota model," a treatment approach developed at the Hazelden Recovery Center in Center City more than thirty years ago. Its key principles include a focus on drug use as the primary problem, not as a symptom of underlying emotional problems; a multidisciplinary approach that addresses the physical, emotional, spiritual, family, and social aspects of the individual; a supportive community; and a goal of abstinence and health.

Those in early recovery in programs based on the Hazelden model live under strict rules. Treatment usually includes individual and group psychotherapy, family therapy, fitness training, relaxation exercises, biofeedback, spiritual counseling, and twelve-step meetings (programs modeled on Alcoholics Anony-

mous that provide peer support for recovering drug users), as well
as formal instruction in the nature of drug dependence and abuse.
The controlled, low-stress environment prepares individuals for
their re-entry into a drug-using world. Aftercare typically consists
of weekly counseling sessions and regular attendance at twelve-
step meetings. Usually, families are involved in all stages of recovery, both with and apart from the user. Those who live far from a
center may participate in intensive sessions at the end of their
family member's stay.

Outpatient programs for substance abuse, offered by freestanding centers, hospitals, and community mental health centers, often run four or five nights a week for four to eight weeks, or in
daily eight-hour sessions for seven or eight days, followed by
weekly group therapy. These programs allow recovering drug users
to continue with their daily lives and to learn to deal with day-
to-day work and family stresses. Mental health professionals in
private practice also offer individually structured outpatient
treatment.

Dealing with underlying psychological conflicts is not enough to
stop drug abuse, nor is resolving psychological problems essential
for living a drug-free life. Nevertheless, psychotherapy can make
an important contribution to recovery. Data indicate that it is of
particular benefit for individuals who are psychologically oriented,
who are married or have a significant other, who are of average or
higher intelligence, who are highly motivated, or who have dual
diagnoses—addiction plus a mental disorder.

Psychotherapy may consist of behavioral and cognitive approaches. One effective behavioral treatment is contingency contracting between the substance abuser and the therapist. If the
agreement is based on negative incentives, the user signs a contract promising to stop taking the drug and gives the therapist a
sealed letter that may reveal an embarrassing secret or make an
irrevocable pledge to give up something important, such as a car
or a large amount of money, if the person breaks the contract. If a
urine test shows that the user is once again on drugs, the therapist opens the letter and the user must comply with the contract.
Alternatively, contracts can be based on positive incentives, such
as vouchers to purchase clothes or other desired items, which are
fulfilled in return for continued abstinence.

A cognitive approach, which emphasizes education, helps to
diminish the frequent guilt and self-loathing that stem from the
sense of losing control. In cognitive-behavioral therapy, persons
identify and record situations and feelings that lead to drug use
and then learn how to avoid such situations or to deal with such
feelings. Social skills training teaches individuals how to handle

everyday situations without the use of drugs. Interpersonal training explores the context of drug use, including the person's relationships with others. (Chapter 27 describes these forms of
psychotherapy.)

Therapy groups provide an opportunity for individuals who have
often been isolated by their drug use to participate in normal social settings. Small groups made up of other drug users can be
especially valuable, because people are usually much more willing
to listen to those who have experienced similar problems than to
those who have not. Because they all share the experience of drug
use, the members can confront one another with frankness and
cut through rationalizations and lies. A professional therapist
keeps members of the group from ganging up on any one person.
Some small groups use role-playing or *psychodrama*, in which
individuals pretend to play other people's roles in the process.
Participation in twelve-step programs for drug abusers, such
as Substance Anonymous, Narcotics Anonymous, and Cocaine
Anonymous, is of fundamental importance in promoting and
maintaining long-term abstinence.

Often persons with substance use disorders do not realize the
impact that drugs have had on their families. Family therapy can
help to bring problems out into the open and deal with family issues related to a member's drug use. Children of individuals who
were frequently high or intoxicated or isolated from other family
members because of their substance abuse or dependence derive
special benefit from this form of therapy.

Relapse prevention   The most common clinical course of substance abuse disorders involves a pattern of multiple relapses over
the course of a lifetime. It is important for people with these problems and their families to recognize this fact. When relapses do
occur, they should be viewed neither as a mark of defeat nor as
evidence of moral weakness. Although painful, they do not erase
the progress that has been achieved, and ultimately they may
strengthen self-understanding. They serve as effective reminders
of potential pitfalls to be avoided in the future.

One key to preventing relapse is learning to avoid obvious cues
and associations that can set off intense cravings. This means
staying away from the people and places linked with past drug
use. Some therapists use conditioning techniques to give former
users a sense of some control over their urge to use the drug. The
theory behind this approach, which is called *extinction of conditioned behavior*, is that with repeated exposure—for example, to
videotapes of dealers selling crack cocaine—the arousal and craving diminish. Although conditioning by itself cannot ward off re-

lapses, it does appear to enhance the overall effectiveness of other concurrent therapies.

Another important lesson that therapists emphasize is that every "lapse" does not have to lead to a full-blown relapse. Users can turn to the skills acquired in treatment—including calling people for support or going to meetings—to avoid a major relapse. Ultimately, they must learn much more than how to avoid temptation: They must examine their entire view of the world and learn new ways to live in it without turning to drugs. This is the underlying goal of the recovery process.

▼
Impact on relationships

Codependence refers to the tendency of the spouses, partners, parents, and friends of individuals who use drugs or alcohol to allow or "enable" their loved ones to continue their drug use and self-destructive behavior. Codependence is discussed in depth in Chapter 10.

Co-Dependents Anonymous, founded in 1986 for "men and women whose common problem is an inability to maintain functional relationships," sponsors support programs throughout the country. Nar-Anon provides groups for people affected by drug abuse. Both organizations are listed in the Resource Directory at the back of the book; local chapters may be found in the white pages of the telephone directory.

If someone you love has a drug problem, get as much information as you can so that you understand what you and your loved one are up against. Denying or minimizing problems is common, and it can be a major obstacle to getting a person one cares about into treatment. If he or she is "in denial," intervention may be necessary. Specially trained intervention counselors work at most chemical dependence units; some offer advice by phone. A typical intervention involves a formal meeting of the substance user with close family members and friends under the direction of a professional counselor. The loved ones confront the drug user with detailed accounts of how the drug abuse has affected or hurt them as well as the user.

Don't expect a drug abuser to quit without help. Substance dependence is an illness that requires professional treatment. Offer your support, but make it clear that you expect the individual to undergo treatment. If he or she agrees to it, make sure that the program is based on a complete evaluation of medical and psychological problems. Abstinence is the goal of the recovery process. A drug user in early recovery should regularly attend support groups, such as Cocaine Anonymous or Narcotics Anonymous, for at least one to two years after rehabilitation. Family members

DO YOU HAVE A DRUG PROBLEM?

The following exercise can identify a possible substance abuse problem in a non-threatening way:

☐ **Keep a diary for two weeks. You may want to use 3″ by 5″ cards or a small notebook.**

☐ **Carry the cards or notebook with you wherever you go and write down everything you take into your body and everything you do.**

☐ **Don't "edit" or reread your diary while you're recording data.**

☐ **At the end of two weeks, read your diary or spread out the cards. Underline or highlight the behaviors that appear again and again. Do they cause you any concern?**

☐ **Consider asking someone else to read your diary and see if he or she spots any worrisome patterns.**

☐ **If there is a potential problem, you might want to try modifying your behavior for one month to reduce or eliminate a substance or habit. During this time, keep a diary and record your feelings as well as what you take in and do. Note any changes in energy, sleep, etc.**

☐ **Ask the people around you if they notice any differences in you.**

☐ **If you are able to modify your behavior over a full month, continue to reduce your substance use or behavior over time.**

☐ **If you can't make changes on your own or feel that it's too hard, get help.**

also should seek help themselves. Most hospitals and chemical-dependence programs offer such support.

▼

Outlook   Whatever the drug, recovery from dependence and abuse is a process of immense inner change that involves every aspect of a person's life. It does not follow a straight, even course; rather, it moves back and forth between denial and awareness, ignorance and knowledge, craving and commitment. It starts with a feeling of great relief, followed by a deep sense of emptiness. Individuals who have abused or become dependent on drugs must form a new identity, stop living in the past or future, give up their search for a quick fix, change the way they relate to family and old friends, find new things to do with the time they previously spent on their drug habit, learn new behaviors, and adopt new attitudes. Through treatment, education, and a re-evaluation of what is truly meaningful, they can find a better way of living.

Although valid statistics are difficult to obtain, substance abuse counselors agree that eventually drug treatment works. In addition, they emphasize that the high likelihood of relapses should not cause undue pessimism. Addiction, after all, is a chronic, progressive, often lifelong illness—not unlike many other medical problems.

"Would one ever place the expectation on patients with diabetes or rheumatoid arthritis to be capable of overcoming their illness through some individual effort on their part?" asks Charles Connors, M.D., a psychiatrist at the Veterans Administration Medical Center in San Francisco. "The answer would certainly be no, but our inclination is to expect just this of patients with substance use disorders. We tend to conceptualize illnesses of addiction differently than medical illness and in so doing often place inordinate expectations on patients to sustain 'abstinence' when, in fact, 'relapse' is the norm, just as 'progression of the illness' is the norm for medical illnesses such as diabetes or rheumatoid arthritis."

Drugs of abuse

The psychoactive substances associated with both dependence and abuse include alcohol (discussed in Chapter 10); amphetamines; cannabis (marijuana); cocaine; hallucinogens; inhalants; opioids; phencyclidine (PCP); and sedative-hypnotic or anxiolytic (anti-anxiety) drugs. Caffeine and nicotine are also discussed in this chapter.

AMPHETAMINES

Amphetamines are stimulants, once widely prescribed for weight control because they are appetite suppressants, that trigger the release of epinephrine (adrenaline), which stimulates the central nervous system. Amphetamines are sold under a variety of names: amphetamine (trade name Benzedrine, street name "bennies"), dextroamphetamine (Dexedrine, or "dex"), methamphetamine (Methedrine, or "meth" or "speed"), and Desoxyn ("copilots"). Related "uppers" include the prescription drugs methylphenidate (Ritalin), pemoline (Cylert), and phenmetrazine (Preludin).

Amphetamines are available in tablet or capsule form. Abusers may grind and sniff the capsules or make a solution and inject the drug. "Ice" is a smokable form of methamphetamine. It is highly addictive and produces an intense physical and psychological high that can last from four to fourteen hours.

"Crank" is the street term for another central nervous system stimulant, propylexedrine, which is less potent than amphetamine. Abusers often extract the drug from the cotton plug of decongestant inhalants and inject it intravenously.

▼

**How amphetamine
users feel**

Amphetamines produce a state of hyperalertness and energy. Users feel confident of their ability to think clearly and to perform any task exceptionally well, although amphetamines do not, in fact, significantly boost performance or thinking. Higher doses make them feel "wired": talkative, excited, restless, irritable, anxious, moody.

Taken intravenously, amphetamines produce a characteristic "rush" of elation and confidence, as well as adverse effects, including confusion, rambling or incoherent speech, anxiety, headache, and palpitations. Individuals may become paranoid, be convinced they are having "profound" thoughts, feel increased sexual interest, and experience unusual perceptions, such as ringing in the ears, a sensation of insects crawling on their skin, or hearing their name called. Crank users may feel high and sleepy or may hallucinate and lose contact with reality.

▼

**Risks and
complications**

Dependence on amphetamines can develop with episodic or daily use. Users typically take amphetamines in increasingly larger doses to prevent "crashing." "Bingeing"—taking high *doses* over a period of several days—can lead to an extremely intense and unpleasant "crash," characterized by a craving for the drug, shakiness, irritability, anxiety and depression, which requires two or more days for recuperation.

Amphetamine intoxication may cause the following symptoms:

- Grandiosity; anxiety; tension; hypervigilance; anger; social hypersensitivity; fighting; jitteriness or agitation; paranoia; and impaired judgment and social or occupational functioning

- Irregular heart rate; dilated pupils; elevated or lowered blood pressure; perspiration or chills; and nausea or vomiting.

- Other possible effects include: weight loss; speeding up or slowing down of physical movement; muscle weakness; impaired breathing; chest pain; confusion; seizures; impaired movements or muscle tone; or even coma.

High doses can cause a rapid or irregular heartbeat, tremors, loss of coordination, and collapse. Amphetamines taken intravenously in high doses can create a sudden increase in blood pressure that can cause very high fever, heart failure, or a fatal stroke.

Smokable methamphetamine, or ice, also increases heart rate and blood pressure; high doses can cause permanent damage to blood vessels in the brain. Other physical effects include dilated pupils, blurred vision, dry mouth, and increased breathing rate. Prolonged use can cause fatal lung and kidney disorders. Injecting

DRUGS OF ABUSE

Amphetamines Speed up physical and mental processes; lessen fatigue; boost energy; create a sense of excitement	**HEALTH EFFECTS** Loss of appetite; blurred vision; headache; dizziness; sweating; sleeplessness; trembling; anxiety; nausea or vomiting; suspiciousness; delusions; hallucinations; confusion; palpitations; jitteriness or agitation; unusual perceptions (such as ringing in the ears or a sensation of insects crawling on the skin); increased heart rate; elevated blood pressure; muscle weakness; impaired breathing or, movements; loss of muscle tone **LONG-TERM RISKS** Dependence; chest pain; heart arrhythmias (disruption of heart rhythm); seizures; malnutrition; skin disorders; ulcers; lack of sleep; depression; paranoia; vitamin deficiencies; brain damage; sexual dysfunction; stroke; high fever; heart failure; violent behavior; coma; fatal overdose
Cannabis (marijuana and hashish) Relax the mind and body; alter mood; heighten perceptions	**HEALTH EFFECTS** Faster heartbeat and pulse; dry mouth and throat; impaired perceptions and reactions; lethargy; nausea; possible hallucinations; panic attacks; decreased motivation **LONG-TERM RISKS** Psychological dependence; impaired thinking, perception, memory and coordination; increased heart rate and blood pressure; impaired fertility; depressed immunity; bronchitis; emphysema; lung cancer
Cocaine and crack Speed up physical and mental processes; create sense of heightened energy and confidence	**HEALTH EFFECTS** Headaches; exhaustion; shaking; sweating; chills; blurred vision; nausea or vomiting; seizures; loss of appetite; impaired judgment; hyperactivity; babbling; speeding up or slowing down of physical activity; impaired breathing; chest pain; impaired movements or loss of muscle tone **LONG-TERM RISKS** Dependence; extreme suspiciousness; violence; damage to nose (if snorted), blood vessels, and heart; blood pressure irregularities; loss of sexual desire; impotence; seizures; chest pain; heart attack; disruptions in heart rhythm; intracranial hemorrhage; damage to liver and lungs (if smoked); hepatitis; HIV infection, skin infections, inflammation of the arteries, and infection of the lining of the heart (if injected)
Hallucinogens (LSD, mescaline) Alter perceptions and produce hallucinations, which may be frightening or pleasurable	**HEALTH EFFECTS** Increased heart rate, blood pressure and body temperature; headache; nausea; sweating; trembling; heart palpitations; blurring of vision; tremors; poor coordination; "bad trips" and irrational acts (LSD) **LONG-TERM RISKS** Disturbing flashbacks; psychological dependence; delusional disorder (with LSD use)

propylexedrine (crank) can lead to convulsions, strokes, and respiratory and kidney failure. Abusers also may develop infected veins and, as with all injected substances, risk infection with the AIDS virus if they share needles.

The long-term effects of amphetamine abuse include: malnutrition; weight loss; skin disorders; ulcers; insomnia; depression; vitamin deficiencies; and, in some cases, brain damage that results in speech and thought disturbances. Sexual dysfunction and impaired concentration or memory also may occur.

DRUGS OF ABUSE

Inhalants Produce temporary feelings of well-being, giddiness, hallucinations	**HEALTH EFFECTS** Dizziness; involuntary eye movements; poor coordination; slurred speech; unsteady gait; lethargy; depressed reflexes; slowed movements; tremors; loss of muscle tone; blurred vision; nausea; sneezing; coughing; nosebleeds; lack of coordination; loss of appetite; decreased heart and breathing rates; loss of consciousness; aggressiveness; impulsiveness; impaired judgment; increased risk for accidents or injuries **LONG-TERM RISKS** Hepatitis; liver failure; kidney failure; respiratory impairment; blood abnormalities; irregular heartbeat; heart failure; destruction of bone marrow and skeletal muscles; stupor or coma
Opioids (opium, morphine, heroin, and synthetic narcotics) Relax the central nervous system; relieve pain; produce temporary sense of well-being	**HEALTH EFFECTS** Restlessness; nausea; vomiting; slowed breathing; weight loss; lethargy; loss of sex drive; mood swings; slurred speech; sweating; impaired judgment; drowsiness; impaired attention or memory. **LONG-TERM RISKS** Dependence; malnutrition; lowered immunity; infections of the heart lining and valves; skin abscesses; congested lungs; hepatitis; tetanus; liver disease; if injected, infections of the heart lining and valves; skin abscesses; hepatitis; tetanus; liver disease; HIV transmission; depression of central nervous system; coma; fatal overdose
Phencyclidine (PCP) Produces changes in perceptions, including hallucinations, and feelings, including delusions of great strength and invulnerability	**HEALTH EFFECTS** Increased heart rate and blood pressure; flushing; sweating; dizziness; painful hypersensitivity to sound; numbness; diminished sensitivity to pain; impaired coordination and speech; stupor **LONG-TERM RISKS** Psychosis; increased danger of injury or harm to others because of impulsivity, aggressiveness, and violence; coma; convulsions; heart and lung failure; ruptured blood vessels in the brain; suicide; death
Sedative-hypnotics and anxiolytic (anti-anxiety) drugs (including benzodiazepines and barbiturates) Slow down the central nervous system; reduce or relieve tension; induce relaxation, drowsiness, or sleep; decrease alertness	**HEALTH EFFECTS** Drowsiness; sleepiness; impaired judgment; poor coordination; slowed breathing; weak and rapid heartbeat; disrupted sleep; dangerously impaired vision; unsteady gait; confusion; irritability **LONG-TERM RISKS** Dependence; stupor; coma; fatal overdose or fatal reaction to sudden withdrawal

People who use amphetamines may develop an acute paranoid psychosis that can be indistinguishable from paranoid schizophrenia: They may see, hear, and feel things that don't exist, have delusions (irrational thoughts or beliefs), and become paranoid (extremely fearful and suspicious) and, sometimes, violent as they battle against "enemies." Delusions often linger for a week or more; occasionally they have been known to last as long as a year. Amphetamine use sometimes leads to delirium, a state of mental disorganization and confusion that also may result in aggressive or violent behavior. Delirium usually develops within twenty-four hours of intake and then gradually resolves.

▼
Withdrawal

When the immediate effects of amphetamines wear off, users experience a "crash," crave the drug, and become shaky, irritable, anxious, and depressed. Withdrawal usually persists for more than twenty-four hours after the cessation of prolonged, heavy use. Its characteristic features include fatigue, disturbing dreams, sleeping much more or less than usual, increased appetite, and speeding up or slowing down of physical movements. Those who are unable to sleep despite their exhaustion often take sedative-hypnotics (discussed later in this chapter) to help them rest, and may become dependent on them as well as the amphetamines. Symptoms usually reach a peak in two to four days, although depression and irritability may persist for months. Suicide is the major risk.

▼
Treating amphetamine dependence

Inpatient hospitalization is often needed for those who use amphetamines intravenously, who are severely depressed or suicidal, or who have developed a paranoid psychosis. Antipsychotic medications can be used to manage the psychotic symptoms (such as delusions, hallucinations, agitation, and confusion) associated with amphetamine intoxication. For those who experience severe depression after withdrawal, antidepressants may be useful. The psychosocial approaches that are a key part of treatment for drug abuse and dependence are essential for recovery and relapse prevention.

CANNABIS PRODUCTS

Marijuana ("pot") and hashish—the most widely used illegal drugs—are derived from the cannabis plant. The major psychoactive ingredient in both is delta-9-THC (delta-9-tetrahydrocannabinol). Almost one in every three Americans over the age of twelve has tried marijuana at least once. Some 12 million use it; more than 1 million cannot control this use.

Different types of marijuana contain different amounts of THC. Because of careful cultivation, the strength of today's marijuana is much greater than that of the pot used in the 1970s; the physical and mental effects are therefore greater. Usually, marijuana is smoked in a cigarette ("joint") or pipe; it may also be eaten as an ingredient in foods (for instance, baked in brownies), although with a less predictable effect. The drug high is enhanced by holding the smoke in the lungs, and experienced smokers learn to hold it for longer periods to increase the amount of drug diffused into the bloodstream. The circumstances in which marijuana is smoked, the communal aspects of its use, and the user's experience can all affect the way a pot-induced high feels.

▼

How cannabis users feel

At low to moderate doses, marijuana typically creates a mild sense of euphoria, a sense of slowed time (five minutes may feel like an hour), a dreamy sort of self-absorption, and some impairment in thinking and communicating. Users report heightened sensations of color, sound, and other stimuli, relaxation, and increased confidence. The sense of being "stoned" peaks within half an hour and usually lasts for about three hours. Even when alterations in perception seem slight, it is not safe to drive a car for as long as four to six hours after smoking a single joint. Some users—particularly those smoking marijuana for the first time or taking a high dose in an unpleasant or unfamiliar setting—experience acute anxiety, which may be accompanied by a panicky fear of losing control. They may believe that their companions are ridiculing or threatening them. The drug may induce a panic attack, a state of intense terror. (Panic attacks are described in depth in Chapter 7.)

The immediate physical effects of marijuana include increased pulse rate, bloodshot eyes, dry mouth and throat, slowed reaction times, impaired motor skills, increased appetite, and impaired short-term memory. High doses intensify all the reactions experienced with low doses and diminish the ability to perceive and to react. They can lead to sensory distortion and, in the case of hashish (a concentrated resin obtained from marijuana flowers), vivid hallucinations and LSD-like psychedelic reactions. The drug remains in the fat cells of the body for fifty hours or more, so individuals may experience psychoactive effects for several days after using marijuana or hashish.

▼

Risks and complications

Dependence or abuse usually develops with repeated use over a long period of time. Typically, individuals smoke more often rather than smoking a larger amount. With chronic heavy use, users may feel a lessening or loss of the pleasurable effect and may develop lethargy, a loss of satisfaction in usual activities, and persistent attention and memory problems. Chronic marijuana use appears to impair thinking, reading comprehension, verbal and mathematical skills, coordination, and short-term memory. Teenagers who smoke pot regularly often lose interest in school and do not remember what they learned when they were high. Some long-term regular users of marijuana may experience "burn-out," a dulling of their senses and responses that is termed *amotivational syndrome.*

Chronic use can also lead to bronchitis, emphysema, and lung cancer. Smoking a single "joint" can be as damaging to the lungs as smoking five tobacco cigarettes. Marijuana smokers absorb almost five times as much carbon monoxide into their bloodstreams and inhale three times as much tar as tobacco smokers.

Marijuana may suppress ovulation and alter hormone levels in female users and may impair the fertility of male users. Frequent use of marijuana during pregnancy can lower infant birth weight and cause abnormalities in the fetus similar to those of fetal alcohol syndrome. Women who smoke pot while pregnant are more likely to have babies with problems such as small head size, irritability, and poor growth.

▼

Treating cannabis dependence and abuse

Marijuana dependence does not cause withdrawal and, in most cases, hospitalization or adjunctive medications are not necessary. Outpatient programs usually resemble those used for alcohol recovery, with group therapy, twelve-step meetings (described in Chapter 10), individual therapy, family therapy, and educational programs. Most programs include urine testing to ensure that the individuals are not continuing to use the drug, which can be detected in urine for as long as thirty days after it was last smoked. Because many marijuana users are adolescents, psychotherapy often focuses on developmental issues, such as poor self-esteem, learning disorders, and family problems, and on depression. Family therapy can be very beneficial.

The most effective approaches emphasize stopping further use of the drug. Training in relapse prevention includes identifying situations that lead individuals to marijuana use and acquiring skills to avoid these situations.

COCAINE

Cocaine ("coke," "snow," "lady") is a white crystalline powder extracted from the leaves of the South American coca plant. Usually mixed with various sugars or with local anesthetics such as lidocaine and procaine, cocaine powder is generally inhaled. When sniffed or snorted (inhaled), it anesthetizes the nerve endings in the nose and relaxes the bronchial muscles of the lungs.

Cocaine can also be dissolved in water and injected intravenously. Because the drug is rapidly metabolized by the liver, the high is relatively brief, typically lasting only about twenty minutes. This means that users commonly inject the drug repeatedly, increasing the risk for infection and damage to their veins. Many intravenous cocaine users prefer "speedballing," the intravenous administration of a combination of cocaine and heroin.

Cocaine alkaloid, or freebase, is obtained by removing the hydrochloride salt from cocaine powder. "Freebasing" is smoking the alkaloid form of cocaine. Crack, pharmacologically identical to freebase, is a cheap, easy-to-use, widely available, smokable, and very potent form of cocaine named for the popping sound it makes when burned. Because it is rapidly absorbed into the bloodstream and large doses reach the brain very quickly, it is particularly dangerous.

▼

How cocaine users feel

A powerful stimulant to the central nervous system, cocaine produces feelings of soaring well-being and boundless energy. Users feel that they have enormous physical and mental ability, yet are also restless and anxious. The euphoria is brief, however, and is followed by a slump into depression. Binges are common, lasting from a few hours to several days.

With continuing use, cocaine users experience less pleasure and more unpleasant effects. Eventually they may reach a point at which they no longer experience euphoric effects and crave the drug simply to alleviate their persistent hunger for it. They think about cocaine constantly, dream about it, spend all their money on it, and borrow, steal, or deal to pay for it. They cannot concentrate on work. They become increasingly irritable and confused. They may also become dependent on alcohol, sedatives, or opioids, which they use to calm down from the drug's after-effects.

Crack dependence develops rapidly. As soon as crack users come down from one high, they want more. Whereas heroin addicts may shoot up several times a day, crack addicts need another "hit" within minutes. Therefore, a crack habit can quickly become more expensive than heroin addiction. Some "crackheads" have thousand-dollar-a-day habits. Police in big cities have traced many brutal crimes and murders to young crack addicts, who often are extremely paranoid and dangerous. Smoking crack doused with liquid PCP, a practice called "space-basing," has especially frightening effects on behavior.

▼

Risks and complications

Cocaine dependence can develop quickly and easily. With repeated use the brain becomes tolerant of the drug's stimulant effects, and users must take more of it to get high. Its grip is strong: Those who smoke or inject cocaine can develop dependence within weeks. Those who snort cocaine may not become dependent on the drug for months or even years. It is thought that 5 to 20 percent of all coke users—a group as large as the estimated total number of heroin addicts—are dependent on the drug.

Users can develop psychiatric or neurological complications. They may become incoherent and paranoid and may experience unusual sensations, such as ringing in the ears, feeling insects crawling on the skin, or hearing their name called. Repeated or high doses of the drug can lead to impaired judgment, hyperactivity, nonstop babbling, the feelings of suspicion and paranoia noted above, and violent behavior.

The physical effects of acute cocaine intoxication include dilated pupils, elevated or lowered blood pressure, perspiration or chills, nausea or vomiting, speeding up or slowing down of physical activity, muscle weakness, impaired breathing, chest pain, and impaired movements or loss of muscle tone.

Although some users initially try cocaine as a sexual stimulant, it does not enhance sexual performance. Both male and female chronic cocaine users tend to lose interest in sex and have difficulty in reaching orgasm. At low doses the drug may delay ejaculation and orgasm and cause heightened sensory awareness, but men who use cocaine regularly have problems in maintaining erections and ejaculating. They also tend to have low sperm counts, less active sperm, and more abnormal sperm than nonusers.

Frequent snorting can irritate and damage the mucous membrane in the nose, cause sinusitis, destroy a user's sense of smell, and occasionally create a hole in the septum (the membrane between the nostrils). Cocaine can damage the liver and cause lung damage in freebasers. Smoking crack causes bronchitis as well as lung damage and may promote the transmission of HIV through burned and bleeding lips. Some smokers have died of respiratory complications, such as pulmonary edema (build-up of fluid in the lungs).

Cocaine use can cause blood vessels in the brain to clamp shut and can trigger a stroke, bleeding in the brain, and potentially fatal brain seizures. It causes the heart rate to speed up and blood pressure to rise suddenly. Its use is associated with many cardiac complications, including arrhythmias, angina (chest pain), acute myocardial infarction (heart attack), and sudden death.

Complications of injecting the drug include skin infections, hepatitis, inflammation of the arteries, infection of the lining of the heart and, if needles are shared, the possibility of transmitting HIV.

The combination of alcohol and cocaine is particularly lethal. When a person ingests both substances, the liver produces a new drug, cocaethylene, which provides even more intense and longer-lasting feelings of euphoria and well-being than cocaine alone. This substance is also more addictive and more deadly, especially in its effects on the heart. Alcohol and cocaine together are second only to the combination of heroin and alcohol in causing substance abuse-related deaths.

Cocaine is extremely dangerous to pregnant women and their

babies, causing miscarriages, developmental disorders, and life-threatening complications during birth. When used early in pregnancy, cocaine can reduce the fetal oxygen supply, possibly interfering with the development of the nervous system. Because cocaine can cause blood vessels in the fetal brain to burst, the fetus may suffer brain damage. Infants born to cocaine and crack users can experience withdrawal and may have major complications or permanent physical disabilities.

▼
Withdrawal

The symptoms of cocaine withdrawal include fatigue, vivid and disturbing dreams, sleeping much more or less than usual, irritability, increased appetite, and physical slowing down or speeding up. This initial crash may last for one to three days after cutting down or stopping use. Some individuals become depressed, paranoid, and suicidal. Symptoms usually reach a peak in two to four days, although depression, anxiety, irritability, lack of pleasure in usual activities, and low-level cravings may continue for weeks. As memories of the crash fade, the desire for the drug intensifies. For many weeks after stopping, individuals may feel an intense craving.

▼
Treating cocaine dependence and abuse

Cocaine dependence is an extremely difficult addiction to overcome. No single treatment or combination of treatments is effective for every user. Outpatient treatment can be effective for some, and has the advantage of allowing individuals to remain in their own environment while learning to deal with everyday stresses and temptations. Although withdrawal is not physically dangerous, hospitalization may be recommended for chronic abusers who have nowhere else to go, develop medical or psychiatric complications, are dependent on other drugs, or have relapsed during outpatient treatment.

Experimental medical approaches for treating cocaine dependence include antidepressant drugs (both tricyclic antidepressants and SSRIs), anticonvulsants such as carbamazepine (Tegretol), bromocriptine (Parlodel, a drug used for Parkinson's disease), and the naturally occurring amino acids tryptophan and tyrosine. However, these agents have demonstrated only limited benefit, and much more research into medical treatments is needed.

Psychotherapy alone almost never solves a cocaine problem, but it can play a significant role in overall treatment. Even individuals who initially begin therapy only to satisfy their families or employers or to avoid threatened legal action can benefit. Therapy helps them to confront their denial, learn about the nature of dependence, reacquaint themselves with a full range of emotions, view

A cokeaholic's tale

By the time he was thirty, Nick was making more than $250,000 a year as a stockbroker in Chicago. He drove an expensive car, wore custom-made suits, and lived in a penthouse condominium with a magnificent view of Lake Michigan. Nick would smile when he thought about making more money than his big brother, Adam. After all, Adam was the one who earned all the A's and won all the awards in school. Yet here Nick was—the "slow" one—with a net worth climbing toward $1 million.

However, Nick's success sometimes left him with a hollow, lonely feeling. When his spirits slumped, Nick had a way of·picking them up: cocaine. Within minutes of snorting a few lines he would feel invincible, certain that he could take on the world and win. With cocaine, he did not need anyone else.

But Nick had always been wary of drug addiction, so he limited his use. "I know what I'm doing," he told himself. "I know how to use it without getting hooked." Then, one night at a party, Nick smoked crack for the first time.

As he inhaled, his heart raced and his breathing quickened. He felt as if he were Clark Kent turning into Superman. Everyone in the room seemed to fade away. Within ten minutes he wanted more crack. Never before had he felt such a craving. At the end of the night he asked his host for the name of his dealer.

Nick tried to limit his crack use, to restrict himself as he had before. But even when he was at his office, caught up in an important transaction, he would find himself thinking about crack. The craving would grow and grow until he could not control it any more.

Nick began smoking crack more often. On a Friday night he'd buy several hundred dollars' worth and invite a woman to spend the weekend with him. Sometimes he and his date would not sleep from Friday through Sunday. The weekends turned into one long high.

Mondays were hell. As the effects of the drug wore off, he could not believe how bad he felt—worse than he had imagined was even possible. He could not stop shaking, could not keep any food down, could not focus his racing mind on anything. Swigging liquor and gulping down tranquilizers to dull the pain, Nick forced himself to go back to work. But all he could think about was crack. In three months he'd spent $50,000 on the drug.

"What's wrong with Nick?" his co-workers would ask. Previously athletic and well-built, he lost sixty pounds and looked emaciated. When he started making crucial mistakes in business transactions, his clients deserted him for more reliable brokers. Worried, his brother badgered him about seeing a doctor. His colleagues, beginning to suspect a drug problem, also urged him to get help.

Finally Nick entered a hospital. He thought he was dying. Every cell in his body seemed to be screaming. The craving for crack was almost unbearable. After the physical crash came a psychological plunge. Nick's money was gone, along with his job, his reputation, his health, and his beloved possessions. The road back seemed impossibly long.

But Nick took the first step. He started to participate in a therapy program as soon as he left the hospital. Slowly rebuilding his self-confidence, he found a new job. In the beginning, almost any problem would make him think about crack, but he would call his therapist instead of buying drugs. One day at a time, he is managing to cope.

themselves as recovering rather than addicted, and develop a plan for avoiding the cues that stimulate cocaine cravings.

Relapse prevention is especially important in helping individuals to explore their ambivalent feelings toward cocaine, minimize high-risk situations, and develop coping strategies. Contracting with a therapist can also be an effective tool (see Chapter 27). Some contracts spell out the worst possible consequences that the therapist would enforce in case of a relapse. Others stress positive rewards for continued abstinence.

Some mental health professionals use interpersonal therapy, a specific approach to brief psychotherapy that focuses on relationships and conflicts with others. (Chapter 27 describes this form of psychotherapy.) The goal is to help individuals accept the need to stop cocaine use, learn to curb their impulsiveness, and recognize the emotional factors that may contribute to relapse.

HALLUCINOGENS

The drugs known as hallucinogens produce vivid and unusual changes in thought, feeling, and perception. The most widely used hallucinogen in the United States is LSD—lysergic acid diethylamide, or "acid"—which was initially developed as a tool to explore mental illness. It became popular among the hippies and flower children of the 1960s and has resurfaced in the 1990s. LSD is taken orally, either blotted onto pieces of paper that are held in the mouth or chewed or along with another substance, such as a sugar cube. The hallucinogen *peyote*, whose active ingredient is mescaline, is much less commonly used in this country. MDMA ("ecstasy") is a common drug of abuse among young adults and teens.

▼

How hallucinogen users feel

LSD produces hallucinations, including bright colors and altered perceptions of reality. Effects from a single dose begin within thirty to sixty minutes and last for ten to twelve hours. During this time there are slight increases in body temperature, heart rate, and blood pressure; sweating, chills, and goose pimples develop. Some users develop headache and nausea. Within thirty to ninety minutes of consumption, mescaline produces vivid hallucinations, including brightly colored lights, animals, and geometric designs, which may persist for twelve hours.

The effects of hallucinogens are strongly dependent on the dose, the individual's expectations and personality, and the setting for drug use. Many users report religious or mystical imagery and thoughts; some feel that they are experiencing profound insights. Usually the user realizes that perceptual changes are caused by the drug, but some become convinced that they have lost their minds. Drugs sold as hallucinogens are frequently mixed with other substances, such as PCP and amphetamines, which can produce unexpected and frightening effects.

Hallucinogens do not produce dependence in the same way as drugs such as cocaine or heroin, and withdrawal is not a problem. Individuals who have an unpleasant experience after trying a hallucinogen may stop using the drug completely; others continue regular or occasional use because they enjoy the effects.

▼

Risks and complications

Physical symptoms of hallucinogen intoxication include dilated pupils, rapid heart rate, sweating, heart palpitations, blurring of vision, tremors, and poor coordination. These effects may last from eight to twelve hours. Hallucinogen intoxication also produces changes in emotions and mood, such as anxiety, depression, fear of losing one's mind, and impaired judgment. Some persons have flashbacks in which they re-experience the effects felt while intoxicated.

LSD can trigger irrational acts. Users have injured or killed themselves by jumping out of windows, swimming out to sea, or throwing themselves in front of cars. Some individuals develop a delusional disorder, in which they become convinced that their distorted perceptions and thoughts are real.

Those having a "bad trip" may blame themselves and feel excessively guilty, tense, and so agitated that they cannot stop talking and have trouble sleeping. They may fear that they have destroyed their brains and will never return to normal. A person who already is depressed may take a hallucinogen to lift his or her spirits, only to become more depressed. Suicide is a real danger.

▼

Treating hallucinogen abuse

Individuals terrified of losing their minds or dying during a bad trip may require professional evaluation and reassurance that the effects of hallucinogens are time-limited and will wear off. Occasionally, anti-anxiety medication may be prescribed. In cases of extreme agitation or great risk for self-injury or suicide, sedation and hospitalization may be necessary.

INHALANTS

Inhalants, or deliriants, are chemicals that produce vapors with psychoactive effects. The most commonly abused inhalants are solvents, aerosols, model airplane glue, cleaning fluids, and petroleum products such as kerosene and butane. Nitrous oxide (laughing gas) and some other anesthetics are also abused. To inhale intoxicating vapors, individuals may soak a rag in the substance, place it against the mouth and nose, and inhale; inhale fumes from a substance placed in a paper or plastic bag; or inhale vapors directly from their containers.

Inhalant use appears to peak during adolescence. Young people, especially those who may not have money for or access to other drugs, are those most apt to try inhalants. Children between the ages of nine and thirteen tend to use inhalants with a group of peers who are likely to use alcohol and marijuana as well. Users are found in all racial, socioeconomic, and gender groups, but the incidence of use is higher among poor minority youth. Many users come from families that have separated or have been affected by alcohol or drug problems. Users often have school difficulties, such as truancy and poor grades, or problems adjusting to work.

▼

How inhalant users feel

Inhalants reach the lungs, bloodstream, and other parts of the body very rapidly. At low doses the person may feel slightly stimulated; at higher doses, less inhibited. Intoxication often occurs within five minutes and can last for more than an hour. Inhalant users do not report the intense rush associated with other drugs, nor do they experience the perceptual changes associated with LSD. However, these substances interfere with thinking and impulse control, so users may act in dangerous or destructive ways.

Often there are visible external signs of use: a rash around the nose and mouth; breath odors; residue on face, hands, and clothing; redness, swelling, and tearing of the eyes; and irritation of throat, lungs, and nose that leads to coughing and gagging. Nausea and headache also may occur.

▼

Risks and complications

Regular use of inhalants leads to tolerance, so that the sniffer needs more and more to attain the desired effects. In children, inhalants used several times a week can cause dependence. Dependent older users may use them many times a day. Those who become dependent on inhalants are likely to have used many different substances as adolescents and to have gradually turned to inhalants as their preferred substance.

Although some young people believe that inhalants are safe to use, this is far from true. Inhalation of butane from cigarette lighters displaces oxygen in the lungs, causing suffocation. Users also can suffocate while covering their heads with a plastic bag to inhale the substance, or from inhaling vomit into their lungs while high.

The symptoms of mild to moderate inhalant intoxication are similar to those of alcohol or sedative intoxication, but with aggressiveness, impulsiveness, and impaired judgment more common. Physical symptoms include dizziness, involuntary eye movements, blurred vision, poor coordination, slurred speech, unsteady gait, lethargy, depressed reflexes, slowed movements, tremor, general muscle weakness, and stupor or coma.

Inhalants can increase the risk for accidents or head trauma. Because users cannot think clearly, they may act aggressively or place themselves in dangerous situations. Chronic heavy users can suffer serious medical complications, such as hepatitis with liver failure, kidney failure, respiratory impairment, destruction of bone marrow and skeletal muscle, and blood abnormalities. Death may occur from depression of the central nervous system or from cardiac arrhythmia; even during first use, there can be instant, fatal heart failure.

OPIOIDS

The opioids include opium (derived from a resin taken from the seed pod of the Asian poppy) and its derivatives morphine, codeine, and heroin, and non-opioid synthetic drugs, such as meperidine (Demerol), methadone, and propoxyphene (Darvon). All act on the central nervous system, and all have similar sleep-inducing and narcotic (pain-relieving) properties. Prescription opioids may be taken orally in pill form or injected intravenously.

Heroin, the most widely abused opioid, is illegal in the United States, although it is used in other countries as a potent painkiller for conditions such as terminal cancer. There are an estimated 400,000 to 600,000 heroin addicts in the U.S., with men outnumbering women addicts by three to one. Heroin users typically inject the drug into their veins. However, purer forms of heroin can be snorted; this has led to a surge in its popularity, especially among more affluent users. Some users dissolve heroin powder and inhale the vapors. Individuals who experiment with whatever recreational drug is new and trendy often prefer "skin-popping" (subcutaneous injection) to "mainlining" (intravenous injection). To try to avoid addiction, some users begin by "chipping," taking small or intermittent doses of the drug. Regardless of the method of administration, tolerance can develop rapidly.

Morphine, used as a painkiller and anesthetic, masks pain by producing mental clouding, drowsiness, and euphoria. It does not decrease the physical sensation of pain as much as it alters the awareness of pain; in effect, the person no longer cares about the pain.

Two semisynthetic derivatives of morphine are hydromorphone (Dilaudid, or "little D"), with two to eight times the painkilling effect of morphine, and oxycodone (Percocet, Percodan, or "perkies"), similar to codeine but more potent. The synthetic narcotic meperidine (Demerol, or "demies") is now probably second only to morphine for use in relieving pain. It is also used by addicts as a substitute for morphine and heroin.

The narcotic codeine is a weaker painkiller and sedative than morphine. It is an ingredient in liquid products prescribed for relieving coughs, and is also available in tablet and injectable form for relieving pain. Propoxyphene (Darvon), a synthetic narcotic, is somewhat less potent as a painkiller than codeine. Although in usual doses it is no more effective than aspirin, it has been one of the most widely prescribed drugs for headaches, dental pain, and menstrual cramps. At higher doses, it produces a euphoric high, which may lead to misuse.

Some people first take a medically prescribed opioid for pain relief or cough suppression, then gradually increase the dose and frequency on their own. They often justify doing so because they are alleviating symptoms, not seeking a high. As dependence develops, they expend increasing time and effort in order to obtain the supply they need, frequently seeking out several doctors to write prescriptions for them.

▼

How opioid users feel

All the opioids relax the user. When injected, they can produce an immediate "rush," or high. Users may feel indifferent, lethargic, and drowsy for two to six hours thereafter, slur their speech, and have difficulty paying attention, remembering, and going about their normal routines.

The primary attractions of heroin ("horse," "junk," "smack," or "downtown") are the euphoria and pain relief it produces. In some people, however, it causes very unpleasant feelings, such as anxiety and fear. Other effects include sensations of warmth or heaviness, dry mouth, facial flushing, and nausea and vomiting, particularly in first-time users.

Some addicts report a "kick" or rush when heroin is injected directly into their veins. Since the effects do not last long—usually only two to four hours—addicts have to "shoot up" two to five times a day.

▼

Risks and complications

Almost all regular users of opioids rapidly develop drug dependence, which can lead to lethargy, weight loss, loss of sex drive, and a continual effort to avoid withdrawal symptoms through repeated drug administration. In addition, they experience anxiety, insomnia, restlessness, and craving for the drug. Users continue taking opioids as much to avoid the discomfort of withdrawal—a classic sign of addiction—as to experience pleasure.

Opioid intoxication is characterized by changes in mood and behavior, such as initial euphoria followed by apathy or discontent and impaired judgment. Physical symptoms include constricted pupils (although pupils may dilate from a severe overdose), drowsiness, slurred speech, and impaired attention or memory.

With large doses of heroin, the skin becomes cold, moist, and bluish. Morphine affects blood pressure, heart rate, and blood circulation in the brain. Both morphine and heroin depress (slow down) the respiratory system; overdoses can cause fatal respiratory arrest. The combination of alcohol and heroin is particularly lethal and is the primary cause of substance abuse-related deaths.

In addition to respiratory depression, opioid poisoning or overdose causes shock or coma and can be fatal. Emergency medical treatment is critical and is often based on drugs called *narcotic antagonists*, which rapidly reverse the effects of opioids when administered intravenously.

Over time, users who inject opioids may develop infections of the heart lining and valves, skin abscesses, and lung congestion. Infections caused by unsterile solutions, syringes, and shared needles can lead to hepatitis, tetanus, liver disease, and HIV transmission. In some cities in the Northeast, 60 to 65 percent of intravenous drug abusers are HIV-positive. The annual death rate among those dependent on opioids is twenty times higher than among other young people, primarily because of physical complications, overdose, suicide, and the violent lifestyle of many users.

▼

Withdrawal   If a regular user stops taking an opioid, withdrawal begins within six to twelve hours and is usually not life-threatening. The intensity of the symptoms depends on the degree of addiction. They may grow stronger for twenty-four to seventy-two hours and gradually subside over a period of seven to fourteen days, although some symptoms, such as insomnia, may persist for several months. Other symptoms include intense craving for the drug, irritability, nausea or vomiting, muscle aches, runny nose or eyes, dilated pupils, sweating, diarrhea, yawning, and fever. Users may plead, demand, or manipulate others in the effort to satisfy their craving and obtain a further supply of the drug.

▼

Treating opioid dependence and abuse   Opioid dependence is a lifelong disorder characterized by recurrent relapses or continued use. It is a very difficult addiction to overcome. Studies demonstrate that only 10 to 30 percent of heroin users are able to maintain abstinence. It is this fact that contributed to the development of a unique, still controversial treatment for opioid dependence: the once-a-day use of methadone, a long-acting synthetic opioid that users can substitute for heroin or other opioids.

Methadone is used in two basic ways to treat opioid dependence. As an opioid substitute for detoxification, it is usually tapered off over a period of twenty-one to 180 days. As a maintenance treatment, methadone has been criticized by some as nothing more than the substitution of a legal opioid for an illegal one. Critics also charge that because methadone maintenance does not have abstinence as its goal, it contributes to the continued use of other drugs, such as cocaine or alcohol. There also is concern, especially by those in law enforcement, that methadone recipients will engage in "diversion," the sale of take-home doses of methadone for profit.

Despite these charges, methadone maintenance remains the mainstay of treatment for opioid dependence and is the most successful treatment presently available. It may also be the most thoroughly studied drug treatment. Research has clearly documented several important positive benefits of methadone maintenance, including decrease in illicit opioid use, decreased criminal behavior, lower risk for contracting HIV infection (through the sharing of needles), and improvements in physical health, employment, and other lifestyle factors. Individuals who have been on methadone maintenance for a long time (often years), have stable relationships and employment, have assimilated themselves into the nondrug culture, and are highly motivated to get off methadone have the best chance for successful detoxification from methadone.

A number of new drug therapies may prove useful in treating opioid dependence. L-α-acetylmethadol (L-AAM) is an opioid that is longer acting than methadone, appears to have less abuse potential, and can be taken three times a week rather than daily. Buprenorphine is a partial opioid blocker, or agonist, which is being studied for use in detoxification and maintenance treatment.

Other medications for opioid withdrawal, such as clonidine (Catapres) and naltrexone (Trexan), are being tried either separately or in combination as outpatient methods of detoxification. Although clonidine, a medication primarily used for hypertension, is not approved by the FDA for detoxification, many outpatient and inpatient treatment centers use it to ameliorate withdrawal symptoms. The side effects of opioids include dry mouth, drowsiness, fatigue, headache, dizziness, sedation, and hypotension (low blood pressure).

Naltrexone prevents opioid-induced euphoria by blocking opioid receptors in the brain and central nervous system. Used on a long-term basis, it may gradually eliminate drug-seeking behavior. It does not produce dependence, causes few side effects, and reduces the likelihood of overdose if opioids are used. Its success rates have varied. Although highly motivated individuals have found it extremely helpful, hard-core addicts are likely to drop out of treatment.

Two of every three detoxified opioid users return to drug use within six months. It is for this reason that methadone maintenance and other emerging opioid substitution treatments play such an important role in the treatment of opioid addiction. Increasingly, individual, group, and family psychotherapy is being recognized as a key component of treatment for opioid dependence. Vocational training also is important to long-term success.

PHENCYCLIDINE

Phencyclidine, or PCP (street names "angel dust," "peace pill," "lovely," or "green"), is an illicit drug manufactured as a tablet, capsule, liquid, flake, spray, or crystal-like white powder that can be swallowed, smoked, sniffed, snorted, or injected. Sometimes it is sprinkled on crack, marijuana (a combination known on the street as "love boat"), tobacco, or parsley, and smoked. PCP was once thought to have value as an anesthetic and was tested under the trade name Sernyl, but its side effects, including delirium and hallucinations, made it unacceptable for medical use.

PCP use peaked in the 1970s, but it remains a popular drug of abuse in both inner city neighborhoods and suburban high schools. According to the National Institute of Drug and Alcohol Abuse, whereas use of other drugs has generally declined, PCP use has increased among teenagers. Often users think that it is the PCP that they take together with another illegal psychoactive substance, such as amphetamines, coke, or hallucinogens, that is responsible for the highs they feel, so they seek it out specifically.

▼

How PCP users feel

In low doses, PCP produces changes—from hallucinations to euphoria to feelings of emptiness or numbness—similar to those produced by other psychoactive drugs. PCP users lack insight and judgment and act without thinking. Many feel aggressive, belligerent, agitated, or impulsive. Higher doses may produce a stupor that lasts for several days, increased heart rate and blood pressure, flushing, sweating, dizziness, and numbness. However, PCP has some effects that are utterly unpredictable. The drug can trigger violent behavior (fighting is common) or irreversible psychosis the first time it is used, or the twentieth, or never. Heavy users develop a craving for PCP and may smoke it two or three times a day.

▼

Risks and complications

Some first-time users feel that PCP is too unpredictable and do not try it again; others quickly become heavy users. Many go on PCP binges, or "runs," that can last for several days. Some people use it daily, often along with marijuana and alcohol. It takes only a short period of occasional PCP use for dependence or abuse to develop.

The behavioral changes associated with PCP intoxication, which can occur within minutes of use, include belligerence, aggressiveness, impulsiveness, unpredictability, agitation, poor judgment, and impaired functioning at work or in social situations. The physical symptoms of PCP intoxication may include involuntary eye movements, repetitive motor movements such as facial grimacing, a painful sensitivity to sound, increased blood pressure or heart rate, numbness or diminished responsiveness to pain, impaired coordination and speech, muscle rigidity, and seizures. Taking large amounts can lead to convulsions, heart and lung failure, coma, ruptured blood vessels in the brain, and death.

Intoxication typically lasts for four to six hours, but some effects can linger for several days. Delirium may occur within twenty-four hours of taking PCP or after recovery from an overdose, and can last for as long as a week.

PCP can trigger an episode of depression or anxiety that may persist for months. Some users feel so restless that they cannot stop talking or fall asleep. Some reproach themselves constantly in fear that they have destroyed their brains and will never return to normal. Those who take PCP to elevate their mood may end up more depressed. Suicide is a definite risk.

Psychotic episodes resulting from PCP use often involve hallucinations, violent behavior, and paranoia. Because of its delusional effects, users may feel they have superhuman strength and abilities; because of its anesthetic effects, they may feel no pain.

▼
Treating PCP dependence and abuse

PCP users with violent or self-destructive behavior may require emergency treatment. Hospitalization is often recommended because of the need for sedation, supervision, and supportive treatment. Anti-anxiety medications, such as diazepam (Valium), are commonly used to treat the anxiety and agitation associated with PCP use. When delusional symptoms, hallucinations, or paranoia are present, antipsychotic medications may be prescribed. Once their condition has been stabilized, PCP users—who often are polysubstance abusers—can begin treatment, as described at the beginning of this chapter. Those who develop major depression or an anxiety disorder after PCP use should receive treatment for these conditions as well.

SEDATIVE-HYPNOTIC AND ANXIOLYTIC DRUGS

Sedative-hypnotic (sleep-inducing) and anxiolytic (anti-anxiety) medications reduce activity and induce relaxation, drowsiness, or sleep. They include the benzodiazepines and the barbiturates.

The benzodiazepines—the most widely used drugs in this category—are commonly prescribed for tension, muscle strain, sleep problems, anxiety, panic attacks, anesthesia, and in the treatment of alcohol withdrawal. They include such drugs as chlordiazepoxide (Librium), diazepam (Valium), oxazepam (Serax), flurazepam (Dalmane), lorazepam (Ativan), chlorazepate (Tranxene), clonazepam (Klonopin), triazolam (Halcion), temazepam (Restoril), and alprazolam (Xanax). Although all act on the central nervous system, they differ widely in their mechanism of action, absorption rate, and metabolism. All, however, produce similar intoxication and withdrawal symptoms.

Benzodiazepines are usually taken by mouth in tablet, capsule, or liquid form. (When used for general anesthesia they are administered intravenously.) These drugs have largely replaced the barbiturates, which were used medically in the past to induce relaxation and sleep, relieve tension, and treat epileptic seizures. Short-acting barbiturates include pentobarbital (Nembutal, or "yellow jackets"), secobarbital (Seconal, or "reds"), and thiopental (Pentothal); they are rapidly absorbed into the brain. The longer-acting barbiturates, such as amobarbital (Amytal, or "blues" or "downers") and phenobarbital (Luminal, or "phennies"), are absorbed slowly into the bloodstream, take a while to reach the brain, and have an effect that lasts for several days.

▼

How users of sedative-hypnotics and anxiolytics feel

In lower doses, these drugs reduce or relieve tension; larger doses can cause a loosening of sexual or aggressive inhibitions. Individuals who use these drugs may experience rapid mood changes, impaired judgment, and impaired social or occupational functioning. High doses produce slurred speech, drowsiness, and stupor. Young people in their teens or early twenties who take sedative-hypnotic or anxiolytic drugs to obtain a high or state of euphoria—sometimes in combination with other drugs—have usually used many illegal substances. Adults often first obtain sedatives, hypnotics, or anti-anxiety medications from a physician who prescribes them for insomnia or anxiety, and then gradually increase the dose or frequency of use on their own, often by seeking prescriptions from several physicians. Although they may justify this continued use because of their symptoms, they become dependent and cannot function normally without the drug.

▼

Risks and complications

All sedative-hypnotic and anxiolytic drugs can produce physical and psychological dependence within two to four weeks. A complication specific to sedatives is cross-tolerance, or cross-addiction, in which users who develop tolerance for one sedative, or become dependent on it, will have tolerance for other sedatives as well.

Individuals with a prior history of substance abuse are at greatly increased risk for abusing this class of drugs if they are prescribed by a physician. However, those who have not abused drugs or alcohol in the past rarely develop an abuse problem with these medications when they are prescribed for legitimate psychiatric disorders.

Intoxication with these drugs can produce changes in mood or behavior, such as inappropriate sexual or aggressive acts, mood swings, and impaired judgment. Physical signs include slurred speech, poor coordination, unsteady gait, involuntary eye movements, impaired attention or memory, and stupor or coma.

The combination of these drugs with alcohol has a synergistic effect that can be dangerous. Thinking and behavior are impaired, and driving is especially hazardous. Alcohol in combination with sedative-hypnotics is potentially lethal, leading to respiratory depression that may result in death.

Regular users of any of these drugs who become physically dependent should not try to cut down on their own or quit abruptly: Stopping suddenly places the user at risk for seizures, coma, and death. It is essential to taper drug use gradually.

In pregnancy, sedative-hypnotic and anxiolytic drugs cross the placenta and cause birth defects and behavioral problems in the infant. Infants born to women who used these drugs during pregnancy may be physically dependent on them and can develop breathing problems, feeding difficulties, disturbed sleep, sweating, irritability, and fever.

▼

Withdrawal   Depending on the degree of dependence, the symptoms of withdrawal from sedative-hypnotic and anxiolytic drugs can range from relatively mild discomfort to a severe syndrome accompanied by seizures. Withdrawal symptoms include malaise or weakness, sweating, rapid pulse, coarse tremor of the hands, tongue, and eyelids, insomnia, nausea or vomiting, temporary hallucinations or illusions, physical restlessness, anxiety or irritability, and a severe syndrome with grand mal seizures. The onset of withdrawal varies, depending on whether the drug is short- or long-acting. It can begin within two to three days with drugs that are eliminated from the body rapidly, such as lorazepam or alprazolam, and may take as long as five or six days to develop if the dependence is on longer-acting drugs, such as diazepam or clonazepam. Symptoms can persist for many weeks. Individuals who have abruptly discontinued the drug after prolonged use may develop delirium or amnesia during withdrawal.

▼

Treating dependence   Detoxification follows the same pattern as with alcohol withdrawal (see Chapter 10). Because stopping suddenly may lead to seizures or even death, the drugs are tapered gradually. In most cases a physician will substitute a longer-acting, less addictive medication for the drug, then gradually decrease the dose of this substitute medication over a period of weeks or sometimes months. Depending on the degree of dependence, the size of the doses that the individual had been taking, and the risk for medical complications, physicians may recommend that initial detoxification take place in a hospital.

Former users may have persistent anxiety and insomnia after detoxification, but they usually do not crave drugs in the same way as individuals recovering from dependence on alcohol or cocaine. Those who develop symptoms of depression after withdrawal or who suffer from underlying anxiety disorders may be prescribed antidepressants.

Young people who have abused sedative-hypnotic or anxiolytic drugs, often in combination with other drugs, often respond best to residential treatment programs that emphasize intensive group therapy. Participation in twelve-step programs is very helpful for people of all ages. For those who have concurrent mental disorders, such as major depression or an anxiety disorder, individual psychotherapy, family therapy, or group therapy, as well as appropriate medication, can be beneficial.

CAFFEINE

Found naturally in sixty-three separate plants, caffeine has been drunk, chewed, or swallowed since the Stone Age. Eighty percent of Americans drink coffee, our principal caffeine source. On average, we drink 3.5 cups a day. Coffee contains 100 to 150 mg of caffeine per cup, tea 40 to 100 mg, cola about 45 mg. Caffeine is also found in a number of medications, in an average amount per dose one-third to one-half the strength of a cup of coffee. Over-the-counter combination pain relievers, such as Anacin, contain 64 mg. Some over-the-counter stimulants contain as much as 200 mg of caffeine.

The effects of caffeine, which has been shown to be addictive, vary. Because it is a stimulant, it relieves drowsiness, helps in the performance of repetitive tasks, and improves the capacity for work. Some athletes feel that caffeine gives them an extra boost that enables them to go farther and longer in endurance events. However, caffeine can also cause anxiety, insomnia, rapid breathing, upset stomach and bowels, and dizziness, and can lead to dependence.

Dozens of studies about caffeine's effects on other medical conditions have created more confusion than consensus. Researchers from the Harvard School of Public Health, who studied 45,589 men aged forty to seventy-five (some of whom averaged six or more cups of coffee daily), found that coffee drinkers seemed no more likely to suffer strokes or heart attacks than the population at large. Medical reports also have cleared caffeine of culpability in causing high cholesterol levels, fibrocystic breast lumps in women, and bladder cancer in smokers.

Although there is no conclusive proof that caffeine causes birth defects, it does cross the placenta. A 1993 study found an increased risk for miscarriage in pregnant women who consumed large amounts, and the U.S. Surgeon General has recommended that pregnant women avoid caffeine or restrict their intake. Some fertility specialists have urged couples trying to conceive to reduce caffeine to increase their chance of success.

It is possible to overdose on caffeine. The characteristic symptoms of caffeine intoxication are restlessness, nervousness, excitement, insomnia, flushed face, increased urination, digestive complaints, muscle twitching, rambling thoughts and speech, rapid heart rate or arrhythmias, physical restlessness, and periods of inexhaustibility. Some people develop such symptoms after as little as 250 mg of caffeine a day; others only with much larger doses. Higher doses may produce ringing in the ears or flashes of light, grand mal seizures, and potentially fatal respiratory failure.

Caffeine withdrawal for those dependent on this substance can cause headaches. Those who must cut back should taper off gradually. One approach is to mix regular and decaffeinated coffee, gradually decreasing the quantity of the former.

NICOTINE

Tobacco use remains the most serious and widespread form of substance abuse and the major cause of preventable deaths in our society. Nicotine—the addictive chemical in tobacco—stimulates the cerebral cortex, the outer layer of the brain that controls complex behavior and mental activity; it also acts as a sedative. Few drugs act as quickly on the brain as does nicotine. It travels through the bloodstream to the brain in seven seconds—half the time of heroin when injected into a blood vessel. Shallow puffs tend to increase alertness, because low doses of nicotine facilitate the release of the neurotransmitter acetylcholine, which makes one feel alert. Deep drags relax the smoker, because high doses block the flow of acetylcholine. Nicotine can also improve memory, help in the performance of certain tasks, reduce anxiety, dampen hunger, and increase pain tolerance.

Nicotine stimulates the adrenal glands to produce adrenaline, increases blood pressure, speeds up the heart rate by fifteen to twenty beats a minute, constricts blood vessels (especially in the skin), inhibits the formation of urine, irritates the membranes in the mouth and throat, and dulls the taste buds so that food does

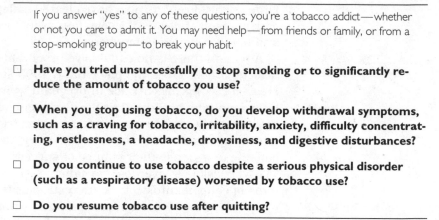

ARE YOU HOOKED ON CIGARETTES?

If you answer "yes" to any of these questions, you're a tobacco addict—whether or not you care to admit it. You may need help—from friends or family, or from a stop-smoking group—to break your habit.

☐ **Have you tried unsuccessfully to stop smoking or to significantly reduce the amount of tobacco you use?**

☐ **When you stop using tobacco, do you develop withdrawal symptoms, such as a craving for tobacco, irritability, anxiety, difficulty concentrating, restlessness, a headache, drowsiness, and digestive disturbances?**

☐ **Do you continue to use tobacco despite a serious physical disorder (such as a respiratory disease) worsened by tobacco use?**

☐ **Do you resume tobacco use after quitting?**

not taste as good as it would otherwise. Nicotine is a major contributor to heart and respiratory diseases, including lung cancer, emphysema, chronic obstructive lung disease, coronary artery disease, and cancers of the mouth, larynx, esophagus, pancreas, and bladder. It also increases the risk for depression.

Nicotine causes dependence by at least three means: providing a strong sensation of pleasure, leading to fairly severe discomfort during withdrawal, and stimulating cravings long after obvious withdrawal symptoms have passed. It reinforces and strengthens the desire to smoke because it acts on brain chemicals involved in feelings of well-being. As with other drugs of abuse, continued nicotine intake results in tolerance, which is why only 2 percent of all smokers smoke just a few cigarettes a day or smoke only occasionally. After a few years of smoking, dependence is so entrenched that the most powerful incentive for continuing to smoke is to prevent withdrawal. For many who smoke heavily, signs of withdrawal, including changes in mood and performance, occur within two hours of their last cigarette.

Quitting   Forty-three million Americans have quit smoking, even though tobacco dependence may be the toughest of all substance use disorders to overcome. One-third of smokers try to quit each year, but fewer than 10 percent succeed. According to therapists, quitting usually is not a one-time event but a "dynamic process" that may take several years and four to ten attempts.

More than 90 percent of former smokers quit on their own—usually after trying other methods—either by throwing away all their cigarettes or by first cutting down. In fact, people who try to do this on their own succeed twice as often as those who enroll in stop-smoking programs, according to a telephone survey of thirteen thousand adult smokers. One characteristic of successful quitters is that they take personal responsibility for their health and see themselves as active participants in health maintenance.

Smokers who quit before the age of fifty cut their risk of dying in the next fifteen years in half, compared with continuing smokers. Even among older, long-time smokers, quitting decreases the risk for heart attack, stroke, lung cancer, chronic lung disease, and cancers of the larynx, esophagus, pancreas, and bladder. After one year without cigarettes, the increased risk for coronary heart disease caused by smoking is cut by about half. After fifteen years the risk is similar to that of people who never smoked. Six to ten years after quitting, the increased risk for lung cancer declines by about 45 percent.

Among the approaches that have helped some smokers are the following:

Going "cold turkey." If you are a heavily addicted smoker, some psychologists recommend a sudden, decisive, and complete break. Smokers who quit "cold turkey" are less likely to light up again than those who gradually decrease their daily consumption of cigarettes, switch to low-tar and low-nicotine brands, or use special filters and holders. You might try to stop for just one day at a time. Promise yourself twenty-four hours of freedom from cigarettes, and when the day is over, make a commitment for one more day. One word of caution: Be sure to reduce your caffeine intake as well. The concentration of caffeine in the blood of individuals who quit smoking but continue to drink the same amount of coffee rises sharply, and this intensifies the symptoms of nicotine withdrawal.

Stop-smoking groups. In this method, a large or small group meets regularly with a leader who conducts sessions designed to change smoking patterns. Perhaps the strongest element in these groups is support from others with the same problem. The American Cancer Society runs about 1,500 stop-smoking clinics of about eight to eighteen members who meet for eight two-hour sessions over a period of four weeks. The cost, if any, is nominal. Courses are also available on many college campuses and through community public health departments.

Many businesses sponsor quit-smoking programs for employees that follow the approaches of professional groups. Motivation is sometimes increased in these programs by attractive incentives, such as lower rates on company-sponsored health insurance.

Aversion therapy. The theory behind aversion therapy is that if you have unpleasant thoughts or are punished every time you have a cigarette, you will finally stop smoking. This approach can involve taking drugs that make tobacco smoke taste unpleasant, undergoing electric shocks, having smoke blown at you, or experiencing rapid smoking—the inhaling of smoke every six seconds until you are dizzy or nauseated, a technique that can be dangerous because it causes rapid heartbeat.

Nicotine gum. A gum containing a nicotine resin that is gradually released as the gum is chewed helps some smokers to break the habit. Each pellet of peppery-tasting nicotine gum delivers about as much nicotine as one cigarette. Absorbed through the mucous membranes of the mouth, the nicotine does not produce the same rush as a deeply inhaled drag, but it does maintain enough nicotine in the blood to diminish withdrawal symptoms. Available with a doctor's prescription, a month's supply costs roughly $120.

Although the gum is lightly spiced to mask nicotine's bitterness, many users have difficulty in becoming accustomed to its unusual taste. Its side effects include mild indigestion, sore jaws, nausea, heartburn, and upset stomach. Because the nicotine gum is denser than regular chewing gum, it may loosen fillings or cause problems with dentures. Drinking coffee or other beverages may block absorption of the nicotine in the gum, and individuals who are trying to quit smoking should not ingest any substance during or immediately before chewing the gum.

Nicotine in any form is harmful, and nicotine gum should *not* be used during pregnancy or by people who are advised to give up smoking because of heart disease. Chewing nicotine is less addictive than smoking, and most people who use it on a temporary basis are able to stop chewing with relative ease. According to some studies, about half of gum users remain nonsmokers a year after treatment. However, 5 to 10 percent transfer their dependence from cigarettes to the gum. When they stop using it, they go through withdrawal, although the symptoms may be milder than with cigarettes.

Nicotine patches. Nicotine transdermal delivery system products, or patches, provide nicotine via a patch attached to the skin by an adhesive. The nicotine is absorbed through the skin. Like nicotine gum, the patch minimizes withdrawal symptoms, such as intense craving for cigarettes. Patches, which cost between three and four dollars each and are available only by prescription, are replaced daily over a period of six to sixteen weeks. Some deliver nicotine around the clock; others, for sixteen hours—during waking hours. Those most likely to benefit are people who smoke more than a pack a day, are highly motivated to quit, and who participate in concurrent counseling programs. The patch is not a cure and in itself does not affect the psychological dependence that makes quitting so difficult. However, when used in combination with counseling, it has been found to be about twice as effective as placebo.

Because nicotine is a powerfully addictive substance, the use of patches for a prolonged period is not advised. Pregnant women and individuals with heart disease should not use them. Patch wearers who continue to smoke or who use more than one patch at a time can experience a nicotine overdose; some individuals have even suffered heart attacks. Occasional side effects include redness, itching, or swelling at the site of the patch application, insomnia, dry mouth, and nervousness.

Breaking the nicotine habit

Here's a six-point program to help you or someone you love toward a smokeless future. (Caution: Don't undertake the quit-smoking program until you have a two- to four-week period of relatively unstressful work and study schedules or social commitments.)

1. Identify your smoking habits. Keep a daily diary (a piece of paper wrapped around your cigarette pack with a rubber band will do) and record the time you smoke, the activity associated with smoking (after breakfast, in the car), and the nature of your urge for a cigarette (desperate, pleasant, or automatic). For the first week or so, don't bother trying to cut down; just use the diary to learn the conditions under which you smoke.

2. Get support. Phone your local chapter of the American Cancer Society, or else get the names of some ex-smokers who can give you support.

3. Begin by tapering off. For a period of one to four weeks, aim at cutting down to, say, twelve or fifteen cigarettes a day; or change to a lower-nicotine brand and concentrate on not increasing the number of cigarettes you smoke. As indicated by your diary, begin by cutting out those cigarettes you smoke automatically. In addition, restrict the times you allow yourself to smoke. Throughout this period, stay in touch, once a day or every few days, with your ex-smoker friend(s) and talk over your problems.

4. Set a quit date. At some point during the tapering period, announce to everyone—friends, family, and ex-smokers—when you're going to quit. Do it with flair. Announce it to coincide with a significant date if possible, such as your birthday or anniversary. Make plans for a celebration of the first day of the rest of your life as a non-smoker.

5. Stop. A week before Q-day, smoke only five cigarettes a day. Begin late in the day, say, after 4 P.M. Smoke the first two cigarettes in close succession. Then, in the evening, smoke the last three, also in close succession, about fifteen minutes apart. Focus on the negative aspects of the cigarettes, such as the rawness in your throat and lungs. After seven days, quit—and give yourself a big reward on that day, such as a fantastic meal or new clothes.

6. Follow up. Stay in touch with your ex-smoker friends during the following two weeks, particularly if anything stressful or tense occurs that might trigger a return to smoking. Think of the person you're becoming—the very person the cigarette ads would have you believe smoking makes you. Now that you are quitting smoking, you are becoming sexier, more sophisticated, more mature, better-looking, and healthier—and you deserve it.

Is it an alcohol dependence or abuse disorder?

Individuals with alcohol dependence or abuse disorders may:

☐ **Drink more or drink for a longer period of time than they desire or intend**

☐ **Attempt, once if not more often, to cut down or control their drinking**

☐ **Spend a great deal of time obtaining alcohol, drinking, or recovering from drinking**

☐ **Frequently become so drunk or feel so bad after drinking that they cannot do their jobs or fulfill their responsibilities at home or work**

☐ **Give up or cut back on important social, work, or recreational activities because of drinking**

☐ **Continue to drink even though they realize that alcohol is causing or worsening physical or mental problems**

☐ **Drink a lot more than in the past in order to achieve intoxication or drink more but feel less intoxicated than in the past**

☐ **Drink in dangerous ways or situations, such as before driving**

☐ **Repeatedly have alcohol-related legal problems, such as drunk driving arrests**

☐ **Continue to drink even though alcohol causes or worsens social or personal problems, such as arguments with a spouse**

☐ **Develop hand tremors or other withdrawal symptoms (nausea or vomiting, headache, sweating, anxiety, restlessness, insomnia, hallucinations, seizures) if they cut down or stop drinking**

☐ **Drink to relieve or avoid withdrawal symptoms**

The more boxes that you or someone close to you checks, the more reason you have to be concerned about alcohol use. This chapter provides information on alcohol dependence and abuse, including their causes and complications, and on seeking help.

10 Alcohol Dependence and Abuse

The chances are that you drink. Most Americans do, at least on occasion. We raise our glasses to toast each other's health. We socialize with cocktails in hand. We knock back a beer while watching a big game. We savor a fine wine or a vintage cognac. For most of us, most of the time, alcohol brings pleasure, not problems.

But this is not always the case. Alcohol abuse and dependence are major public health problems that cost the American economy more than $90 billion a year. No illness other than heart disease causes more disability and premature death. No mental or medical disorder touches and torments the lives of more families. However, with treatment, individuals with alcohol-related disorders can return to full, satisfying, and productive lives.

Alcoholism is a chronic, progressive, and potentially fatal illness, not a failure of willpower. Like other diseases, this complex problem causes many symptoms and can lead to serious complications. The *Diagnostic and Statistical Manual of Mental Disorders, Fourth Edition (DSM-IV)*, defines alcoholism as a *substance dependence disorder* (see Chapter 9), in which individuals develop a strong craving for alcohol because it produces pleasurable feelings or relieves stress or anxiety. Over time they experience physiological changes that lead to *tolerance* of its effects; this means that they must consume larger and larger amounts in order to achieve intoxication. If they abruptly stop drinking, they suffer *withdrawal*, a state of acute physical and psychological discomfort.

Alcohol abuse—a separate disorder—involves continued use of alcohol despite awareness of social, occupational, psychological, or physical problems related to drinking and/or drinking in dangerous ways or situations (such as before driving).

Understanding alcohol and its effects

Ethyl alcohol, or ethanol, the type of alcohol in alcoholic beverages, is a central nervous system depressant—a fact that individuals drinking to "drown their sorrows" often do not realize. Low doses affect the regions of the brain that inhibit or control behavior, so people feel "looser" and become more outgoing and talkative. Continued drinking gradually dulls the responses of the brain and nervous system and leads to sleep or unconsciousness. Alcohol's effects are particularly dangerous and deadly when combined with other nervous system depressants, such as sleeping pills or anti-anxiety medications. Taken together, they may cause a person to stop breathing, and the combination can be fatal.

Unlike drugs in tablet form, alcohol is absorbed quickly into the bloodstream through the walls of the stomach and upper intestine. A typical drink reaches the bloodstream in fifteen minutes and rises to peak level in about an hour. The liver converts about 95 percent of the alcohol to carbon dioxide and water. The remaining 5 percent is excreted unchanged, mainly through urination, respiration, and perspiration.

The rate of alcohol absorption depends on how strong a drink is; whether there is food in the stomach; the drinker's size, weight, sex, age, and race; and a family history of alcoholism. Women have smaller amounts of a stomach enzyme that neutralizes alcohol and therefore feel its impact much more quickly and severely than men. Many Asians have high levels of an enzyme that is not very effective at removing acetaldehyde, the initial by-product of alcohol metabolism. After drinking only a small amount, they may develop flushing of the skin, sometimes along with nausea.

According to the *DSM-IV*, intoxication consists of "clinically significant maladaptive behavioral or psychological changes," such as inappropriate sexual or aggressive behavior, mood changes, and impaired judgment and social and occupational functioning. Alcohol intoxication, which can range from mild inebriation to loss of consciousness, is characterized by at least one of the following: slurred speech, poor coordination, unsteady gait, abnormal eye movements, impaired attention or memory, stupor, or coma.

The best indicator of intoxication is the amount of alcohol in the blood, or blood-alcohol concentration (BAC), expressed as a percentage. A BAC of 0.05 percent indicates approximately five parts

RECOGNIZING THE WARNING SIGNS OF ALCOHOLISM

☐ **Experiencing the following symptoms after drinking: frequent head-aches, nausea, stomach pain, heartburn, gas, fatigue, weakness, muscle cramps, or irregular or rapid heartbeat**

☐ **Needing a drink in the morning to start the day**

☐ **Denying any problem with alcohol**

☐ **Doing things while drinking that are regretted afterward**

☐ **Dramatic mood swings, from anger to laughter to anxiety**

☐ **Sleep problems**

☐ **Depression and paranoia**

☐ **Forgetting what happened during a drinking episode**

☐ **Changing brands or going on the wagon to control drinking**

☐ **Having five or more drinks a day**

alcohol to 10,000 parts other blood components. Most people reach this level after one or two drinks and typically experience relaxation, euphoria, and a sense of well-being. If they continue to drink past this level, intoxication develops, and they gradually lose control of speech, balance, coordination, and emotions.

The U.S. Department of Transportation has called on states to set 0.08 percent—the level reached by a 150-pound man after three mixed drinks—as the blood alcohol concentration level at which a person can be cited for drunken driving. In the past, 0.1 percent was often the legal limit. At a BAC of 0.2 percent, individuals may pass out. At a BAC of 0.3 percent, they may lapse into a coma; at 0.4 percent, they can, in rare cases, die.

For some people, even very low blood alcohol concentrations can cause a headache, upset stomach, or dizziness. These reactions often are inborn. Those who are unusually fatigued or who have a debilitating physical illness may also have a low tolerance to alcohol and respond inappropriately to small amounts. Tolerance can also diminish with advancing age. People who have suffered brain damage—often as a result of head trauma or encephalitis—may lose tolerance for alcohol, temporarily or permanently, and may behave abnormally after drinking small amounts.

▼

How common are alcohol dependence and abuse?

Alcohol dependence and abuse are among the most common mental disorders. The recent National Comorbidity Survey indicates that 23.5 percent of Americans may become dependent on or abuse alcohol in the course of a lifetime, and 9.7 percent experience these disorders during the course of a year. According to the American Psychiatric Association, 10 million adults and 3 million children under the age of eighteen are alcoholics. Others estimate the total as high as 22 million.

The National Council on Alcoholism describes alcohol as the number-one drug problem among the nation's youth. At all ages, men are two to five times more likely than women to abuse alcohol. Drinking in men usually begins in the late teens or the twenties. Women tend to start at a later age, are less likely to stop without help, and often have a history of depression. By middle age, they develop as many alcohol-related health, social, occupational, and personal problems as men.

▼

What causes alcohol dependence and abuse?

Although the exact cause of alcoholism is not known, certain factors—including biochemical imbalances in the brain, heredity, cultural acceptability, and stress—seem to play a role in the disease. Alcoholism usually develops slowly, over the course of five to fifteen years of heavy drinking.

Genetic factors may account for part of the vulnerability to alcoholism. Scientists who are working toward mapping the genes responsible for addictive disorders have not yet been able to identify conclusively a specific gene that puts people at risk for alcoholism, but epidemiological studies have shown evidence of the role of heredity. The identical twin of an alcoholic is twice as likely as a fraternal twin to have an alcohol-related disorder. The incidence of alcoholism is four times higher among the sons of white alcoholic fathers, regardless of whether they grow up with their biological or adoptive parents. The sons of alcoholic fathers have characteristic changes in brain wave activity. There also seems to be a genetic vulnerability to alcoholism in women. Based on a study of 1,030 pairs of twins, researchers concluded that at least half of alcoholism in women may be the result of genetic factors. Both men and women with a family history of alcoholism tend to start drinking heavily at an earlier age and develop more severe social and medical consequences than those without such a history.

Mental health professionals have developed different theoretical models for alcoholism. Although these models are chiefly used by researchers and clinicians, they offer individuals with drinking problems and those close to them some insight into various personality and drinking patterns.

According to one long-established model, there are two primary types of alcoholics. *Type 1*, or milieu-limited, alcoholics usually begin heavy drinking, often in response to setbacks, losses, or

Is it alcohol dependence (alcoholism)?

According to the DSM-IV, a diagnosis of substance dependence is based on three or more of these criteria occurring during any twelve-month period:

■ *Tolerance,* as defined by either
1. **A need for markedly increased amounts of alcohol to achieve intoxication or desired effect, or**
2. **Markedly diminished effect with continued drinking of the same amount of alcohol as in the past**

■ *Withdrawal,* as manifested by
1. **Characteristic symptoms, including at least two of the following: sweating, rapid pulse, or other signs of autonomic hyperactivity; increased hand tremors; insomnia; nausea or vomiting; temporary hallucinations or illusions; physical agitation or restlessness; anxiety; or grand mal seizures, or**
2. **Drinking to avoid or relieve these symptoms**

■ **Consuming larger amounts of alcohol or over a longer period than was intended**

■ **Persistent desire or unsuccessful efforts to cut down or control drinking**

■ **A great deal of time spent in activities necessary to obtain alcohol, drink it, or recover from its effects**

■ **Important social, occupational, or recreational activities given up or reduced because of alcohol use**

■ **Continued alcohol use despite knowledge that alcohol is likely to cause or exacerbate a persistent or recurring physical or psychological problem**

Adapted from the Diagnostic and Statistical Manual of Mental Disorders, 4th Edition. *Used with permission.*

other external circumstances, after the age of twenty-five. They can abstain for long periods of time, and they often feel loss of control, guilt, and fear about their alcoholism. They also have characteristic personality traits: They tend to be anxious, shy, pessimistic, sentimental, emotionally dependent, rigid, reflective, and slow to anger. Because alcohol reduces their anxiety level, it serves as a positive reinforcer for continued drinking and contributes to the development of alcohol dependence.

Type 2, or male-limited, alcoholics are close male relatives of an alcoholic man and become heavy drinkers before the age of twenty-five. They drink regardless of what is going on in their lives, have a history of frequent fights and arrests, and do not usually experience guilt, fear, or loss of control over their drinking. Unlike Type 1 alcoholics, they are impulsive and aggressive risk-takers, curious, excitable, quick-tempered, optimistic, and independent. Alcohol reinforces their feelings of euphoria and pleasant excitement. Often they abuse drugs as well as alcohol. Some researchers have challenged this categorization, noting that Type 2 alcoholics actually may have antisocial personality disorder. (Chapter 21 discusses the personality disorders.)

Newer research on male and female alcoholics classifies alcoholics as *Type A* or *Type B*. Type A alcoholism is characterized by later onset, fewer childhood risk factors, less severe dependence, fewer alcohol-related physical and social consequences, fewer symptoms of other mental disorders, and less interference with work and family. Type B alcoholism is linked with childhood and familial risk factors, begins at an earlier age, involves more severe dependence and abuse of other substances, leads to more serious consequences, and often occurs together with other mental disorders. Type B alcoholics are more inclined to experiment with other drugs and are more anxious, younger, and of lower occupational status than Type A alcoholics.

Stress and traumatic experiences can trigger heavy drinking even in those with no family predisposition to alcoholism. Many people start drinking heavily as a way of coping with or "treating" psychological problems. About half of all individuals who abuse or are dependent on alcohol also have another mental disorder. Alcoholism is linked most often with depressive and anxiety disorders, and men and women with these problems may begin to drink in an attempt to alleviate their anxiety or depression. Individuals with schizophrenia may use alcohol to ease social anxiety, insomnia, and other symptoms.

Whatever the reason that causes individuals to start drinking, some continue drinking out of habit. With continued drinking they gradually develop tolerance and need to drink increasing amounts of alcohol to obtain the same effect. Those with severe alcoholism may be able to drink huge quantities without experiencing the effects this amount would have on others.

Alcoholism is also associated with the abuse of other psychoactive substances, including such drugs as marijuana, cocaine, heroin, amphetamines, and various anti-anxiety medications. Adults under the age of thirty and adolescents are most likely to use alcohol plus several drugs of abuse, such as marijuana and cocaine. Middle-aged men and women are more likely to combine alcohol with benzodiazepines, such as anti-anxiety medications or sleeping pills, which may have been prescribed for them.

▼
**How alcohol
dependence and
abuse feel**

In the early stages before alcohol dependence or abuse develops, individuals may have a few quick drinks before a party to reduce social anxiety; alcohol gives them a sense of well-being and confidence. When they go out, they may order doubles. When alcohol

Is it alcohol abuse?

According to the DSM-IV, a diagnosis of substance abuse is based on one or more of these criteria occurring at any time during a twelve-month period:

■ **Recurrent alcohol abuse resulting in a failure to fulfill major role obligations at work, school, or home (e.g., missing work or school)**

■ **Recurrent alcohol use in situations in which it is physically hazardous (e.g., before driving)**

■ **Recurrent alcohol-related legal problems (e.g., drunk driving arrests)**

■ **Continued alcohol use despite persistent or recurring social or interpersonal problems caused or exacerbated by alcohol (e.g., fighting while drunk)**

■ **No current or past alcohol dependence, as defined in the *DSM-IV***

Adapted from the Diagnostic and Statistical Manual of Mental Disorders, 4th Edition. *Used with permission.*

isn't available they feel uncomfortable. A common pattern is to gradually "up" their limits on drinking, from a drink before dinner to two, three, four, or more over the course of the day. In time, they may start drinking at lunch, or take a surreptitious drink in the morning because they cannot wait for that first drink. They choose friends who drink and activities that involve alcohol. Although they may physically tolerate an increasing amount of alcohol, they show a progressive lack of control, which eventually leads to drunkenness and blackouts (a kind of amnesia in which the drinker continues to function but remembers nothing later).

Individuals dependent on alcohol feel a *need* to drink. This compulsion, rather than any absence of willpower, is the key to alcoholism. As the disease progresses, alcohol becomes the means they use to alter mood—to calm down, to cheer up, to feel sociable with others, to ward off loneliness when by themselves.

Yet alcoholics do not feel that they are drinking too much or have a problem with alcohol. The reason is the powerful defense of *denial*, which enables them to convince themselves that they are not alcoholics so that they can continue to drink. In fact, they may try to cut down or stop, perhaps by switching brands or kinds of alcohol—another sign of their denial. They blame job problems, an unhappy marriage, or personal difficulties for their increasing problems related to alcohol. They cannot see that the drinking is the cause, not the result, of their difficulties.

Alcoholics also drink because they feel tired, anxious, or depressed, even though large amounts of alcohol produce or exacerbate fatigue, anxiety, and depression. As their self-esteem plummets and their self-loathing grows, they may snap irritably at everyone around them and become angry or even violent. Physical symptoms can develop, including digestive problems, minor hand tremors, and increased tolerance.

In the later stages, alcoholics become consumed by their addiction. They drink because they feel they must, despite their doctors' warnings or their family's pleas. Even if they cannot keep their first drink down in the morning, they have another, and another. They often lose their jobs; their partners leave them; they develop severe health problems—yet they keep drinking.

▼

Seeking help   Denial that you or someone close to you has a problem is the keystone of alcoholism. Asking the following questions may help:

- Do you find yourself drinking more alcohol or drinking over a longer period of time than you had intended?

- Have you wanted or tried to cut down or control your drinking, but failed?

- Do you spend a great deal of time doing whatever you must to get alcohol and drink as much as you want?

- Have you given up or cut down on activities at work or home or with others because of your alcohol use?

- Have you continued drinking even though you realize that your alcohol use is creating or worsening a physical or mental problem?

- Do you have to drink a lot more to feel the way a few drinks used to make you feel in the past?

- Can you drink more and more without getting drunk?

- Regardless of how much you drink or the problems drinking has caused, do you deny being an alcoholic?

- If you cut down or stop drinking, do your hands shake? Do you develop nausea or vomiting, headache, sweating, anxiety, restlessness, or insomnia? Have you ever experienced hallucinations or blackouts?

- Do you drink to relieve or avoid these withdrawal symptoms?

If you or someone close to you answers "yes" to several of these questions, the problem may be alcohol dependence, or alcoholism. Even if this does not seem to be the case, ask the following:

- Are you often drunk or do you feel so badly after drinking that you cannot do your job or fulfill your responsibilities at home or work?

- Do you drink in dangerous ways or situations, such as before driving or operating machinery?

- Have you had repeated alcohol-related legal problems, such as being arrested for drunk driving?

- Do you continue to drink, even though alcohol causes or worsens social or personal problems, such as family arguments?

If you answer "yes" to any of these questions, the problem may be alcohol abuse. Talk to your doctor or a mental health professional about your drinking.

▼

Risks and complications

Chronic heavy drinking adversely affects virtually every organ system in the body, including the brain, the digestive tract, the heart, muscles, blood, and hormones. In addition, because alcohol interacts with many drugs, it can increase the risk for harmful interactions and potentially lethal overdoses. Among the major risks and complications are:

Liver disease. Because the liver is the organ that breaks down and metabolizes alcohol, it is especially vulnerable to damage. Chronic heavy drinking can lead to alcoholic hepatitis (inflammation and destruction of liver cells) and, in the 15 percent of people who continue to drink beyond this stage, cirrhosis (irreversible scarring and destruction of liver cells). The liver eventually may fail completely.

Cardiovascular system. Heavy drinking can weaken the heart muscle (causing cardiac myopathy), increase blood pressure, and increase the risk for stroke. Both heavy drinking and the combined use of alcohol and tobacco greatly increase the likelihood of damage.

Cancer. Heavy alcohol use may contribute to cancer of the liver, stomach, and colon, as well as malignant melanoma, a deadly form of skin cancer. Alcohol in combination with tobacco use also increases the risk for cancer of the mouth, tongue, larynx, and esophagus. Several major studies have implicated alcohol as a possible risk factor in breast cancer, particularly in young women, although the degree of risk remains unclear.

Brain damage. Chronic brain damage resulting from alcohol consumption is second only to Alzheimer's disease as a cause of cognitive deterioration in adults. Long-term heavy drinkers may suffer memory losses and may be unable to think abstractly, recall names of common objects, or follow simple instructions.

Vitamin deficiencies. Alcoholics often tend to have very poor nutrition. Alcoholism is associated with vitamin deficiencies, especially thiamine (B_{12}), which may be responsible for certain diseases of the neurological, digestive, muscular, and cardiovascular systems. Lack of thiamine caused by alcoholism may result in Wernicke's syndrome, a serious disease marked by a "clouding" of consciousness and paralysis of the nerves of the eye. Korsakoff's syndrome, a rare form of amnesia caused by an alcohol-associated thiamine deficiency, is characterized by disorientation, memory loss, confabulation, and hallucinations.

Digestive problems. Alcohol triggers the secretion of acids in the stomach, which irritate the mucous lining and cause gastritis. Chronic drinking may result in peptic ulcers (sores or craters that pierce the stomach lining) and bleeding from the stomach lining.

Reproductive and sexual dysfunction. Alcohol interferes with male sexual function and fertility through direct effects on the hormone testosterone and the testicles. Half of alcoholic men have increased levels of female hormones that lead to breast enlargement and a feminine pubic hair pattern. Damage to the nerves in the penis by heavy drinking can lead to impotence. In women who drink heavily, a drop in female hormone production may cause menstrual irregularity and infertility.

Fetal alcohol syndrome. Alcohol consumption during pregnancy can lead to physical and mental defects in the fetus. About one of every 750 babies is born with fetal alcohol syndrome (FAS), which is characterized by low birth weight, small head circumference, flattened facial features, jitters, poor muscle tone, and sleep disorders. They suffer sluggish motor development, failure to thrive, short stature, delayed speech, and lifelong mental impairment. The risk for FAS is greatest if a pregnant woman drinks three ounces or more of pure alcohol (the equivalent of six or seven cocktails) a day. Consumption of smaller quantities of alcohol can lead to fetal alcohol effects (FAE), including low birth weight, irritability in the newborn, and permanent mental impairment. Because no one knows how much—if any—alcohol is safe during pregnancy, the National Institute of Alcohol Abuse and Alcoholism recommends that pregnant women not drink at all.

Accidents and injuries. Alcohol may contribute to almost half of the deaths caused by car accidents, burns, falls, and choking. Nearly half of those convicted and jailed for criminal acts committed these crimes while under the influence of alcohol.

Higher mortality. The mortality rate for alcoholics is two to three times higher than that for nonalcoholics of the same age. The leading alcohol-related cause of death is injury, chiefly in auto accidents involving a drunk driver. The second leading cause of alcohol-related deaths is digestive disease, most notably cirrhosis of the liver. In addition, alcohol plays a role in about 30 percent of all suicides. Alcoholics who attempt suicide may have other risk factors, including major depression, poor social support, serious medical illness, and unemployment.

Withdrawal dangers. Withdrawal from alcohol can be life-threatening when accompanied by problems such as grand mal seizures, pneumonia, liver failure, or gastrointestinal bleeding.

▼
Treating alcohol dependence and abuse

The first phase of treatment focuses on detoxification, the gradual withdrawal of alcohol from the body. For 90 to 95 percent of alcoholics, withdrawal symptoms are mild to moderate. They include sweating, rapid pulse, elevated blood pressure, hand tremors, insomnia, nausea or vomiting, malaise or weakness, anxiety, depressed mood or irritability, headache, and temporary hallucinations or delusions.

Those who have been heavy drinkers for prolonged periods may develop more severe symptoms, including seizures or alcohol withdrawal delirium, commonly known as *delirium tremens*, or DTs. This condition is characterized by agitated behavior, delusions, rapid heart rate, sweating, vivid hallucinations, hand tremors, and fever. It is most likely to develop in chronic heavy drinkers who also suffer from a physical illness, fatigue, depression, or malnutrition. The symptoms usually appear over several days after heavy drinking stops. Individuals often report terrifying visual hallucinations, such as seeing insects all over their bodies. With treatment, most cases subside after several days, although delirium tremens has been known to last as long as four to five weeks. In some cases, complications such as infections or heart arrhythmias prove fatal.

The decision whether to treat an alcoholic as an inpatient in a medical or psychiatric hospital or a freestanding residential facility not associated with a hospital, or as an outpatient, depends on many factors, including the presence of medical problems, co-existing mental disorders, severe withdrawal symptoms such as DTs or seizures, co-addiction to other substances, past history, and available support.

For inpatients, health professionals provide careful monitoring and medical treatment to prevent potentially fatal withdrawal reactions. Withdrawal is treated with medications (usually benzodiazepines) to ameliorate the symptoms and to prevent or halt seizures or DTs. These drugs are then gradually withdrawn over a period of several days or weeks.

Treatment of the psychological aspects of alcohol dependence usually begins at the same time as detoxification. In inpatient and residential programs, treatment usually includes individual and group psychotherapy, family therapy, exercise, relaxation techniques, spiritual counseling, and AA meetings, as well as formal instruction about the nature of alcoholism. Those with another mental disorder, such as depression, receive appropriate care.

Outpatient treatment for alcoholism is the best option for the majority of individuals with mild withdrawal symptoms. Daily visits, conscientious follow-up, and evaluation for any possible complications are essential to this approach. Individuals who are highly motivated and have good social support, who have not had recent prolonged drinking binges, who are not addicted to more than one substance, and who can arrange daily visits to a doctor during the initial phase of withdrawal are most likely to benefit.

A doctor's tale

A burly bear of a man, Will had been a football hero in high school and college. He married the prettiest, brightest cheerleader and headed for medical school. "I wasn't just an M.D.; I was an M. Deity," he says. "I became a surgeon. I saved people's lives. I felt there wasn't anything I couldn't do."

Will and his wife were eager to have a family, but their first child— a girl—died at birth. Their son, born a year later, became the light of their life. He died of a rare infection when he was eight. Will's wife, crushed by grief, began to drink heavily. Will took her to the most expensive alcoholism treatment centers in the country. She'd recover, come home, then suffer a relapse. "I kept trying to fix everything up and make it right," Will recalls. "I figured that if I could cut the cancer out of someone's lung or stomach, why couldn't I save the people I loved?"

Work became everything to Will. He became chief of surgery at his hospital and an officer in national medical organizations, but his success couldn't keep his marriage together. He and his wife divorced, and Will gave up the big house and fancy cars he'd loved. In time, he started seeing Gina, a woman who worked as an administrator at his hospital. When they married, Will felt he was getting a fresh chance.

Will took Gina skiing the first year they were married. In a nasty fall he fractured his leg and wrenched his back. For months, he had to strap himself into a brace to operate. Even painkillers didn't bring total relief. "I'd come home feeling so bad that I'd take another pill and wash it down with a drink," he says. "I didn't think twice about it. I was in pain. I thought I had a legitimate reason for every pill and every drink I took."

Will started to mix stronger drinks and more of them. In the evening, he'd sit in an oversized chair, his bad leg propped up, a bottle of scotch never far from his hand. On weekends he'd mix up Bloody Marys at ten in the morning. Gina tried to talk to him about his drinking, but he waved her away. "I'm a goddamn doctor," he roared. "Don't tell me what to do."

As Gina pulled away from him, doctoring became the only thing Will cared about. Although he never drank before surgery, his partners noticed a difference. He refused weekend call, and if they called him at home, he had a hard time focusing on what they were discussing. Agonizing about what to do, they telephoned Gina, who agreed it was time for an intervention.

With the help of a former physician and recovering alcoholic who had started a special program for impaired physicians, the group sat down with Will. They catalogued incident after incident in which he had been drinking and how his be-havior had affected each of them. By the end of the session, Will realized that he had no choice: Either he would have to give up drinking or end his career.

The next month Will entered an inpatient treatment program designed for health professionals. "I sat in a room with people I couldn't fool—doctors, nurses, alcoholics all—and they would sense my faking and confront me," says Will. "The hardest thing was just admitting to myself and then to others that I am an alcoholic." After four weeks Will moved to a halfway house, where he continued day-long counseling and group therapy. He also attended daily AA meetings.

Going back to his practice several months later wasn't easy. "I kept wondering if my colleagues would accept me," he says. "But the first day I had surgery scheduled, one of the nurses came up and said, 'I'm so proud of you.' Everyone was pulling for me." As a special crusade, Will has devoted himself to talking to health professionals about drug and alcohol problems. "It's not easy to get up in front of a group of medical students or doctors and say, 'I used to be just like you: I thought I had some sort of immunity to alcohol and drug problems because I'm a doctor. I was wrong. They can happen to anyone, no matter how smart or successful you are. They can happen to you.'"

After detoxification and stabilization, whether in an inpatient or an outpatient setting, individuals are usually advised to continue treatment in an outpatient program that emphasizes relapse prevention and uses a combination of group therapy, individual supportive therapy, marital or family therapy, and regular AA attendance. The initial phase of treatment is usually intensive, running for three to five hours a day, three to five days a week, for four to twelve weeks. Some programs provide continuing outpatient care, usually on a weekly basis, for several years. Antabuse (disulfiram), a medication described below, can be a useful adjunctive treatment, especially in early recovery.

Once abstinence is achieved in the first months of recovery, persons are strongly encouraged to continue their progress through long-term, even lifelong, participation in AA. In addition to a formal outpatient program and AA attendance, those with emotional or psychiatric problems may need longer-term individual psychotherapy and/or treatment with medication. Some therapists draw up a "contingency contract" with the person that spells out the type and frequency of treatment, the consequence that must be paid for relapsing (such as disclosing an embarrassing secret or giving up something of great value), the involvement of significant others, and the acceptance of the goal of abstinence.

Participating in a small group with other alcoholics is of special value because, having been through similar experiences, the members are able to recognize lies and excuses and to confront one another honestly. A professional therapist can keep members of the group from ganging up on one individual. Some small groups use role-playing or psychodrama, in which the participants pretend to play other people's roles (such as the long-suffering spouse) to illuminate characteristic behaviors.

MEDICATION

The drug disulfiram (Antabuse), given to deter drinking, causes nausea, vomiting, and other acute symptoms when alcohol is consumed. It acts by interrupting the decomposition of alcohol by the liver, leading to a build-up of acetaldehyde, a toxic substance that enters the bloodstream and is responsible for the symptoms. Antabuse causes no reaction unless alcohol is drunk, and its side effects are usually mild: drowsiness, bad breath, skin rash, and temporary impotence.

If individuals taking Antabuse drink *at all* or consume foods with any alcoholic content, they become very ill. They must avoid foods cooked or marinated in wine, as well as cough syrup or mouthwash preparations containing alcohol. Some persons have experienced reactions to the alcohol in after-shave lotion. Drinking a large amount of alcohol with Antabuse is extremely dangerous; fatalities have occurred. Because this drug causes such unpleasant reactions, it can be an effective deterrent to drinking. However, since it does not reduce the craving for alcohol, psychotherapy and support groups remain a necessary part of treatment.

Anti-anxiety and antidepressive drugs are sometimes useful in early treatment for alcoholism and for those with underlying mental disorders. Several medications, including the selective serotonin reuptake inhibitors (SSRIs), such as fluoxetine (Prozac), sertraline (Zoloft), and paroxetine (Paxil), the anxiolytic medication buspirone (BuSpar), and the opioid agonist naltrexone (Trexan), are being studied as medical interventions to reduce cravings or prevent relapses. Vitamin supplements, especially thiamine and folic acid, can help to overcome some nutritional deficiencies.

ALCOHOLICS ANONYMOUS

Founded more than fifty years ago in Akron, Ohio, Alcoholics Anonymous (AA) has grown into an international organization that includes about two million members and 185,000 groups around the world. AA is based on the belief that alcoholics who recognize that they have a disease can become and remain sober through acceptance of their powerlessness over alcohol and the support of other recovering alcoholics. The steps and traditions of AA emphasize self-honesty, sobriety, humility, self-care, and group support.

Many studies have found AA to be the most effective means of overcoming alcoholism and maintaining abstinence; the emphasis on spirituality and peer support may be the reasons why. AA instills the message that recovery from alcoholism truly takes place one day at a time throughout a lifetime. Acknowledging the power of alcohol, it offers support from others struggling with the same illness, from a sponsor who is available at any time of the day or night, and from meetings that are held every day of the year.

The average age of entry into AA is thirty; about 60 percent of the members are men. Members come from a wide range of ages, occupations, nationalities, and socioeconomic classes. Increasingly, AA offers specialized meetings for gay, atheist, HIV-positive, and professional individuals with alcohol problems.

AA meetings may be "open" (for members and nonmembers) or "closed" (only for members). Some feature speakers or focus on one of the twelve steps. Most meetings last about an hour and a half and follow a similar format: Someone reads the twelve steps or the AA preamble, and a discussion follows, usually on a topic picked from AA literature. One person speaks at a time, often sharing personal experiences. Such "shares" are fairly brief and can deal with any aspect of addiction or recovery. No one is re-

WHAT TO DO IF A LOVED ONE IS AN ALCOHOLIC

Here are some *dos* and *don'ts* from Al-Anon for dealing with a loved one who is an alcoholic.

DO:	DON'T:
☐ **Forgive**	☐ **Be self-righteous**
☐ **Be honest with yourself**	☐ **Try to push anyone but yourself**
☐ **Be humble**	☐ **Keep bringing up the past**
☐ **Take it easy (tension is harmful)**	☐ **Keep checking up on your alcoholic**
☐ **Play (find recreation and hobbies)**	☐ **Wallow in self-pity**
☐ **Keep on trying whenever you fail**	☐ **Make threats you don't intend to carry out**
☐ **Learn the facts about alcoholism**	☐ **Try to dominate, nag, scold, complain, or lose your temper**
☐ **Attend support group meetings, such as Al-Anon**	☐ **Be overprotective**
☐ **Pray**	☐ **Be a doormat**

quired to speak. Near the end of the meeting, a collection basket is passed and people contribute whatever they choose. Meetings close with the Lord's Prayer, the Serenity Prayer ("God, grant me the serenity to accept the things I cannot change, the courage to change the things I can, and the wisdom to know the difference"), or another AA-approved prayer.

AA uses slogans ("One day at a time"; "Progress not perfection") that serve as useful and helpful reminders of a better way to live. People are advised to attend AA meetings every day when they first begin recovery; most groups advocate "ninety meetings in ninety days." A sponsor, recommended for each new member, establishes a unique relationship with him or her, serving as a special friend and guide through the program of recovery. To be eligible to be a sponsor, individuals must have been "in recovery" themselves for some time, usually at least a year.

As recovery progresses, many attend one or two meetings a week. "Working" the program means reading about alcoholism, writing about one's experiences and feelings, and providing support and help to others.

Alternatives to AA include Women in Sobriety and Secular Organizations for Sobriety (SOS), which was established in 1986 for people who find themselves uncomfortable with the emphasis on spirituality in AA. Some people do not accept the concept of a Higher Power—which is a key part of AA's philosophy—or object to prayers during the meeting. Like AA, SOS holds confidential meetings and views recovery as a one-day-at-a-time process.

FAMILY THERAPY

A person's alcoholism is sometimes a symptom of a poor family relationship or marriage. Family therapy deals both with alcohol dependence and any underlying problems. Even when there is no pre-existing problem, alcoholism itself can have a powerfully destructive effect. For this reason, families need help, not only in understanding their relationships but also in recovering from the damage that has been done and in dealing with codependence (see "Impact on Relationships" section below).

RELAPSE PREVENTION

Relapses are so common that occasional returns to drinking can be viewed as an expected event in the course of the disease of alcoholism. According to some estimates, more than 90 percent of those recovering from substance use will use alcohol or drugs in any one twelve-month period after treatment. Some people go on a single binge; others return to their old pattern of alcohol use. Increasingly, treatment programs focus on relapse prevention and include the development of coping strategies, learning the techniques that make it easier to live with alcohol cravings, and rehearsal of various ways of saying "no" to offers of a drink.

Self-help As they create a new alcohol-free lifestyle, individuals recovering from alcohol dependence and abuse can do a great deal to ease the adversities they face. Exercise provides many benefits; it releases tension, enhances self-image, and reduces mild depression. Stress-reduction techniques, such as those described in Chapter 29, can help in coping with the desire to drink. Continuing participation in AA can be critical, as are lifestyle changes, particularly developing a network of nondrinking friends, removing alcohol from the house, and avoiding cocktail parties and bars.

Impact on relationships Alcoholism shatters families and creates unhealthful patterns of communicating and relating. Separation and divorce rates are high among alcoholics. Another common occurrence is *codependence*, a term used to described the behavior of close family members or friends who act in ways that "enable" their spouses, parents, or friends to continue their self-destructive behavior.

Codependent spouses of alcoholics follow a predictable pattern of behavior: While trying to control the drinkers, they act in ways that enable the drinkers to keep drinking. If an alcoholic finds it hard to get up in the morning, his wife wakes him up, pulls him

ARE YOU CODEPENDENT?

If you're involved with someone with an addictive behavior, read through the following list of characteristics of codependence. If you identify with some of the statements, you may wish to visit a self-help group in your area:

☐ **I find myself "covering" for another person's alcohol or drug use, eating, or work, gambling, sexual escapades, or general behavior.**

☐ **I spend a great deal of time talking about and worrying about other people's behavior/problems/future instead of living my own life.**

☐ **I have marked or counted bottles, searched for a hidden "stash," or in other ways monitored someone else's behavior.**

☐ **I find myself taking on more responsibility at home or in a relationship, even when I resent it.**

☐ **I ignore my own needs in favor of meeting someone else's.**

☐ **I'm afraid that if I get angry the other person will leave or not love me.**

☐ **I worry that if I leave a relationship or stop trying to control the other person, that person will fall apart.**

☐ **I spend less time with friends and more time with my partner/parent/child in activities that I wouldn't normally choose.**

☐ **My self-esteem depends on what others say and think of me, or on my possessions or job.**

☐ **I grew up in a family where there was little communication, where expressing feelings was not acceptable, and where there were either rigid rules or none at all.**

out of bed and into the shower, and drops him off at work. If he is late, she makes excuses to his boss. By helping him evade his responsibilities, his wife is helping him to continue drinking.

Such behavior is harmful because it reinforces denial. Alcoholic individuals do not feel out of control or powerless over alcohol because the persons closest to them are constantly protecting them from the consequences of their actions. Every crisis—a missed deadline, a forgotten appointment, a child's disappointment when a parent doesn't come to an important event—should be viewed as a chance for the individual to recognize the impact alcohol is having. If family members allow their loved one to experience the consequences of drinking, the person may be able to arrive at the moment of truth concerning alcohol.

Like alcoholics, codependents try to rationalize or deny their own behavior, often using excuses: "The reason I stayed home was to catch up on my reading, not to keep an eye on my partner."

In time, the worlds of the alcoholic and the codependent become smaller and smaller, with the codependents losing sight of everything but their loved one. They feel that if they can only solve this person's problems, everything will be fine.

Codependents often need help in acknowledging their own feelings and needs. National self-help organizations, such as Al-Anon, help adult family members to recognize dysfunctional behaviors in their relationships and to start looking at their own problems. Similar self-help groups, such as Alateen, provide support for the teenaged children of alcoholics. These organizations also help family members to cope with their loved one's alcoholism.

Alcohol strongly affects the children in a family. According to the literature on adult children of alcoholics, growing up with an alcoholic parent leads youngsters to assume certain roles. The adjuster or "lost child" does whatever the parent says. The responsible child or "family hero" typically takes over many household tasks and responsibilities. The acting-out child or "scapegoat" causes problems at home or in school. The "mascot" disrupts tense situations by focusing attention on himself or herself, often by clowning. Regardless of which roles they assume, the children of alcoholics are prone to learning disabilities, eating disorders, and addictive behavior.

The consequences of their parents' drinking may haunt children long after they have grown up. Adult children of alcoholics are more likely to have difficulty in solving problems, identifying and expressing feelings, trusting others, and being intimate. In addition to being at increased risk for addictive behaviors and disorders, they are more likely to marry individuals with a substance use disorder and to keep on playing the roles assumed in childhood.

Because the impact of alcoholism can be so enduring, support groups—such as Adult Children of Alcoholics, Children of Alcoholics, and Adult Children of Dysfunctional Families—have spread throughout the country over the last decade. These organizations provide adult children of alcoholics with a mutually supportive group setting in which to discuss their childhood experiences with alcoholic parents and the emotional consequences they carry into adult life. Through such groups or other forms of therapy, individuals may learn to move beyond anger and blame, to see the part that they themselves play in their current unhappiness, and to create a healthier and happier future.

▼

Outlook   Recovery from alcoholism is a lifelong process of personal growth and healing. The first two years are the most difficult, and relapses are extremely common. About 70 percent of those who obtain formal treatment stop drinking for prolonged periods. Even

Young children of alcoholics

According to federal estimates, more than seven million children have at least one alcoholic parent. The National Clearinghouse has prepared information packets for these children, spouses, and helpers, such as teachers and club leaders. Here is a sampling of tips:

FOR CHILDREN

☐ Talk about your feelings with a close friend, relative, teacher, pastor, or others. Talking to someone can make you feel less alone.

☐ Try to get involved with fun things at school or near where you live. This can help you to forget about problems at home and to feel better about yourself.

☐ Don't feel guilty or ashamed about the problem at home. Alcoholism is a disease, and diseases are nobody's fault.

☐ Don't pour out or try to water down a parent's alcohol. You didn't make the drinking problem start, and you can't make it stop. What your parent does is not your responsibility or your fault—so give yourself a break!

FOR PARTNERS

☐ When children go off to be alone during or after a parent's drinking episode, seek them out and comfort them. Try to avoid letting them go to sleep under upsetting conditions. If this does occur, talk to them at the first opportunity.

☐ Avoid putting your oldest child in the position of being a confidant or surrogate parent. This places too much strain on a youngster and may anger your spouse.

☐ Avoid pressuring children, either verbally or with your actions, to take sides in conflicts with your spouse. Youngsters usually want their parents to behave in ways that do not force them to take sides. If they are pressed to do so, they face even more problems.

☐ Don't use your children's opinions about drinking or the alcoholic parent to "get at" your partner. This approach places youngsters in a bad position, and they may not be willing to share their feelings with you in the future.

For more information, see the Resource Directory's listings of support organizations.

---

without treatment, 30 percent of alcoholics are able to stop drinking for long periods. Persons most likely to remain sober after treatment have the most to lose by continuing to drink; they tend to be employed, married, and upper middle class.

Most recovering alcoholics experience urges to drink, especially during early recovery. These urges are a natural consequence of years of drinking and diminish with time. Mood swings are common during recovery, and individuals typically describe themselves as alternately feeling relieved or elated and then discouraged or tearful. Such disconcerting ups and downs also decrease over time. Patience—learning to take "one day at a time"—is crucial.

The vulnerability to alcohol never goes away entirely. Years after their last drink, many ex-alcoholics, painfully aware of alcohol's power, describe themselves as "recovering," not recovered.

Is it an eating-related problem or disorder?

Individuals with an eating-related problem or disorder may:

☐ **Diet frequently or constantly be concerned about weight**

☐ **Repeatedly go on binges or eat unusually large amounts of food**

☐ **Find it hard to control how much they eat**

☐ **Repeatedly eat much more rapidly than usual, eat until uncomfortably full, or eat even when not hungry**

☐ **Eat throughout the day rather than at regular mealtimes**

☐ **Eat alone due to embarrassment about how or how much they eat**

☐ **Lose at least 15 percent of ideal weight**

☐ **Be extremely fearful of gaining weight or becoming fat, even if underweight**

☐ **Have a distorted body image; feel fat even when very thin or emaciated**

☐ **Miss at least three menstrual cycles (in women of childbearing age)**

☐ **Regularly induce vomiting or use laxatives to prevent weight gain**

☐ **Binge and purge at least twice a week for three months**

☐ **Feel significant distress or impaired ability to work, function, or relate to others normally because of their eating behavior**

The more boxes that you or someone close to you checks, the more reason you have to be concerned about eating behavior. This chapter provides information and insight about unhealthful eating patterns and more serious eating disorders, and guidance on diagnosis and treatments.

11

Eating-Related Problems and Disorders

We eat to live. However, eating rarely is as simple as this sounds. Throughout much of history—and even today in many parts of the world—people have struggled to get enough food. Now, with a plentiful array of dietary choices available in our society, eating too much has become a common health problem. According to the National Center for Health Statistics, one in every four Americans—some 34 million adults—weighs 20 percent or more than what is considered ideal.

Ironically, as average weights have increased, the quest for thinness has become a national obsession. In a society in which "slimmer" is seen as "better," anyone who is less than lean may feel like a failure. Individuals, especially young women who are overweight, are embarrassed by their appearance, or simply overwhelmed by feelings of inadequacy, often assume that they would be happier, sexier, or more successful in thinner bodies.

Although abnormal and unhealthful eating behaviors seem to be increasing, they are not new. The ancient Romans gorged themselves at huge feasts and then forced themselves to vomit. For centuries, pious men and women starved and purged for religious reasons. Anorexia nervosa was first identified more than a hundred years ago by William Gull, an English physician, who described it as a disorder of starvation in pursuit of thinness.

It was not until 1980, however, that anorexia nervosa and other eating disorders were recognized as mental as well as medical problems. Increasingly, therapists are viewing eating disorders along a continuum that includes extreme dieting, frequent eating binges, and vomiting or using laxatives to "purge" the calories consumed. This chapter describes the complete spectrum of unhealthful and potentially dangerous eating behaviors.

Hunger and appetite

Why do you wake up in the morning ravenous or feel your stomach rumbling in the middle of the afternoon? The simple answer is hunger: the physiological drive to consume food. More than a dozen different signals influence and control our desire for food. Researchers at the National Institutes of Health (NIH) have discovered appetite receptors within the hypothalamus region of the brain that specifically respond to hunger messages conveyed by neurotransmitters. Hormones, including insulin and stress-related epinephrine (adrenaline), may also stimulate or suppress hunger. Even the size of our fat cells can affect the degree of hunger we tend to feel. (Many overweight people have fat cells two to 2.5 times larger than normal.)

Appetite usually begins with the apprehension of the unpleasant sensation of hunger. We learn to avoid hunger by eating a certain amount of food at certain times of the day. However, hunger isn't the only trigger of appetite. In one classic experiment, psychologists bought bags of high-calorie goodies—peanut butter, marshmallows, chocolate-chip cookies, salami—for their test rats. The animals ate so much on this "supermarket diet" that they gained more weight than any laboratory rats ever had before. The snack-food regimen that caused these rats to gain excessively was particularly high in fats. Biologists speculate that creamy, buttery, or greasy foods may cause internal changes that increase appetite and, consequently, weight.

Satiety is the feeling of fullness and relief from hunger that we achieve by eating. It is thought that each of us may have an unconscious control system for regulating appetite and satiety to keep our body fat at a predetermined level or setpoint. If our fat stores fall too low, our appetite gnaws at us, so we eat more. Conversely, appetite subsides once we eat.

The neuropsychiatry of hunger and appetite is complex. The neurotransmitter serotonin has been shown to produce feelings of fullness. Low doses of another brain messenger, dopamine, stimulate eating, whereas higher doses inhibit it. Various neuropeptides, such as corticotropin-releasing factor, also may play a role. In addition, several peptides are released from the digestive tract by ingested food and may signal the brain to stop or restrict eating. The best known of these is cholecystokinin (CCK), which often is low in individuals with anorexia nervosa or bulimia nervosa.

Obesity

Obesity, a medical rather than a mental disorder, is characterized by excessive accumulation of fat in the body, usually 20 percent or more above "desirable" weight. There is no single or simple cause for this often-chronic problem. Heredity, metabolism, developmental factors, environment, activity level, and lifestyle all appear to play a role. A very fat parent is more likely to have a fat child than one who is only slightly overweight. Twins end up with similar body weights regardless of whether they grew up in the same family or were reared apart. Although scientists do not know precisely how heredity exerts its influence, it is believed that it may affect the way individuals metabolize food. Some overweight people who eat very little have very low metabolic rates. They burn up relatively few calories and retain the excess as fat.

Some obese people have a high number of fat cells, others have large fat cells, and the most severely obese have both more *and* larger fat cells. Whereas the size of fat cells can increase at any time in the course of a person's life, the number is set very early, possibly as the result of genetics and overfeeding in infancy. Once formed, fat cells persist, so that when obese people lose weight, their fat cells shrink but the total number remains the same.

Obesity tends to accompany a sedentary lifestyle. Physical activity constrains or prevents obesity by increasing caloric expenditure, moderating appetite and decreasing food intake, and increasing metabolic rate. By comparison, individuals who rarely exercise are much more likely to become obese.

Emotions can play a role in weight problems. Just as some people reach for a drink or a drug when upset, others cope by overeating. In general, however, people do not become obese because they are psychologically troubled. However, the converse is sometimes true since obesity can lead to mental disorders, such as depression. Obesity also increases the likelihood of a variety of physical disorders, including high blood pressure, stroke, high cholesterol, heart disease, diabetes, breast cancer (in postmenopausal women), gallbladder disease, upper respiratory problems, arthritis, gout, skin disorders, menstrual irregularities, ovarian abnormalities, complications of pregnancy, and, in extreme cases, early death. Overweight people who take over-the-counter appetite-reducing medications, such as phenylpropanolamine, may develop side effects such as irritability and nervousness.

People who are moderately or mildly obese can lose weight

through different approaches, including behavioral modification (monitoring food intake, altering eating style, avoiding eating "triggers," and similar strategies), cognitive therapy (changing thoughts or beliefs that lead to overeating), and support groups (such as Overeaters Anonymous). For severe obesity, medical treatments, including surgery to bypass the stomach, may be necessary to overcome the danger to health and life.

Unhealthful eating behaviors

Many eating-related problems are not true mental disorders, although individuals with these problems may suffer emotional consequences and can benefit from therapy. Teenagers and young adults often experiment with various eating patterns, such as frequent dieting, binge eating, and vomiting to avoid weight gain. Behaviors such as these, which are far more common than full-blown eating disorders, are not in themselves psychiatric illnesses, but they increase the likelihood for development of more dangerous eating patterns and can be early warnings of potentially serious problems, so they should not be ignored.

At any given time, more than 25 percent of adults in this country are trying to lose weight, and millions of others are trying to keep off the weight they lost. Most dieters cut back on food not because they want to *feel* better but because they want to *look* better. Individuals who drastically reduce their food intake and make weight loss a major part of their lives may be jeopardizing their physical and psychological well-being.

DANGEROUS FORMS OF DIETING

Any diet that involves a major reduction in calories (to fewer than 800 calories a day) or a pattern of rapid weight loss followed by weight gain ("yo-yo dieting") can undermine health by causing serious vitamin and mineral deficiencies and lead to other unhealthful eating behaviors, such as starving, bingeing, and purging. Young women are particularly likely to diet in potentially harmful ways. Although they may not develop the severe malnutrition and other symptoms, such as amenorrhea, associated with anorexia nervosa (described later in this chapter), their weight loss can cause physical symptoms, including weakness and sensitivity to cold. Although technically they do not yet have anorexia nervosa, they are at increased risk for developing it.

Individuals who are constantly dieting and struggling to keep their weight as low as possible typically think they know a great deal about nutrition, yet many of their beliefs about food and weight are misconceptions or myths. Some, for instance, eat only protein because they mistakenly believe that complex carbohydrates, including fruits and breads, are fattening.

Many have difficulty identifying their feelings (the same is true of individuals with anorexia nervosa) and, rather than acknowledging that they are anxious, angry, or bored, they focus on food and their fear of fatness. Their weight control regimens become ways of coping with any stress in their lives.

Sometimes nutritional education alone can help to change abnormal eating behaviors. However, many avid dieters deny that they have a problem with food and may need counseling (which they usually agree to only at their family's insistence) to prevent complications. Most therapists recommend a combination of nutritional, cognitive, behavioral, and psychodynamic approaches.

The initial focus is on nutrition and eating patterns. Individuals are instructed to record everything they eat, including time, location, exactly what and how much they consume, and their feelings at the time they are eating. The therapist reviews this record, not to criticize or provoke guilt, but to help identify unconscious patterns, such as a link between anxiety about an upcoming event and skipping a meal.

For dieters who are significantly underweight, a nutritionist may develop a well-balanced diet to restore weight at the rate of one or two pounds a week. Individuals usually need repeated reassurance that they will not become overweight. Therapy for such persons, particularly younger women, may include their families, who also benefit from education about the impact that relationships and interactions can have on eating behavior.

Eventually—usually after three to six months—therapy focuses more on the chronic dieter's thoughts and feelings. Cognitive techniques (described in Chapter 27) help individuals learn to identify, challenge, and correct their misconceptions about food. The process of struggling with uncomfortable feelings, psychological conflicts, and developmental challenges leads to greater insight, self-confidence, and coping skills that can help in all aspects of daily living. The prognosis for those who obtain help is excellent, even though relapses are common, particularly under stress.

COMPULSIVE EATING

Compulsive eating—losing control over when, what, or how much a person eats—is not uncommon, especially among young women. It is not a mental disorder, although some of those affected eventually develop bulimia nervosa and induce vomiting or use laxatives to avoid weight gain. Others continue to overeat and to feel intensely guilty and ashamed afterward.

Individuals who eat compulsively typically feel unable to stop eating. They may eat much more rapidly than others, eat until they are uncomfortably full, eat large amounts of food even when they are not hungry, eat throughout the day with no planned mealtimes, eat alone because of embarrassment over how much they consume, and feel disgust or depression after overeating. Some binge; others snack continuously.

Some mental health professionals describe compulsive eating as an addiction. Compulsive eaters often crave sweet, sugary foods, become preoccupied with eating them, eat them to change their mood or avoid their problems, and continue overeating in spite of harmful consequences, including obesity. If they cut back or eliminate such foods, they report withdrawal symptoms, such as irritability, depression, fatigue, insomnia, nausea, headaches, and severe mood swings.

Women are more likely to eat compulsively than men. According to Overeaters Anonymous (OA), founded in 1960 by three women who got together to talk about food and weight, many women who eat compulsively view food as a source of comfort against feelings of inner emptiness, low self-esteem, and fear of abandonment.

Recovery from compulsive eating can be challenging because people with this problem cannot give up their "substance" entirely; after all, everyone must eat. However, they can learn new eating habits and ways of dealing with underlying emotional problems. A survey by OA, which has more than nine thousand groups around the world, found that most of its members joined to lose weight but later felt that the most important benefit of membership was their improved emotional, mental, and physical health. As one OA member put it, "I came for vanity but stayed for sanity."

BINGE EATING

Binge eating is the rapid consumption of an abnormally large amount of food in a relatively short time; it often occurs in compulsive eaters. Persons with binge-eating *disorder* typically eat a larger than ordinary amount of food during a relatively brief period, feel a lack of control over eating, and binge at least twice a week for a six-month period. During most of these episodes, they experience at least three of the following:

- Eating much more rapidly than usual
- Eating until they feel uncomfortably full
- Eating large amounts of food when not feeling physically hungry
- Eating large amounts of food throughout the day with no planned mealtimes

- Eating alone because they are embarrassed by how much they eat and by their eating habits
- Feeling disgusted with themselves, depressed, or very guilty after overeating.

Although bingeing is not in itself a mental disorder, repeated bingeing that causes serious distress or impairment may be. The *DSM-IV* includes binge eating as an "eating disorder not otherwise specified." Research studies have found that individuals with this problem may spend up to several hours eating and consume 2,000 or more calories in a single binge—more than many people eat in a day. After such binges, they do not induce vomiting, use laxatives, or rely on other means (such as exercise) to control weight. They simply get fatter. As their weight climbs, they become depressed, anxious, or troubled by other psychological symptoms to a much greater extent than others of comparable weight.

Estimates suggest that about 2 percent of Americans—about 5 million people—may have binge-eating disorder. It is most common among young women in college and, increasingly, in high school. As many as 10 to 15 percent of individuals enrolled in diet programs may have this problem, which could explain their difficulty in keeping their weight under control. Often they lose excess pounds, and then regain them—over and over again.

Persons who binge-eat may require professional help in changing their behavior. Treatment is similar to the approach used for extreme dieters and includes education, behavioral approaches, cognitive therapy, and psychotherapy. As they recognize the reasons for their behavior and begin to confront the underlying issues, these individuals usually resume normal eating patterns.

CRAVINGS AND PICA

A food craving is an intense desire for a specific food. Some people may crave certain substances because of a nutritional need. Pregnancy is one period in which this can occur; for instance, the often-reported craving for pickles may be the result of a pregnant woman's body needing salt to maintain a proper fluid balance. Cravings also may be rooted in brain chemistry. Some researchers speculate that certain foods stimulate the release of specific neurotransmitters in the brain.

Cravings can occur at different times or in specific places. Some women crave sweets before or during their periods. Persons with seasonal affective disorder (discussed in Chapter 5) typically crave more carbohydrates during winter, when they are most depressed, and find that this craving eases with the arrival of spring. Most food cravings are normal and harmless. The association of a place with a particular food can induce a craving, such as a yearning for a hot dog at a ballpark—a perfectly understandable behavior. Sometimes, however, cravings may be symptoms of undetected illness. Constant thirst can be an early sign of diabetes; a desire for ice may be a symptom of anemia.

Pica is a craving for a single food or for substances not commonly regarded as food, such as clay or starch. Some researchers believe that there is a link between pica and nutritional deficiencies, particularly a lack of iron, zinc, or calcium; any such lack should, of course, be corrected. But whether or not a nutritional deficiency is involved, ingesting substances other than food can cause serious medical complications, including lead and mercury poisoning and intestinal perforation and obstruction. Behavioral therapy, using techniques such as overcorrection (such as forcing individuals to spit out the substance, wash out their mouth, brush their teeth, and wipe their lips every time they put something they shouldn't in their mouths), can help to eliminate the behavior.

Anorexia nervosa

Anorexia means loss of appetite, but most individuals with anorexia nervosa are, in fact, hungry all the time. For them, food is an enemy—a threat to their sense of self, identity, and autonomy. In the distorted mirror of their mind's eye, they see themselves as fat or flabby even at a normal or below-normal body weight. Some simply feel fat; others think that they are thin in some places and too fat in others, such as the abdomen, buttocks, or thighs. The refusal to maintain a normal body weight is a key characteristic of anorexia nervosa, along with fear of weight gain and a distorted perception of body size or shape.

Individuals with anorexia nervosa lose weight primarily by reducing total food intake and avoiding high-calorie foods or by eating a very restricted variety of food. Neither dieting nor weight loss eases their intense fear of fatness, and it is common for them to become increasingly concerned about losing control and putting on weight. They may weigh themselves several times a day, measure various parts of their body, check mirrors to see if they look fat, and try on different items of clothing to see if they feel tight. By the time most people with anorexia seek psychiatric treatment, they weigh less than 85 percent of the normal weight for individuals of their sex and height. Even then, they wish they were thinner. Women with anorexia stop menstruating. This usually occurs after a significant amount of weight has been lost, although in about 20 percent it develops before body weight falls dramatically.

In "restricting type" anorexia, individuals lose weight by dieting, fasting, or exercise. In "binge eating/purging type" anorexia, they engage in binge eating, purging (through self-induced vomiting, laxatives, diuretics, or enemas), or both.

▼

How common is anorexia nervosa?

The incidence of anorexia nervosa seems to have increased in most developed countries over the last three decades. An estimated 0.5 to 1 percent of young women in their late teens and early twenties develops anorexia, but according to the American Psychiatric Association's Work Group on Eating Disorders, cases are increasing among males, minorities, women of all ages, and possibly preteens.

Anorexia usually develops between ages ten and thirty, peaking at ages fourteen and eighteen; the mean age at onset is seventeen. Ninety percent of those with anorexia nervosa are women.

▼

What causes anorexia nervosa?

There have been many hypotheses about the complex factors that may interact and lead to this disorder. Family patterns and heredity play a role. Anorexia is more common among close relatives of those with anorexia than among the general population. Sisters of women with anorexia, especially identical twins, face a risk of developing this disorder that is many times what might be expected in the general population. There is also a higher than expected frequency of depressive disorders among the close relatives of those with anorexia nervosa and of obsessive-compulsive disorder in the mothers of anorexic individuals.

Complex neurochemical abnormalities may be involved, such as disturbances in the hypothalamus, a part of the brain that plays an important role in the production and regulation of hormones. Individuals with anorexia often have increased cortisol production and higher than normal levels of corticotropin-releasing factor (CRF) in their cerebrospinal fluid. There may be abnormalities in levels of dopamine, serotonin, and norepinephrine—neurotransmitters that influence appetite and satiety—and in cholecystokinin (CCK), a peptide found in the brain and digestive tract that affects feelings of fullness. It is not clear, however, whether these neurochemical divergences from the norm are a cause or a consequence of this disorder.

Anorexia nervosa may also be a response to a personal loss or a sign of a driven, perfectionist personality. Often young people with this problem have above-average grades and an unwarranted fear of failure. Many therapists have noted that individuals with anorexia, regardless of age, report feeling ineffective and helpless. Some psychological theorists have speculated that a teenage girl may starve herself because of a fear of her budding sexuality. By

drastically reducing her weight, she prevents or stops menstruation and breast development. A thin body comes to symbolize all
that is good, whereas fatness or loss of control over eating epito-
mizes all that is bad. In time, those with anorexia may place so
much value on thinness that they cannot recognize the dangers
to their health.

The psychiatrist Hilde Bruch, a pioneer in the study of the
causes of anorexia nervosa, speculated that girls who diet excessively and those who develop anorexia often have no insight or
awareness of their feelings, needs, or wants. From very early in
life, they may have grown and developed by always reacting to the
needs and expectations of others, and they may feel inadequate
and incompetent as they approach the age of independence. In
some cases, starvation may serve as a way of creating an identity
and asserting independence.

About one-third of those who develop anorexia are mildly overweight and cut back on food just to lose a few pounds. In other
cases, individuals of normal weight begin to diet because they
think they will look more attractive or to gain some professional
advantage. Sometimes illness, stress, or surgery may trigger the
process. But unlike those who stop dieting when they reach a
target weight or who try to regain weight lost when ill, some people
continue to be preoccupied with weight loss.

Other external factors can also play a part in the development
of the disorder, as when parents first encourage and reward a
young girl who diets to get rid of her "baby fat." Only when her
dieting becomes extreme do they criticize it, yet by this point she
may be more convinced than ever that she needs to lose weight—
often, at least in part, because our culture, which places a high
premium on beauty and thinness, reinforces a vulnerable girl's
conviction that she is indeed too fat.

▼

**How anorexia
nervosa feels**

Even if they lose 25 percent of their body weight and appear painfully thin, individuals with anorexia *feel* fat. Because they believe
that thinness is absolutely essential for happiness and well-being,
they justify extreme eating behavior, such as refusing adequate
nourishment, as necessary. No matter how much their weight
drops, they still do not feel thin. Often they are convinced that
parts of their bodies—their thighs, for example—are fat or flabby.
In addition to dieting, they may induce vomiting and use large
quantities of laxatives and diuretics, which speed up water loss.
They may devote hours every day to demanding exercise routines,
running many miles and then working out in a gym.

When family or friends urge them to eat, they argue and refuse
food. In their heart of hearts, they *know* that they are fat and un-

desirable. Only when they lose more weight do they feel any gratification, mastery, or sense of accomplishment. Feelings such as these may be especially powerful in those who are unhappy with other parts of their lives, as adolescents often are. Yet persons with anorexia often deny any emotional problems and do not talk about their feelings as much as they demonstrate them through their behavior. They are often unable to identify emotions and thoughts or to express in words what they truly feel and think.

Anorexia nervosa feels physically and psychologically painful. Most therapists agree that malnutrition is a primary reason. As individuals lose large amounts of weight, they become very sensitive to cold. They are chronically constipated; their blood pressure drops; fine hair (lanugo) may grow on their bodies. Fingernails become brittle; hair and skin turn dry. A lack of adequate vitamin C leads to gum infections. They find it hard to sleep. Their sexual desire disappears. As anorexia progresses, many of those affected become indifferent or irritable, withdraw from others, become depressed, and no longer can function normally at school or work.

Like prisoners of war and others who have been starved, those with anorexia become preoccupied with food. They collect recipes, prepare elaborate meals for others, hide food around the house, or carry large quantities of candy in their pockets and purses. Food is always on their minds, although the most they do is nibble on a few low-calorie foods. At meals they may cut what is on their plate into tiny pieces, move it around, or try to hide it in their napkins or pockets. Some refuse to eat with others or in public. Others develop compulsive and ritualistic behaviors, such as frequent hand washing, constant house cleaning, or obsessive studying.

▼

Seeking help   Most people with anorexia nervosa insist that they do not have a problem or minimize its severity. Almost always, their alarmed parents or friends are the ones who insist that they see a therapist. If you suspect that someone close to you may have anorexia, these are the questions that should be asked:

- Has the individual lost at least 15 percent of ideal weight? Does he or she refuse to maintain a normal body weight?

- Is the person extremely fearful of gaining weight or becoming fat, despite being underweight?

- Does the person have a distorted body image and feel fat even when emaciated, or deny how severely underweight he or she is?

- Has an adolescent girl or a premenopausal woman missed at least three menstrual cycles?

Individuals with anorexia usually resist therapy because they fear that they will be forced to gain weight and get fat. They may argue against whatever treatment is recommended. However, most do respond when relatives, friends, and the therapist emphasize the positive benefits of treatment, such as relief of troubling symptoms like insomnia or depression, increased energy, and an improved sense of well-being.

A complete physical examination is essential. In addition to low body weight, emaciation, and medical symptoms, anorexic individuals may have abnormal heart rhythm, liver function, hormone levels, or blood chemistries, especially low glucose, which contribute to irritability, depression, confusion, and emotional volatility. Therapists may use standardized self-assessment questionnaires for eating disorders, in addition to conducting a comprehensive, detailed psychiatric evaluation and taking a complete history of the individual's height and weight at various ages, food intake, beginning of food restriction, frequency of bingeing, and other related eating behaviors. For preteens and teens, therapists also interview parents and possibly school counselors.

▼

Risks and complications   Anorexia nervosa is a serious threat to mental and physical health. More than half of those with this disorder also suffer from dysthymia or major depression (see Chapter 5). About 10 percent develop obsessive-compulsive disorder, an anxiety disorder described in Chapter 8. Menstrual periods stop in women; testosterone levels decline in men. Adolescents do not undergo normal sexual maturation, such as breast development, and may not reach their anticipated height.

Even individuals who look and feel reasonably healthy may have subtle or hidden abnormalities, including heart irregularities and arrhythmias that can increase the risk of sudden death. Women who do not menstruate for six months or more may suffer possibly irreversible weakening and thinning of their bones. Osteoporosis is a long-term complication of anorexia nervosa.

Other possible complications include anemia, impaired kidney function, infertility, hormonal imbalances, electrolyte disturbances, and abnormalities in digestion and metabolism. Those who vomit regularly may experience erosion of their dental enamel, scars or calluses on their hands from using them to induce vomiting, and the other medical complications associated with bulimia described later in this chapter. They are more likely to have impulse control problems and to abuse alcohol or drugs.

Anorexia nervosa can have long-term effects and shorten a person's life span. The long-term mortality rate among those admitted for treatment at university hospitals is 10 percent. The most common causes of death are starvation, suicide, and electrolyte imbalances.

▼

Treating anorexia nervosa

Often, the greatest challenge in treating anorexia nervosa is convincing individuals with this problem that they need help and that treatment can work. Even when they realize that they are jeopardizing their health, they tend to fear that treatment will make them worse—that is, fatter. They need repeated reassurance that they will not become overweight and that they can and will find more healthful and more satisfying ways of coping with their lives.

Most therapists agree that malnutrition is the direct cause of many of anorexia's physical and mental symptoms, including medical problems, preoccupation with food, hoarding, bingeing, indifference, irritability, depression, and other changes. "Refeeding" to restore normal weight relieves or removes most of these symptoms, although full recovery can take a long time.

The APA's Work Group on Eating Disorders has developed practice guidelines for the treatment of anorexia nervosa, which include medical, behavioral, cognitive, psychodynamic, and family therapy. For those who are severely underweight (more than 15 percent below ideal weight), the first goal is to correct the effects of malnutrition and to restore weight to normal, for both medical and psychological reasons. In addition to serious physiological complications, starvation impairs a person's ability to think clearly and to relate to others normally. Obsessed with food, unable to sleep, depressed and irritable, anorexic individuals may act inappropriately or immaturely and are incapable of insight and perspective.

Unless and until they return to a healthful weight, psychotherapy does little, if any, good.

In the past, therapists would identify a "target weight" for those with anorexia. However, because there are different views about ideal body weight, many specialists in eating disorders prefer to rely on standardized tables that give healthy ranges of body mass index (BMI), figures based on weight divided by height. As they work toward a target BMI, anorexic individuals should gain weight slowly and steadily—about one-quarter of a pound a day.

A return to normal menstrual cycles usually lags behind the return to a normal body weight. Marked psychological improvement often occurs at about the same time that menstrual cycles resume. Many therapists vary their approach at different stages of therapy. Initially, they may rely on cognitive-behavioral techniques to change eating behaviors and to help maintain a healthful weight. As treatment progresses, they may use psychodynamic approaches to enhance insight, promote maturity, and help build effective coping skills.

HOSPITAL-BASED TREATMENT

In the past, many, if not most, individuals with anorexia were hospitalized, often for several months. This is no longer the case, largely because of changes in insurance reimbursement for hospitalization and the trend toward shorter inpatient stays. In severe cases, however, inpatient treatment remains essential.

Depending on age and medical status, individuals initially may be hospitalized on a psychiatric, medical, or pediatric-adolescent unit. The first priority in hospital treatment is medical stabilization and "re-feeding," often with liquid dietary formulas that are nutritionally balanced, easily digested, and likely to cause less anxiety because they are viewed more as medicine than food. In rare, life-threatening cases of extreme malnourishment, individuals may require feeding through a tube directly into the stomach. However, this therapy is considered both risky (potential dangers include heart failure and severe fluid retention) and controversial.

Inpatient and partial hospitalization programs, which offer daytime treatment only, utilize cognitive-behavioral and psychodynamic approaches. Either a psychiatrist or another physician may oversee the medical aspects of care, while a different therapist, who may or may not be a psychiatrist, handles psychological treatment. Most health care teams also include nurses, social workers, occupational therapists, and dieticians.

Nutritional counseling, which may include an analysis of current diet, identification of needed nutrients, and an individualized eating plan, is essential. Because people with anorexia often fear certain foods (usually those containing fat), a dietician may draw up a meal plan that relies mainly on foods that cause little anxiety and then gradually introduce feared foods.

Bringing a person back to normal weight is not a cure. Recovery will not occur until underlying psychological conflicts—poor self-esteem, fear of fatness, obsession with thinness, dependency, immaturity, distorted perceptions, difficulty separating from parents—are dealt with through therapy. When affected persons suffer from major depression or an obsessive-compulsive disorder, these conditions must be treated.

Once individuals get their weight within a normal range, they begin preparing for eating in real-world situations. (Initially, hospital day programs and inpatient units may provide all meals.) Staff members may accompany them to a restaurant or join them in a family meal at home to help relieve anxiety about eating. Before a program is completed, therapists may negotiate a behavioral contract with patients and their families to ensure that they work together to deal with any problems.

After-care following partial or full hospitalization can take many forms: intensive psychotherapy, structured monitoring of weight and eating, family therapy, or all three. Signs of relapse include significant weight loss, inability to regain lost weight, worsened binge eating or purging, or serious depression.

COGNITIVE-BEHAVIORAL THERAPY

Increasingly, therapists are combining behavioral and cognitive approaches to anorexia nervosa, with promising results. Often the thoughts and beliefs of those with the disorder are as distorted as their behavior—at least in part because of the mental effects of starvation.

Cognitive therapy offers strategies to deal with distorted beliefs and faulty reasoning. One approach is education about the effects of starvation, weight control, nutrition, and societal attitudes and influences. Another technique is to ask individuals to write down their thoughts and beliefs about food, eating, and weight. The therapist then works to recognize and correct reasoning errors. Commonly encountered themes are:

- *All-or-nothing thinking:* Anorexic individuals tend to see foods as either good (low-calorie) or bad (fattening). To them, a weight gain of only a pound seems a step toward obesity.

- *Extreme sensitivity to others' possible disapproval:* For example, anorexic individuals may believe that complete strangers will notice if they eat a forbidden food.

- *Magical thinking:* Anorexic individuals may anticipate severe punishment if they eat more than they planned or fail to exercise as much as usual.

- *Generalizing:* Anorexic individuals may think that fatness equals incompetence or that weight loss brings happiness.

In therapy, persons learn to become more aware of illogical reasoning or distorted thoughts and to see the connection between their beliefs and their behaviors. Gradually they learn to substitute more realistic and appropriate interpretations and to modify the assumptions that can lead to self-destructive behavior.

Behavioral methods include keeping a food diary and noting any problem behaviors (such as bingeing or vomiting). This helps individuals to recognize the triggers for these behaviors and therefore avoid them. They also learn how many calories to consume for slow weight gain and how to set weight goals. At home, they may be asked to remain with a friend or family member after each meal and not to weigh themselves. Instead, they are weighed weekly at a clinic or the therapist's office.

Training in assertiveness, social skills, and problem solving helps many individuals to develop healthier coping mechanisms for dealing with stress. A written contract between individuals and their families, which specifies goals (such as maintaining normal weight) and reinforcements (such as a loss of privileges for losing weight) also can be helpful.

PSYCHODYNAMIC PSYCHOTHERAPY

Psychotherapy helps persons with anorexia to deal with their inner confusion and their misconceptions about their feelings, needs, self-worth, and ability to control their lives. Its goal is to bring about greater understanding of the role the illness plays in their lives so that they can find other ways of coping that eliminate the need for anorexia.

Initially, this therapy mainly helps individuals to accept weight gain without anxiety or fear. In time, it helps them to recognize that their abnormal eating behaviors are a smokescreen for unresolved psychological conflicts that may be the result of a loss, family conflict, developmental challenges, or a lack of a coherent sense of identity.

Anorexic individuals struggle constantly for control. Because they often feel controlled by others, they despair of being able to influence them or resist their influence, and may become stubborn and negative. Therapy can help them to recognize and understand their true fears, to acknowledge their feelings of powerlessness, helplessness, and ineffectiveness, and to deal with conflicts.

With the therapist's help, they can learn to stop basing their self-worth on external references and pursue their own goals—something they may never have considered possible.

FAMILY THERAPY

As explained in Chapter 27, family therapy always involves looking at the family as a system, tracing its roots in the past, unlocking secrets, and assessing the dynamics among family members. Because most individuals who develop anorexia nervosa are young and are living at home with their parents and siblings, family therapy is critical.

Eating disorders seem particularly likely to develop in emotionally troubled families, particularly those in which at least one person suffers from depression, alcoholism, or an eating disorder. Eating, body shape, and weight often tend to be major topics in family communication. Marital problems are common; indeed, a teenager's anorexia may keep together parents who might otherwise divorce. Family therapy helps to identify the factors that may be sustaining their child's anorexia or interfering with recovery and to unravel both the causes and course of the anorexia. It can deal with hidden issues, such as excessive emphasis on appearance, and help parents to allow their child greater independence.

Although they should be supportive, parents should not let a child's anorexia dominate daily life or dictate eating patterns for the entire family. Providing a special low-calorie diet, for instance, may only reinforce the illness, and discussing the disorder, particularly at mealtimes, often increases the child's anxiety.

The goals of family therapy vary. For younger individuals, the family may strive to learn to live together more comfortably, whereas an older adolescent or young adult may need help in breaking away. Ideally the therapist helps to find ways for everyone in the family to benefit, rather than trying to "cure" one person at the expense of another.

In one report on eighty individuals with anorexia nervosa or bulimia nervosa, family therapy proved more supportive and beneficial than one-to-one therapy for those under the age of nineteen. Most therapists offer both family and individual sessions.

GROUP THERAPY

Group therapy is not considered a primary approach to anorexia nervosa although groups can be a useful part of inpatient or outpatient programs. The structure of the group is crucial, and most members should be similar in terms of age and maturity. Some anorexic individuals may be so withdrawn, nonverbal, or depressed that they cannot participate until their condition improves.

Initially, a group may focus on educating its members about the disorder and may provide nutritional counseling, focusing on proper dietary habits, meal planning, and food choices. But groups can provide much more than information. In the group setting, individuals can observe the illness in their fellow members, see how they act and react, and develop better social skills. Because participants often have great insight into how others with anorexia feel and behave, the group offers the opportunity to discuss common problems, such as perfectionism, self-control, and rigidity. Members who are making progress in terms of both weight and outlook serve as valuable role models for those who worry that they will become fat or depressed.

MEDICATION

Psychiatrists have tried various medications in treating anorexia nervosa, but with the exception of antidepressants, there have been few controlled studies and little is known about their effectiveness. At most, medication should play a secondary role in a comprehensive treatment approach. For emaciated individuals receiving intensive inpatient treatment, cyproheptadine, an antihistamine, has shown some small benefit in increasing weight gain, especially in those with no history of bulimia. Some psychiatrists prescribe anti-anxiety agents for use before meals, but many therapists prefer behavioral strategies for pre-eating apprehensiveness.

Controlled studies have shown that tricyclic antidepressants do not improve weight gain, and malnourished individuals seem more likely to develop side effects, including dangerous cardiac arrhythmias. There have been reports from uncontrolled studies that low doses of fluoxetine (Prozac) help some—but not most—individuals in gaining and maintaining weight.

Because of the calcium loss and increased risk of osteoporosis that occur when women stop menstruating, those with anorexia nervosa may be given replacement hormones (estrogen and progesterone). This approach is not advised for teenagers unless they have not resumed menstruating after at least a year of treatment.

RELAPSE PREVENTION

Anorexia nervosa tends to be a chronic, recurring problem, and individuals who have returned to normal weight must realize that they may need maintenance treatment. Relapse prevention techniques similar to those developed for alcoholics (described in Chapter 10) can help them to identify high-risk situations that are likely to trigger overeating or purging.

▼

Self-help   In anorexia nervosa, the compulsion to restrict food and lose weight takes on a life of its own and becomes irresistible. On their own, those with this disorder cannot force themselves to eat more or exercise less. Only with comprehensive treatment can they begin to learn healthful eating patterns and practical coping skills.

There is, however, one very effective self-help aid: a diary. Individuals may begin by keeping a detailed record of their food intake and eating behavior, writing down their thoughts and beliefs about food and weight, trying to identify what they are feeling and thinking, and putting all this into words. This is very hard for them to do initially, but as they improve with treatment they become increasingly capable of such insight.

▼

Impact on relationships   Anorexia nervosa creates emotional upheaval in families. By starving themselves, adolescents and young women may be both asserting their independence and expressing their anger, and home life can become a power struggle between parents who urge their child to eat and the child who refuses to do so.

Parents often fluctuate between denying the problem, blaming each other, and feeling guilty. When nothing they try—begging, threatening, bribing, cajoling—works, they can feel increasingly frustrated and helpless. Those who become demoralized may need to get away temporarily to restore their own internal reserves; a respite can be of great help. They also benefit from counseling, information, support, help in problem solving, and preparation for living with their child after treatment. As has been noted above, family therapy can be a critical element in the treatment of this disorder.

For married individuals with anorexia nervosa, therapy should always involve spouses. Often the partner is unconsciously reinforcing the disorder or may deny other problems in the relationship by focusing solely on the anorexia.

▼

Outlook   According to the APA Work Group on Eating Disorders, four-year follow-up studies show that about 44 percent of individuals who receive treatment have a "good" outcome, that is, a return to normal or near-normal weight and a resumption of menstruation. As many as two-thirds continue to be preoccupied with food and weight, however, and many go on to develop bulimia or experience dysthymia, social phobia, obsessive-compulsive symptoms, and substance abuse. Mortality rates for those treated for anorexia nervosa continue to be high for more than twenty years after diagnosis.

Individuals with less severe symptoms tend to have the best

outcomes. Those who are older, have had anorexia for a long period of time, have previously been admitted to psychiatric hospitals, had childhood or personality difficulties before developing anorexia, and have severely disturbed relationships with family members are less likely to do well.

Bulimia nervosa

Individuals with bulimia nervosa go on repeated eating binges and rapidly consume large amounts of food, usually sweets, stopping only because of severe abdominal pain, a need to sleep, or an interruption. Those with "purging type" bulimia induce vomiting or take large doses of laxatives to relieve guilt and control their weight. In "nonpurging" bulimia, individuals use other means, such as fasting or excessive exercise, to compensate for binges. Bulimia is much more common than anorexia, although there is great overlap between the two. Unlike those with anorexia nervosa, bulimics tend to be of more or less normal weight. However, the medical complications of this disorder are also serious and can be life-threatening.

"Trendy" or experimental bulimia is common among certain college and high school groups. Young women who try bingeing and purging don't necessarily have a psychiatric disorder; often they engage in vomiting for a few months to a year and then stop when their social or living situation changes. For those who seek help, education, group therapy, and cognitive-behavioral treatments are very effective.

▼
How common is bulimia nervosa?

Bulimia nervosa is fairly common among young women. According to the *DSM-IV*, 1 to 3 percent of adolescent and young adult females develop bulimia; among males, this disorder is about one-tenth as common. The average age for developing bulimia is eighteen, with a range between twelve and thirty-five. Individuals who were obese as adolescents may be more likely to develop bulimia as adults.

About one-fourth to one-third of those with bulimia have had a previous history of anorexia. Persons who develop this problem often have obese parents and a higher than expected incidence of major depression among their close relatives.

▼
What causes bulimia nervosa?

Bulimia nervosa usually begins after a rigid diet that lasted from several weeks to a year or more and that may or may not have been successful. Strict dieting may affect brain chemistry in such a way as to disrupt the normal mechanisms for appetite and satiety. Semi-starvation sets off a binge; bingeing leads to purging. Once dieters realize that vomiting reduces the anxiety triggered by gorging, they no longer fear overeating. When this happens, bingeing may become more frequent and severe until, in time, it becomes an all-purpose way of coping with stress. However, the driving force in this disorder may not be the eating but the vomiting, since it is likely that individuals would not overeat if they couldn't vomit afterwards.

Obesity in adolescence may increase the likelihood of bulimia in adulthood. Persons who had been extremely obese may start bingeing and vomiting to keep their weight down. Although they may want to stop, they prefer bulimia to severe obesity. Normal-weight bulimics may have a history of anorexia; although their weight is now normal, they continue to binge and purge.

Biological abnormalities also may play a role, although it is not clear whether they are a cause or a consequence of repeated bingeing and purging. According to researchers at the NIH and Duke University, individuals with bulimia, like those with anorexia, have low levels of the peptide cholecystokinin (CCK). Because of this deficiency, they don't feel satisfied after a meal and may binge to reach satiety. The cycle of bingeing and purging can also wreak havoc on other biological controls that keep weight at a certain level.

Since bulimia, like anorexia nervosa, tends to develop in late adolescence, it may be linked to difficulties in making the transition to adulthood. Family conflicts, such as feeling torn between two parents, may also lead a young woman to turn to bulimia as a way of coping. The disorder appears to have some association with life stresses, such as going away to school or getting a job.

Although the great majority of bulimic individuals feel unhappy and disappointed because they feel out of control of their eating patterns, bulimia also may be a symptom of primary depression. About 20 to 30 percent of those with this problem are chronically depressed; others have experienced previous episodes of depression. Anxiety disorders can also coexist with bulimia. Personality studies comparing women with bulimia and those with alcohol or drug abuse disorders have shown similarly elevated scores for depression, as well as for anger and rebelliousness.

Other problems often found in bulimic persons include alcohol abuse, difficulty tolerating frustration, problems with interpersonal relationships, and impulsive behaviors. Some abuse amphetamines or over-the-counter medications to reduce appetite and lose weight. Others shoplift or steal food, clothing, jewelry, and other items, or give in to the impulse to cut themselves.

The families of persons with bulimia have a higher than usual incidence of depression, alcoholism, drug abuse, and obesity. A significant percentage of bulimic individuals—estimated to be from a quarter to a half—may have been victims of incest, sexual molestation, or rape, but this correlation has been challenged.

▼

How bulimia nervosa feels

The lives of people with this disorder revolve around food. Although most are within a normal weight range, they are enormously concerned about weight and repeatedly try to control it by dieting, vomiting, or using laxatives and diuretics. They gain and lose pounds rapidly as they alternate between binges and purges. Conflicts about eating dominate their lives. Most do not eat regular meals and do not feel full at the end of a normal meal. They prefer to eat alone and at home because of shame and guilt.

Binges can become an intense preoccupation. Bulimic individuals may be in a frenzy to leave work in order to get home and binge. Their binges are carefully planned, and anything that interferes with these plans creates great anxiety and further perpetuates the binge-purge cycle. Typically, they choose high-calorie, sweet-tasting foods, such as cake or ice cream, that they can gobble down as rapidly as possible with little chewing. The typical binge lasts for an hour or two, and once they start eating they cannot stop. In a frenzied state, they may look for more food to continue the binge, stopping only because they are interrupted or cannot physically eat any more. Once the binge is over, they feel ashamed, self-critical, and depressed. Purging eases the physical pain of their distended stomachs and often reduces remorse and anguish. Usually individuals stick a finger down the throat; some learn to vomit at will. A smaller number take laxatives after a binge, and some may fast for a day or exercise excessively.

▼

Seeking help

Bulimia may continue off and on for many years, with binges alternating with periods of regular eating. Most people with bulimia look normal and are of more or less normal weight, although even when their bodies are slender their bellies protrude, stretched by frequent binges. In general, they manage to function normally despite their bulimia, although in extreme cases they may spend every waking moment planning binges, buying food, and then bingeing and purging.

If you think that you or someone close to you may have bulimia, here are the questions that should be asked:

- Do you frequently eat abnormally large amounts of food in a brief period of time and feel a lack of control over what or how much is eaten?
- Do you regularly rely on self-induced vomiting or laxatives to prevent weight gain?
- Have eating binges occurred two or more times a week for at least three months?

Is it bulimia nervosa?

According to the DSM-IV, a diagnosis of bulimia nervosa should be based on these criteria:

- Recurrent episodes of binge eating, characterized by:
  1. Eating, in a discrete period of time (e.g., within any two-hour period), an amount of food that is definitely larger than most people would eat in a similar period of time and similar circumstances, and
  2. A sense of lack of control during the episode (e.g., a feeling that one cannot stop eating or control what or how much one is eating)
- Recurrent inappropriate behavior to prevent weight gain, such as self-induced vomiting, misuse of laxatives, diuretics, or other medications, fasting, or excessive exercise
- Binge eating and compensatory behaviors both occur, on average, at least twice a week for three months.
- Self-evaluation is unduly influenced by body shape and weight.
- The disturbance does not occur exclusively during episodes of anorexia nervosa.

Adapted from the Diagnostic and Statistical Manual of Mental Disorders, 4th Edition. *Used with permission.*

Dentists are often the first to detect bulimia because they notice damage to teeth and gums, including erosion of the tooth enamel, from the stomach acids in vomit. Other medical signs of bulimia include scrapes and calluses on the back of the hand (the so-called Russel's sign), which is the result of scraping the hand against the teeth while trying to induce vomiting. Another telltale indication is the person's excusing herself during or after a meal to go to the bathroom, where she forces herself to vomit.

In evaluating individuals for bulimia, therapists usually use standardized diagnostic questionnaires in addition to completing a comprehensive psychiatric examination and history of various eating behaviors. They ask about food intake, preferences, attitudes about eating, the person's view of how symptoms developed, and the extent of binge eating, vomiting, and other forms of purging. In addition, they look for any signs of other psychiatric disorders, such as substance abuse, depression, or impulsive behavior such as shoplifting or self-mutilation. A physical examination is critically important to assess health status and need for medical care.

▼

Risks and complications

Bulimic individuals may consume 5,000 calories or more in a single binge, but the purging that follows is what causes serious harm. The stomach acids in vomit commonly irritate the gums and erode tooth enamel, leading to cavities. Repeated vomiting robs the body of essential nutrients and fluids, causing dehydration and electrolyte imbalances. Potassium depletion (hypokalemia) impairs the ability of the heart and other muscles to function and can trigger cardiac arrhythmias and, occasionally, sudden death. Other complications include muscle spasms in the hands and feet, palpitations, irritation and bleeding of the esophagus and stomach, and digestive tract disorders. The use of ipecac, a drug that induces vomiting, can cause generalized muscle weakness and lead to sudden death from cardiac failure.

Many people falsely believe that using laxatives or diuretics speeds weight loss and frequently use these preparations. In fact, taking laxatives and using diuretics actually lead to rebound fluid retention, perpetuating the feeling of being bloated and reinforcing the purging cycle. There are serious complications of laxative abuse, including constipation and rectal prolapse, as well as the rare condition of cathartic colon, which is a surgical emergency. Complications of diuretic and laxative abuse, like those of repeated vomiting, include dehydration and electrolyte imbalances and the risk of dangerous cardiac arrhythmias.

Even when their weight and physical health seem normal, individuals with bulimia may suffer the psychological effects of starvation, including mood swings, fatigue, and depression. They also have higher than normal rates of anxiety disorders, bipolar illness (manic depression), and personality disorders. Many have symptoms of dissociation (see Chapter 18), report sexual difficulties, or engage in self-destructive impulsive behaviors, such as shoplifting, promiscuity, or self-mutilation.

▼

Treating bulimia nervosa

Most therapists use a combination of approaches, including nutritional counseling; psychodynamic, behavioral, and cognitive therapy; individual, group, and family psychotherapy; and medication. There have been many more studies of treatments for bulimia than of treatments for anorexia nervosa. The first choice of treatment has usually been cognitive-behavioral therapy, although in a recent study, interpersonal therapy, which focuses on relationships and social interactions (see Chapter 27), proved to be as effective initially as cognitive-behavioral treatment, and more effective in maintaining improvement on follow-up. The use of antidepressants alone, without concurrent psychotherapy, is not considered effective.

COGNITIVE-BEHAVIORAL THERAPY

According to the APA's guidelines on treatment of eating disorders, the combination of cognitive and behavioral approaches has proved very effective in treating bulimia, at least from the short-term standpoint. This approach modifies the person's distorted views about shape, weight, dieting, and vomiting to control weight, and leads to greater overall improvement compared with other short-term psychotherapies.

The basic principle of cognitive-behavioral therapy is that bulimia is maintained by reinforcers, such as the pleasure of eating or the reduction of anxiety after vomiting. The first step in treatment is usually self-monitoring by recording of all eating episodes. Individuals may resist doing this because they are ashamed of how much they eat and how abnormal their eating patterns are, but the therapist provides reassurance that monitoring and confronting abnormal behavior are essential to recovery.

A record of how much they eat, what types of food they choose, how often they binge, and the circumstances and feelings associated with binges and vomiting or laxative abuse, enables individuals and their therapists to analyze eating habits and the situations in which problems arise. Common triggers for bingeing and purging include feelings of hunger, stress, negative emotions, specific sites, being at social events in which they feel uncomfortable, or irrational thoughts, such as feeling that, since they already "blew" their diets by having a scoop of ice cream, they might as well eat all the ice cream in the container.

Once they recognize these high-risk circumstances, individuals can learn to avoid them or to change the way they handle them to avoid abnormal eating. Those who binge when cramming for a test, for example, might arrange to study with a friend. Since bulimics often gobble food while watching TV or reading, they are taught to eat only in a set place, such as the dining table, and to eat slowly, putting down their fork or spoon between mouthfuls. High-risk foods are introduced gradually into the diet, beginning with those least likely to lead to a binge. They are not banned, because they tend to be favorites, and avoiding them entirely increases the risk of relapse.

Since many individuals binge under stress, stress management techniques—problem-solving skills, assertiveness training, tips for effective communication, and relaxation methods—can be very helpful. If the bulimia provides positive benefits, such as extra attention from the family, these persons may have to learn better ways to achieve the same payoffs.

One behavioral technique used to prevent vomiting is response prevention. After eating, the individual is placed in a situation in which she cannot vomit—for example, she may be required to remain in the presence of others after eating. Another is to have the person bring foods she usually binges on to the therapist's office and eat as much as she wishes; the therapist stays with her until

'Pudge' and the Friday night pig-outs

Nina's childhood nickname was 'Pudge.' "I loved sweets," she recalls, "And I ate so many of them that I looked like the Campbell's Soup kid, with chubby cheeks that everyone loved to pinch." As Nina entered her teens, her other friends all suddenly seemed to develop thin, shapely bodies. "It's just baby fat," her mother would say when Nina worried about her formless figure. "It'll melt off as you get older and taller."

Nina couldn't wait that long. She went on a strict low-fat, low-calorie diet. Every day she portioned out what she would eat into tiny servings. Within a month, she had shed twenty pounds. Everyone complimented her on her new figure, including boys who had never looked at her before. But as Nina returned to her old eating habits her weight climbed back up. By the time she went away to college, she'd lost and gained the same twenty pounds several times.

During her frantic first semester on her own, Nina never seemed to stop eating. Someone at the dorm was always calling out for pizza. Parents would send "Care" packages stuffed with goodies. At the library Nina would munch on candy bars during study breaks. During Christmas vacation her mother baked all her favorites, and Nina came back to school determined to diet. She tried a slow, sensible approach, but it was frustrating watching others eat the treats Nina loved. "How can you eat so much and stay so skinny?" she asked one of the girls on her floor. "Come on," her friend said. "I'll show you my secret." She led Nina to the bathroom, where she leaned over a toilet, expertly stuck her index finger down her throat, and threw up.

Soon Nina was doing the same. All week long she kept thinking about what she'd eat in what she thought of as her "Friday night pig-out." She hoarded chips and cookies, stole extra pieces of cake from the cafeteria, and early in the evening bought a half-gallon of ice cream at the local store. If asked to go out with friends, she'd say no. She couldn't imagine how she'd make it through the week without having her binge to look forward to. Alone in her room, she would eat and eat and eat as fast as she could, hardly even taking time to chew. She stopped only when it was physically impossible to put another bite in her mouth. Feeling bloated and disgusted, she'd go to the bathroom and force herself to vomit. Almost always she'd feel better immediately.

Nina kept bingeing and purging throughout her years at college. Her dentist was the first one to suspect a problem. "I've seen the same kind of erosion of tooth enamel and gum irritation in lots of young women with bulimia," she told Nina. "Take my advice: Go talk with a therapist." Nina, who had been troubled by feelings of anxiety and depression, decided to talk to one of the counselors at the student health center. That's where she learned about eating disorders.

The counselor recommended a therapist who used a cognitive-behavioral approach. As part of her homework, Nina had to record everything she ate, whether she induced vomiting, and how she felt at the time. Together with the therapist, she reviewed the situations that had triggered bingeing or purging and developed a plan to avoid high-risk circumstances, such as making certain she arranged to go out with others on Friday night. Nina also worked on re-examining her beliefs about her body, her relationships, and the role of food in her life.

Within three months Nina was able to greatly reduce her bingeing-purging pattern. But five years after graduation, a man she'd been seeing for three years broke up with her. Depressed and distressed, she returned to the comfort of "pigging out." Knowing that she needed help, she consulted a psychiatrist, who prescribed fluoxetine (Prozac) as well as brief psychotherapy to deal with underlying issues troubling her. Within a month Nina was bingeing much less often. Nevertheless, she now realizes that when times get tough she's likely to be tempted to bury her troubles with food. "But I'm not 'Pudge' anymore," she says. "I've learned there are better ways to cope with stress."

the urge to vomit diminishes. Sometimes the therapist and the patient draw up a contract that sets target goals, such as a reduction in bingeing. Rewards, including praise from the therapist or spending money that once went for food on a special indulgence after reaching a certain goal, provide reinforcement for the progress an individual makes.

At the same time, therapists also focus on faulty assumptions that lead to bizarre eating patterns, such as the belief that dieting and weight control are essential for happiness or well-being, and other erroneous ways of thinking, such as the following:

- Irrational thoughts, such as "I've gained two pounds. I have no alternative but to binge and vomit."

- All-or-nothing thinking, such as "If I have one cookie, I'll eat the whole box."

- Black-or-white thinking, such as believing that thin is good and being overweight is bad or that certain foods are good and others are bad.

PSYCHODYNAMIC PSYCHOTHERAPY

Usually, bulimic individuals binge and purge not only because of a fear of fatness but also because these behaviors provide gratification and a sense of control. They may see thinness or these forms of control over their eating as something they can work toward and achieve, unlike less certain goals, such as a career or a satisfactory relationship. Sometimes weight control is the only way in which persons who are extremely dissatisfied with other areas of their life can bolster their abysmally low self-esteem.

Initially, bulimic individuals may have no insight into the psychological origins of their eating behavior and may resist any suggestion to change. Over time, therapists help them explore psychological problems, such as a lack of self-esteem, personal ineffectiveness, poor impulse control, perfectionism, dependency issues, and negative body image. Ideally, psychotherapy changes self-concept as well as eating patterns so individuals can come to understand the psychological purpose bulimia has served.

In mild cases, brief goal-directed psychotherapy can help bulimic individuals to resume normal eating patterns and to restructure their lives and relationships. In severe cases, changes come slowly, and additional forms of therapy, such as family therapy or medication, may be needed.

NUTRITIONAL COUNSELING

Nutritional instruction is an important part of any treatment program for bulimia nervosa. Because their normal sensations of fullness, appetite, and hunger tend to be disturbed, these persons are initially told to disregard these sensations until they re-learn normal eating patterns. Although improvement begins within weeks on a regular schedule of modest meals, their bodies take months to readjust fully.

Individuals learn about symptoms, associated problems, medical complications (which improve along with eating behaviors), and weight regulation, so that they may recognize that recurrent bingeing and purging can cause metabolic disturbances, irritability, depression, and sleep disturbances. They also discover that neither vomiting nor laxatives are effective ways of reducing or controlling body fat, since vomiting usually does not retrieve everything they have eaten and laxatives have a minimal effect on absorption of calories. They are asked to eat only three planned meals a day, perhaps with one snack. Skipping meals is forbidden because regular eating decreases the urge to binge. Those within 10 percent of ideal weight may go on a maintenance diet, whereas those who are overweight aim for very gradual weight reduction so that they can lose weight without bingeing and purging.

GROUP THERAPY

Group therapy can be beneficial. A recent analysis of forty studies of this approach concluded it was of "moderate efficacy," with greater and more long-lasting improvement when it was combined with other forms of therapy. Groups that include nutritional counseling and management and that require more frequent sessions early in treatment may be more helpful than those that do not. Some groups place more emphasis on education to correct distorted ideas about food, weight, and dieting; others stress self-monitoring and progressive goal setting.

FAMILY THERAPY

The families of bulimic individuals need education about the nature and medical seriousness of bulimia and about the factors that may be helpful for treatment. Family therapy can also help to resolve long-buried issues, such as the extent to which unresolved conflicts may be contributing to the bulimia, and can show the family how to deal with these issues through direct negotiations. Those who receive caring support from their families during these sessions often feel less isolated and demoralized.

The relationship with a spouse often affects bulimic behavior patterns. Marital therapy is potentially very beneficial, especially for couples whose relationships have suffered because secretiveness about bulimia has interfered with intimacy.

MEDICATION

Selective serotonin reuptake inhibitors (SSRIs), such as the antidepressant fluoxetine (Prozac), have shown specific antibinge
activity independent of their antidepressant effects. Some psychiatrists consider a trial of Prozac or another SSRI part of the state
of the art of treatment for bulimia. Individuals often notice a
significant decrease in their desire to binge and purge within two
to four weeks. Bingeing may even stop completely. Relapses are
not uncommon, however, and some individuals appear to benefit
from long-term treatment with Prozac.

There have been few studies comparing psychotherapy with
medication; in general, a combination of medication and psychotherapy is considered most effective in the long run. In addition
to the SSRIs, other antidepressant medications, including certain
tricyclic antidepressants and monoamine oxidase (MAO) inhibitors,
have consistently proved more effective than placebos, especially
for individuals who also have symptoms of depressive, anxiety,
obsessive, or impulse disorders. Psychiatrists usually prescribe
the same doses of tricyclics and MAO inhibitors as for depression,
although Prozac seems more effective in higher doses.

In most studies comparing medication with supportive psychotherapy (described in Chapter 27), those who took medications experienced fewer and less severe binges, less preoccupation with
food, a greater sense of well-being, and decreased depression. In
small studies, women who have taken medication in combination
with psychotherapy had the most long-lasting relief.

HOSPITAL-BASED TREATMENT

Hospitalization is rarely necessary, but there are exceptions. These
include individuals at risk for potentially deadly arrhythmias because of serious electrolyte imbalances and dehydration, those
who have suffered acute distension of the stomach resulting from
binge eating, and those with tears of the esophagus (which are
rare) because of self-induced vomiting. Severe depression may also
require hospitalization if the person is at risk for suicide. Other
indications are severe alcohol or drug abuse (which must be
treated first or, if possible, simultaneously with the bulimia).

The first goal of both inpatient and partial hospitalization treatment (in which individuals live at home while undergoing a treatment program) is to halt the binge-purge cycle and re-establish
normal eating behavior. Individuals who receive regular, balanced
meals of sufficient calories to maintain their weight learn to accept
the feeling of having food in the stomach and to resist the impulse
to purge. Once they learn or re-learn normal eating behavior, the
focus shifts to interpersonal relationships and development of

social skills. Many bulimic persons have been isolated for so long that they must re-learn how to interact with others.

Before they complete a treatment program, individuals must have stopped bingeing and purging, resumed and maintained normal eating patterns, and shown significant psychological improvement. The prospect of ending this stage of treatment can be extremely frightening because it means leaving the relative safety of the program. It can help for a bulimic individual to first test the waters by going out for a meal with family and friends and seeing if newly learned coping techniques work. If these fail, as often happens, the staff can help the person to understand why and to develop alternative strategies to handle a situation differently.

RELAPSE PREVENTION

Individuals with bulimia nervosa are at highest risk for relapse in the initial months after successful treatment. They may be able to control their eating for a while but then fall back into previous patterns, especially during times of stress. During treatment, they and their therapists should prepare, discuss, and write out a plan of action to use when the danger of recurrence arises. This makes people less likely to overreact to an occasional binge and to use it as an excuse to return to their old eating behaviors. Dealing with problems such as low self-esteem and poor communication and interpersonal skills helps to prevent relapses. Although there are no long-term follow-up studies, relapse prevention with antidepressants, usually Prozac or another SSRI, may help some individuals in controlling the desire to binge and purge.

▼

Self-help   As noted above, cognitive-behavioral therapy uses extensive "homework" and teaches many useful coping skills, including keeping a diary and planning meals in advance. Some people find that twelve-step groups (described in detail in Chapter 10), such as Overeaters Anonymous, which is modeled on the Alcoholics Anonymous approach, can help. This group participation gives them a sense of connectedness with others who have similar problems, and makes round-the-clock support available at times of stress or possible relapse.

Some therapists have questioned the value of groups that focus exclusively on abstinence without also educating individuals about nutrition and eating behavior, or that serve as the sole initial treatment for bulimia. They also challenge the negative beliefs, such as "once a bulimic, always a bulimic," that are common in some of these groups, because most bulimic individuals who obtain professional help do recover from this disorder, even if they experience occasional lapses. However, self-help groups may be useful in the prevention of relapses.

▼

Impact on relationships

Bulimia nervosa is more likely to develop in families characterized by eating or emotional disturbances, including depressive disorders, alcoholism, obesity, anorexia nervosa, or parental binge eating. For bulimic individuals of normal weight, the family dynamics are often similar to those in cases of anorexia nervosa. Discovery of a person's bulimic behavior often generates great family turmoil and intense blaming and criticism. Parents may use a child's eating disorder to avoid dealing with their own marital problems, and family therapists can help family members sort out such issues.

In addition to psychological difficulties within their families, bulimic individuals almost always have problems in interpersonal relationships. Because they devote a great deal of time to concealing their behavior, they may isolate themselves from social situations. Over time, relationships with friends may also deteriorate. In severe, chronic bulimia, an individual may be unable to function at school or work because her life revolves around food.

▼

Outlook

Individuals usually show signs of improvement within two to four months of treatment. About 70 percent of those who complete treatment programs improve, reducing their bingeing and purging by anywhere from 50 to 90 percent. Persons with milder symptoms who can be treated as outpatients have a better prognosis than those with disabling symptoms who require hospitalization. Follow-up studies have documented sustained improvement for up to six years, although some symptoms, such as occasional bingeing, may persist, particularly during times of stress.

As the APA's Work Group on Eating Disorders notes, "Little is known about the natural history or long-term outcome of bulimia"—especially untreated bulimia. Some individuals have reported a "spontaneous" 25 to 30 percent reduction in their bingeing and purging over a period of one to two years. However, there are no scientific studies indicating whether such improvements occur often or prove to be long-lasting.

Is it an adjustment or a stress disorder?

Individuals with an adjustment or a stress disorder may:

- ☐ Develop emotional or behavioral symptoms after a stressful event or major life change in the previous three months

- ☐ Feel greater than expected distress or impairment as a result of these symptoms

- ☐ Be involved in or witness a traumatic event that threatens life or safety and that triggers intense fear, helplessness, or horror

- ☐ Feel emotionally numb or detached, or lack emotional responsiveness

- ☐ Become less aware of their surroundings

- ☐ Sense themselves or their environment as strange, unreal, or dreamlike

- ☐ Be unable to recall an important aspect of the traumatic event

- ☐ Re-experience a trauma in various ways, such as recurrent images, upsetting dreams, or flashbacks

- ☐ Feel extreme distress triggered by anything that symbolizes, resembles, or precipitates a memory of the traumatic event

- ☐ Deliberately avoid any person, place, or activity that reminds them of the trauma

- ☐ Have difficulty sleeping, be restless or irritable, have problems concentrating, be hyperalert, have exaggerated responses to sudden sounds

- ☐ Show less interest or participate less in significant activities

- ☐ Feel detached or estranged from others

- ☐ Be incapable of certain emotions, such as tender feelings

- ☐ Sense that they will not live a normal life span

- ☐ Feel great distress or impairment in work, studying, relating to others, or engaging in their usual activities

The more boxes that you or someone close to you checks, the more reason you have to be concerned about adjustment and stress-related disorders. This chapter provides information and insight about these disorders and guidance on seeking help.

12

Adjustment and Stress Disorders

Life happens. Cars crash. Companies fold. Loved ones become ill or die. Money runs out. A spouse has an affair. Such upheavals always take a toll, and it is normal for individuals in such situations to feel sad, tense, angry, overwhelmed, or incapable of coping with the ordinary demands of daily living. Such feelings and behaviors usually subside with time. The stressful event fades into the past, and those whose lives it has affected come to terms with its lasting consequences. But some individuals do not adapt; instead, they remain extremely upset and unable to function as they once did. This condition is called an *adjustment disorder.*

In other circumstances, the source of stress is a traumatic event in which individuals are caught up in or exposed to situations that threaten their lives and safety or those of others: natural disasters, airplane crashes, rape, kidnapping, street shootings, combat. People who survive such traumas normally experience strong emotional aftershocks, such as feeling very sad, frightened, guilty, ashamed, or angry. About 30 percent of the survivors of a disaster develop some psychiatric symptoms. Sometimes these symptoms are so severe and distressing or persist for so long that they interfere with normal functioning. In such cases, the problem may be an *acute stress disorder* or *posttraumatic stress disorder.*

Mental disorders triggered by stress may be much more prevalent than had previously been thought, and traumatic experiences may be a particularly common risk factor for women. In the

National Comorbidity Survey, published in 1994, 12 percent of women reported that a traumatic experience, most often rape or sexual molestation, had resulted in psychiatric problems.

Adjustment disorders

The term *adjustment disorder* refers to an out-of-the-ordinary response to a stressful event or situation. In *acute* adjustment disorders, symptoms last for less than six months. In *chronic* adjustment disorders, they persist for a longer period.

Adjustment disorders are categorized according to their dominant emotional and behavioral symptoms. The most common are:

- *Adjustment disorder with depressed mood,* characterized by sadness, tearfulness, and feelings of hopelessness

- *Adjustment disorder with anxiety,* characterized by nervousness, worry, and jitteriness

- *Adjustment disorder with mixed anxiety and depressed mood,* in which individuals experience a combination of anxiety and depression

- *Adjustment disorder with disturbance of conduct,* in which the primary sign of a disturbance is violation of societal norms and rules, such as fighting or vandalism

- *Adjustment disorder with mixed disturbance of emotions and conduct,* in which symptoms of depression, anxiety, or both, and conduct problems occur

- *Unspecified,* in which individuals may develop maladaptive responses, such as withdrawal or physical complaints.

▼
How common are adjustment disorders?

Anyone can have difficulty in adapting to a life crisis, but people may be much more vulnerable at certain times, as, for example, when first leaving their parents' home or after retiring from a long and gratifying career. Age is also a factor. The thirty-year-old who is laid off may be less devastated than the sixty-year-old who faces great difficulty getting another job. A childless young woman is likely to find it much more upsetting to undergo an emergency hysterectomy than a middle-aged mother with three children.

Most people who seek treatment for adjustment disorders are in their twenties. Adolescents tend to "act out" their difficulty in handling stress by skipping school, not doing homework, shoplifting, vandalizing, or engaging in other antisocial behavior. Adults are more likely to become depressed or anxious.

Adjustment disorders are also common among the elderly, who often react strongly to stressors that younger individuals might shrug off, such as an angry encounter on the subway. Correct diagnoses are not always made in such cases. An older person who becomes withdrawn after moving into a nursing home might be seen as demented rather than as having an adjustment disorder.

▼
What causes adjustment disorders?

Psychosocial stressors can take many forms: global events, such as a war or widespread famine; national events, such as the assassination of a political leader; regional events, such as an earthquake; large group events, such as strikes or racial discrimination; small group events, such as loss of a hard-fought basketball championship; and personal events, such as illness or the betrayal of a friend. The impact of any of these situations depends on the meaning they have for a particular individual. No two people may respond to the same situation in the same way.

The key to understanding stress responses is not the nature of the stressor but the way individuals react to stress. Some people collapse, whereas others manage to cope. Why? Each person may simply have a different psychological "breaking point," depending on the intensity of stressors, underlying personality, and temperament. Age, gender, and physical well-being can also be factors.

Any event or combination of circumstances can lead to an adjustment disorder. The stressor does not have to be extreme; even a seemingly minor event, such as the news that an ex-spouse has remarried, may cause great psychological pain.

Some people who develop adjustment disorders experience a single stressful life crisis, such as a divorce; others go through a period of several simultaneous stressors, such as family illnesses in combination with financial problems. Stressors may recur at certain times every year (for example, the Christmas crush for a toy store owner or the anniversary of a child's death), or they may be continuous (such as the pressures of caring for several small children or living with an alcoholic spouse). Specific developmental events (such as leaving home, getting married, having a child, losing a job, or retiring) can also trigger adjustment disorders. Sometimes an entire community, such as the residents of a town hit by a devastating flood or hurricane, develops emotional symptoms.

▼
How an adjustment disorder feels

After being fired, a copywriter is unable to sleep, feels jumpy all the time, irritable, and angry. A college student whose boyfriend breaks up with her cannot concentrate during lectures. A woman who suffered a miscarriage weeps uncontrollably when she sees a baby at a mall or in the park. An individual identified as HIV-positive continues to seek out new sex partners and does not practice safe sex. A parent who loses custody of a child withdraws from everyone, refusing to leave the house.

Each of these reactions is understandable for a brief period.

However, if such reactions become so intense or last so long that they create great internal misery or interfere with normal functioning, they can be signs of an adjustment disorder.

The feelings associated with an adjustment disorder vary greatly. If anxiety is the primary problem, individuals worry and fret, feeling nervous and jittery most or all of the time. In an adjustment disorder with depression, the emotions associated with major depression predominate: sadness, tearfulness, helplessness, hopelessness, despair. Some people experience a combination of anxious and depressed feelings.

In contrast to the fleeting feelings of sadness or anxiety that are common after any traumatic event, adjustment disorders involve more persistent and distressing emotions. Whereas most people come to terms with setbacks, those who develop adjustment disorders do not feel better or find life easier to deal with as time passes. Usually their symptoms begin within three months of the stressful occurrence. If the stressor is a specific event, such as being fired, the disorder usually lasts only a few months. If the stressor persists, however, as in a chronic illness, it may take longer for an individual to come to terms with it.

The severity of a stressor does not determine the severity of an adjustment disorder. People who are particularly vulnerable may find it extremely difficult to cope even with a mild stressor, as when their car is broken into and a tape deck stolen. Others will have only minor difficulty adjusting to a much greater trauma, such as the loss of their home in a fire.

▼

Seeking help The problem for individuals reeling from the impact of a trauma or a life crisis lies in trying to sort out which feelings are normal under the circumstances and which are not. If you suspect that an adjustment disorder may be troubling you or someone close to you, these are the questions that should be asked:

- Did your emotional or behavioral symptoms develop after a stressful event or life change in the previous three months?

- Do these symptoms cause much greater distress than might be expected, considering what happened?

- Do the symptoms interfere significantly with your ability to work, study, relate to others, or carry on your usual activities?

- Have your symptoms persisted for more than six months?

If you or someone close to you answers "yes" to these questions, the problem may be an adjustment disorder, and professional help may be of benefit.

Is it an adjustment disorder?

According to the DSM-IV, a diagnosis of an adjustment disorder should be based on these criteria:

■ Development of emotional or behavioral symptoms in response to an identifiable stressor that occurred within the previous three months

■ These symptoms are clinically significant, as shown by either:
1. Marked distress in excess of what would be expected from exposure to the stressor, or
2. Significant impairment in social, occupational, or academic functioning

■ No other mental disorder accounts for the symptoms.

■ Bereavement is not responsible for the symptoms.

■ Symptoms do not persist for more than six months after the termination of the stressor or its consequences.

Adapted from the Diagnostic and Statistical Manual of Mental Disorders, 4th Edition. *Used with permission.*

A thorough physical examination and a careful, comprehensive history may be necessary to determine whether the problem is a normal and expectable reaction to stress or an adjustment disorder. Mental health professionals also check for other psychiatric problems, such as depression or a personality disorder, that may worsen under stress. Sometimes individuals have both a personality disorder and an adjustment disorder.

▼

Risks and complications

If unrecognized and untreated, an adjustment disorder may lead to other mental disorders, such as major depression or an anxiety disorder. Teenagers coping with the normal upheavals of adolescence may be vulnerable to lingering problems if they do not get help with unexpected or especially difficult transitions. There is an increased risk for suicide, especially in the elderly.

▼

Treating adjustment disorders

There is no specific treatment for an adjustment disorder, although the goal is always the same: improving an individual's ability to adapt. The primary means to this end is talking. Putting painful fears and feelings into words reduces the pressure caused by the stressor and enhances the individual's ability to cope. Ordinarily, time helps to ease the pain or difficulty of coping with a stressful situation. When the impact of a crisis is more intense or persistent, supportive therapy can help.

Brief psychotherapy can help a person to understand the significance of what has happened, put it into perspective, deal with it in a more healthful way, or in cases in which the source of

Getting adjusted

Kathryn thought that people had to have something terrible happen to make them feel bad. "I should be happier than ever," she told herself. Her husband, Stuart, had been transferred from Cleveland, their home town, to a better-paying job in San Diego. They'd bought a California-style house with everything she'd ever wanted, right down to wraparound decks and a pool. But three months after the move, Kathryn developed a case of the blues that she just couldn't shake.

Stuart was totally wrapped up in his new job, working longer hours than ever. Their two teenaged sons had discovered surfing and spent every free moment at the beach. Although Kathryn had built a thriving catering business in Cleveland, the thought of starting from scratch in a bigger city frightened her. And although everyone in the neighborhood waved and wished her a good day, she hadn't made a single new friend. She spent her days lying next to their pool or staring blankly at the TV. All she could think of was the little Cape Cod house they'd left behind—the home where their children had grown—and the friends who were as much a part of life as the air she breathed.

When an old friend from "back home" called, Kathryn poured out her misery. "What's wrong with me?" she sobbed. "I must be crazy!" Her friend reassured her that she had good reason to be sad. She'd left behind a lifetime of friends and memories, and she hadn't found anyone or anything to replace the severed connections in her life. "Kath," said her friend, "you're not the type to mope around. Why don't you just get out there and start making the most of it?"

Kathryn realized her friend was right: She'd been through a major life change and had lost many important relationships in her life. She couldn't move back to Cleveland or bring back her old life. But there were two things she could do something about: her isolation from others and her inactivity.

Living in one of the country's most beautiful areas, Kathryn decided to take advantage of it. At first, it was all she could do to pull herself out of the house and go for a walk. Her strolls, which gradually grew longer and took her further from home, made her curious. She checked books on local history out of the library and began reading about the Spanish mission and the old town of San Diego. She began attending lectures and slide shows sponsored by the city's historical society. When one of the women she met asked her to volunteer as a guide, she was flattered.

As she felt more sure of herself, Kathryn sat down with her husband and expressed her worries that they were growing apart. Together they blocked out some weekends when they could plan some just-for-us trips. By the time her old friend came out to visit, Kathryn was delighted to show off her new city.

stress is ongoing, as in caring for an elderly parent, adapt to it more effectively. Specific recommendations may include confronting difficult issues individuals may have been avoiding, keeping a journal of symptoms and ways of coping with them, learning stress reduction techniques, and joining self-help groups. In some cases, as when a spouse's substance use or infidelity is the source of stress, family therapy may be helpful.

Through group therapy that involves people with similar problems, individuals can learn more about their problem, gain a fresh perspective on it, face emotional issues, release pent-up feelings, become less sensitive about thorny issues, and feel less isolated.

In their sessions, group members come to realize that, given the circumstances with which they are dealing, their feelings are entirely normal—even such black emotions as desperation, hopelessness, guilt, or fear. Most individuals continue to attend group sessions until they feel that they can cope adequately with their life circumstances.

Although medication may be prescribed to relieve specific symptoms, psychiatric drugs are not considered a primary treatment for an adjustment disorder. When needed, they should be used as a supplement to psychotherapy, in the lowest possible dose, and for the briefest possible time. Thus, a psychiatrist may prescribe a sleeping pill for a few nights for a distraught young man who has lost his job and whose insomnia is interfering with his ability to function during the day—but the man takes the medication only for those few nights and continues therapy. When used properly, medication enhances rather than interferes with psychotherapy.

In the past, physicians often routinely prescribed anti-anxiety drugs, such as the benzodiazepines (the group of medications that includes Xanax and Valium), for individuals with adjustment disorders and anxiety, often for extended periods of time. This practice is neither effective nor appropriate. If they are needed, anti-anxiety drugs, which can make extremely agitated individuals more comfortable, should be used only for a limited time.

▼
Self-help   Recognizing that you have been through or are facing unusual stress is the first step. The stress management techniques described in Chapter 29 may help. Take extraordinarily good care of yourself, paying special attention to diet, sleep, and exercise. Talk through your feelings with a close friend or someone, such as a minister, whom you respect and trust. Find out if there are any self-help or support groups for people coping with similar problems, and attend their meetings. For many people, religion provides support and comfort in times of difficulty and crisis.

▼
Impact on relationships   Sometimes the loved ones of those with adjustment disorders may be dealing with the impact of the same stressor. A move or the birth of a baby, for example, affects the entire family. Persons who adapt quickly may be baffled by and unsympathetic to those who do not bounce back as rapidly. Spouses and children may resent their emotional unavailability. Family therapy can help everyone to understand how the stressful event has altered their relationships and what they can do about these changes.

▼
Outlook   Adjustment disorders do improve with time, and the prognosis, particularly for adults, is good. Adolescents may have a more difficult time getting back on track. In several follow-up studies, most of the adults were completely well five years later, but a significant percentage of teenagers continued to struggle with a range of personal problems and mental disorders.

Acute stress disorder

Some individuals who have survived an unusually frightening experience or event develop symptoms that are more severe than those of an adjustment disorder, but they are not suffering from posttraumatic stress disorder (described later in this chapter). Recognized for the first time as an official psychiatric disorder in the *DSM-IV*, acute stress disorder is classified as an anxiety disorder and does produce some classic anxiety-related symptoms. However, many of its other symptoms are "dissociative"; that is, they involve an altered sense of identity, memory, or perception. (Chapter 18 discusses dissociative disorders.) By definition, the symptoms of acute stress disorder occur within one month of exposure to an extremely traumatic stressor, last for at least two days, and resolve within four weeks.

▼
How common is acute stress disorder?   Most persons who experience or witness a traumatic event, such as a natural disaster, physical assault, accident, or combat, develop symptoms. The more severe the traumatic stressor, the greater the likelihood that symptoms will occur. In studies of survivors of disasters, such as the firestorm in Oakland, California, in 1991 and the Loma Prieta earthquake in the San Francisco Bay area in 1989, a quarter to a third developed symptoms such as emotional numbing and an inability to feel deeply about anything.

▼
What causes acute stress disorder?   Acute stress disorder is a reaction to events that involve actual or threatened death or serious injury or that threaten the physical integrity of the individual or others. Overwhelmed by fear or helplessness, people may develop dissociative symptoms, such as numbing or detachment, as a psychological defense. "It may well be that dissociation works well at the time of trauma," says David Spiegel, M.D., professor of psychiatry and behavioral sciences at Stanford University and a leading expert on dissociation, "but if the defense persists too long, it interferes with the working through necessary to put traumatic experience into perspective."

Is it acute stress disorder?

According to the DSM-IV, a diagnosis of acute stress disorder should be based on these criteria:

■ Exposure to a traumatic event in which:

1. The person experienced, witnessed, or was confronted with an event or events involving actual or threatened death or serious injury, or a threat to the physical integrity of the person or of others, and

2. The person's response involved intense fear, helplessness, or horror

■ Either while or immediately after experiencing the distressing event, the individual develops at least three of the following dissociative symptoms:

1. A subjective sense of numbing, detachment, or absence of emotional responsiveness

2. A reduction in awareness of surroundings (e.g., being in a daze)

3. Derealization (the environment seems unreal or dream-like)

4. Depersonalization (feeling detached, as if one were an outside observer of one's own mental processes or body, or feeling like an automaton)

5. Dissociative amnesia (inability to recall an important aspect of the trauma)

■ Persistent re-experiencing of the traumatic event in at least one of the following ways: recurrent images, thoughts, dreams, illusions, flashbacks, or a sense of reliving the experience; or distress when exposed to reminders of the traumatic event

■ Marked avoidance of thoughts, feelings, conversations, activities, places, or people that arouse recollections of the trauma

■ Marked symptoms of anxiety or increased arousal, such as difficulty sleeping, irritability, poor concentration, hypervigilance, exaggerated startle response, or motor restlessness

■ The disturbance causes significant distress or impairment in social, occupational, or other important areas of functioning or prevents the individual from performing some necessary task, such as obtaining necessary medical or legal assistance or mobilizing personal resources by telling family members about the traumatic experience.

■ Symptoms last for a minimum of two days and a maximum of four weeks and occur within four weeks of the trauma.

■ The disturbance is not due to the physiological effects of a substance (drugs of abuse or medication), a medical condition, a brief psychotic disorder [see Chapter 17], or exacerbation of a mental or personality disorder.

Adapted from the Diagnostic and Statistical Manual of Mental Disorders, 4th Edition. *Used with permission.*

▼

How acute stress disorder feels

At the time of the traumatic event or immediately after it, people feel intense fear, helplessness, or horror. The suddenness of the trauma and loss of control over what is or might be happening to their bodies sometimes leads them to experience themselves or their surroundings in a different way. Many feel detached or have a sense of psychological numbing. They may feel that they are in a daze, not fully aware of where they are or what is going on around them. The environment may become dreamlike or unreal. Some see themselves as observers watching their own bodies or listening in on their own thoughts. Others feel less than fully human, more like automatons or robots. Afterwards, individuals may not be able to remember where they were, what happened when, or how they felt or reacted at the time of the experience.

Within four weeks of the traumatic event, they may also begin to re-experience it repeatedly. Distressing images or thoughts may intrude into their consciousness. They may have vivid, upsetting dreams and nightmares. Some have disturbing illusions or flashbacks, or feel they are reliving the experience. Many become upset when they confront reminders of the trauma and may do everything possible to avoid places, people, activities, objects, thoughts, or feelings that might trigger recollections of what happened.

Individuals with acute stress disorder typically develop various symptoms of anxiety as well, such as problems in sleeping, irritability, poor concentration, a sense of hyperalertness, physical restlessness, and an extreme reaction when startled, as by an unexpected noise. They may find it hard to enjoy activities that they once found pleasurable and feel guilty resuming their usual routine. Some feel hopeless and despairing.

▼

Seeking help

Individuals with acute stress disorder are often so distressed and dazed that they cannot seek help for themselves. Some seem unusually calm, which friends and family may misinterpret as an indication that they made it through the trauma in good shape. If you suspect that someone you know may be suffering from this disorder, these are the questions that should be asked:

- Has the person experienced or witnessed a traumatic event that was extremely frightening or horrifying?

- During or after the trauma, has the person described or shown signs of emotional numbing, detachment, or a lack of any emotional response?

- Does the person seem to be in a daze or unaware of his or her surroundings?

- Does the person describe him- or herself or the environment as different, changed, unreal, or dreamlike?

- Is the person unable to recall an important aspect of the trauma?

- Has the person been re-experiencing the trauma in recurrent images, thoughts, dreams, illusions, or flashbacks?

- Does the person become very upset by reminders of the trauma and go to great lengths to avoid anything that might trigger such memories?

- Does the person have noticeable symptoms of anxiety, such as difficulty in sleeping, restlessness, irritability, poor concentration, or hyperalertness?

If the answer to these questions is "yes," the problem may be acute stress disorder. You should arrange for the individual to see a mental health professional as soon as possible. Early treatment can prevent long-term problems.

▼

Risks and complications

Acute stress disorder causes significant distress and interferes with a person's ability to work, study, relate to others, or maintain usual routine and social activities. It also can keep individuals from necessary tasks. Persons with acute stress disorder are at increased risk of developing *posttraumatic stress disorder* (PTSD), a more persistent disorder described later in this chapter.

▼

Treating acute stress disorder

Individuals with an acute stress disorder benefit from the same approaches that can help in PTSD, described on page 280. Initially, they need protection, consolation, assurance of safety, and assistance with decisions and plans. The greatest help of all may be the support of those closest to them.

Supportive psychotherapy with a focus on working through emotional responses to trauma or stress is also beneficial. With training in self-hypnosis, persons can induce a pleasant sense of floating lightness to replace their distressing feelings. Relaxation techniques, such as progressive muscle relaxation and biofeedback, can also help. If a person is unable to get much-needed rest, benzodiazepine sleeping pills may be prescribed either for a single night or for a week or so until normal sleep patterns return.

▼

Self-help

As soon as possible—preferably before going to sleep the night after the trauma—it helps to talk about what happened with an empathic person or with someone who has shared the same or a similar experience. This enables people to begin to deal with what has just occurred. In group sessions, which should also begin soon after the trauma, they can share views and experiences. Self-care techniques, such as relaxation and self-hypnosis, are useful, and social rituals, such as a memorial service when someone has died or a funeral for accident victims, can help those who survived to come to terms with the meaning of the loss.

▼

Impact on relationships

Sometimes individuals who have survived a trauma are so upset or stunned that they do not tell family members or friends what has happened. A young rape victim, for example, may not confide in her parents because she fears they may blame or condemn her. Once those close to the person learn what their loved one has been through, they can help by ensuring that he or she obtains appropriate treatment, and by encouraging discussion—repeatedly, if need be—about the traumatic event.

▼

Outlook

Although little is known about this recently recognized disorder, mental health professionals believe that with early intervention to help the person acknowledge, confront, and put into perspective a traumatic experience, most individuals can recover and will not suffer long-term problems.

Posttraumatic stress disorder

Posttraumatic stress disorder (PTSD) is an intense, persistent, extremely distressing response to an event that threatened a life or safety. Although it was first designated as a psychiatric disorder in 1980, this syndrome had been recognized much earlier, particularly during wartime. PTSD gained its greatest attention after the Vietnam War, when large numbers of American veterans developed troubling symptoms after returning home.

But combat is by no means the only experience that can forever change the way in which people view themselves and their world. A woman may be brutally raped. A man may survive an airplane crash that killed most of the other passengers. A child may be kidnapped. A teenager may be shot in a drive-by shooting. A family may see their home destroyed by a fire or flood. Coming to grips with the impact of such experiences always requires time to accept what has happened and to work through the painful implications.

In PTSD, the reaction goes beyond such normal responses and includes intrusive thoughts and feelings and the denial or avoidance of upsetting emotions. Individuals with PTSD re-experience their terror and helplessness again and again in their thoughts or dreams. To block this psychic pain, they avoid anything associated with the trauma. Those who have been mugged, shot, or raped may be afraid to venture out by themselves. Some with the disorder enter a state of emotional numbness and are no longer able to respond to people and experiences the way they once did, especially in showing tenderness or affection.

▼

How common is PTSD?

PTSD can occur in childhood, adolescence, or adulthood. In epidemiological studies, the lifetime prevalence has ranged from 1 to 14 percent. Up to 30 percent of disaster victims may develop PTSD. Most of the men with PTSD have experienced combat; most of the women have been raped or physically assaulted.

Individuals who have had previous psychiatric problems or have experienced previous traumas, such as childhood abuse, may be especially vulnerable, possibly because of a greater sensitivity induced by the traumatic experience. Those who have few social supports are also more likely to develop PTSD. Individuals exposed to the most shocking or terrible aspects of a disaster—such as watching others burn to death or removing the bodies of the wounded or dead—are more prone to PTSD than those who were spared such experiences.

▼

What causes PTSD?

The conditions or events that lead to PTSD would be profoundly distressing to anyone. They include natural disasters (floods, hurricanes, earthquakes) and accidents (car or airplane crashes, large fires, the collapse of physical structures), although both of these kinds of stressors are less likely to induce the disorder than are those that violate an individual's self-esteem and sense of integrity as a person: torture, rape, and personal assaults (sexual abuse, shootings, muggings, robbery). The trauma of discovering a serious threat or harm to a close friend or relative, such as finding out that a child has been kidnapped or killed, can cause PTSD. The disorder tends to be more severe and longer lasting when the stressor is not an act of fate or bad luck but instead involves deliberate human malice.

Acts of violence or destruction (bombing, hijackings, or combat) can lead to PTSD. So can certain physical conditions that cause damage to the brain, such as head injury. The death of a loved one, particularly under violent circumstances, can also cause PTSD, although most bereaved people do not develop the disorder even though, as part of the normal process of mourning, they may feel guilt, fear of dying, shame, and sadness.

Some researchers believe that traumatic events produce the

Is it post-traumatic stress disorder?

According to the DSM-IV, a diagnosis of posttraumatic stress disorder should be based on these criteria:

■ **Exposure to a traumatic event in which:**

1. **The person experienced, witnessed, or was confronted with an event or events that involved actual or threatened death or serious injury, or a threat to the physical integrity of self or others, and**

2. **The person's response involved intense fear, helplessness, or horror (in children, may be distressed or agitated behavior)**

■ **Persistent re-experiencing of a traumatic event in at least one of the following ways:**

1. **Recurrent and intrusive distressing recollections of the event, including images, thoughts, or perceptions (in children, repetitive play expressing themes or aspects of the trauma)**

2. **Recurrent, distressing dreams of the event (in children, frightening dreams without any recognizable content)**

3. **Acting or feeling as if the traumatic event were recurring, including a sense of reliving the experience, illusions, hallucinations, and dissociative flashback episodes, including those that occur upon awakening or when intoxicated (young children may reenact the trauma)**

4. **Intense psychological distress at exposure to internal or external cues that symbolize or resemble the traumatic event**

5. **Physiological reactivity when exposed to such cues**

■ **Persistent avoidance of stimuli associated with the trauma and numbing of general responsiveness as indicated by at least three of the following:**

1. **Efforts to avoid thoughts, feelings, or conversations associated with the trauma**

symptoms of PTSD by causing changes in brain chemistry and in levels of stress-related hormones. From a behavioral perspective, PTSD may be a conditioned response to a certain stimulus, as when, for example, the sound of a helicopter provokes the physiological and psychological experience of being in combat.

PTSD also may stem from the difficulty involved in grasping and assimilating a traumatic experience. During a catastrophe or serious crisis, too much occurs too quickly for the mind to absorb completely what has happened and to deal with its emotional implications. The traumatic perceptions, which appear to enter the memory in a way that causes them to retain a nightmarish vividness for years or even decades thereafter, take so much time to process that they may return again and again as intrusive images. Each time they return, they set into motion the information processing needed to understand and to come to grips with a trauma.

2. Efforts to avoid activities, places, or people that arouse recollections of it
3. Inability to recall an important aspect of the trauma
4. Markedly diminished interest or participation in significant activities
5. Feeling detached or estranged from others
6. Restricted range of feelings (e.g., an inability to feel love)
7. A sense of a foreshortened future (not expecting to have a career, marriage, children, or a normal life span)

■ Persistent symptoms of increased arousal (not present before the trauma), as indicated by at least two of the following:
    1. Difficulty falling or staying asleep
    2. Irritability or outbursts of anger
    3. Difficulty concentrating
    4. Hypervigilance
    5. Exaggerated startle response

■ Symptoms persisting for more than one month

■ Clinically significant distress or impaired social, occupational, or other important areas of functioning as a result

PTSD may be acute (with symptoms lasting less than three months) or chronic (lasting three months or more) or have a delayed onset (with symptoms not developing for at least six months after the trauma).

Adapted from the Diagnostic and Statistical Manual of Mental Disorders, 4th Edition. *Used with permission.*

▼

How PTSD feels   PTSD can develop in stages. Immediately or soon after the trauma, individuals may feel greater anxiety, respond more intensely than others to the trauma, and become obsessed or preoccupied with it. After four to six weeks of this mounting distress, they begin to feel helpless and out of control and to re-experience the trauma, with intensely vivid recollections intruding on their dreams or waking thoughts. Increasingly, their lives focus around the traumatic event, and they may change their lifestyle, personality, and social relationships. Some begin to avoid certain places or situations. Many persons become extremely irritable and are afraid of losing control of their tempers. Survivors who have committed violent acts, such as combat veterans, may be so fearful of their potential for violence that they try to stifle angry feelings. However, their suppressed rage may periodically explode.

Many individuals show signs of psychic numbing, as if they were in a state of emotional anesthesia. They feel cut off from others, uninterested in activities they once enjoyed, and incapable of certain emotions, particularly those associated with intimacy, tenderness, and sexuality. Physiologically, they are always agitated. They may not be able to fall asleep or stay asleep, in part because of recurrent nightmares in which they relive the trauma. They jump at the slightest sound. During the day, they are always on guard and may have difficulty concentrating or completing tasks. Over time, PTSD can become chronic, with individuals feeling despondent and demoralized by symptoms they can neither understand nor control.

Not all cases of PTSD follow this course. Sometimes symptoms do not develop for months or even years. (This is more likely to happen after a major catastrophe rather than an "ordinary" accident.) Some individuals with PTSD completely forget an important part of the traumatic event, a condition called *dissociative amnesia*. Others relive parts of the trauma and behave as if it were occurring at that moment. Symptoms may worsen at anniversaries or during situations that resemble or symbolize the trauma.

Whatever its course, persons with PTSD describe themselves as fearful of a repetition of the trauma or of sharing the fate of others who died or were injured. They may feel rage at those responsible, resentment toward those who were not harmed, shame over their own helplessness, remorse over what they thought or did during the event, and guilt because they survived and others did not.

Children who live through a trauma, such as witnessing a schoolyard shooting, may not talk at all or may refuse to discuss what happened, but this does not mean they cannot remember what occurred. Younger children may have distressing dreams of the event that change over time into generalized nightmares of monsters or other threats. Young children typically relive the trauma through repetitive play. They also may develop a variety of physical symptoms, such as stomachaches and headaches. Many youngsters no longer think of the future in the way they once did; some no longer expect to live a long time, get married, or have families or careers of their own.

At all ages, symptoms of depression and anxiety are common. Adults may act impulsively, suddenly changing their place of residence, disappearing without explanation, or switching to an unconventional lifestyle. Some develop the symptoms of a physically induced mental disorder, such as failing memory, difficulty in concentrating, frequent mood shifts, headache, and vertigo.

▼

Seeking help   Many people who have had a traumatic experience put off seeking help because they expect to feel upset, given the circumstances, and do not realize that care is advisable. However, the sooner that trauma survivors seek and receive psychological help, the better they are likely to fare.

If you or someone close to you has experienced or witnessed a traumatic event that was extremely frightening and upsetting, PTSD may be a problem. If you suspect that this is so, these are the questions (organized into groups) that should be asked:

- Have you been repeatedly re-experiencing the trauma in various ways, such as in recurrent images, distressing dreams, or flashbacks?
- Do you feel extremely upset by anything that symbolizes, resembles, or reminds you of the traumatic event?
- Do you try to avoid thinking or talking about the trauma?
- Do you avoid any activities, places, or people that could remind you of it?
- Are you unable to remember an important aspect of the trauma?

- Have you lost interest or reduced your participation in major activities in your life?
- Do you feel detached or estranged from others?
- Do you feel incapable of certain emotions, such as tenderness or loving feelings?
- Do you sense that you will not live a normal life span, marry, or have children or a career?

- Have you had difficulty in falling or staying asleep, irritability or outbursts of anger, difficulty in concentrating, or jumpiness?

- Have your symptoms persisted for more than a month?
- Have they caused you great distress or interfered with your ability to work, study, relate to others, or engage in your usual activities?

If the answer to at least one of the questions in each group is "yes," the problem could be a response to the trauma you or the person close to you endured. It is wise to seek professional help as soon as possible rather than to wait for further symptoms to develop or to turn to self-destructive ways of coping, such as drinking or drug use.

In evaluating survivors of traumatic life experiences, mental health professionals must differentiate between normal stress responses, acute stress disorder, and PTSD. Individuals with PTSD respond more intensely than others, becoming panicky, exhausted, or incapable of movement. Instead of normal denial, they withdraw, turn to drugs or alcohol, act impulsively, or consider suicide. They feel distracted, pressured, or confused, and develop physical symptoms. Unable to work through their feelings (as normally happens during the process of bereavement, for example), they become anxious and depressed and unable to work or love. Therapists also look for signs of anxiety disorders, depression, or another mental disorder; these problems may develop along with PTSD and also require treatment.

▼

Risks and complications

Individuals who have recently been through a trauma are at higher risk of accidents because they cannot concentrate, their attention wanders, and they may overreact to a sudden sound or movement. They should avoid driving, operating dangerous machinery, and any tasks that demand alertness for safety.

PTSD can lead to phobias about certain situations or activities that resemble or symbolize the original trauma. Frequent mood swings, depression, and guilt may lead to substance abuse, self-defeating behavior, or suicidal actions. Other complications can include aggression and violence, as well as their consequences. Nevertheless, despite the common misconception that PTSD may lead combat veterans to commit crimes, one study found that only those who had committed criminal acts before their military service committed similar offenses afterward.

▼

Treating PTSD

Individuals with PTSD may require different types of help at different stages. During the first days after the trauma, protection, reassurance of safety, help with decisions and plans, and the support of those closest to them can be most significant in easing their distress. Simple companionship—even that of a pet—can make a difference.

MEDICATION

Benzodiazepine sleeping pills may be prescribed either for a single night or for a week or so until normal sleep patterns return. Small doses of anti-anxiety drugs can ease intense feelings of distress or panic during the day. These medications are not recommended for long-term use and are usually prescribed on an as-needed basis.

In various reports, antidepressant medications have shown to be effective in reducing nightmares, flashbacks, panic attacks, and episodes of anxiety. However, most psychiatrists feel that medication should be prescribed only as part of a treatment plan that includes working through traumatic memories in psychotherapy. Some report that drug treatment has a positive impact on psychotherapy, boosting motivation and easing distressing symptoms. Individuals with PTSD who develop a major depression may benefit from antidepressant medication.

PSYCHOTHERAPY

Brief psychotherapy, usually consisting of twelve to twenty sessions, is recommended for most cases of PTSD. (Long-term therapy has not proved any more effective.) The first step in therapy is the recounting of the events that occurred before, during, and after the trauma, with the person elaborating on the bare facts and adding personal meaning and interpretations to them. The therapist works to build an alliance, a solid working relationship, with the person so that he or she feels safe enough to reappraise the implications of what has happened. As individuals achieve greater awareness and their trust in the therapist increases, they are able to confront and then assimilate thoughts about the trauma that they may have blocked. This process continues until the final sessions, when they prepare for the end of the therapy and the work they must continue on their own.

Hypnosis, which helps enhance control over dissociative states and experiences, can be especially beneficial in individuals with PTSD, who tend to be excellent subjects. (Chapter 27 discusses hypnosis.) Enhanced feelings of control are especially important, since the loss of physical control is the core of trauma. This is often symbolically re-experienced as a loss of mental control over traumatic memories. The intensity of traumatic experience, with its strong central focus, is similar to hypnosis, and the state of focused attention in hypnosis can be used to retrieve traumatic memories, face them, and view them in a clearer or broader perspective. For example, an assault victim may say, "Yes, he tried to kill me, but I fought him off, and I survived." This is the difference between merely reliving trauma and working it through: Individuals learn to transform the memory, making the uncomfortable emotions associated with it more bearable.

When therapists utilize hypnosis, many people can recall memories that may have been pushed out of consciousness and see them from a new point of view. One way of doing this is with a "split-screen" technique, in which individuals project an image of the traumatic event on one-half of an imaginary screen. On the other half of the screen they project an image of what they did to protect themselves or to survive. This can make very painful life events easier to think about, accept, and bear. In a hypnotic trance, individuals can remember as much of the traumatic event as they wish, when they wish, rather than desperately trying not to recall what happened. In this way they come to recognize that once they have dealt with their memories and put them into perspective, they can leave them behind. Various behavioral techniques, including cognitive therapy, systematic desensitization, and relaxation training, also have proved useful.

After the rape

Alice never saw his face. That night, as she walked into the parking garage, she remembers feeling nervous. The seminar she'd been attending had run late, and there were few cars left. As she fumbled with her car keys, the man grabbed her from behind. He stuck something vile into her mouth and pinned her against the car. When she struggled to get free, he began banging her head—again and again—against the roof of the car. The pain was excruciating, and Alice could feel blood oozing down her forehead. She thinks she must have blacked out for a few minutes. The next thing she remembers was the man's weight on top of her as he thrust himself into her. She lay there limply, feigning unconsciousness, through the endless minutes. When he finally stood up, he reached for her purse, then kicked her, over and over, in the head and back. She lay there, whimpering with pain, until she heard voices—a man and woman chatting—and called for help. At the hospital, the rape counselor kept saying the same thing: "It's over. You're alive. You're going to be okay. It's over."

These words became Alice's mantra. She repeated them to herself at the police station, in the shower at home, the next morning when she woke up and felt the terror flood back into her body. She called in sick for a few days and, wrapped in an old fuzzy robe, stayed in her apartment watching back-to-back movies on television. She told a few very close friends what had happened and went to one meeting of a support group for rape victims. But listening to the stories of other women, resonating with their pain, was more than she could bear. She left early and never returned.

For a few weeks she went through the motions of her usual routine. She tried to stay busy, to be around people, to push the ugly memories of the rape out of mind. But every time she'd read about a rape or see someone attacked on television or in a movie, her heart would start pounding and she would be unable to think about anything else. When any of the men she had been dating called, Alice made excuses to avoid seeing them. In time she stopped going out at all during the evenings, and since just approaching her car made her tremble, she almost never drove anywhere.

Six months after the rape, Alice couldn't understand why she still felt so shaky and irritable. When the rape counselor called and asked how she felt, Alice described herself as numb, not really feeling anything at all, at least during the day.

At night she would wake up screaming from intensely vivid nightmares—always of the man, the garage, the pain, the rape. Then the flashbacks started. She'd be sitting at her desk, reading a newspaper, walking down the street, and something—a scene, a sound, a smell—would trigger a flood of memories. Suddenly she was back in the garage, reliving the rape.

Alice was desperate when she called a therapist with extensive experience in helping trauma victims. One of the techniques that she suggested was hypnosis. After teaching Alice how to induce a hypnotic trance, she had her conjure up a split screen. On one side, she visualized the rape. In the other, she focused on what she did to protect herself and survive, such as feigning unconsciousness. This process helped to restore Alice's shattered sense of control by enabling her to face her memories, put them in perspective, and, after several months of therapy, leave them behind. "I'll never forget what happened," she says. "But I've been able to put the past in the past so it no longer has such power over me or my future."

▼

Self-help   Often talking about what happened with an empathic person or someone who has shared the experience, ideally, before going to sleep on the actual day the trauma occurred, can help an individual begin to deal with the trauma. Group sessions, preferably beginning as soon as possible after the trauma, enable individuals to share views and experiences. When there has been a death or deaths, societal rituals can provide a meaningful context for what has happened. A funeral for accident victims, for example, can help those who survived to deal with their conflicting feelings of relief that they did not perish and of guilt because others did.

Support groups made up of others who have experienced a similar trauma (such as parents of murder victims, combat veterans, families of individuals who committed suicide) are especially helpful in providing empathy, understanding, and encouragement. Self-care techniques, such as relaxation, are also useful during and after psychotherapy or counseling.

▼

Impact on relationships   After the trauma, loved ones can provide invaluable help by offering consolation, assuring individuals that they are safe and protected, and helping with decisions and plans that need to be made. Such support can make more of a difference to the person's mental and emotional condition than anything else. In the weeks and months after the trauma, love and acceptance remain critically important but can be more difficult for affected individuals to accept because, as they try to stifle painful memories and feelings, they unconsciously damp down their normal emotional responses. Feelings related to tenderness, affection, love, and sexuality are the hardest for those with PTSD to acknowledge and express. Their closest friends and family members may feel rejected and helpless. For them, talking with a counselor or attending support groups can provide insight and foster greater understanding of a loved one with PTSD.

▼

Outlook   Without recognition and treatment, PTSD can last as long as thirty or forty years, with symptoms intensifying during periods of stress. When identified and treated, more than half of affected persons achieve complete recovery within three months. The odds of recovery are best when symptoms develop soon after the trauma, when the individual had previously been in good psychological condition, when there are strong social supports, and when there are no other mental or medical disorders. Aggressive early treatment is best. Treatment is very effective because it helps individuals with PTSD to increase their control over anguishing memories and feelings. In time, they come to accept what happened, however horrible, as a tragic reality of the past that does not have to shape their future.

Is it a sexual dysfunction?

Individuals with a sexual dysfunction may:

- ☐ **Experience a decline in sexual pleasure or feel less satisfied with a sexual relationship**
- ☐ **Feel less interested in sexual activity or fantasy than previously**
- ☐ **Experience a numbing or lessening of usual sexual responses**
- ☐ **Feel distress, frustration, or anxiety as a result of a sexual problem**
- ☐ **Have difficulty in an intimate relationship because of a sexual problem**
- ☐ **Not achieve orgasm during intercourse**
- ☐ **Feel repeated or persistent discomfort, burning, irritation, or pain before, during, or after intercourse**
- ☐ **Become preoccupied with a special sexual fantasy**
- ☐ **Not be able to attain or maintain an adequate erection throughout sexual activity (for men)**
- ☐ **Be unable to control or delay ejaculation (for men)**
- ☐ **Experience decreased vaginal lubrication that interferes with sexual intercourse (for women)**
- ☐ **Experience involuntary spasms of the vaginal muscles that make penetration by a penis difficult or impossible (for women)**

The more boxes that you check, the more reason you have to be concerned about sexual dysfunction. It may be helpful to discuss your feelings with your sexual partner and to consider consulting your primary physician, a mental health professional, or a sex therapist.

13 Sexual Dysfunctions

From birth to death, we are sexual beings. Sexuality is an integral part of who we are, how we see ourselves, and how we relate to others. The giving of oneself to another—sharing thoughts, feelings, experiences, sexual pleasure—touches the essence of what it means to be a human being. For this reason, of all of our involvements with others, sexual intimacy can be the most rewarding. But although sexual expression and experience can provide intense joy, they also can involve enormous distress.

Normal sexual behavior

Human sexuality is as rich, varied, and complex as life itself. The pioneers in defining and describing human sexuality, William Masters and Virginia Johnson, first studied more than eight hundred individuals in their laboratory during the 1950s. They discovered that sexual response is a well-ordered sequence of events with a predictable pattern. As they proved, sexual response is always the same, whether the means of stimulation is masturbation, intercourse, or oral-genital sex, and whether the partners are of the same or different sexes.

SEXUAL RESPONSE

The four stages of human sexual response are:

Appetitive. Desire is the essential component of this phase of sexual response. The trigger may be a thought, a touch, a look, or a fantasy. Visual cues, such as the sight of his partner naked, appear to be more stimulating for a man; a woman responds more to tactile stimuli, such as a tender caress.

Excitement. In this stage, sexual excitement builds and causes physiological changes. In men, blood rushes to the genitals. As the penis fills, valves in the veins keep the blood from flowing out. Because these blood vessels are wrapped in a thick sheath of tissue, the penis becomes erect. The testes lift. Women respond to stimulation with vaginal lubrication. The clitoris becomes larger, as do the vaginal lips (the labia), the nipples, and later the breasts. The vagina lengthens and the uterus lifts, increasing the free space in the vagina. The color of the penis, vagina, and labia changes. Breathing and heart rate increase; blood pressure rises. The penis increases further in both length and diameter. The lower third of the vagina swells. During intercourse, the vaginal muscles grasp the penis to increase stimulation for both partners.

Orgasm. Orgasm is remarkably similar in men and women. Both experience three to twelve pelvic muscle contractions approximately four-fifths of a second apart and lasting up to sixty seconds. Both undergo other muscle contractions and spasms, as well as increases in breathing and pulse rates and in blood pressure. Both can sometimes have orgasms with no involvement of the genitals— from kisses, stimulation of the breasts or other parts of the body, or fantasy alone. The major difference at orgasm is that men ejaculate (discharge semen).

The process of ejaculation in men requires two separate events. First, the vas deferens, the seminal vesicles, the prostate, and the upper portion of the urethra contract. The man perceives these subtle contractions deep in his pelvis just before the point of no return, which therapists refer to as the point of "ejaculatory inevitability." Then, seconds later, muscle contractions force semen out of the penis via the urethra.

In women, orgasm is triggered by the clitoris, the primary sensory sexual organ in the female. When stimulation reaches an adequate level, the vagina responds by contracting. Although it sometimes seems that vaginal stimulation alone can set off an orgasm, the clitoris is almost always involved—at least indirectly— during full penetration. There is no evidence that there is a vaginal, as distinct from a clitoral, orgasm.

Resolution. This stage brings a sense of general relaxation and well-being. The sexual organs of both partners return to their normal, nonexcited state. Heightened skin color quickly fades after orgasm, and the heart rate, blood pressure, and breathing rate soon return to normal. The clitoris resumes its normal position and appearance very shortly thereafter, whereas the penis may remain partially erect for up to thirty minutes.

After orgasm, the male enters a refractory period, during which he is incapable of another orgasm. This period lasts from minutes to days, depending on age and on the frequency of previous sexual activity. Some women may have a refractory period after orgasm, but others do not and can have several orgasms. If either partner does not have an orgasm after becoming highly aroused, resolution may occur much more slowly and may be accompanied by a sense of discomfort.

SEXUAL CONCERNS

No one is born knowing about sex. Everyone learns by doing and, as in almost any activity, the initial attempts are often awkward. Even sexually sophisticated individuals experience occasional failures or unsatisfactory experiences, perhaps caused by fatigue, stress, or alcohol. These can lead to problems because of anxiety that things will not go well the next time.

Understanding sexual needs and behaviors can be difficult because of widespread myths and misinformation. There is no truth behind the misconceptions that men are always capable of erection, that sex always involves intercourse, that most partners experience simultaneous orgasms, or that people who truly love each other always have satisfying sex lives. Similarly, there is no single standard for how often sexual activity should occur, how sex organs should look, how long an erection should last, or how orgasm should feel.

Cultural and childhood influences can affect our attitudes toward sex. Even though America's traditionally puritanical values have eased, our society continues to convey mixed messages about sex. Some children, repeatedly warned of the evils of sex, never accept the sexual dimensions of their identity. Others— especially young boys—may be exposed to macho attitudes toward sex and therefore may feel that they need to engage in sex to prove their virility. Young girls may feel confused about media messages that encourage them to look and act provocatively and by a double standard that blames them for leading boys on.

In addition to such concerns, virtually everyone has individual worries. A woman may feel self-conscious about the shape of her breasts; a man may worry about the size of his penis; both partners may fear not pleasing the other. Most often, individuals wonder about what is "normal." Yet the concept of sexual normalcy differs greatly among different times, cultures, and racial and ethnic groups. In certain times and places, only sex between a husband and wife has been deemed normal. In other times and places, "normal" has been applied to any sexual behavior—alone or with others—that does not harm others or produce anxiety and guilt.

Sexual concerns can affect the relationship between partners and contribute to sexual difficulties. The most frequent of these difficulties are insufficient foreplay, a lack of enthusiasm for sex, and an inability to relax. In a survey of one hundred well-educated, happily married couples, 40 percent of the men reported a problem with erection or ejaculation at some point in their lives. Of the women, 63 percent said they had had problems of arousal or orgasm. About half of the men and three-quarters of the women reported other difficulties, such as diminished desire.

Sexual dysfunctions

Sexual dysfunction is a disruption of any phase of sexual response. The causes may be anatomical, biological, or psychological. Heterosexual, homosexual, and bisexual individuals may develop sexual dysfunctions, which are common, particularly in mild forms. A key difference between a difficulty and a dysfunction lies in the way an individual or a couple feels and responds to a situation. Some people become very upset almost as soon as they encounter any sexual difficulty; others become concerned only after repeated or prolonged difficulties. When a dysfunction develops in either partner, ultimately it will affect both. A man who is anxious about pleasing his partner may not be able to maintain an erection; his partner may become so preoccupied with this difficulty that she cannot relax and achieve orgasm; and her lack of sexual satisfaction adds to his anxiety and the erectile problem.

Most sexual dysfunctions occur during sexual activity with a partner; a few occur during masturbation; some are limited to certain situations or partners. A sexual dysfunction may develop suddenly after years without any problems, last for a brief time, recur over a longer period, or become chronic.

Because sexuality is an important part of an individual's identity and activity, sexual dysfunctions can cause a great deal of distress. Until recently, many individuals were reluctant to seek help or talk over their concerns with a physician or therapist, but this reticence appears to be fading. A few decades ago most men and women did not seek help, if ever, until their forties; today they are most likely to seek help in their late twenties and early thirties.

A sexual dysfunction can occur anywhere in the sexual response sequence. Either partner may lose interest in sex or fail to respond to sexual stimulation. A man's penis may not become erect; a woman's vagina may not become moist. A man may lose his erection while attempting to penetrate; the woman's vaginal lubrication may dry up. Some men and women become aroused, enjoy the plateau stage, but then are unable to achieve orgasm. One or both partners may feel that the sexual activity is too prolonged or too brief.

Many factors can contribute to sexual dysfunction. Physical conditions, illnesses, injury, and pain can impair sexual desire and response. (The table below lists some medical conditions and medications that can affect sexual functioning.) Anxiety, allergies, depression, muscle spasms, obesity, ulcers, irritable colon, cancer, and other ailments can all have an effect. Common substances, including alcohol and medications used to treat high blood pressure, affect sexual performance. Individuals who use illicit drugs have a high incidence of sexual dysfunction. In one study of several hundred men and women with sexual problems, about a third had mental disorders, including anxiety, depression, and personality disorders. Victims of sexual trauma, such as incest, child molestation, or rape, may experience continuing sexual difficulties.

Knowledge, attitudes, and feelings about sex also play a role. Misinformed or ignorant about sex, some partners may have poor sexual skills and not provide adequate stimulation. Some people have excessively high personal expectations for sexual performance or are unusually sensitive to real or imagined rejection by a sex partner. Others, consciously or not, feel anxious about sex-

MEDICAL CONDITIONS AND MEDICATIONS THAT CAN AFFECT SEXUAL FUNCTIONING

- ☐ **Injury**

- ☐ **Neurological illnesses (e.g., multiple sclerosis, spinal cord lesions, and neuropathy)**

- ☐ **Endocrine diseases (e.g., diabetes mellitus, hypothyroidism, hyperthyroidism, pituitary disorders, and other hormonal imbalances)**

- ☐ **Cardiovascular conditions**

- ☐ **Genitourinary problems (e.g., Peyronie's disease, urethral, pelvic, or vaginal infections, cystitis, endometriosis, vaginitis, or uterine prolapse)**

- ☐ **Pain**

- ☐ **Substance abuse (including use of alcohol, cocaine, and opiates)**

- ☐ **Antihypertensive medications (including diuretics, methyldopa, clonidine, beta blockers, reserpine, and guanethidine)**

- ☐ **Steroids**

- ☐ **Estrogens**

- ☐ **Cimetidine**

- ☐ **Antipsychotic agents (including thioridazine, chlorpromazine, and fluphenazine)**

- ☐ **Antidepressants (including tricyclics, monoamine oxidase inhibitors, serotonin reuptake inhibitors, and trazodone)**

uality, often because of a puritanical upbringing or because they are fearful of not satisfying a partner.

The quality of the relationship between partners also can affect their sexual satisfaction. Poor communication about feelings and preferences can make it difficult to establish a mutually gratifying sexual relationship. A man may not be sensitive to a woman's need for tenderness and affection. A woman may interpret a man's difficulty in maintaining an erection as a sign that she is not attractive. Often sex becomes a symbol or pawn as couples deal with issues of closeness, dependency, control, or fear of abandonment. Partners may harbor unexpressed resentment or feel caught in a power struggle both in and outside the bedroom. Other events—pregnancy, the birth of a child, children leaving home, guilt about an affair—may also lead to sexual dysfunction.

Sometimes one person's sexual problems may mask the other's. If a man is impotent, a woman need not worry about her ability to achieve orgasm; someone whose partner feels little desire may be pleased not to have to respond to sexual demands. Sometimes both partners, unsure of how close they want to be, use a loss of desire or satisfaction to keep their emotional distance. By providing emotional support and interpreting behavior, therapists can help partners recognize and overcome barriers to sexual pleasure by exploring their motives, fantasies, anger, and fears.

Often more than one factor contributes to a sexual dysfunction. For example, diabetes may cause occasional erection problems in a man, whose anxiety about being able to perform may then lead to a loss of sexual desire. Similarly, a woman who experiences diminished vaginal lubrication after menopause may find intercourse painful; her concern about pain may interfere with her ability to become aroused and to have an orgasm.

Sexual dysfunctions can affect other aspects of a person's life and self-image. Some individuals feel that they are not living up to their idea of what "normal" men or women should do; others feel depressed, anxious, guilty, ashamed, or frustrated. Many become so focused on every nuance of their responses that they begin *spectatoring*—constantly monitoring themselves and their sex partners. This can further impair sexual performance and satisfaction.

SEX THERAPY

Modern sex therapy, pioneered by Masters and Johnson in the 1960s, views sex as a natural, healthy behavior that enhances a couple's relationship. Their approach emphasizes education, communication, reduction of performance anxiety, and sexual exercises that enhance sexual intimacy.

Today most sex therapists, working either alone or with a partner, have modified Masters and Johnson's approach. Instead of an intensive two-week program, most see couples once a week for eight to ten weeks. Weekly sessions have proven more convenient, more economical, and equally effective. The focus of sex therapy is on correcting dysfunctional behavior, not on exploring underlying psychodynamics.

Contrary to a common misconception, sex therapy does not involve sexual activity in front of therapists. The therapist may review psychological and physiological aspects of sexual functioning and evaluate the couple's sexual attitudes and ability to communicate. The core of the program is the couple's "homework"—a series of exercises, carried out in private, that enhance their sensory awareness and improve nonverbal communication.

The initial exercise is *sensate focusing*, in which partners explore each other's bodies except for the genitals, caress each other, and tune in to their sensations and fantasies. They are not allowed to attempt intercourse; the goal is learning to give and receive pleasure. The partners are encouraged to talk openly about sexual needs and wishes. In the next stage, genital touching is allowed. The partners can assume positions for intercourse, but cannot actually have intercourse until the last phase of treatment. They may be asked to keep a diary in which they report on each session. At weekly meetings, the therapist offers advice, information, and reassurance.

Individuals respond in many different ways to sex therapy. Some people feel guilty about sexual fantasies or jealous of their partner's fantasies. Often treatment upsets the equilibrium in a precarious relationship. Even in a healthy relationship, the partner may have adapted to the problem and may be fearful of any change. Therapists use psychodynamic techniques to deal with such issues. Some people feel that the exercises are mechanical or boring; therapists may interpret this response as a possible sign of hostility toward the partner, fear of rejection, performance anxiety, or fear of losing affection or control if the partner overcomes his or her sexual problem.

Most sex therapists work primarily with couples. However, individual therapy can be successful for those who do not have a partner or do not want the partner to participate, or if the partner refuses. Sometimes simple information and reassurance are effective for a man who suddenly develops a dysfunction. Men in committed relationships may be given behavioral assignments to complete with a partner who will not come to the sessions. Single men without partners may be helped by assertiveness training, permission to fantasize, masturbation exercises, and instructions in how to change habits that lead to avoidance of sexual activity. Women with difficulty in achieving sexual excitement and orgasm have been successfully treated without their partner's active par-

ticipation in therapy. They learn techniques for fantasy and masturbation and ways to transfer their new skills to partners.

Although sex therapy does work, therapists do not agree on
how often or to what extent. Masters and Johnson reported success in 60 percent of cases of primary impotence, 70 percent
for secondary impotence, 97 percent for premature ejaculation,
and 80 percent for female orgasmic disorder. In a more recent
follow-up study of couples who underwent training in sensate
focusing, 60 percent felt continued improvement after three or
four years; 25 percent still had serious problems; 15 percent
had ended their relationships and found new partners.

OTHER TREATMENTS FOR SEXUAL DISORDERS

Sex therapy is not likely to work if the underlying problem stems
from the relationship between the partners; from a mental disorder, such as depression; from sexual trauma; or from unconscious
fears that impair a person's capacity to feel loving and lovable. In
such instances, different forms of therapy, such as individual psychotherapy or couples therapy, may be more effective. Couples
therapy usually does more to improve a couple's sex life than sex
therapy does to improve a marriage.

Behavioral therapy   The basic assumption in behavior therapy is
that sexual dysfunction is a learned maladaptive behavior. The
basic techniques, originally developed to treat phobias, aim at
helping a patient to overcome fear of sexual interaction. The
therapist may set up a series of anxiety-provoking situations,
ranging from the least to the most threatening. The thought of
kissing, for example, might provoke mild anxiety, and intercourse
a near panic. Through a standard program of systematic desensitization, the person first fantasizes about the least anxiety-
provoking situation and progresses to the one that produces the
most anxiety. Medication, hypnosis, or special training in muscle
relaxation may be used to help master anxiety. At home, the partner, following the same technique as the therapist, may provide
the person with situations of ever-increasing stimulation.

Assertiveness training helps to teach individuals to express
their sexual needs openly and without fear. When it is used in
combination with sex therapy, the focus is on helping them learn
to make sexual requests or to refuse unreasonable demands.

Psychodynamic sex therapy   This lengthier approach, which inte-
grates sex therapy with psychodynamic and psychoanalytically
oriented psychotherapy, allows time for the learning or relearning
of sexual satisfaction in the context of day-to-day living. It is par-

ticularly useful when a sexual dysfunction is associated with other mental or emotional problems. In therapy sessions, the individual can deal with such issues as difficulty in trusting a partner, fear of intimacy, or aggressive or hostile feelings.

Group therapy Therapy groups provide a strong support system for individuals who feel ashamed, anxious, or guilty about a particular sexual problem. They can help to counteract myths about sex; correct misconceptions; provide accurate information on sexual anatomy, physiology, and behavior; and enhance self-esteem and self-acceptance in the supportive setting of others with similar problems.

Hypnosis Hypnosis focuses on the particular sexual dysfunction that causes anxiety, enabling an individual to gain control over this problem. The therapist meets with the person and assesses his or her hypnotizability. During a hypnotic trance, the person learns to deal with the anxieties triggered by sexual encounters.

Most therapists also teach relaxation techniques to use before sexual relations. The combination of these methods to alleviate anxiety enables the individuals to respond more fully to pleasurable stimulation. Hypnosis helps to remove psychological impediments to vaginal lubrication, erection, and orgasm.

Medication Because many psychiatric problems can lower sexual desire and affect sexual functioning, appropriate medications can help. In addition, psychiatric drugs may be used as part of therapy. For example, anti-anxiety agents may help very tense individuals to relax during sex exercises, although these medications sometimes can have sexual side effects. On occasion, drugs such as the tricyclic antidepressants are used to prolong sexual response in conditions like premature ejaculation. Testosterone, a male sex hormone that affects the libido, is sometimes used for sexual desire disorders in men who have a demonstrated low testosterone level.

Self-help Basic communication techniques, alone or in combination with therapy, can enhance the quality of a couple's sexual relationship. Among the guidelines offered by mental health professionals are:

- Remember that your feelings are neither wrong nor right. They simply *are*.
- Use an "I" statement, such as "I really enjoy making love, but I'm so tired right now that I won't be a responsive partner. Why don't we get the kids to bed early tomorrow so we can enjoy ourselves?

- Remember that neither you nor your partner can always explain your feelings.

- When your partner is talking, do not dismiss what he or she is saying as crazy, irrational, or selfish.

- If your partner has temporarily lost interest in sex, express concern and ask what the two of you might do to make things better. Don't blame yourself.

- Speak up if something hurts during sex. Be specific.

- If you would like to try something different, say so. Practice saying the words first if they embarrass you. If your partner feels uncomfortable, don't force the issue, but do try talking it through.

- Set aside time for a regular sex discussion. Take turns bringing up topics. Mention special pleasures or particular problems.

- If you want to request changes or tackle a touchy topic, start with positive statements. Let your partner know how much you enjoy having sex, and then express your desire to enjoy lovemaking more often or in different ways.

- Encourage small changes. If you want your partner to be less inhibited, start slowly, perhaps by suggesting sex in a different room or place.

Sexual desire disorders

Like every other aspect of a committed, ongoing relationship, sex evolves and changes over time. The red-hot sexual chemistry of the early stages of intimacy invariably cools down. Sexuality, like personality, is dynamic and changes throughout life. However, partners may not be able to acknowledge and adapt to these changes or, even after being together for a long time, may not feel sufficiently at ease with each other in terms of their sex life to discuss any anxieties they may have.

Sexual desire is a biological urge that varies among individuals and over the life cycle. One partner who is less interested in sex than the other does not necessarily have abnormally low desire; a partner who is more interested in sex is not necessarily "oversexed." Problems of sexual desire are the most common reasons people turn to sex therapists and marriage counselors.

REDUCED SEXUAL DESIRE DISORDER

Reduced (hypoactive) sexual desire disorder is a persistent or prolonged lessening or loss of sexual desire and sexual fantasies. However, occasional periods of diminished sexual desire and activity are not uncommon. In one group of one hundred couples in stable marriages, 8 percent had intercourse less than once a month. In another group, one-third reported not having sex for periods averaging eight weeks. Temporary sexual droughts like these are not considered a problem unless they are upsetting to either partner.

To some individuals, sex may become so fearful and repugnant that they avoid all or almost all sexual contact. This problem, *sexual aversion disorder*, is usually considered to be a specific phobia (see Chapter 7) and is treated with behavior modification and sex therapy.

▼

How common is reduced sexual desire?

About 20 percent of the population may experience a reduced sexual desire disorder at some point in their lives. This problem occurs equally in men and women, often in individuals who have not had previous arousal or orgasm problems.

▼

What causes reduced sexual desire?

Relationship problems are the primary cause of lowered sexual desire, although many other factors, including age, personality characteristics, and past experiences, can also contribute to it. Among young married couples who had not had sex for at least two months, the most common reason for stopping or reducing sexual activity is marital conflict. The men blame a variety of social factors: recent immigration, religion, a wife's working or not working. The women focus on the relationship itself, mentioning problems in dominance, decision making, and showing affection.

Severe stress—as with a recent move, a new baby, a high-pressure job—can short-circuit normal sexual response. In such cases, couples who try to unwind by drinking or using anti-anxiety drugs may make the problem worse because these substances further dampen sexual responsiveness. Desire also can be affected when one partner is having an affair or hiding a secret, such as a plan to divorce. Sometimes, one partner in a relationship finds that sexual desire wanes after a more enduring commitment is made, such as becoming engaged or marrying. Problems within the sexual relationship itself can diminish desire; the partners may not agree about the timing or kind of sexual activity they enjoy or may not provide adequate stimulation for each other.

Some people—women more often than men—may be born with a poorly developed sexual appetite. Prolonged abstinence in itself can suppress sexual desire. Other factors include sexual abuse as a child or sexual trauma, such as rape; sexual dysfunction in one partner that leads to a loss of desire in either or both of them, perhaps because of a sense of helplessness; and unconscious fears of sex. Because they have been exposed to early, powerful antisexual messages, some individuals have difficulty in accepting the sexual dimensions of their identity and may be unaware of these difficulties until they fall in love and marry. People who have homosexual impulses and consider these unacceptable may suppress all sexual feelings or avoid sexual contact.

Freud traced low sexual desire to unresolved oedipal conflicts or, for men, a fear of castration. Another explanation is a childhood trauma, such as rejection or abuse, that has created a fear of intimacy and consequent pain. The problem in such cases is not the partner but rather the unresolved issues of the past.

Physical problems, including almost any major illness, can affect desire directly and indirectly. Surgery that affects body image (such as mastectomy, hysterectomy, prostatectomy, or ileostomy), and drugs that depress the central nervous system or decrease testosterone levels, can lessen sexual desire. In a small percentage of men, the problem is a deficiency in male hormones. Mental disorders, such as depression, anxiety, and psychosis, may impair desire.

▼

How reduced sexual desire disorder feels

A desire problem can develop after the honeymoon or after the couple's silver anniversary. Sometimes perfectly healthy couples, with no physical impairment, simply become bored with sex, despite the fact that they love each other and find each other attractive and enjoyable. Desire difficulties play a complex role in a couple's mental and emotional life.

A husband may lose interest in sex after being laid off from his job. As the weeks or months pass, his wife gives up trying to make sexual overtures. When he gets a new position and begins feeling good about himself again, she may be the one who has lost any desire for sexual intimacy. Similarly, new parents who had been advised not to engage in sexual activity for several weeks after childbirth may find themselves so exhausted by the stresses of parenthood that months go by before they initiate sex. At that point, the wife may be distracted by concern about whether the baby is sleeping, the husband may worry about hurting her or about the tenderness of her breasts if she is nursing, and both may find themselves thinking about sex as more of a chore than a pleasure.

Couples with good relationships and the ability to talk through their problems usually deal with such temporary sexual slumps on their own. Other situations are more daunting. One partner may lose sexual desire after learning about an affair the other had with a close friend before their marriage. In another couple, a spouse who has gained a substantial amount of weight may interpret the other's loss of desire as a reaction to his or her changed

Is it reduced (hypoactive) sexual desire disorder?

According to the DSM-IV, a diagnosis of hypoactive sexual desire disorder should be based on these criteria:

■ Persistent or recurring deficiency or absence of sexual fantasies and desire for sexual activity

■ Does not occur exclusively during the course of another mental disorder and is not caused by drugs of abuse, medications, or a medical condition

■ Causes marked distress or interpersonal difficulty

Adapted from the Diagnostic and Statistical Manual of Mental Disorders, 4th Edition. Used with permission.

appearance. If the lack of desire persists or if either partner becomes increasingly upset about it, the couple may not be able to get their sex life back on track without help.

▼

Seeking help

If you feel that a lack of sexual desire may be a problem for you or your partner, these are questions that should be asked:

- Are you less interested in sexual activity than before?
- Have you also lost interest in sexual fantasy?
- Have you been upset by this change?
- Has your diminished interest in sex caused problems in your relationship with your partner?

If you answer "yes" to these questions, discuss your concerns with your partner and consider consulting a mental health professional experienced in sex therapy. Therapists take into account many factors in diagnosing this problem, including a person's age, physical condition, and relationships.

▼

Treating reduced sexual desire

The couple often begins by working with a therapist toward a hypothesis about the cause of the problem. This process may require medical workups as well as a discussion of each partner's sexual history, possible psychological conflicts, and an assessment of the overall relationship. The therapist may see partners alone, as a couple, or both.

If the problem is not physical, the most effective approach combines cognitive therapy (to deal with misconceptions, for example, that two people in love always want to have sex at the same time and in the same way); psychodynamic therapy to deal with unconscious conflicts and fears; behavioral treatments, such as communication and sensate focusing exercises; and marital therapy to deal with issues such as how each partner uses sex to gain control in the relationship. The goal is to come to grips with specific dilemmas so that one or both partners can admit fears, reveal any secrets, or make some other needed change. In therapy, they discuss what each partner likes and learn new techniques for giving and receiving sexual attention and pleasure. A man who has lost sexual desire may be told to masturbate to demonstrate to himself that erection, excitement, and ejaculation are still possible.

If the underlying problem is the relationship between partners, couples therapy is often recommended. Such therapy can enhance intimacy and lead to a new appreciation of the partners' motivations and behavior. Thus, a husband may have interpreted his wife's lack of interest in sex as a personal rejection. In therapy, she may be able to explain that she often feels exhausted and tense because of the demands of their young children. She may see him as pressuring her to have sex at awkward times or as rushing toward climax before she can become aroused. From his perspective, he may try to ejaculate quickly because he feels she just wants to get sex over with. With a therapist's help, each partner can find a more positive way of interpreting why each does certain things. They both come to see the lack of desire as a way of coping with a difficult situation. Even after relatively brief couples therapy, sexual desire may improve dramatically, as long as the partners continue to deal with the underlying issues.

If a sexual identity problem is the source of diminished desire in a married couple, the spouse may be shocked to discover that his or her partner is homosexual or bisexual. Often the heterosexual spouse becomes concerned about his or her own sexual identity and attractiveness. In this difficult situation, therapy may focus on the spouse's reaction to the information and education about sexual development and orientation.

If the problem is physical, medical treatment focuses on the underlying condition. Even then, a therapist can help by fully explaining the nature of the problem, what is possible sexually, and how the couple can enhance their abilities to relate to each other.

▼

Self-help If the problem stems from stress, busy schedules, or daily demands, couples should review their priorities together. If they want to give sex a higher priority in their relationship, they should make a conscious effort to do so. One possibility is to make "dates" for sex. At first the idea of deliberately setting aside a time for sex may seem too calculated and businesslike, but it need not be. One sex therapist compares it to "lighting the pilot light so the furnace has time to warm up." Creating a sexy atmosphere (music, soft lights, a glowing fire, a setting other than the bedroom) can also help to ignite the spark of desire.

Sometimes deliberately deciding *not* to have intercourse for a while (a key element of sex therapy) works wonders. During this time, partners kiss, hug, touch, and massage each other, not as a prelude to sex, but as pleasures in themselves. Popular self-help books that address the problem of sexual boredom may suggest new approaches. What happens out of bed also affects what happens in bed. The more time two people spend enjoying themselves (dining out, going to movies, playing tennis), the more they will enjoy each other sexually.

Impact on relationships

Sexual desire problems are intertwined with other issues in a relationship. Sometimes they are the cause of misunderstanding and conflict; sometimes they are a consequence. Often couples or marital counseling can help partners to unravel the spoken and unspoken issues between them. If one partner thinks that the other is "undersexed" or "oversexed," counseling can help both to understand each other's needs and work out compromises. At times, however, one partner—often the one who complained most about the lack of sexual desire—resists therapy, perhaps because he or she does not feel free to talk in front of the other. A skillful therapist can deal with such barriers.

Outlook

Disorders of desire have proven to be extremely complex and challenging. Today, mental health professionals feel that success depends chiefly on the therapist's basic style and skills at psychotherapy, including tact, timing, and creativity, and on the partners' desire to preserve the relationship, their understanding of the cause of the problem, their ability to talk rather than act out their conflicts, and their basic honesty with each other.

SEXUAL AVERSION DISORDER

The primary characteristic of this disorder is an extreme aversion to and avoidance of genital sexual contact with a partner. Individuals with this persistent or recurrent problem experience emotional distress—ranging from moderate anxiety to strong disgust or fear—or encounter great difficulties in their intimate relationships. Some are particularly repulsed by certain aspects of sexual

Falling out of the habit

Back when Sam and Lynne were dating, they couldn't seem to get enough of each other. When they were apart they fantasized about being together. When they were alone they couldn't stop touching, kissing, hugging, or holding onto each other. The red-hot passion of their courtship cooled somewhat over the first five years of their marriage, but they continued to have an active sex life, making love two times a week.

Then baby Bonnie was born. "I went into some sort of hormonal shut-down," says Lynne. "I became totally sexless." After months of getting up at night to nurse, Lynne was so exhausted that the only thing she wanted to do in bed was sleep. Sam, fatigued himself, was sympathetic. The couple managed to have sex occasionally, although even then they always seemed to be listening for the baby's cry.

Just before Bonnie's first birthday, Sam injured his back playing softball. He spent weeks immobilized in bed, and had to take painkillers and wear a brace for a long time afterward. Struggling to get through each day, Sam and Lynne both felt stretched to the limits. Sex seemed almost irrelevant, a luxury that had to take a low place on their priority list for a while.

By the time Bonnie was two, life had turned another corner. Lynne was rested and energetic. Sam's back was better. The daily grind was no longer such a burden. And yet weeks, even months, would pass without Lynne and Sam making love. "What scared me wasn't that we weren't doing it anymore," says Lynne, "but that I didn't even want to. I'd lost any semblance of desire." Sam complained that whenever he'd tried to initiate sex, Lynne always had a reason not to. "After a while, we got out of the habit of making love," he says.

On their seventh anniversary, Sam and Lynne arranged for a sitter and went to a hotel for the night. That's when they realized that it had been more than three months since they'd had sex. Still in love, still committed to their marriage, they began to talk about what they might do to resurrect what had once been such a joyous part of their relationship.

When she got back home, Lynne bought some books that talked about sexual desire and sex therapy. "I realized that we weren't alone, that lots of couples go through the same experience," she says. "I also learned that you can't just wait for sexual interest and feelings to come back on their own, because they may not. You have to take action

and behave in sensual ways. The feelings will follow."

Rather than focusing only on their jobs or their child, Sam and Lynne began refocusing their energy and attention on each other, not just during romantic evenings and special occasions but on a day-to-day basis. They traded neck rubs every night. They left flirty messages on each other's answering machines. Some nights they would set the alarm early to allow extra time in the morning for a snuggle. Occasionally one would lock the bathroom door and join the other in the bath or shower. They kissed more and complimented each other often. When they were alone, they practiced some of the basic techniques of sex therapy, such as sensate focusing and sharing fantasies.

As Sam and Lynne began to spend more time relating to each other, not simply as Mom and Dad or as householders juggling their many obligations, but as a man and a woman, their sexual interest rekindled. "For me, it was like getting back part of my old self and feeling sexual again," says Lynne. "I can see how easily couples fall out of the habit of making love, but my advice is not to let too much time pass before you make each other your top priorities again."

activity, such as fluids produced by the genitals, while others find any aspect of sex, including hugging and kissing, repugnant. In order to avoid sexual encounters, individuals with this disorder may avoid potential partners or sexual situations. Some devote all their time and energy to work or other activities; others may travel, neglect personal hygiene and appearance, or go to bed early. In severe cases, a sexual situation may trigger a panic attack, which may include feelings of terror and physical symptoms, such as dizziness and difficulty breathing.

Treatment of sexual aversion disorder aims to diminish the individual's fear and avoidance of sexual activity. Among the approaches that have been used successfully are systematic desensitization and the specific anxiety-lowering techniques employed by sex therapy.

EXCESSIVE SEXUAL DESIRE

An unknown number of individuals suffer from another extreme: excessive (hyperactive) sexual desire. This problem is not recognized as a true mental disorder. However, some therapists view it as a sexual addiction, characterized by a compulsive drive for sex. For individuals with this problem, sex is more than a normal pleasure: It is a need that must be met, even at the cost of their careers and marriages. Even therapists who challenge the concept of sexual addiction acknowledge that some people become preoccupied with sex, cannot control their sexual desire, and may act in potentially harmful ways for the sake of sexual satisfaction.

Anyone can develop excessive sexual desire. Those who are affected may engage in behaviors that include masturbation, phone sex, pornography, strip shows, affairs, anonymous sex with strangers, prostitution, exhibitionism, voyeurism, child molestation, incest, and rape. They get relief from distressing feelings, such as restlessness, inadequacy, or worthlessness, only through sex (either masturbation or with a partner). Once the sexual high ends, the same negative feelings overwhelm them, and they are driven, once more, to have sex.

Some of the characteristics exhibited by those whom some therapists describe as sexual "addicts" include:

- A sexual preoccupation that interferes with a normal sexual relationship with a spouse or a lover
- A compulsion to have sex repeatedly within a short period of time and to engage in sexual behavior that results in feelings of anxiety, depression, guilt, or shame
- A great deal of time away from family or work in order to look for partners or to engage in sex
- Use of sex to avoid facing personal or professional problems.

Individuals with this problem often were physically and emotionally abused as children or have family members who abuse drugs or alcohol. They typically are unable to control their compulsion for sexual activity, which they continue despite the dangers, including the risk of contracting sexually transmitted diseases. Their lives are dominated by recurrent erotic images and sensations. Many masturbate ten or more times a day and cannot concentrate on learning and work or develop normal relationships.

No one knows whether abnormally intense sexual desire stems from a biological abnormality or psychologic factors. Men, who seem more likely to develop this problem than women, have been treated with medroxyprogesterone acetate (Depo-Provera), an intramuscular medication that lowers testosterone and can dramatically lessen the frequency and intensity of erotic imagery, masturbation, and other sexual behavior.

Some therapists believe that sexual excitement may protect individuals with excessive sexual desire from painful emotions. Rather than experiencing anger or fear, they act out sexually. If they cannot engage in sex, they may develop major depression, anxiety, or rage.

Because excessive sexual desire is a controversial and not universally accepted diagnosis, there has not been extensive research on various approaches to this problem. Psychotherapy can help individuals deal with the shame that both triggers and follows sexual activity. Several organizations, such as Sexaholics Anonymous and Sexual Addicts Anonymous, offer support from people who share the same problem.

Sexual arousal disorders

Sexual arousal is a combination of psychological and physiological responses to a sexually stimulating situation. A *sexual arousal disorder* exists when a man or woman repeatedly fails to respond to sensations—sights, sounds, smells, touches, tastes—and fantasies that normally trigger sexual excitement.

FEMALE SEXUAL AROUSAL DISORDER

In women, a sexual arousal disorder is characterized by the repeated lack of the physical signs of sexual excitement: vaginal lubrication and swelling. In diagnosing this problem, therapists focus on these symptoms. However, women often are less concerned with vaginal lubrication and other physiological aspects of sex than they are with feeling physically aroused and responsive. Even if their physiological responses are completely normal, they may not find sex appealing or gratifying, and this lack of enjoyment is their primary sexual complaint.

An arousal disorder can be hard to distinguish from problems of sexual desire or orgasm. It may occur in every sexual situation, or only with certain partners or under certain circumstances. If a woman consistently fails to become aroused, she may be unable to achieve orgasm and eventually may lose sexual desire.

▼
How common is female sexual arousal disorder?

No one knows how common this problem actually is, but women probably fail to become aroused at least as often as men. However, some sex therapists feel that sexual arousal disorder is rare except as part of either reduced sexual desire or an orgasmic disorder. In one study of couples described as relatively happy, one-third of the women said they found it hard to maintain sexual excitement.

▼
What causes female sexual arousal disorder?

Psychological issues can affect sexual arousal, just as they can interfere with desire or orgasm. Performance anxiety, sexual guilt, conflicting feelings about her partner, fear of pregnancy, or fear of orgasm may all contribute to a woman's lack of arousal. Sometimes a woman concerned with her sexual response may begin spectatoring—obsessively observing her every reaction—which interferes with spontaneous pleasure.

Hormonal changes during a woman's menstrual cycle can affect her responsiveness. Postmenopausal estrogen deficiency may lead to problems with vaginal lubrication and pain during intercourse. Other conditions that can affect lubrication include certain neurological disorders and medications, including antihistamines that "dry up" various mucous membranes in the body.

▼
How female sexual arousal disorder feels

In situations that most women would find sexually stimulating, those with this problem describe themselves as feeling numb or as if their feelings of sexual excitement had been shut off. Often this problem occurs along with, and may be a symptom of, reduced sexual desire or difficulty in achieving orgasm.

▼
Seeking help

If you suspect that sexual arousal disorder may be a problem, these are the questions that should be asked:

- Have you felt a numbing or lessening of your usual sexual responses?

- Have you noticed changes in vaginal lubrication?

Is it female sexual arousal disorder?

According to the DSM-IV, a diagnosis of female sexual arousal disorder should be based on these criteria:

- Persistent or recurrent inability to attain or maintain an adequate lubrication and vaginal swelling until completion of the sexual activity

- Does not occur exclusively during the course of another mental disorder and is not caused by drugs of abuse, medications, or a medical condition

- Causes marked distress or interpersonal difficulty

Adapted from the Diagnostic and Statistical Manual of Mental Disorders, 4th Edition. *Used with permission.*

- Has a lack of lubrication interfered with sexual intercourse?
- Has this problem occurred repeatedly or persisted for a long time?
- As far as you can tell, does this problem seem unrelated to any physical illness or the use of medication, drugs, or alcohol?
- Has this problem caused significant distress or problems in your relationship with a sexual partner?

If you answer "yes" to these questions, the problem may be a sexual arousal disorder or another form of sexual dysfunction. You may want to talk over your feelings with your partner and consider consulting a health professional with experience in sexual disorders, or a sex therapist.

Treating female sexual arousal disorder

Sex therapy, particularly sensate focusing exercises that enhance sexual awareness and responsiveness, and relaxation techniques (described in Chapter 29) are most effective in helping women overcome an arousal disorder.

Self-help

Some couples do not realize that women require almost continuous physical or psychological stimulation to maintain arousal and lubrication. Greater attention to foreplay, intimacy, and a romantic atmosphere can help.

Impact on relationships

This problem may lead to other sexual dysfunctions, including problems with orgasm, and may cause difficulties in a woman's intimate relationships. A partner may interpret a woman's lack of sexual arousal as a sign of rejection or sexual inadequacy. Both partners may find it hard to talk about this problem and may pull away from each other.

Outlook   Treatments for female sexual arousal disorder, which may include sex-therapy exercises, behavioral therapy, and couples counseling, are highly effective.

IMPOTENCE

Impotence, officially termed *male erectile disorder*, refers to a man's inability to attain an erection and have intercourse. Men with primary impotence have never had intercourse. Those with secondary impotence have had intercourse successfully in the past but can no longer do so, or can have intercourse in certain situations, such as with a prostitute but not with a wife.

How common is impotence?   Although estimates vary, as many as 20 to 40 percent of American men may suffer from an erectile disorder at some point in their lives. Primary impotence, which is rare, affects about 1 percent of men under the age of thirty-five. About 8 percent of young men in the United States and Europe report secondary impotence, and the incidence increases steadily with age. According to sex researcher Kinsey's studies, more than 75 percent of men over the age of eighty are impotent.

What causes impotence?   Psychological factors, such as anxiety about performance, may cause about half of all erectile disorders; physical illness, such as diabetes, accounts for an increasing percentage as men grow older. Alcohol, drugs, and stress can also lead to erection difficulties.

Freud traced impotence to an inability to reconcile feelings of affection with feelings of desire; he theorized that some men can function sexually only with women they see as degraded. Fear, anxiety, anger, or moral restraint can interfere with a man's ability to achieve erection. Other psychodynamic factors that may contribute are an inability to trust, feelings of inadequacy, or a sense of sexual undesirability.

In an ongoing relationship, impotence may reflect problems in communication, particularly if the man cannot express his needs or anger directly. Some men become impotent after a stressful event, such as divorce or the death of a spouse, child, or parent. In widowed and divorced men, an erectile difficulty may reflect

Is it male erectile disorder (impotence)?

According to the DSM-IV, a diagnosis of male erectile disorder (impotence) should be based on these criteria:

- Persistent or recurrent inability to attain or maintain an adequate erection until completion of sexual activity

- Does not occur during the course of another mental disorder and is not caused by drugs of abuse, medications, or a medical condition

- Causes marked distress or interpersonal difficulty

Adapted from the Diagnostic and Statistical Manual of Mental Disorders, 4th Edition. *Used with permission.*

feelings of guilt or apprehensiveness about starting another sexual relationship.

Normal aging affects sexual response. As they get older, men take longer to become sexually excited and have erections less often. Erections during REM sleep (the period of vivid dreaming), which are almost continuous in teenaged boys, occur only 20 percent of the time in men over sixty. However, only 30 percent of sixty-five-year-old men report chronic erection problems.

Whereas erection problems are not a universal consequence of aging, fear of impotence may be. Masters and Johnson speculated that all men over the age of forty worry about loss of virility with advancing age. Yet any decline in sexual excitement is less likely to be a function of aging than to be related to the lack of availability of a sex partner, illness, physical changes, drugs, surgery that affects nerves and blood vessels, or endocrine disorders that cause low testosterone levels or other hormonal imbalances.

One-fourth of impotent men over the age of fifty have diabetes, which damages the nerves and arteries; more than half of men with diabetes become impotent. Atherosclerosis—a build-up of fatty plaque within the blood vessels—may narrow arteries and damage veins in the penis. Prostate surgery, liver disease, obesity, and loss of physical fitness can all affect erectile capacity.

Many drugs can affect erectile ability, including antidepressants, anti-anxiety and antipsychotic medications, alcohol, opiates, antihistamines, diuretics, and drugs that lower blood pressure, especially beta-blockers. Even cigarettes can create erection problems for men sensitive to nicotine.

Men with primary impotence are more likely to have an associated mental disorder and a possible underlying physiological abnormality. They experience far fewer complete or nearly complete erections during sleep and do not demonstrate the significant surges in testosterone during sleep that occur in other men.

▼

How impotence feels

Erection problems tend to be self-perpetuating. After one episode, a man may become so anxious about another that he is distracted and cannot become aroused. Each time he tries, his anxiety increases. He starts spectatoring, or self-monitoring, and may expect a problem. In one study, 94 percent of men with erectile disorders reported anxiety related to intercourse, particularly about failure. Most men suffer a loss of self-esteem and a sense of helplessness.

▼

Seeking help

If impotence may be a problem, these are the questions that should be asked:

- Have you repeatedly been unable to attain or maintain an adequate erection throughout sexual activity? (Some therapists suggest seeking help if a man fails to have an erection more than once in every four attempts to have sex.)
- Has this problem persisted for some time?
- Does this problem, as far as you know, seem unrelated to any physical illness or use of medication, drugs, or alcohol?
- Has this problem caused you great distress or anxiety?
- Has it created difficulties in your intimate relationships?

If you answer "yes" to these questions, you may want to discuss your concerns with your partner and consider consulting a health professional with experience in sexual disorders. Many men initially see a primary physician or urologist, who may refer them to a sex therapist.

To make a diagnosis and find out if the problem is psychological or physiological, physicians and therapists ask a man whether he has erections at times when he does not plan to have intercourse, morning erections, spontaneous erections during sleep, or erections with masturbation or other partners. Laboratory tests can measure blood flow and blood pressure in the penis. To assess the responsiveness of the blood vessels, the physician may inject the drug papaverine into the penis. If the arteries are normal, this drug usually produces an erection.

Nocturnal penile tumescence monitoring (described in Chapter 15) can determine whether or not a man is having normal erections during sleep; if erections occur, the problem is probably not physical. Other possible tests include: glucose tolerance for diabetes; tests for liver disease, pituitary tumors, calcium abnormalities, or hypothyroidism; measurements of different hormones; and assessment of possible alcoholism or depression.

▼
Treating impotence

Sex therapy for erection problems usually consists of prohibition of any attempts at intercourse, frank discussion concerning sexual activities, and sexual exercises to increase physical intimacy. As part of their homework, a couple sets aside at least two one-hour sessions a week when they are rested and unrushed. The exercises begin with exploration of each other's bodies, except for the breasts and genitals, and alternately giving and receiving sensual pleasure. In the next phase of sex therapy, the partners explore each other's genitals or breasts. The man, who focuses on his personal pleasure rather than on his partner's arousal, is encouraged to fantasize and to share his fantasies with his partner. Once he is comfortable talking with his partner, he is instructed to masturbate almost to orgasm. Some men first stimulate their partners to orgasm, either manually or orally. Eventually, the man inserts his penis into his partner's vagina with minimal thrusting; he then thrusts to orgasm while lying on his back; finally he has intercourse with his partner lying on her back.

Therapists provide reassurance by informing men that erectile problems are quite common and are usually time-limited. Most men can understand the concept of a vicious cycle of failure and performance anxiety and the need to interrupt this cycle by focusing on pleasure. Some therapists use erotic films and literature, but there is no evidence that these are necessary or effective. Sex therapy for impotence usually involves twelve to fourteen sessions, although it does not always take that many to resolve the problem. If there is no progress in five or six sessions, the program probably will not be successful. The most common barrier to such progress is marital conflict, and couples therapy may be advised.

Group therapy, hypnotherapy, and systematic desensitization can all help to reduce anxiety about sexuality. Psychoanalysis is not considered a treatment for impotence, but psychotherapy can sometimes help to ease intrapsychic conflicts that may be contributing to performance anxiety. Since alcohol and drug use can affect a man's erectile ability, it can be helpful to cut down on or eliminate alcohol, cigarettes, and any drugs of abuse. When impotence is a side effect of medication, a physician may reduce the dosage or suggest an alternative drug that provides similar therapeutic benefits.

Men with physically caused impotence should seek help from their primary physicians and the appropriate specialists. Many new treatments have been developed in recent years, including vacuum devices that increase blood flow to the penis to induce erection; injections of papaverine into the penis; vascular reconstruction (grafts of arteries from the lower abdomen bypassing narrowed branches of the main artery leading to the penis to restore blood flow); and penile implants, some inflatable, some permanently semi-rigid. Some therapists may suggest implants for men with psychologically induced impotence if they are older than fifty, have had erection problems for more than two years, and have not improved during sex therapy. Both a man and his partners should always obtain as much information as possible about implants so that they will have realistic expectations of the man's performance and are aware of possible risks and complications, such as decreased or altered sensation.

Testosterone is not considered an effective or appropriate treatment for impotence. Topical medications, such as nitroglycerin patches, may help by relaxing smooth muscle in the penis. Oral medications, such as yohimbine (a substance found in the bark of the yohimbine plant and sometimes used for hypertension), have been tried, with some reports of improvement.

▼
Impact on relationships

Impotence can lead to other sexual dysfunctions, such as a loss of desire, and can create problems in a man's relationship with his spouse or sexual partners. In married couples, a man's erection problems often follow a familiar pattern: The husband, fearing failure, avoids all physical intimacy; even a tender hug reminds him of his inadequacy. His wife, sensitive to his emotional distress, tries not to pressure him in any way. Eventually, however, she begins to resent his withdrawal. The emotional distance between the partners widens, and they become less likely to share moments of emotional or physical intimacy, until they find themselves living in an atmosphere of pain and resentment. Some couples never discuss their feelings. In others who try to talk through the problem, recriminations may force them into an angry silence.

Some women interpret their partner's erection problem as evidence of rejection. The anger and pain they feel make it harder for the couple to try to solve the problem. Like their husbands, women need to be able to relax sufficiently to experience full arousal and regain self-confidence. Talking these concerns through with a therapist can be of enormous benefit.

▼
Outlook

Impotence may occur once or rarely, or persist or recur over long periods. Sometimes a single session with a urologist or psychiatrist, who explains that impotence can have behavioral as well as biological causes and usually improves with time, is helpful.

Some researchers have found that simple reassurance or marital therapy is as effective as sex therapy. When problems persist, however, sex therapy can help to decrease performance anxiety and spectatoring by shifting attention away from fear of failure to the enjoyment of sensory pleasure. Often sex therapy helps even when the problem stems, at least in part, from a physical condition such as cardiovascular disease or diabetes. Even without treatment, 15 to 30 percent of men with psychologically caused impotence improve. The long-term outlook for men who seek help for impotence is very good, especially if their partners are willing to participate in treatment. Men whose problems develop quickly and have a clear cause have a better prognosis than those whose difficulties begin more insidiously or those who delay seeking treatment for several years.

Orgasmic disorders

By simplest definition, orgasm is a peak experience of sexual pleasure. Individuals describe a sense of suspended sensation, throbbing, release, and warmth that spreads through the genitals. The average time for a woman's sexual arousal to climax is about thirteen minutes; a man's is about two-and-a-half minutes. Orgasmic disorders include problems in achieving orgasm and in the timing of orgasm.

FEMALE ORGASMIC DISORDER

Women who cannot achieve orgasm by masturbation or intercourse may have an orgasmic disorder. However, women vary widely in their responses to different types of sexual stimulation. About 90 percent of those who are sexually active have experienced orgasm. About 30 to 45 percent have orgasm during intercourse, most with simultaneous direct stimulation of the clitoris.

Women tend to reach orgasm more easily and in response to a wider range of sexual stimuli as they grow older and more sexually experienced. For many, the peak years of sexual enjoyment are their thirties and forties; some first achieve orgasm during intercourse at this time. The reason may be a lessening of inhibitions, greater comfort in a marriage, and the absence of very young children at home. In addition, since a man typically requires a longer period of foreplay to achieve an erection as he grows older, the woman may have more time to become aroused.

After menopause, vaginal lubrication is lighter and takes longer to appear, and muscle contractions during orgasm are less intense and frequent. However, sexual desire, arousal, and orgasm do not necessarily decline with age. The level of a woman's sexual activity as she grows older depends more on the availability of a sexual partner, previous sexual behavior, and responsiveness than on age alone.

Some women have never experienced orgasm. This problem is called a *primary orgasmic disorder*. Women with a secondary orgasmic disorder have experienced at least one orgasm, regardless of the circumstances or means of stimulation, but can no longer achieve orgasm, whether under certain circumstances or in all forms of sexual activity.

Women's orgasms have long been a controversial subject. Freud argued that vaginal orgasms in response to intercourse were a sign of sexual maturity, as opposed to clitoral orgasms. This belief was held for a long time, but modern research has shown that a woman's orgasm is the same whether it is triggered by clitoral or vaginal stimulation, and that the clitoris is the primary sensory organ in orgasm.

Sex therapist and researcher Helen Singer Kaplan has described a continuum of female orgasmic response. At one end is "the rare woman" who can reach orgasm without genital stimulation; then women who climax during intercourse without simultaneous clitoral stimulation; women who require additional clitoral stimulation during intercourse; women who achieve orgasm with clitoral stimulation but not during intercourse; women who cannot reach orgasm with a partner but can with solitary masturbation; and, finally, women who have never reached orgasm.

▼

How common is female orgasmic disorder?

The estimated incidence of primary lack of orgasm ranges from 5 to 12 percent of sexually active women. An estimated 30 percent of women have a secondary orgasmic disorder. Primary orgasm problems are more common among young, unmarried women than among older, married women.

▼

What causes female orgasmic disorder?

Inadequate foreplay can cause this problem. Since women's needs for stimulation vary greatly, ten minutes or less of foreplay can be sufficient for orgasm in some women, while others may require twenty minutes or more. However, some women never reach orgasm even when foreplay is longer.

Sometimes medications—including anticholinergics, clonidine, methyldopa, tricyclic antidepressants, and monoamine oxidase inhibitors—can interfere with a woman's arousal and orgasm. Other problems, such as a sex-related phobia or anxiety, may play a role. Psychological factors—fears of getting pregnant, sexual rejection, or vaginal injury, or hostility toward a partner—can also sabotage sexual satisfaction. Some women may unconsciously inhibit their excitement because of concern about losing control or because of cultural and societal restraints. On the basis of a puritanical upbringing or strict religious beliefs, they may feel that sexual pleasure is somehow wrong or immoral. Strong sexual urges may make them feel so anxious or guilty that they cannot relax and accept their sexual impulses.

▼

How female orgasmic disorder feels

In terms of overall psychological well-being, researchers have found little difference between women who have orgasmic disorders and those who do not. However, women with this problem may have high levels of anxiety or guilt related to sex. In sex therapy these women tend to report more performance anxiety, spectatoring, and detachment during sexual situations. Some have very few or very negative sexual fantasies. In some cases they feel ambivalent about intimacy or intercourse or may be holding back anger or resentment of their partner. After sexual activity, some women with orgasmic disorders experience uncomfortable symptoms, such as lower abdominal pain, itching, vaginal discharge, a sense of increased tension, irritability, or fatigue.

▼

Seeking help

If the problem may be an orgasmic disorder, these are the questions to consider in deciding whether to seek help:

- Do you become sexually aroused but find it difficult to achieve orgasm?

- Does it take what seems to you to be a very long time to achieve orgasm?

- Are you unable to achieve orgasm through direct clitoral stimulation with a partner present?

- Does this problem happen repeatedly, or has it been occurring for a long time?

- As far as you can tell, is this problem unrelated to a physical illness, mental disorder, or the use of alcohol or drugs?

- Does it cause you anxiety, anger, frustration, or other forms of distress?

- Does it interfere with an intimate relationship?

If you answer "yes" to these questions, you may want to talk over your concerns with your partner and consider seeing a sex therapist. In making a diagnosis of orgasmic disorder, the therapist takes into account a woman's age, sexual experience, and the adequacy of the sexual stimulation she receives.

Is it female orgasmic disorder?

According to the DSM-IV, a diagnosis of female orgasmic disorder should be based on these criteria:

- **Persistent or recurrent delay in or absence of orgasm after a normal sexual excitement phase**

- **Does not occur exclusively during the course of another mental disorder and is not caused by drugs of abuse, medications, or a medical condition**

- **Causes marked distress or interpersonal difficulty**

Adapted from the Diagnostic and Statistical Manual of Mental Disorders, 4th Edition. *Used with permission.*

▼ Treating female orgasmic disorder

Brief sex therapy, based on the techniques developed by Masters and Johnson, has proved very successful. The goal is to enable a woman to relax and accept her own sexual needs. The therapist may start by encouraging her to fantasize, have sexual daydreams, or read erotic literature. During homework sessions, she practices sensate focusing (as described on page 291), masturbation, clitoral stimulation by herself or her partner or with her partner present, and Kegel exercises (tightening and relaxing the muscles around the vagina). Some women need reassurance that they will not lose control during orgasm or require information about differences in the way orgasm may feel. Once women are able to experience orgasm through self-stimulation, they can teach their partners the most effective and pleasurable ways of stimulating them. Both partners can learn various sexual positions that allow stimulation of the clitoris during vaginal intercourse.

Group therapy is highly effective in teaching women who have never had an orgasm about masturbation. In women with secondary orgasmic disorder, the emphasis is on communication techniques, whether as a couple or in a group (either of all women or including male partners).

Women who have serious underlying problems that interfere with their sexual functioning may benefit from long-term individual psychotherapy. Couples therapy may help those with marital problems. Some therapists prescribe anti-anxiety drugs to help women with high anxiety levels or phobias about sex respond better to sex therapy.

▼ Self-help

For many women, learning more about their own bodies can make an enormous difference in the enjoyment of their sexuality. There

are excellent self-help books available. Many recommend a graduated program of genital self-examination, sexual fantasy, and self-
stimulation, either by hand or with an electric vibrator. In many
communities, support groups provide a forum for women with
sexual dysfunctions, including orgasmic disorders, to advise and
reassure one another and share similar problems.

Women who specifically want to achieve orgasm or multiple
orgasms during intercourse should talk with their partners about
the type and duration of stimulation they need. Some are more
likely to experience orgasm when they are on top or in a position
that allows them or their partner to stimulate the clitoris. This
has been called a *bridge maneuver*, because the woman may then
begin to experience orgasm during intercourse without manual
stimulation.

**Impact on
relationships**   An orgasmic disorder can lead to problems of sexual desire, affect
a woman's self-image, and create tension in intimate relationships
and marriages.

Outlook   More than 90 percent of women who try self-help programs achieve
orgasm through masturbation, and more than three-quarters
through stimulation by a partner. Sex therapy is also highly effective in helping women to relax, enjoy their own sexuality, and
achieve orgasm.

PREMATURE EJACULATION

Premature ejaculation is a problem of timing. A man who experiences normal arousal reaches orgasm earlier than he or his partner desires, usually before penetration or immediately or very soon
after entering the vagina.

Masters and Johnson defined premature ejaculation as the inability to control ejaculation long enough to satisfy a responsive
partner at least 50 percent of the time. By this definition, premature ejaculation may occur during sex with some women but not
with others. Most mental health professionals do not use a specific
time frame to define this problem but instead take into consideration the man's age, sex partner, and the frequency and duration
of intercourse.

**How common is
premature
ejaculation?**   About 35 percent of men who seek help for sexual dysfunctions
have premature ejaculation. In one group of one hundred white,
happily married couples, 36 percent of the men expressed dissat-

isfaction because they ejaculated too quickly. This problem is more common among college-educated men than among those with less education, and may be related to their concern for partner satisfaction.

▼
What causes premature ejaculation?

Chronic premature ejaculation often begins with a man's first sexual encounters, which may occur in adolescence in situations in which he fears he might be discovered (as in the back seat of a car), so that he learns to achieve orgasm quickly. Other factors that can contribute include sexual inexperience, ignorance, or awkwardness; high excitement; sexual and social inhibitions; religious or moral concerns; fear of not performing well, of being punished, of displeasing a partner, or of being ridiculed; concern about pregnancy or disease; return to a regular partner after a long absence; and intercourse less often than once a month.

There are no known physical causes for premature ejaculation, such as drugs or illness. Masturbation does not cause premature ejaculation, although many people believe this to be the case. Sexual abstinence and marital stress make premature ejaculation worse. The problem is self-perpetuating: The more often it happens, the more likely it is to happen again.

▼
How premature ejaculation feels

A single episode of premature ejaculation may be embarrassing. If the problem persists, it typically becomes more and more upsetting. A man yearning for tenderness, touching, and some physical closeness may ejaculate at the sight of his partner nude or during an affectionate caress. Eventually he may avoid any genital contact because he may ejaculate even with a partial erection or a flaccid penis.

Young men who develop premature ejaculation can feel anxious, guilty, and ashamed. Although the prospect or even the thought of intercourse can be upsetting, they may become preoccupied with sex. A married man with this condition may have an affair to see if the problem is "my wife or me." If his wife finds out, or if he contracts a sexually transmitted disease, marital problems can worsen. Other men avoid all sexual encounters or desperately search for cures, such as ointments, pills, or mechanical devices.

▼
Seeking help

In considering whether the problem might be premature ejaculation, these are the questions that should be asked:

- Do you repeatedly ejaculate before you want to?

Is it premature ejaculation?

According to the DSM-IV, a diagnosis of premature ejaculation should be based on these criteria:

■ **Persistent or recurrent ejaculation with minimal sexual stimulation before, upon, or shortly after penetration and before the person wishes it**

■ **Causes marked distress or interpersonal difficulty**

Adapted from the Diagnostic and Statistical Manual of Mental Disorders, 4th Edition. *Used with permission.*

- Do you find it impossible to control or delay ejaculation?
- Is this problem causing you great anxiety and worry?
- Is it interfering with an intimate relationship?

If you answer "yes" to these questions, talk over your concerns with your partner. Some men do not realize they have a problem. Some believe that the real difficulty is not that they are too quick to climax but that their partners are too slow. These men may not seek help until their partners complain. Even if they do not feel dissatisfied personally, many men will seek treatment if they realize that a longer erection will enhance pleasure for themselves and their partners. As part of a general medical assessment, a physician may perform some medical tests, including urinalysis, a complete blood count, and assessment of various hormone levels.

▼

Treating premature ejaculation

Sex therapy is the treatment of choice for this disorder, although some couples may also require and benefit from marital therapy. Treatment begins with the man's complete sex history, particularly how long he has been troubled by premature ejaculation; his partner's reaction; his sexual experiences and fantasies; any feelings of shame and guilt; his dating and social activity; his approach to intercourse; his thoughts during intercourse; and any methods he has tried in an effort to resolve the problem. As the man reviews his sexual history, the therapist may point out certain events, often including initial sexual experiences in adolescence, that may have led to the development of the problem. The therapist may reassure him that it is common and emphasize that he can learn to sustain his erection longer.

Couple-based sex therapy consists of four to six sessions, beginning with practicing nongenital sensual awareness and pleasure for both partners. The couples proceed to breast and genital stroking, caressing, and ultimately to intercourse, usually beginning with the woman on top.

The two basic behavioral approaches to premature ejaculation are the *squeeze technique* and the *stop-start program* (also known as the *pause program*). In the squeeze technique, either partner stimulates the erect penis until the man senses impending ejaculation. At this point, the woman squeezes the penis at the place where the head meets the shaft for up to five seconds, then releases it for thirty seconds. She continues this procedure until the erection subsides. The couple repeats this process several times. Eventually it raises the man's threshold for the feeling of ejaculatory inevitability. He becomes more aware of his sexual sensations and more confident about his control.

In the stop-start technique, the man lies on his back while his partner strokes his penis. He focuses on the pleasurable feelings and the sensations that precede the urge to ejaculate. When he feels that he is about to ejaculate, he signals his partner to stop stimulation. He should stop and start at least four times before ejaculation.

In another variation on this technique, the man squeezes the area between his scrotum and anus firmly with his second and third fingers for four seconds. With practice, relaxation, and full body pleasuring and touching, this also improves his mastery. Group meetings with men with similar problems can be helpful in dealing with myths, macho attitudes, early sex pressures, and personal distress.

Some physicians have tried medications, including antidepressants and androgens (male sex hormones), to cure this problem, but there is no evidence of their effectiveness.

▼

Self-help   To delay orgasm, some men try to distract themselves by thinking of other subjects, such as sports. Others masturbate before intercourse, taking advantage of the refractory period during which a man cannot ejaculate again. Others bite their lips or dig their nails into their palms; the usual results of this are bloody lips or scarred palms. Some men try special anesthetic creams on the penis, but these rarely work after the first or second application, and they dull sensation for the woman as well.

Sometimes a man may respond to an occasional episode of premature ejaculation with low-key humor and reassurances for his partner. In such cases, the simplest treatment is a second attempt at intercourse the same evening, because a second erection lasts longer and may restore the man's confidence. During the second episode of love-making, preferably in a secure, comfortable setting, he can focus his attention on his partner rather than his performance.

The key to better control of ejaculation is learning to sense the feelings that precede ejaculation and recognizing the point of ejaculatory inevitability. The penile squeeze technique, which can be used during masturbation or with a partner, can lead to greater skill and confidence in extending the duration of erection. By practicing at home in a relaxed state of mind, a man can master the process of lessening and then regaining an erection, giving him greater control and reducing his anxiety about premature orgasm.

▼
Impact on relationships

Premature ejaculation, because it is so frustrating and embarrassing for both partners, can lead to erection problems for the man and loss of sexual desire for both. The interaction between the partners after premature ejaculation is crucial. If the woman responds with criticism or quickly pulls away to wash, switch on the television set, or turn her back to him, the man's feelings of failure and shame may be intensely painful.

The exercises that are the essential part of sex therapy can initially make both partners feel vulnerable. Each exposes very private aspects of his and her identity in the course of this process, and looks to the other for acceptance and understanding. If these responses are conveyed, working together to overcome the problem can create a sense of trust and tenderness that brings the partners closer.

▼
Outlook

Sex therapy is highly successful for premature ejaculation, even when the problem has persisted for as long as twenty years. Most men develop some control over their erections within two to ten weeks; within several months their control is excellent. One major sex therapy center, the Loyola University Sexual Dysfunction Clinic, reports that up to 90 percent of men improve. Premature ejaculation may recur but usually improves with home practice or one or two additional sessions with a therapist. The condition may also improve naturally after the age of fifty.

MALE ORGASMIC DISORDER

In this condition of inhibited or retarded ejaculation, a man has great difficulty in achieving ejaculation during intercourse—if he succeeds at all. Usually he cannot reach orgasm during vaginal intercourse but can do so with other types of stimulation, such as masturbation.

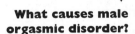

Is it male orgasmic disorder?

According to the DSM-IV, a diagnosis of male orgasmic disorder should be based on these criteria:

■ **Persistent or recurrent delay in or absence of orgasm after a normal sexual excitement phase during sexual activity**

■ **Does not occur exclusively during the course of another mental disorder and is not caused by drugs of abuse, medications, or a medical condition**

■ **Causes marked distress or interpersonal difficulty**

Adapted from the Diagnostic and Statistical Manual of Mental Disorders, 4th Edition. *Used with permission.*

▼

How common is male orgasmic disorder?

There is little available research on the incidence of male orgasmic disorder. According to various estimates, this dysfunction may occur in 4 to 10 percent of men.

▼

What causes male orgasmic disorder?

Most temporary cases of retarded ejaculation are caused by alcohol. Fifty percent of alcoholic men have sexual performance problems; 10 percent have inhibited or absent ejaculation. Illicit drugs also may have an effect.

Orgasmic problems can also have physiological causes, including prostate surgery, spinal cord disorders, Parkinson's disease, hormonal abnormalities, diabetes, and certain medications, including the antihypertensive guanethidine monosulfate, methyldopa, and the phenothiazines.

This problem also can stem from psychological factors, including anxiety; sexual inhibitions or a belief that ejaculation is messy, dirty, or sinful; worry about urinating during coitus; or a fear of intimacy, loss of control, pregnancy, or parenting. Some boys, taught stringent religious prohibitions against masturbation to orgasm, condition themselves to stop or delay ejaculation and continue to do so in adulthood.

▼

How male orgasmic disorder feels

Men with a primary orgasmic disorder have never experienced orgasm during intercourse. They have often been reared in a rigid, puritanical background in which sex is seen as "dirty," or they may have conscious or unconscious incest wishes and problems in intimacy that inhibit their becoming close to anyone. Men with secondary orgasmic disorder have experienced orgasm during intercourse but no longer can do so. Some may feel unacknowledged hostility toward their partner or toward all women. In others who are in a committed relationship, this problem may develop as the man's way of coping with real or imagined changes in the relationship that he finds threatening, such as plans for pregnancy or demands by his partner for greater commitment. Depending on the circumstances, a man may feel frustrated or embarrassed by this problem.

Seeking help

In considering if the problem may be orgasmic disorder, these are the questions that should be asked:

- Have you repeatedly found it difficult to achieve an orgasm during vaginal intercourse?
- Does it consistently take longer for you to reach orgasm than you would like?
- Do you feel your usual level of sexual excitement and arousal during sexual activity?
- As far as you can tell, is this problem unrelated to a physical condition, a mental disorder, or the use of medication, alcohol, or illicit drugs?
- Has this problem caused you distress or anxiety?
- Has it created difficulty in your intimate relationships?

If you answer "yes" to these questions, you may want to discuss your concerns with your partner and consider seeking professional help. You may want to see your primary physician or a urologist first, since this problem requires a thorough medical examination that checks for physical illness as well as the effects of alcohol, medication, or illicit drugs.

Treating male orgasmic disorder

Men with this dysfunction are advised to abstain from alcohol. Sex therapy, the most frequently used treatment for this problem, usually consists of four to six weekly visits. Each session deals with physical, sexual, and marital factors, and the therapist explores each partner's feelings about sinfulness, sharing, closeness, pleasing each other, and impregnation. The couple is given permission and encouragement to enjoy affection and sexual fantasies and feelings. They also learn relaxation techniques, such as slow breathing or "thinking of floating or gliding" during sexual activity.

The couple regularly practices sex exercises at home, and goes through successive phases of sensate focusing, nongenital stimulation, and genital caressing. The man is instructed to masturbate while his partner is in the house and later with his partner in the same room. Eventually she stimulates him, with his hand over hers so she can feel how much pressure he requires. After a few weeks of this, he is allowed to masturbate only when she is present. Finally, she may be instructed to sit astride him and stimulate him, eventually putting his penis in her vagina when he reaches the point of ejaculatory inevitability. Together with the therapist, the partners discuss the sexual role reversal, with an active female and passive male.

Medications are sometimes used to reduce anxiety. For example, a man may take an anti-anxiety drug an hour before intercourse if he is fearful that slow breathing and relaxation will not calm him down sufficiently. Once men successfully ejaculate during intercourse, they quickly overcome their anxiety.

▼

Self-help
About 25 percent of men with an orgasmic disorder who abstain from alcohol for about four weeks require no other treatment. A sex therapy technique that can be practiced at home is masturbation to ejaculation as quickly as possible while the man fantasizes that his penis is inside his partner's vagina.

▼

Impact on relationships
Male orgasmic problems can create or reflect severe conflict in an ongoing relationship. The woman, who may blame herself or feel anxious about finding a solution to the problem, may be even more upset than her partner. Depending on the circumstances and the issues facing the couple, the man's self-esteem may be affected, and he may find it hard to express his feelings of inadequacy or shame.

▼

Outlook
Although there have been few follow-up studies, sex therapy is believed to be highly effective in treating this dysfunction. In one seven-week program, eleven of sixteen men with retarded ejaculation progressed from ejaculation through a partner's stimulation to ejaculation during intercourse.

Sexual pain disorders

Pain is a subjective symptom. One individual may be highly sensitive to hurting sensations that another can tolerate with ease. Some people who feel pain during sex endure it for the sake of physical closeness and sexual release. For others, pain may be a welcome reason to avoid all sexual or affectionate contact.

DYSPAREUNIA

Dyspareunia (pain during intercourse) is persistent or recurring pain associated with intercourse, whether before, during, or after it. Although women are far more likely to develop this problem, often because of a lack of lubrication or vaginismus (discussed later in this chapter), it occurs in men as well, who report sensations of tearing, burning, throbbing, and heavy, shooting pain in the genitals before, during, or after ejaculation.

▼

How common is dyspareunia?

As noted previously, dyspareunia is much more common in women than in men and often coincides with vaginismus (discussed later in the chapter). The overall incidence of dyspareunia is not known.

▼

What causes dyspareunia?

In women, the problem may be lack of arousal. If her partner insists on going ahead with intercourse regardless of her readiness, the woman may become increasingly apprehensive about sex, which makes the problem worse. Sometimes rupture of the hymen in a young woman, which most often occurs during manual stimulation or her initial use of tampons, may be so painful that it leads to fear of penetration thereafter.

Various medical conditions can lead to pain during sexual activity, including infections such as herpes or trichomoniasis; disorders of the external genitals, such as scarring after trauma; endometriosis; ovarian cysts; and prolapsed uterus. Chronic musculoskeletal or neurological conditions can also cause pain during sex. Certain medications, including the tricyclic antidepressants imipramine and protriptyline, have been associated with pain during intercourse. Postmenopausal women may suffer dyspareunia because of thinning of the vaginal walls and reduced lubrication. Of women who seek help at sex therapy clinics because of dyspareunia, 30 to 40 percent have some pelvic physical condition, such as vaginitis (infection), endometriosis, and episiotomy scars.

Various physical conditions can cause dyspareunia in men. Gonorrhea can cause burning or sharp penile pain during ejaculation. Prostatitis or a herpes lesion can cause pain in the tip of the penis during sex. Some men report painful ejaculation after vasectomy, prostatectomy, urethral obstruction, or urethritis. Men with severe cardiac or respiratory disease may experience chest pain, shortness of breath, or intense chest pain at climax. Some men develop an orgasmic headache before or right at the time of climax. In Peyronie's disease, which mainly affects men between the ages of forty and sixty, scar tissue forms inside the penis for un-

<table>
<tr><td>

Is it dyspareunia?

According to the DSM-IV, a diagnosis of dyspareunia should be based on these criteria:

</td><td>

■ Persistent or recurrent genital pain in either a man or a woman before, during, or after sexual intercourse

■ The disturbance is not caused exclusively by vaginismus or lack of lubrication, a mental disorder, drugs of abuse, medications, or a medical condition.

■ Causes marked distress or inter-personal difficulty

Adapted from the Diagnostic and Statistical Manual of Mental Disorders, *4th Edition. Used with permission.*

</td></tr>
</table>

known reasons (it is not believed to be related to infection, tumor, contagious disease, or sexual practice) and causes curvature of the penis that makes intercourse difficult.

Younger men may experience a feeling of congestion in their testicles if sexual arousal does not culminate in orgasm; young teens may experience testicular torsion (twisting) during sexual arousal. Priapism, a prolonged painful erection of the penis with no associated sexual excitement, is a rare but potentially danger-ous condition and requires immediate medical treatment. In rare cases, men who have suffered pain during sex can develop muscle spasms in the perineum (the area between the anus and the geni-tals) and experience pain or a burning sensation with any kind of sexual arousal or attempt at genital manipulation.

▼

How dyspareunia feels

Dyspareunia can take the form of burning, irritation, or intense pain. Some people feel so psychologically helpless about stopping the pain that they don't even try, and live with the problem for years before seeking help; others avoid intercourse.

▼

Seeking help

If dyspareunia may be a problem for either partner, these are the questions that should be asked:

• Do you feel repeated or persistent discomfort before, during, or after intercourse?

• Do you experience burning, irritation, or pain?

• As far as you know, is this problem not the result of a lack of lubrication, a physical condition, a mental disorder, or the use of alcohol or drugs?

- Has this problem caused you anxiety or distress?
- Do you avoid sexual intimacy because of the possibility of pain?
- Has it created difficulties in your relationships?

If you answer "yes" to these questions, discuss your feelings with your partner. Individuals often deny this problem, even though it may cause them soreness, repeated infection, and other problems. Often partners never mention pain during sex until some other dysfunction, such as an arousal or orgasmic disorder, leads them to seek treatment.

▼

Treating dyspareunia

Treatment depends on the cause. If the problem is physical, a physician should treat the underlying disorder; a mental health professional may help to deal with its emotional or marital impact. If lack of sexual arousal is the problem, sex therapy has proved helpful.

For men who develop an orgasmic headache at the time of climax, self-relaxation techniques or small doses of a benzodiazepine such as lorazepam (Ativan) before intercourse can be helpful. The curvature of the penis caused by Peyronie's disease can be treated by various methods, including surgery.

▼

Impact on relationships

Dyspareunia can greatly impair a couple's sexual relationship. If one partner avoids sex because of pain, the other may feel rejected. If the partner who experiences pain endures it without seeking help, he or she may feel resentful. The condition can have an enormous impact on self-image and can lead to other sexual dysfunctions, such as a loss of desire.

▼

Outlook

The prognosis depends on the underlying cause of the problem and the couple's willingness to get treatment.

VAGINISMUS

Vaginismus is an extreme form of painful intercourse in which involuntary contractions of the muscles of the outer third of the vagina are so intense that they partially or totally close the vaginal opening, preventing the insertion of the penis. Its incidence is not known.

Vaginismus may be primary (lifelong) or secondary (acquired). Women with primary vaginismus have always had muscle spasms and difficulty with penetration, starting with first intercourse.

Women with acquired vaginismus have had pain-free intercourse in the past.

▼

What causes vaginismus?

The most common cause is a woman's fear that vaginal penetration will be painful. Although each woman may have a unique reason for this fear, there have usually been childhood experiences that associated pain with penetration of various kinds, including injection needles, painful or frightening dentistry, frequent throat cultures, or one or more urethral dilatations without anesthesia.

One of the most common experiences that women with vaginismus report is difficulty inserting tampons when they first began menstruating. A girl's uterus and vagina are small at the age of menarche, and the insertion of a tampon may rupture the hymen, causing pain. Girls who repeatedly try but fail to insert a tampon may come to believe they are anatomically abnormal. Later they may try again, but because their previous experience has made them tense and apprehensive, their vaginal muscles may tighten involuntarily, making the vaginal opening too small for insertion of a tampon.

A small percentage of teenage girls have a strand of tissue that bisects the vaginal opening. They can insert a tampon successfully by pushing the strand to one side, but removal may require strenuous pulling, which causes sharp pain and bleeding. The result is a lasting association between an object in the vagina and severe pain.

Other experiences with genital trauma—accidental injury to the vulva when riding a bicycle or climbing a fence, difficult pelvic exams in the early years, or excision of a boil on the labia—can also lead to an association of sexual activity with pain, depending on the girl's emotional response to the trauma and the amount of reassurance that parents and health professionals are able to provide.

Vaginismus can occur after sexual trauma, such as rape. Childhood sexual abuse, particularly vaginal penetration by a finger, object, or penis, can increase the likelihood of vaginismus. Alternatively, a medical condition, such as endometriosis, may be responsible. Women also appear to be more vulnerable during the months after childbirth and at the time of menopause, when hormonal changes may lead to discomfort during intercourse.

From a psychodynamic view, vaginismus may stem from a conflict between a woman's conscious wish to have intercourse and her unconscious effort to prevent the penis from entering her body. Some women, particularly small women who grow up continuing to think of themselves as fragile little girls with tiny bodies, may see a penis as a huge and threatening weapon.

<table>
<tr><td>

Is it vaginismus?

According to the DSM-IV, a diagnosis of vaginismus should be based on these criteria:

</td><td>

■ **Recurrent or persistent involuntary spasm of musculature of the outer third of the vagina that interferes with sexual intercourse**

■ **The disturbance is not better accounted for by a mental disorder or a medical condition.**

■ **Causes marked distress or inter-personal difficulty**

Adapted from the Diagnostic and Statistical Manual of Mental Disorders, 4th Edition. *Used with permission.*

</td></tr>
</table>

Another important factor is ambivalence about sexual intercourse. Some young women, who may not feel ready for sex but want to assert their independence, may try intercourse only to find that their tight vaginal muscles make penetration difficult or impossible. Sometimes the pain of first intercourse is so severe that women develop vaginismus during subsequent attempts. Anxiety may also stem from religious or cultural prohibitions, fear of pregnancy or disease, concern about being discovered in sexual activity or becoming promiscuous, or confusion about sexual identity.

A woman's feelings about her partner can be a factor, especially if she is angry, feels she is being used sexually, or mistrusts his caring and commitment. A partner's sexual skill—or lack of it—may create or worsen a woman's anxiety. If she is already anxious, she may become more fearful if a man's penis is unusually large. Some women who feel emotionally abused by their partners may unconsciously develop vaginismus as a protest.

▼

How vaginismus feels

Vaginismus occurs in differing degrees. In mild cases, although the pain or discomfort during penile insertion (which is often described as burning) subsides after thirty to sixty seconds or may continue, intercourse is possible. Some soreness may persist afterward. Moderate vaginismus involves pain and discomfort plus difficulty inserting the penis, which may only partially penetrate the vagina. Severe vaginismus occurs when a muscle spasm completely blocks penetration; even pressure against the vaginal opening is painful.

Most women with vaginismus respond similarly to all attempts at vaginal penetration, whether by a tampon, finger, speculum, or penis. Sometimes, however, the condition occurs only with sex or with sex with a specific partner.

Seeking help   If the problem may be vaginismus, the questions that should be asked are:

- Do involuntary, repeated spasms of the vaginal muscles make penetration by a penis difficult or impossible?
- Does penetration, when possible, cause pain, discomfort, or a burning sensation?
- Does this problem recur often or has it persisted for a while?
- As far as you know, is this problem not related to any physical condition or mental disorder?
- Does it cause you anxiety or distress?
- Do you avoid sexual activity or intercourse because of this problem?
- Does it cause difficulty in your relationships?

If you answer "yes" to these questions, you should consult a gynecologist. Vaginismus can only be conclusively diagnosed by a pelvic examination. Typically, the muscles tighten as the examiner places a hand on the woman's inner thigh or touches her genital area, although she may be unaware of this contraction. Whenever possible, the partner should be present for the pelvic examination, because seeing the muscles tighten helps to ease his feelings of rejection.

Treating vaginismus   A variety of treatments have been used in overcoming vaginismus: the insertion of dilators of progressively greater widths into the vagina, individual psychotherapy, relaxation training, anti-anxiety drugs for relaxation, hypnosis, and surgery.

Sometimes all that is needed is the use of fingers or dilators to desensitize the woman to vaginal penetration. Some therapists suggest that she insert the tip of her finger or a tampon into her vagina while stroking her genitals gently. Dilators of graduated sizes can also be used, either in a therapist's office or the patient's home, to enlarge the vaginal opening. During the weeks of dilator treatment, there should be no other vaginal penetration, including tampons if they trigger muscle tensing. Relaxation training or hypnosis also can help a woman to relax.

When the couple ultimately attempts intercourse, they start with the woman on top so that she can be in control of insertion and motion and stop if there is pain. They proceed to slow motions and finally to full ones. Since many women with this problem also have problems becoming aroused, concurrent sex therapy may focus on relaxation, sensory awareness, and stimulation.

Psychotherapy alone may be effective when the cause of vaginismus stems from psychological or interpersonal factors and when the fear that penetration will hurt is not deeply entrenched. Hypnosis and the use of medication to induce relaxation can succeed on their own or in combination with dilators. Surgery is recommended only in case of a very thick, tight hymen.

▼

Self-help   Many women with vaginismus are extremely tense. Various relaxation techniques, such as progressive muscle relaxation and transcendental meditation, can be useful. Some women feel more relaxed after soothing themselves with a warm bath, listening to music, or focusing on relaxing images. Kegel exercises (tightening and relaxing the muscles around the vagina) can also be helpful.

▼

Impact on relationships   Vaginismus profoundly affects the way a man and woman relate to each other sexually. A woman with this condition may develop other sexual dysfunctions, such as loss of desire or arousal and orgasmic disorders. A man may develop erectile problems or premature ejaculation as a result of his concern about hurting his partner.

Therapy itself can also affect the relationship. It is helpful to be aware that sometimes, as a woman begins to have success inserting dilators, her partner may become anxious about her increasing autonomy and assertiveness or her potential sexual demands once she can have intercourse comfortably.

▼

Outlook   Most therapists report success in most or all cases. In the rare instances in which treatment does not work, the reason often is another sexual problem, such as inhibited sexual desire.

Paraphilias

The key element of a paraphilia is a recurrent, sexually arousing fantasy that involves sexual urges or acts focused on inanimate objects or nonconsenting partners. Paraphilias do not conform to generally accepted views of what is normal and acceptable in a specific place and time, and they may cause harm to the individual or others. Some practices, such as bondage or cross-dressing, are considered a disorder only if they become the exclusive or preferred means of sexual excitement and orgasm, or if the behavior involves any form of sexual activity with children or, with adults, is not consensual. Over time, a paraphilia may become the central preoccupation of a person's life.

TYPES OF PARAPHILIAS

Recent studies indicate that many individuals have several paraphilias, and that more than half develop these conditions before age eighteen.

Exhibitionism   Exhibitionism occurs only in men and involves repeated exposure of the genitals to a stranger (almost always a girl or woman). This disorder, as with other paraphilias, may take the form of sexual urges, fantasies, or actual activity. Men may expose themselves to assert their masculinity, although they unconsciously feel castrated and impotent. Usually exhibitionists are not dangerous and do not attempt sexual activity with the person to whom they expose themselves. They may do this out of an urge to shock or surprise a stranger, or may fantasize that the person will become sexually aroused by the exposure.

Fetishism   Fetishism involves the use of inanimate objects intimately linked with a person's body (underwear, shoes, stockings, boots) to obtain sexual excitement. The fetishist, who is almost always a man, may use this object himself to induce sexual arousal or may ask a partner to wear it during sex. He may choose items, such as panties or bras, that he finds sexually arousing, and masturbate while holding, rubbing, or smelling them. Some men are unable to achieve an erection or orgasm without such stimulation. Fetishism usually begins by adolescence and tends to be chronic.

Frotteurism   In frotteurism, a man touches, fondles, or rubs his penis against the buttocks or breasts of a fully clothed woman unknown to him. It occurs in men, usually between the ages of fifteen and twenty-five, who are typically very lonely and passive. They select an attractive woman and press against her buttocks or touch her breasts in a crowded place, such as on a bus or subway. As they do this, they may fantasize about being involved in an exclusive, caring relationship with the woman. The woman may initially think that this contact is accidental because she cannot imagine that anyone would attempt sexual molestation in public.

Pedophilia   Pedophilia consists of repeated sexual urges, fantasies, or activity involving children aged thirteen or younger. Adults

PARAPHILIAS

☐ **Exhibitionism.** Exposing the genitals to an unwilling observer

☐ **Fetishism.** Obtaining sexual pleasure from an inanimate object or an asexual part of the body, such as the foot

☐ **Frotteurism.** A male's rubbing against or fondling a fully clothed woman's breasts or buttocks as she stands next to him

☐ **Pedophilia.** Repeated sexual urges, fantasies, or activity involving children age thirteen or younger

☐ **Sexual masochism.** Obtaining sexual gratification by suffering physical or psychological pain

☐ **Sexual sadism.** Becoming sexually aroused by inflicting physical or psychological pain

☐ **Transvestism.** Becoming sexually aroused by wearing the clothing of the other sex

☐ **Voyeurism.** Obtaining sexual gratification by observing people undressing or involved in sexual activity

with this disorder may be of the same or opposite sex as the child and may or may not be related. The great majority of pedophiles—95 percent—are heterosexual. Some have previously been involved in exhibitionism, voyeurism, or rape. Many were themselves victims of sexual abuse as children.

A single sexual act with a child is not necessarily pedophilia; it may be an aberration, the consequence of marital problems, recent loss, or intense loneliness, in which the child serves as a substitute for an adult partner who is not available. In rare cases, sexual acts with children are the result of the person's mental retardation, a psychiatric disorder, or alcohol intoxication. Records show that at the time of an incident, half of pedophilic adults have consumed an excessive amount of alcohol.

Individuals with pedophilia may undress a child, expose themselves, masturbate, fondle the child, perform fellatio or cunnilingus, or—much more rarely—penetrate the child's vagina, mouth, or anus with fingers, objects, or penis. Some try to rationalize their acts by stating that such acts are educational or sexually pleasurable for the child or that the child was sexually provocative. They may limit pedophilic activity to their own children, stepchildren, or relatives, or may find children outside the family. Some work to win the child's trust and affection; others threaten the child in order to keep their behavior secret. Pedophiles may go to great lengths to gain access to children, such as dating or even marrying the mother of a child who attracts them or even abducting children from strangers. Many are drawn to both boys and girls; others are attracted to one sex or the other, or to a child of a certain age. Usually pedophilia begins in adolescence, although its onset can occur as late as middle age. Stress may increase the intensity of pedophilic activity. The disorder tends to be chronic, especially in those attracted to boys.

Sexual masochism Sexual masochism involves urges, fantasies, or experiences in which the source of sexual excitement comes from being voluntarily beaten, bound, humiliated, or otherwise made to suffer. Some people have masochistic fantasies in which they imagine being tied up or shamed during sex or masturbation but never act on their imaginings. Such fantasies are considered a problem only if they cause the person great distress. Others may actually mutilate themselves, stick themselves with pins, or hurt themselves in other ways. About 30 percent of sexual masochists also have sadistic fantasies and are known as *sadomasochists*.

Masochistic sexual activities can also occur with a partner, and include bondage, blindfolding, paddling, spanking, whipping, beating, electrical shocks, cutting, and humiliation, such as verbal abuse, being urinated or defecated on, being forced to crawl and bark like a dog, or being dressed in diapers and treated like a baby.

One particularly dangerous form of sexual masochism is masturbation and sexual fantasy through *hypoxyphilia*—sexual arousal by oxygen deprivation. To reduce the supply of oxygen a boy or man may tie a noose around his neck, put a plastic bag over his face, or use a chemical (such as volatile nitrite) that sends blood away from the brain. As a rule, he stops the activity before losing consciousness, but each year one or two individuals in the United States, England, Australia, and Canada die as a result of this practice.

Masochism, which is more common among men, may stem from destructive fantasies turned against the self or from an inability to experience sexual pleasure unless punishment follows. Masochistic sexual fantasies often begin in childhood and are first acted on during the teens, either alone or with partners. Persons tend to repeat the same masochistic act over the years, although some increase its severity over the course of time or during periods of stress.

Sexual sadism Sexual sadism involves urges, fantasies, and activity in which the primary source of sexual excitement is the psychological and physical suffering of a victim. It is named after the Marquis de Sade, an eighteenth-century French writer repeatedly imprisoned for his violent acts against women. Most people with this paraphilia are men.

The sexual sadist wants complete control over a terrified victim or a consenting partner who willingly suffers pain or humiliation and is sexually aroused by this suffering. Sexual activities include dominance, restraint, blindfolding, paddling, spanking, whipping, pinching, beating, burning, electrical shocks, rape, cutting or stabbing, strangulation, torture, or mutilation.

It is thought that sadism in men may be a defense against fears of castration; a man does to others what he fears might be done to him. Some individuals with this problem have an underlying schizophrenic disorder. Sadistic fantasies often develop in childhood, and individuals may begin acting on them by early adulthood. Sadists may continue their activity with nonconsenting partners until arrested. Usually, the severity of their acts increases over time and may involve sexual assault, rape, injury, or even murder.

Transvestic fetishism Transvestic fetishism involves fantasized or actual dressing in female clothes by heterosexual men during masturbation or intercourse. When not dressed in women's clothes, transvestite men are unremarkable in appearance and occupation, and their primary sexual preference is usually heterosexual. Some are lonely and are troubled by guilt or depression; others are sociable members of a transvestite subculture. Transvestic fetishism can involve a single item of clothing, such as underwear, or an entire wardrobe, including jewelry and makeup.

Transvestic fetishism begins in childhood or early adolescence, but a man does not appear cross-dressed in public until adulthood. Many men with this problem report that they were punished or humiliated in boyhood by being dressed in girls' clothing. With increasing age, some are no longer sexually aroused by dressing in women's clothes, although they may do so again during periods of stress.

Voyeurism Voyeurism involves observation of an unsuspecting person who is naked, disrobing, or engaging in sexual activity. The voyeur does not attempt any sexual activity with those he observes. It is the act of looking alone that provides sexual excitement, which may lead to orgasm, either by masturbating while watching or later while recalling the scene and fantasizing about having sex with the person. Voyeurism, which may become a person's exclusive sexual activity, usually begins before the age of fifteen and tends to be chronic.

▼

How common are paraphilias?

Little is known about the frequency of these disorders. Pornography and paraphernalia associated with paraphilias constitute a major commercial business, suggesting that they are common. Paraphilias are almost exclusively male, except for sexual masochism, and even that is twenty times more common in men than in women. Often individuals have three to five different paraphilias, either at the same or at different times in their life. More than half begin before the age of eighteen, peak between the ages of fifteen and twenty-four, and gradually decline. Paraphilias are rare in men fifty or older, except for those that occur with a partner or in private.

▼

What causes paraphilias?

According to psychoanalytic theory, people who develop paraphilias have never completed the normal developmental process toward heterosexual adjustment. They may choose one paraphilia over another either to cope with the threat of castration by the father or separation from the mother. Other theories trace paraphilias to early experiences that condition or socialize a child into committing a particular act. Thus, a child whose first sexual experience is molestation may be predisposed to growing up as an abuser or victim of abuse. Individuals may also model their behavior on that of others whom they see carrying out paraphilic acts either personally or in the media.

By the time young people realize that their interests and urges induced by their fantasies are considered abnormal, they may have become conditioned to these fantasies for sexual arousal. If they continue to use them during masturbation, the fantasies become linked with orgasm and the arousal produced by the paraphilia intensifies.

Paraphilias may also be the result of a delusion, dementia, mental retardation, or other psychiatric problems. Some studies suggest that there is an association between paraphilias and certain biological abnormalities such as seizures, hormone imbalances, chromosomal irregularities, or altered brain waves.

▼

How paraphilias feel

Often people with paraphilias do not consider themselves ill or deviant. Many claim that they feel no distress because of their behavior and say that the only problem is the reaction of others. A minority report extreme guilt, shame, and depression because their unusual sexual activity is socially unacceptable or because they themselves regard it as immoral.

Some individuals with paraphilias never act on their sexual urges and failures. There are great differences in the degree to which a person requires the fantasy central to his paraphilia in order to achieve sexual excitement. Those who act on their paraphilia are more likely to be under severe stress, to use drugs or alcohol, and to have antisocial personality traits.

In some instances, the unusual behavior, such as exhibitionism, may become the major sexual activity in the person's life.

Some individuals select an occupation, develop a hobby, or volunteer for work that brings them into contact with desired stimuli (such as women's shoes or lingerie). They may read books, collect photographs, purchase films, or view tapes depicting their paraphiliac fantasies. Some seek out the services of prostitutes or others who provide specialized services, such as bondage and domination or cross-dressing. Others act out fantasies with unwilling victims. Certain paraphilias, such as sexual masochism, can result in serious injury; others, such as pedophilia, may lead to arrest and imprisonment.

▼

Seeking help

Because most individuals with paraphilias do not feel upset by their behavior, they seek treatment only when their behavior brings them into conflict with sexual partners or society. Diagnosis is based on a detailed sexual history and psychiatric evaluation.

▼

Treating paraphilias

Both medication and various forms of psychotherapy have been used to treat paraphilias, depending on the particular type. Medication has been used primarily for individuals with pedophilia or exhibitionism. In countries other than the United States (where legal issues restrict such uses), drugs that block or decrease the levels of male sex hormones, such as medroxyprogesterone acetate (MPA) and cyproterone acetate (CPA), have been given to sex offenders since the late 1960s. These drugs decrease libido and halt the individual's pattern of compulsive sexual behavior, although relapse usually occurs as soon as the medication is discontinued. More recently, some psychiatrists have experimented with fluoxetine (Prozac) as a potentially useful treatment for individuals with voyeurism, exhibitionism, pedophilia, and frotteurism.

Behavioral therapies have been extensively used. Therapists try to disrupt the learned pattern by various means, including negative stimuli, such as electric shocks or noxious odors, that the person administers to himself when he feels a sexual urge. Cognitive techniques focus on faulty beliefs, such as a pedophile's interpretation of a child's docility as an expression of sexual desire. Relaxation training may help to reduce the anxiety and stress that can trigger paraphiliac behavior. Group therapy can also be helpful in confronting faulty thinking and rationalizations.

For some individuals, psychodynamic psychotherapy provides an opportunity to understand the dynamics and events that caused the paraphilia to develop and to become aware of the daily events that cause them to act on their impulses. Although it can offer the person useful insights, it is rarely effective as the sole form of therapy.

Impact on relationships

About half of those who seek treatment for paraphilias are married. Their marital and sexual relationships may suffer if their spouses become aware of their unusual activity or refuse to tolerate it. Often a person with a paraphilia cannot engage in reciprocal, affectionate sexual activity and may develop other sexual dysfunctions, such as inhibited arousal or orgasm.

Outlook

The prognosis for paraphilias depends on the age of onset, frequency, the presence of concurrent substance abuse, and the individual's feelings of guilt or shame. The outlook is best in those who have experienced normal intercourse in the past and are highly motivated to change.

Is it an attention disorder?

Adults with attention disorders may:

☐ **Be restless and irritable**

☐ **Not be able to concentrate on a focused activity like reading**

☐ **Be distractable, forgetful, absent-minded**

☐ **Find it difficult to wait; become extremely irritated when standing in line or stuck in traffic**

☐ **Experience frequent mood swings**

☐ **Be disorganized and have difficulty finishing projects or chores**

☐ **Find it hard to solve problems or manage time**

☐ **Be impulsive or reckless; make rash decisions**

☐ **Have low tolerance for stress; be easily overwhelmed by ordinary hassles**

☐ **Be clumsy**

☐ **Have a poor body image**

The more boxes that you or someone close to you checks, the more reason you have to be concerned about a possible attention disorder. This chapter can provide information on seeking help and on understanding and overcoming this problem. (Chapter 26 discusses attention disorders in children.)

14

Attention Disorders in Adults

They are studies in perpetual motion, squirming constantly, incapable of sitting still. They interrupt when others talk, don't get along with their peers, hate waiting for anyone or anything. Derailed by the smallest distraction, they cannot stick with a task long enough to finish it. When faced with frustration, they explode into furious rages. For them and for their loved ones, daily life can be exhausting and exasperating.

These fidgety, impulsive people fit the classic description of hyperactive youngsters, but there is one big difference: They are grown-ups. Little more than a decade ago, mental health professionals assumed that what is now termed *attention-deficit/hyperactivity disorder* (AD/HD)—the most common psychiatric diagnosis in childhood—was strictly kid stuff. They were wrong. About half of youngsters with AD/HD do *not* outgrow their restless, often reckless ways at puberty but continue to have attention problems in adolescence. Half of these individuals—25 percent of all children who develop AD/HD—continue to have the condition as adults, and even more may have some lasting symptoms.

AD/HD, a term that has replaced *minimal brain dysfunction* and *hyperactivity*, refers to a spectrum of difficulties in controlling motion and sustaining attention. Its primary symptoms—hyperactivity, impulsivity, and distractibility—are less obvious in adults than in youngsters. Rather than scooting around a room, grown-ups with attention problems may tap their fingers or jiggle their feet. Some appear calm and organized on the surface but cannot concentrate long enough to finish reading a paragraph or follow a list of directions. Others, on a whim, go on buying sprees or take wild dares. Such behavior does not happen only at some times or in some circumstances; it is chronic and pervasive, meaning that it goes back for as long as the individuals can remember and affects every aspect of their lives.

▼

How common are attention disorders in adults?

In all, 1 to 2 percent of adult men and women in the United States, perhaps as many as 5 million, have problems in sustaining attention or controlling their movements and impulses. These problems are even more common in children, affecting 3 to 10 percent of youngsters, about three-quarters of them boys.

In adulthood, men and women seem equally prone to attention problems. It is possible that boys, who usually develop more visible (and vexing) symptoms, have been more readily diagnosed than girls, whose symptoms may be more subtle. It is also possible that attention problems may develop later in females than in males.

▼

What causes attention disorders?

AD/HD may stem from an abnormality in brain functioning. Using sophisticated brain-imaging techniques, researchers at the National Institute of Mental Health (NIMH) have measured metabolic activity in the brains of adults who have had symptoms of AD/HD since childhood and who have at least one child with the disorder. The resultant images, when compared with those of normal volunteers, show that these individuals metabolize glucose, the brain's main energy source, at a slower rate, particularly in the regions of the brain that regulate movement and attention.

Vulnerability to this problem may be inherited. AD/HD tends to run in families and is more common among close relatives of people with this disorder than in others. Approximately one-third of children diagnosed with AD/HD have a parent or sibling with the same problem. In other cases, it is thought that something may have gone amiss during pregnancy, probably during the second trimester, that affects the development of specific areas of the brain.

Despite years of controversy, there is no proof that food allergies, additives, sugar, head injury, or fluorescent lights cause AD/HD. However, preliminary findings from ongoing studies do suggest that a thyroid disorder may account for a small fraction of AD/HD cases.

▼

How attention disorders feel

Individuals with attention disorders live in a confusing, often frustrating world. Their thought processes are different from others, and they can be very easily distracted. On the way from an office building to the post office on the corner, for example, they may forget their objective, wander into a store, and impulsively buy an expensive coat or watch. As long as they are working or talking one to one (as during an interview or while working at a computer), they may do perfectly well; but when they have to wait in line, do chores, attend meetings, or wait for a delayed flight, they become enormously aggravated.

Men and women who grew up before the late 1960s and early 1970s, when attention problems were first widely recognized in children, may have always sensed that something was wrong but never knew what. Unaware of attention problems, their teachers may have viewed them as underachievers. Their subsequent employers may have thought or may still think of them as goof-offs, and their families may remember them as difficult, demanding youngsters who grew up to be irresponsible adults.

"I always thought I was stupid," says a thirty-eight-year-old man, who blames his undiagnosed attention disorder for the loss of several jobs, his poor credit rating (he kept forgetting to pay bills and taxes), and the break-up of his first marriage. Like many others, he finally discovered his real problem when his son was diagnosed with AD/HD. His reaction, like that of many parents who find out that they, too, have attention disorders, was enormous relief at finally discovering what had caused problems for him all his life.

While children with AD/HD find it hard to filter out extraneous noises or activities, adults report what some describe as "an internal distractibility." They fail to pay close attention to details, make careless mistakes, find it hard to focus, sustain attention, keep track of several projects at the same time, or to organize their thoughts coherently. Just like youngsters with AD/HD, they may act or speak without thinking. Some rush into decisions or business ventures without taking the time to weigh potential disadvantages. Because of this tendency, others may assume they are immature or have poor judgment.

Adults with attention disorders can lead successful lives, although they are less likely to achieve this in more conventional ways. In fact, the individuals with undiagnosed AD/HD who make their way into therapists' offices with their children are usually the luckier ones. Through determination, talent, or sheer grit, they have found ways to cope, perhaps by going to the gym every night to sweat away their restlessness or by pushing themselves to work harder and longer merely to keep up with everyone else. Some

The man who couldn't sit still

When Jeff, his wife Melanie, and their son, Colin, spent the Thanksgiving holidays with Jeff's parents, his mother watched as Jeff repeatedly hopped up and down from the dinner table, restlessly flipped through the channels on the TV, and scattered magazines he'd started reading around the house. One moment Jeff was helping his Dad clear some shrubs; the next he was driving to the local mall. He and Colin would start building a tower, then race off to play catch. "I can't believe it," Jeff's mother finally declared. "You're thirty-two years old, and you still can't sit still. You're as bad as Colin."

She was right. Jeff no longer scooted around the house constantly the way Colin did, but he too was a study in perpetual motion. Even when he did manage to stay in one place for a time, he'd tap his fingers or jiggle his feet. "Colin's teacher thinks he may be hyperactive," said Melanie. "Maybe Jeff is too."

Everyone laughed, but Jeff knew that his attention problems weren't anything to joke about. As a youngster, he had struggled through school, trying to be good but never managing to behave like his classmates. He'd been kept behind one year, and he had needed special tutoring in reading and writing. His teachers sent home notes complaining that Jeff interrupted when others were talking, didn't get along with his peers, and was so easily distracted that he couldn't stick with a task long enough to finish it.

When he finished high school, Jeff swore he would never enter a classroom or pick up a textbook again. Personable and hardworking, he found it relatively easy to find a job. The problem was keeping one. He couldn't sit behind a desk for more than a few minutes at a time. The smallest frustration could set off a tirade. If he had to read complicated instructions, his attention would wander after a paragraph or two. Driving around on service calls, he'd grow frustrated if caught in traffic.

For a few years, Jeff seemed to be going nowhere fast. After a hard day at work—and every day seemed hard—he'd unwind by drinking or smoking marijuana. He would get intensely involved with a woman, but then his fiery temper would lead to arguments, and they'd break up. Melanie was different. She worked as a floral arranger in a shop that hired Jeff as a delivery man. Calm and quiet, she would spend hours creating beautiful bouquets and displays. Jeff would watch her delicate fingers and listen to her soothing voice and somehow feel calmer himself.

Melanie was the one who suggested that Jeff try going into retail sales. "With your energy, you'd be a natural," she said. Jeff took a job at a bustling consumer electronics store. Working the floor, chatting with customers, and ringing up sales suited him, although he constantly had to struggle to keep his impatience and temper in check. Every evening he'd go to a gym and work out until he had sweated himself into a state of quiet exhaustion. After his marriage to Melanie, he worked even harder to focus his energies.

Jeff was the one who took Colin to a child psychiatrist, at his teacher's suggestion, for evaluation for possible hyperactivity and attention problems. As he described his son's behavior, he said, "I used to be the same way—as a matter of fact I still am." When the psychiatrist said that she suspected that Jeff might have an attention disorder, something clicked in his mind. "I knew she'd hit the nail on the head. I'd always thought there was something wrong, but no one had ever been able to tell me what it was before. Everything she said made sense."

Jeff and his son started taking stimulant medications and going for individual psychotherapy. Both needed the same daily low doses of the drug. It did not make them feel high; rather, they found it made it easier to concentrate and control their physical restlessness. Finally capable of focusing his attention for prolonged periods, Jeff began taking night courses. Eventually, he'd like to get a degree in business and become a manager. In the meantime, he is happy to be less impulsive, less short-tempered, and more organized. "Now that I know what the problem is I can meet it head-on and deal with it," Jeff says. "After all these years, I finally know what it's like to function like a grown-up."

have chosen jobs, such as retail sales or taxi driving, that do not demand sustained concentration. In one study that followed more than a hundred boys with AD/HD into their twenties, a smaller than normal number completed college or graduate school, and a much higher than expected percentage went into business for themselves.

For some adults, however, the inability to focus or control impulses is a serious handicap. They drift from job to job and place to place, never really settling down. Their relationships tend to be short and stormy. Their lives often become a jumble of dead-ends, wrong turns, frustrations, and failures. They are more prone to abuse alcohol or drugs, to get into accidents or trouble with the law, to develop other mental disorders, and to commit suicide.

There is one major difference between adults who were diagnosed and treated for attention disorders or hyperactivity as children and those who were first identified as having AD/HD as adults. Those who have been struggling with an unknown difficulty all their lives, and who may have been ostracized, criticized, or ridiculed as stupid or lazy, tend to have much lower self-esteem and to feel more depressed than those who knew the nature of their problem from childhood.

▼

Seeking help Most adults with this problem initially seek treatment for other reasons. Many have developed other problems, such as anxiety or depression. Some are troubled by constant money woes or difficulties in sustaining a relationship. Others have managed to find a good job or win a promotion but want help in getting along with others or feeling in better control. Parents with a child who has been diagnosed with an attention deficit disorder may recognize similar symptoms in themselves and seek help at that point.

If you suspect that you or someone close to you might have an attention problem, these are the questions that should be asked:

- Are you chronically restless? Are you unable to settle down and read or concentrate on paperwork?

- Are you easily distracted? Is your mind often somewhere else? Are you forgetful?

- Do you have problems finishing tasks? Are you disorganized? Do you switch haphazardly from one project or chore to another? Do you have constant difficulty in managing your time?

- Are you easily provoked or constantly irritable?

- Are you impulsive or reckless? Do you make decisions with little reflection or too little information? Do you go on rash buying sprees or make foolish investments?

- Do you begin and end relationships abruptly?
- Are you easily hassled? Do you overreact to stress? Is your life in a state of constant crisis?

Many people might answer "yes" to at least a few of these questions. However, if you or someone close to you answers "yes" to many or most of them, the problem may be an attention disorder. Since these symptoms can also have other causes, it is important to undergo a complete evaluation by a mental health professional.

Because there is no clear-cut method for detecting attention disorders, diagnosis can be difficult. A careful, comprehensive history is critical. One key question is when the first symptoms appeared. AD/HD almost always begins before the age of seven. Researchers have developed a rating scale, based on recollections of childhood such as poor concentration, daydreaming, fidgeting, and not achieving up to potential. If such behaviors began recently or occur only in certain circumstances, the probable cause is another emotional condition. The primary cause of restlessness, impulsivity, and distractibility in adults is anxiety. The second most common cause is agitated depression, which makes people extremely restless.

Many adults with attention problems have several of the symptoms listed in the table on the opposite page, rather than the complete AD/HD syndrome. A key consideration in determining the need for treatment is the extent to which these symptoms interfere with their ability to function normally, to perform adequately at work, and to engage in satisfying relationships.

▼

Risks and complications

Attention disorders take a toll on mental health. People with these problems have a higher than normal incidence of anxiety disorders, mild depression, and mood swings. They also tend to abuse alcohol or drugs, but not in the typical way. Rather than trying to get high or euphoric, they reach for a drink or a drug to become more calm and focused. Teens and young adults with AD/HD experience four times as many car accidents and are more than four times as likely to be at fault in the accident as other young drivers, according to recent studies by University of Massachusetts researchers.

▼

Treating attention disorders

Adults with AD/HD benefit from the same therapy as children with this disorder. The most successful approaches involve a combination of medication, psychotherapy, and appropriate academic or vocational education.

<table>
<tr><td>

Is it an attention-deficit/ hyperactivity disorder?

</td><td></td></tr>
</table>

Is it an attention-deficit/ hyperactivity disorder?

According to the DSM-IV, a diagnosis of AD/HD is based on the following criteria, which occur frequently and have persisted for six months or longer:

■ *Inattention,* **as indicated by at least six of the following:**

1. **Failure to give close attention to details or making careless mistakes**
2. **Difficulty sustaining attention**
3. **Not seeming to listen when spoken to directly**
4. **Failing to follow through on instructions and finish a task**
5. **Avoidance, dislike of, or reluctance to engage in activities requiring sustained mental effort**
6. **Losing things necessary for a task or activity**
7. **Easily distracted**
8. **Forgetful**

OR

■ *Hyperactivity-impulsivity.* While the physical restlessness and fidgeting associated with childhood AD/HD often stop or lessen in adulthood, some individuals remain unusually active. They or their family members may report that they cannot sit still at the movies or at a restaurant. They often act as if "driven by a motor," are constantly on the go, or talk excessively. Just like youngsters with AD/HD, they may act or speak without thinking. Some rush into decisions or business ventures without taking the time to weigh potential disadvantages. Because of this tendency, others may assume they are immature or have poor judgment.

■ **A history of inattentive or hyperactive-impulsive symptoms prior to age seven**

■ **Some impairment in two or more settings (such as work and home) as a result of the symptoms**

■ **Clear evidence of significant impairment in social, occupational, or academic functioning**

■ **Symptoms are not better accounted for by another mental disorder, such as a mood disorder, anxiety disorder, dissociative disorder, personality disorder, or a psychotic disorder, such as schizophrenia.**

Adapted from the Diagnostic and Statistical Manual of Mental Disorders, 4th Edition. *Used with permission.*

MEDICATION

The primary medications—methylphenidate (Ritalin), dextroamphetamine (Dexedrine), and pemoline (Cylert)—are stimulants that would produce a high-intensity rush of euphoria in most people. In those with AD/HD, however, they have a paradoxical effect, aiding in concentration and reducing restlessness. Most adults need the same daily low doses that children do, do not feel high, do not take more than they need, and do not become tolerant to the therapeutic effects of the medications.

"We are not sedating or tranquilizing people; we are making them normal," says psychiatrist Larry Silver, M.D., of Bethesda, Maryland, a leading expert on AD/HD. "It's like giving insulin to diabetics." The most common side effects of stimulants are difficulty in falling asleep and loss of appetite. Adjustments in dosage and timing can ease such reactions. Some people report stomachaches or headaches. Much rarer is the development of tics, which go away once the drug is discontinued. About 60 to 80 percent of adults improve after taking stimulants. When stimulants don't work, tricyclic antidepressants, such as Norpramin, Pamelor, and Tofranil (described in Chapter 28), sometimes do.

The length of time that adults must continue to take medication varies. Some need it only until they finish school or learn coping strategies. Others take it for many years but eventually find ways to manage without it. Many report that medication makes them less short-tempered, less distractible, less impulsive, less moody, less vulnerable to stress, and more organized and responsive to others. "It offers me the same sense of continuity and control that most other people seem to have to begin with," says one man.

PSYCHOTHERAPY

Because AD/HD can sabotage self-esteem as well as relationships, individual and family therapy may also be important. "Therapy helps undo past patterns," says Silver. "A marriage may be shaky because of the person's impulsivity or financial problems. Both partners may have to learn better ways to deal with each other."

EDUCATION

Medication also makes it possible for adults with AD/HD to participate in and benefit from psychotherapy, general counseling, vocational rehabilitation, and academic retraining. "It frees them up to get on with their lives," Silver notes. "As many as 70 to 80 percent of adults with AD/HD have learning disabilities, and there are just as many resources and opportunities for them as there are for kids." If they are having trouble on the job, men and women with AD/HD may need training. Time-management courses often help to make their lives less chaotic.

Impact on relationships   The distractibility, impulsivity, and irritability common in attention disorders can interfere with an individual's ability to form long-lasting intimate relationships. Some men and women develop a pattern of getting involved in relationships very quickly and breaking them off almost as rapidly. Friends and relatives may become irritated because these individuals do not seem to pay attention, remember things they were supposed to do, or follow through on promises. Once their partners begin treatment, spouses often say that the differences are so dramatic that they now feel as though they are married to a different person.

▼

Outlook   With treatment, most adults with attention disorders report a dramatic improvement in their mood, concentration, and frustration levels. Some finish school, get promoted, and give up self-destructive behavior. Symptoms of other mental disorders, such as depression, also may improve. Even when the changes are smaller, they still can add up to a sizable boost to an individual's self-image and confidence.

Is it a sleep disorder?

Individuals with a sleep disorder may:

- [ ] **Have difficulty falling or staying asleep**
- [ ] **Not feel refreshed or restored by sleep**
- [ ] **Be extremely drowsy in the daytime**
- [ ] **Be unable to resist daytime sleep attacks and lose muscle control during them**
- [ ] **Experience vivid hallucinations or be unable to move major muscles while waking up or falling asleep**
- [ ] **Have a mismatch between their work schedules and usual sleep-wake times because of travel or shift work**
- [ ] **Not be able to fall asleep or wake up at typical or desired times**
- [ ] **Have extremely frightening dreams**
- [ ] **Suddenly wake up screaming in the night, with no recollection of a bad dream**
- [ ] **Repeatedly sleepwalk, with no memory of the episode the next day**
- [ ] **Feel great distress or interference with usual routines, relationships, and performance at work or school due to sleep difficulties**

The more boxes that you or someone close to you checks, the more reason you have to be concerned about sleep difficulties, especially if problems persist for more than a month. This chapter provides information on the most common sleep disorders and guidance on obtaining appropriate treatment.

15   Sleep Disorders

O n any given night, one in three people has a problem falling or staying asleep. According to the National Commission on Sleep Disorders Research, 40 million men, women, and children have chronic sleep problems; another 20 to 30 million occasionally have difficulty getting the rest they need.

Mental health professionals define sleep disorders as persistent disturbances in the quantity or quality of sleep that interfere with an individual's ability to function normally for a month or more. The primary types are:

- *Insomnia:* A problem in falling asleep, staying asleep, or feeling rested after sleep
- *Hypersomnia:* A problem involving too much sleep or extreme daytime sleepiness
- *Circadian rhythm sleep disorders:* Problems in falling asleep or staying awake at appropriate times
- *Parasomnias:* Problems that occur during sleep.

Primary sleep disorders are not related to any medical or mental disorder. *Secondary* sleep disorders are symptoms of physical or mental illness, stress, drug or alcohol use, work shifts, or travel.

Normal sleep

A normal night of sleep consists of several distinct stages and types of sleep. Stage 1 is a twilight zone between full wakefulness and sleep. The brain produces irregular, rapid electrical waves; muscles relax; breathing is smooth and even. In stage 2, brain waves are larger and are punctuated with occasional sudden bursts of electrical activity. In stages 3 and 4, the brain produces slower, larger waves, sometimes referred to as *delta* or slow-wave sleep.

After about ninety minutes in the four stages of quiet sleep, the brain shifts into a more active state, characterized by rapid eye movement (REM) and called REM sleep. (The four stages of quiet sleep are referred to as non-REM, or NREM, sleep.) The brain waves produced during REM resemble those of waking more than those of quiet sleep. The large muscles of the torso, arms, and legs cannot move during REM, although the fingers and toes may twitch. Breathing is quick and shallow; blood flow through the brain speeds up; men have partial or full erections. This is the time of vivid dreaming.

During the course of a night's rest, adult sleepers spend about 75 percent of their time in NREM sleep and 25 percent in REM. In the early part of the night the deep stages of NREM sleep are longer. They grow progressively shorter through the night, and REM periods lengthen. The first REM period is usually less than ten minutes long; later REM periods last fifteen to thirty minutes. A typical night consists of four or five cycles of NREM and REM sleep.

Sleep needs and patterns change over the course of a lifetime. From infancy to adulthood, total sleep times decrease by more than half. Adults average 7.5 hours of sleep a night. More is required during illness or during periods of increased stress, mental challenge, or physical exertion. Some women find that their sleep patterns change at different times in their menstrual cycles.

Total sleep time gradually diminishes with age; many elderly men and women sleep only six hours. The quality of sleep changes over time as well. Periods of very deep sleep and of REM sleep dwindle steadily from childhood into adulthood. At all ages, some people seem to be natural "short sleepers," who need less than six hours of rest a night to feel energetic the following day. "Long sleepers," who tend to have more REM periods during sleep, may sleep ten hours or more a night.

Recognizing the differences between normal and abnormal sleep often depends on subjective judgment. Only the individual can say whether he or she is getting enough sleep to feel alert and energetic during the day. Each person seems to have an innate sleep "appetite" that is as much a part of genetic programming as hair color, height, and skin color. Although the average sleep time is 7.5 hours a night, the "normal" range can be anywhere from five to ten hours. One or two people in one hundred can get by with just five hours; another small minority needs twice that amount.

Insomnia

Insomnia is a lack of sleep so severe that it interferes with a person's ability to function normally during the day. Whereas most people fall asleep within thirty minutes of getting into bed, others toss and turn for an hour or more. Some awaken frequently in the night, cannot sleep long enough to feel alert and energetic the next day, or do not feel rested even if they have no apparent difficulty in falling or staying asleep.

Most often insomnia is transient, typically occurring before or after a major life event, such as a wedding, a move, or the start of a new job, and lasting for three or four nights. During periods of prolonged stress, such as a divorce or the illness or death of a loved one, transient insomnia may persist for several weeks. On the other hand, chronic or long-term insomnia may persist for months or years.

▼

How common is insomnia?

Each year an estimated 15 to 30 percent of adults seek professional help because of insomnia. About 30 percent of them have a chronic problem. Insomnia can begin at any age, but the likelihood increases with age. Younger people are more likely to have problems falling asleep; those who are older complain more of difficulty staying asleep or of waking too early.

▼

What causes insomnia?

In primary insomnia, sleeplessness itself is the problem. Researchers speculate that certain individuals may have subtle physiological abnormalities in the sleep-wake control centers in the brain that disrupt their rest from infancy. This lasts throughout their lives, and they tend to be extremely light sleepers, easily disturbed by noise, temperature, or worry. They often recall that they were poor sleepers as youngsters.

Secondary insomnia is a symptom of something else that is wrong: stress, physical pain, discomfort or illness, another sleep disorder, lifestyle habits, such as irregular hours, or excitement or worry about a particular event. Sometimes acute sleep difficulties turn into chronic ones. Although most people who are apprehensive about a major event or upset by a life crisis and cannot sleep return to normal sleep patterns after a night or two, some continue to have sleep difficulties even after the stressful situation has eased. Increasingly anxious and exhausted, they try harder and harder to get more sleep, but end up feeling frustrated. Each night of poor sleep reinforces their worry about not sleeping, and their sleep problems may persist for weeks, months, or even years.

Such *learned* or *behavioral* insomnia afflicts about 15 percent of those with chronic insomnia who seek help at sleep disorders centers. Individuals with learned insomnia typically fall asleep when they are not trying to, for example, while reading or watching a movie, and sleep better anywhere but in their own beds—on the sofa, at a hotel, in a sleep laboratory.

About one-third of those with insomnia have an underlying mental disorder, usually depression or an anxiety disorder. Depressed individuals have characteristic changes in their sleep patterns, including a shorter than usual time from sleep onset to REM, an abnormally long first REM period, and greater than usual eye movements during REM. Insomnia also may occur in individuals with anxiety disorders, including posttraumatic stress disorder, obsessive-compulsive disorder, Alzheimer's disease, and schizophrenia.

Almost any medical illness, injury, or surgical procedure that produces discomfort or pain can cause insomnia. Minor symptoms such as sore muscles, heartburn, fever, or cough can disturb sleep for a few nights. Chronic illnesses, such as asthma or disorders of the heart, lungs, kidneys, liver, pancreas, and digestive system, can create long-term difficulties. Even when pain subsides and other symptoms disappear, sleep may remain elusive. The table on the opposite page lists substances that can disrupt sleep.

Sometimes sleep is disturbed by leg pains and movements during the night, called *nocturnal myoclonus*, or by a condition known as "restless legs," characterized by discomfort in the lower limbs as a person is trying to fall asleep. Often individuals with these problems awaken during the night and have to get up and walk around. They may complain of both insomnia and excessive daytime tiredness.

Many substances, including alcohol, drugs of abuse, and prescription medications, can disrupt sleep. Sleeping pills also can be a culprit. People who take sleeping pills for two weeks or more and then stop typically find it hard to fall asleep—this is called *rebound insomnia*—and have very vivid, frightening dreams once they do. An estimated 20 percent of all cases of insomnia are complicated by withdrawal reactions from sleeping pills. Sleep usually returns to normal several weeks after the medication is stopped. Insomnia also can be a problem during withdrawal from amphetamines, cocaine, or pain medications.

SUBSTANCES THAT CAN CAUSE INSOMNIA

☐ **Caffeine-containing products**	☐ **Methyldopa**
☐ **Nicotine**	☐ **Steroid preparations**
☐ **Alcohol**	☐ **Thyroid medications**
☐ **Nasal decongestants**	☐ **Anti-arrhythmic drugs**
☐ **Appetite suppressants**	☐ **Antihypertensive drugs (some)**
☐ **Asthma medications (epinephrine, theophylline, etc.)**	☐ **Medications containing scopolamine**

Individuals with what is called "insomnia complaint without objective findings" report poor sleep even though they have no history of using medications, drugs, or alcohol, and tests show no evidence of a disorder or abnormality. Very few, if any, are faking their complaints. It may be that sleep studies are simply not sophisticated enough to detect the true cause of this problem. Sleep specialists have observed that when these persons are wakened from stage 2 sleep, they can often report what has passed through their minds in the previous half-hour, as if their thought processes had not stopped during sleep. Treatment, either with behavioral strategies or the brief use of medication, can improve sleep.

▼

How insomnia feels

People with insomnia suffer not just during the night but during the day as well. Sleep loss can lead to irritability and difficulty in remembering and concentrating. Fretting about their sleepless nights, chronically poor sleepers may become totally preoccupied with getting enough rest. Their worry about not sleeping makes them tense and unable to relax.

Not everyone with insomnia appears or feels anxious. However, many report vague feelings of apprehension or distressing thoughts that keep them awake. Their insomnia may worsen during times of stress and improve during vacations. People who can trace their sleep difficulties back to childhood typically do not think or talk in psychological terms and do not like to talk about or analyze their insomnia.

▼

Seeking help

If you suspect that insomnia may be a problem for you or someone close to you, these are the questions that should be asked:

- Have you been having problems falling or staying asleep?
- Do you wake up not feeling rested, regardless of how much you sleep?
- Are you so tired that you cannot function normally during the day?
- Have your sleep problems persisted for a month or longer?
- Have you been very upset about them?

If you answer "yes" to most of these questions, the problem may be insomnia. You should consult your primary physician, a psychiatrist, or a sleep specialist. You may be asked to keep a sleep diary, in which you record bedtimes, wake-up times, time asleep, and daily naps for a week or two, and to follow the self-help guidelines on page 357. In some cases your doctor may suggest polysomnography, which can detect underlying abnormalities affecting your sleep. The box on the opposite page describes the most common sleep evaluation tests.

▼
Risks and complications

Insomnia affects the way a person feels and functions. Although it rarely causes major life difficulties, the solutions that those desperate for rest may turn to—alcohol, over-the-counter or prescription sleeping pills, stimulants to enhance alertness during the day—can create serious complications, including drug dependence.

▼
Treating insomnia

The treatment of insomnia is highly individualized. In the long term, behavioral approaches to sleep problems have proven as effective as medication, without the risks associated with drug use. However, individuals must practice these behavioral techniques regularly for several weeks before they begin to see improvement. Among the most helpful are:

Relaxation therapy. Audiotapes providing instruction in progressive muscle relaxation, diaphragmatic breathing, hypnosis, meditation, and biofeedback can help individuals who have temporary sleep difficulties. Chronically poor sleepers usually need to work with an experienced trainer to learn how to relax, particularly when they are preparing for sleep.

Cognitive therapy. Techniques that shift a poor sleeper's mind away from anxiety-inducing thoughts and fears can help the person fall asleep. Specific approaches depend on the individual's needs. For instance, those who cannot "turn off" their racing minds may be told to read in bed until they drift into sleep. Those who constantly check the time may have to remove clocks from the bedroom. Those who find themselves thinking about daytime worries

Sleep tests

Sleep disorders centers around the country, certified by the Association of Sleep Disorders Centers, offer the specialized equipment and technical experts required to diagnose certain sleep disorders and other psychiatric problems. Health care plans, including Medicare, usually cover the charges. The most commonly used tests are:

☐ **Polysomnography.** This is a night-long recording of various mental and physical functions, including brain waves, muscle tension, heart rhythm, and breathing, made by a device called a polysomnograph. This test requires no injections, incisions, or X-rays. The only discomfort is the slight initial irritation of electrodes, which are placed in pairs on the skin, usually over an ointment that creates a better seal. Electrodes at the corner of the eyes measure eye movement; those on the scalp detect brain waves; those on the chest measure heartbeats;

those on the legs record movements. A temperature-sensitive device taped just below the nostrils records breathing rate and volume of inhaled air. A belt around the lower chest monitors the diaphragm. The electrodes relay signals through a central line to the polysomnograph, which converts them into electrical impulses that appear as wavy lines on continuous sheets of paper. A computer analyzes these data and a trained polysomnographer interprets them to determine if there is a problem.

☐ **REM latency.** Normal adults usually have their first REM period about ninety minutes after falling asleep. If they enter REM earlier, this shortened "REM latency" may be a sign of a mental disorder, including depression or narcolepsy. Therapists can assess REM latency in a sleep laboratory. An electroencephalograph (EEG) records the brain waves characteristic of REM, and an electromyograph (EMG)

evaluates muscle tone to see whether it is reduced.

☐ **Nocturnal penile tumescence.** During REM, a man's penis becomes partially or fully erect. A sleep test for the purpose of measuring the stiffening (or *tumescence*) of the penis is particularly helpful in determining whether a man's impotence is caused by physiological or psychological factors. If there is a physiological problem, the penis does not become erect during REM. If the problem is psychological, erections do occur.

☐ **Multiple sleep latency test.** This daytime test is a way of analyzing excessive daytime sleepiness. At two-hour intervals, an individual is hooked up to a polysomnograph and allowed to nap. Individuals with a hypersomnia disorder, such as narcolepsy, typically fall asleep very quickly and enter REM sleep within minutes. (Two episodes of daytime sleep with REM periods confirm that the problem is narcolepsy.)

can try various "refocusing" techniques, such as memory games like trying to remember state capitals or counting backward from a certain number.

Stimulus control therapy. This approach is specifically tailored for people with learned insomnia. At night, they go to bed only when they are so tired they feel they can fall asleep easily. If this does not happen, they must get up, leave the bedroom, and engage in some quiet activity until they are very sleepy, at which point they can return to bed. If they still do not fall asleep easily, they again leave the bedroom, repeating the process as often as necessary. In the morning, they must get up at their usual time and avoid any daytime naps. During the first night of this therapy, some people spend as much time out of bed as in it. As they become more fa-

Is it primary insomnia?

According to the DSM-IV, a diagnosis of primary insomnia should be based on these criteria:

■ **Difficulty falling or staying asleep or nonrestorative sleep for at least one month**

■ **The sleep disturbance or daytime fatigue causes significant distress or impairment in social, occupational, or other important areas of functioning.**

■ **Does not occur exclusively during the course of a circadian rhythm sleep disorder, narcolepsy, a breathing-related sleep disorder, or a parasomnia**

■ **This disorder does not occur exclusively during the course of another mental disorder, such as a major depressive or generalized anxiety disorder.**

■ **This disorder is not due to the direct effects of a substance (drugs of abuse or medication) or medical condition.**

Adapted from the Diagnostic and Statistical Manual of Mental Disorders, 4th Edition. *Used with permission.*

tigued, however, they find it easier to fall asleep when in bed, and when this happens they no longer associate their beds with poor sleep. This treatment typically requires several weeks and the encouragement of a supportive therapist during what can be a frustrating process.

Sleep restriction therapy. In this form of therapy, individuals first fill out sleep logs that record their judgments of how much time they spend in bed and how much time they actually sleep. They are then allowed to stay in bed only as long as they have indicated they usually sleep. Thus, someone who has reported sleeping for only four of the eight hours he or she spends in bed would have to get up after four hours and could not nap in the course of the day. Once people spend at least 90 percent of their allotted time in bed in actual sleep, they earn an additional fifteen minutes in bed. Like stimulus control therapy, this approach makes individuals extremely sleepy, which eventually makes it easier for them to fall asleep in bed. However, some people become so tired during the day that they cannot maintain the program long enough for it to be effective.

Sleeping pills may be used for a specific, time-limited problem, always with a physician's approval and supervision. The American Sleep Disorders Association has stated officially that the use of benzodiazepines, the most commonly used sleeping pills (hypnotics) in the United States, is warranted as a time-limited treatment for transient insomnia and as an occasional adjunctive treatment for chronic insomnia that persists despite treatment of the underlying conditions. According to its position statement, "the benzodiazepine hypnotics are preferred over barbiturates and other

PERSONAL VOICE

Sleepless nights

Nate never slept well in the final stages of a take-over battle. By day, he was a consummate deal-maker, always cool and in control. At night, when he got into bed, the figures would keep racing through his mind. He'd get up and pour himself a drink, sometimes two. He would then nod off, only to waken a few hours later with his head filled with ideas. Once the negotiations were over, Nate would take a long weekend off and sleep most of it away.

But weeks after losing one particularly nasty take-over fight, Nate found that he still wasn't resting easily. Each night he'd get into bed and replay the entire process, second-guessing his every move, trying to figure out why things had gone wrong. Over time his sleeping problems began to take a toll on his daytime performance. Colleagues commented on how haggard he looked. His wife worried about his health. Nate called his internist, who prescribed some sleeping pills.

The medication helped. Nate would pop a pill and get a few hours of badly needed rest. But after a couple of weeks the pills no longer seemed to be working. He started taking two instead of one. Once again, he was able to sleep—but only for a while. Not wanting to risk taking an even higher dose, Nate stopped the pills completely. The next night he was up for hours and, when he finally did fall asleep, his dreams were filled with bizarre, often gruesome scenes.

Convinced that he would never get a good night's sleep again, Nate began taking what he called "a little siesta" on the sofa in his office in the afternoon. If he missed this nap, he'd often fall asleep watching television in the evening. Yet whenever he got into bed, nothing happened. He'd lie there for hours wondering if he would sleep at all. The only times that he did sleep well were when he was out of town on a business trip.

Nate's wife, whose own sleep was suffering because of his insomnia, called a local sleep disorders center and made an appointment for him. The sleep specialist at the center explained the effects that alcohol and sleeping pills have on normal sleep, and he talked about what he thought was Nate's real problem: "learned" insomnia.

"You've conditioned yourself to go to bed expecting you aren't going to be able to sleep, and it becomes a self-fulfilling prophecy," the specialist said. He outlined a treatment plan that would require Nate to get out of bed whenever he hadn't fallen asleep within ten or fifteen minutes, and would eliminate all naps, as well as the use of alcohol. Nate agreed to try.

The first night he stayed up reading until midnight. Although exhausted when he got into bed, Nate was still awake ten minutes later. He got up and read before making his way back to bed. Once again, he couldn't fall asleep. It was 4 A.M. before Nate finally nodded off. The next night was a little better, as was the next, and the next. After several weeks, Nate was sleeping well.

The sleep specialist encouraged Nate to continue to follow some basic guidelines. He no longer chugged coffee all hours of the day and evening. He stopped napping and cut down on alcohol. What also helped Nate deal with both sleep and stress was a regular exercise program for the early evening that released the tensions of the day and got his body in shape for a good night's rest.

central nervous system suppressants currently available in the U.S. The scientific literature clearly demonstrates that the benzodiazepines are safe and effective for the treatment of insomnia when used appropriately. The lowest effective dose should be used for the shortest period of time."

The main benefits of the benzodiazepines are that they speed the onset of sleep, reduce nighttime awakenings, and extend total sleep time. The disadvantage is that after about two weeks almost all sleeping pills tend to lose their effectiveness. In addition, different sleeping pills have different durations of action. Some remain in the body long enough to have a hangover effect and dull various reactions the next day. Others are more rapidly metabolized. People may develop tolerance and increase their doses in order to replicate the drug's initial effectiveness. When this happens, if the medications are discontinued abruptly, individuals typically develop anxiety and rebound insomnia. Careful tapering of dosages over the course of a few nights can prevent these problems.

The elderly, whose bodies metabolize these medications more slowly, are more prone to side effects, including daytime confusion, impaired memory, difficulty driving and performing other tasks, and an increased risk of falling. A National Institute of Health (NIH) consensus conference on treating sleep problems in the elderly recommended that clinicians consider sleeping pills only after a thorough assessment of possible causes of insomnia, improvements in sleep hygiene, and behavioral treatments. If these efforts are unsuccessful, sleeping pills are recommended, but only in low doses and for short periods of use.

Other dangers of benzodiazepines include the possibility of fatal overdoses, especially when combined with alcohol or other drugs that act on the central nervous system; harmful interactions with other prescription medications; interference with breathing, especially in people with chronic respiratory problems; impaired daytime coordination, memory, driving skills, and thinking; disruption of normal sleep stages; potential damage to the kidneys, liver, and lungs; confusion, hallucinations, and other psychiatric disturbances, especially in the elderly; possible birth defects in the fetus if taken during pregnancy; and difficulty in awakening in case of a nighttime crisis.

The most recent advance in sleep medication is a nonbenzodiazepine called zolpidem (Ambien). It has minimal effects on normal sleep stages, and thus far there has been no evidence that people become tolerant or addicted to it. It works quickly, and its effects last for only a few hours. (See Chapter 28 for more information on sleep medications.)

Antihistamines, which are usually the main ingredient of over-the-counter (OTC) sleep products, do not put people to sleep; they simply make them groggy, which may help some tense individu-

How to get a good night's sleep

☐ **Keep regular hours, especially for getting out of bed.** A consistent wake-up time helps to regulate your internal biological clock.

☐ **Cut down on stimulants, such as coffee and colas.** Remember that caffeine can linger in the body for six to eight hours, so stop sipping by late afternoon.

☐ **Don't use alcohol as a sedative.** It undermines the quality of sleep and leads to awakenings in the second half of the night.

☐ **Exercise regularly.** Aerobic activities, such as walking, swimming, or jogging, can burn off tension and reduce stress. But don't work up a sweat in the evening, when you should be winding down.

☐ **Use your bed for sleeping and sex only.** If you curl up in bed to pay bills or catch up on work, you may associate it with stress rather than rest.

☐ **Develop a bedtime routine.** A regular pre-bedtime ritual, such as a bath, relaxation or deep-breathing exercises, or yoga, can help ease the transition from day to night.

☐ **Remember that quality matters more than quantity.** Try to get as much sleep as you need, not more. The longer people remain in bed, the shallower and more fragmented their sleep becomes.

☐ **Schedule a regular worry time earlier in the day to think about issues in your life.** It sometimes helps to write down concerns and possible solutions so they don't crowd into your mind as you're trying to sleep.

☐ **Create a soothing sleep environment.** Turn down the lights. Use earplugs or a machine that produces soothing sounds, such as white noise, rain, or surf. Try to avoid keeping the room temperature either too warm or too chilly.

als to fall asleep sooner. They are just as likely to cause daytime drowsiness and disturbances in memory as prescription medications. If taken in very high doses, OTC sleeping pills can produce nausea, vomiting, hallucinations, delirium, and convulsions.

▼
Self-help

Lifestyle habits have a major impact on how an individual sleeps. Caffeine, nicotine, and alcohol can all undermine good sleep. Irregular hours, late meals, or a lack of exercise can also make falling or staying asleep more difficult. Relaxation techniques, such as simple yoga exercises or progressive muscle relaxation (described in Chapter 29), can help people to unwind before bedtime.

Ideally, everyone should try to get as much sleep as needed to feel alert and energetic, and no more. The longer people stay in bed, the shallower and more fragmented their sleep is. The sleep environment can also make getting a good night's sleep more difficult, particularly if it is too bright, noisy, or warm.

▼
Impact on relationships

Insomnia usually takes some toll on the way in which individuals relate to others, by making them more irritable and distracted. Because they lack energy, they may not participate in or enjoy family activities and may spend more time alone.

Outlook In general, two-thirds of those with chronic insomnia improve with treatment. The success of behavioral treatments for insomnia depends largely on individual motivation. Those who devote the necessary time to practicing these procedures over a period of several weeks generally report better sleep and greater satisfaction in the long run than those who rely on sleeping medications.

Hypersomnia

Over the course of a lifetime, 1 to 2 percent of all people develop hypersomnia (excessive sleep). Most people who experience profound sleepiness and involuntary sleep periods during the day have a breathing-related problem or narcolepsy, described later in this chapter. However, hypersomnia can also be caused by physical illnesses, such as iron-deficiency anemia, hypothyroidism, or chronic fatigue syndrome; substance abuse, particularly marijuana dependence; and medications, including antihypertensives, antihistamines, allergy drugs, certain antibiotics, such as tetracycline, and methysergide, a drug used to prevent severe migraines. It also can be caused by tolerance to or withdrawal from stimulants such as amphetamines, caffeine, and cocaine. Regular use of alcohol and other depressants can also lead to hypersomnia. In some people, sleeping much more than usual may be their way of responding to stress or may reflect a general lack of purpose in their lives.

Mental disorders can lead to excessive sleep or sleepiness. Adolescents, young adults, and those with atypical depression (described in Chapter 5) tend to sleep more when depressed. Those with somatoform disorders, borderline personality disorder, or schizophrenia may complain of extreme tiredness despite normal amounts of sleep. "Sleep binges" may occur in individuals (mostly males in their teens and twenties) with Kleine-Levin syndrome, a rare disorder affecting certain control centers in the brain.

BREATHING-RELATED SLEEP DISORDERS

About 50 to 60 percent of men and women who seek help at sleep disorders centers for excessive daytime sleepiness have a breathing-related disorder. The most common is a potentially serious condition called *sleep apnea.* Translated from the Greek words meaning "no" and "breath," apnea is exactly that: the absence of breathing for a brief period. People with apnea may stop breathing for ten- to sixty-second periods dozens or even hundreds of times during the night.

<table>
<tr>
<td>

Is it primary hypersomnia?

According to the DSM-IV, a diagnosis of primary hypersomnia should be based on these criteria:

</td>
<td>

■ **Excessive sleepiness for at least one month, as evidenced by either prolonged sleep episodes or daytime sleep episodes occurring almost daily**

■ **Significant distress or impairment in social, occupational, or other important areas of functioning**

■ **The disorder is not better accounted for by insomnia, does not occur exclusively in the course of another sleep disorder, and cannot be accounted for by an inadequate amount of sleep.**

■ **Does not occur exclusively during the course of another mental disorder**

■ **The disturbance is not due to the direct effects of a substance (drugs of abuse or medication) or medical condition.**

Adapted from the Diagnostic and Statistical Manual of Mental Disorders, 4th Edition. *Used with permission.*

</td>
</tr>
</table>

How common are breathing-related disorders?

Breathing-related disorders typically begin in middle age and become more common with advancing years. About one-quarter of Americans over the age of sixty-five have a breathing-related disorder. These disorders are much more common in men, especially those who are overweight and suffering from hypertension.

What causes breathing-related disorders?

Breathing-related disorders can have various causes. In most cases of sleep apnea, an obstruction in the upper airway, such as flabby throat muscles or a large tongue, blocks the flow of air to the lungs. Obesity greatly increases the likelihood that this will happen. In cases of central sleep apnea, the problem is a malfunction of the respiration control centers in the medulla of the brain. Other common causes of breathing-related problems are ear, nose, and throat disorders (such as large tonsils and adenoids); upper airway abnormalities; neurological diseases such as polio and myasthenia gravis; respiratory problems; and heart disease.

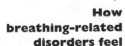

How breathing-related disorders feel

People with breathing-related sleep disorders often have no idea what is wrong. They are usually extremely sleepy during the day, even though they think they have had a normal night's sleep. Many wake up with morning headaches and spend the entire day struggling to stay awake. Some become so weary that they fall asleep while eating, driving, or talking to others. Long naps, also interrupted by breath stoppages, make them feel groggier rather than more alert. Many with a severe breathing disorder are ex-

Is it a breathing-related sleep disorder?

According to the DSM-IV, a diagnosis of breathing-related sleep disorder should be based on these criteria:

- Sleep disruption leading to excessive sleepiness or insomnia

- Disturbed sleep judged to be due to a sleep-related breathing disorder, such as sleep apnea

- The disturbance is not better accounted for by another mental disorder and not due to the direct effects of a substance (a drug of abuse or a medication) or medical condition.

Adapted from the Diagnostic and Statistical Manual of Mental Disorders, 4th Edition. *Used with permission.*

tremely irritable and often confused, and have difficulty thinking, concentrating, and remembering during the day.

One telltale sign of a breathing-related sleep disorder is extremely loud snoring or gasping for air. The brain, which receives a signal that the body needs oxygen, rouses the sleeper just enough so that he sucks air in loudly and vigorously. As he struggles to breathe, he also may flail his arms and legs.

▼

Seeking help   If you suspect that a breathing-related sleep disorder may be a problem for you or someone close to you, these are the questions that should be asked:

- Are you extremely tired during the day?

- Are you aware of any abnormalities in your breathing that occur during your sleep, or has a sleeping partner or member of your family noticed extremely loud snoring, kicking or flailing, or gasping for air?

- Are you having difficulty functioning normally during the day? Have you noticed problems in concentrating or thinking?

- Has this problem persisted for a month or longer?

If you answer "yes" to most of these questions, the problem may be breathing related. You should consult your primary physician, who may refer you to a sleep specialist. A polysomnogram (described on page 353) is essential in diagnosing this disorder.

It typically shows dozens or hundreds of breath stoppages, lasting for ten seconds or longer, during sleep.

▼

Risks and complications

Severe breathing-related sleep disorders can create physical and psychiatric complications, including headaches, hypertension, depression, and impotence, and impair thinking, perception, memory, communication, and the ability to learn new information. Chronically low levels of oxygen can affect the heart and lungs and may cause cardiovascular changes, including arrhythmias. Over time, sleep apnea may increase blood pressure, and its ultimate effects on the heart and lungs may be life-threatening.

▼

Treating breathing-related disorders

In some cases of breathing-related problems, weight loss, abstaining from sedating medications, and training the person not to sleep on his or her back can greatly improve these conditions. Various medications, such as tricyclic antidepressants, that reduce REM periods, when severe apneas tend to occur, may be helpful.

In moderate to severe cases, one effective approach is *continuous positive airway pressure* (CPAP), which delivers room air under pressure. Each night, sleepers place small masks or prongs over their noses. These are hooked up to a machine on the bedside table that pushes a continuous supply of room air (heated and humidified, if desired) directly into the upper throat. This minute amount of air pressure prevents the airway from collapsing during respiration. In one study, CPAP totally eliminated breath stoppages. CPAP devices have become increasingly lightweight and portable, allowing persons to take them along when traveling. A newer device called BiPAP lowers the air pressure during exhalation, which makes breathing more comfortable than with standard CPAP equipment.

In the past, in severe cases of obstructive sleep apnea, surgeons would create a permanent opening in the windpipe (a tracheostomy) for air to enter. Although this procedure did lessen daytime sleepiness, about 30 percent of those who underwent this surgery developed serious complications and discomfort. A newer procedure, called *uvulo-palato-pharyngoplasty,* literally resculpts the upper airway by removing the tonsils and soft tissues of the throat. In a survey of individuals with sleep apneas at six medical centers, about half who had undergone this operation had a 50 percent reduction in their disorder.

Central sleep apnea, which is less common than obstructive

sleep apnea, is usually treated with CPAP, respiratory stimulants, or a diaphragmatic pacemaker, a device implanted in the diaphragm that stimulates it to contract as in normal breathing.

▼

Self-help   Because obesity greatly increases the risk of apnea, losing weight can dramatically reduce breathing stoppages during sleep and can even overcome mild cases of sleep apnea. It is also helpful in cases of moderate to severe apnea; one study of fifteen overweight men found that those who lost an average of twenty pounds had fewer episodes, slept better, and felt more alert during the day.

A change in sleep position also helps. By lying on their sides instead of their backs, individuals with mild to moderate apnea can dramatically reduce the number of times they stop breathing during the night, possibly because their tongues are less likely to fall backward and block the airway. A pillow placed at the small of the back and held in place by a belt around the waist can help to keep sleepers on their sides. Tongue-restraining devices may make a difference for those who have apnea only when they lie on their backs.

People with a breathing-related sleep disorder should avoid alcohol, anti-anxiety drugs, and sleep-inducing medications, all of which can depress respiration and put them in greater danger during sleep.

▼

Impact on relationships   The family often helps to diagnose a breathing-related sleep disorder by recognizing the characteristic nighttime pattern of silences followed by snorts, loud snoring, gasps, and jerky movements. Family members also may notice mood changes in the person, such as increased irritability or confusion.

▼

Outlook   Many people with a breathing-related sleep disorder suffer for years before their problem is identified. Once recognized and treated, the prognosis is good. Sometimes self-help measures alone, such as weight loss, are effective. About 60 percent of those who try CPAP adapt and improve with long-term therapy. Those who cannot tolerate CPAP often opt for surgery.

NARCOLEPSY

Narcolepsy, a term that literally means "sleep seizure," is characterized by sudden, frequent, irresistible attacks of REM sleep that occur throughout the day. About three-quarters of those with narcolepsy develop other characteristic symptoms, including:

■ *Cataplexy,* a sudden loss of muscle tone that may cause drooping of the jaw or head, weakness of the knees, or total collapse, usually triggered by excitement or intense emotion

■ *Hypnagogic phenomena,* such as hallucinations or realistic perceptions either of sights or sounds that occur in the semiconscious state between wakefulness and sleep

■ *Sleep paralysis,* the inability to move for several minutes after waking.

▼

**How common is
narcolepsy?**

Narcolepsy affects about 200,000 to 500,000 Americans and is equally common in men and women. It usually begins in adolescence or young adulthood.

▼

**What causes
narcolepsy?**

Although the exact cause of narcolepsy is not known, sleep researchers describe it as a disorder of the sleep-wake control mechanisms within the brain that interferes with both daytime wakefulness and nighttime sleep. Narcolepsy has a hereditary component, and there is one chance in twenty that the children of a narcoleptic parent will develop the problem. It can also develop after an illness or injury that causes brain damage, such as a brain infection or head trauma.

▼

**How narcolepsy
feels**

Narcolepsy is a chronic disease that can affect every aspect of a person's life. In addition to sleep attacks, individuals may lose muscle tone whenever they feel strong emotion. One woman became weak whenever she began to scold her child; a stockbroker would collapse into sleep while negotiating a big trade. Some people with this problem experience *automatic behavior;* that is, even though asleep, they continue a routine activity, such as washing dishes or driving, and wake only after cutting themselves with a knife or driving off the road.

At night, people with narcolepsy experience unusual symptoms, such as hallucinations that can be very frightening. Some wake up but find themselves unable to move a muscle—an extremely uncomfortable condition. As the narcoleptic's symptoms worsen, night wakening may increase. About 15 to 30 percent develop some degree of involuntary leg movements and apnea during nighttime sleep. With aging, people with narcolepsy may have extremely fragmented sleep at night.

▼

Seeking help

The average person with this disorder spends ten years before the problem is correctly identified. If you suspect that narcolepsy may

Is it narcolepsy?

According to the DSM-IV, a diagnosis of narcolepsy should be based on these criteria:

■ **Irresistible attacks of refreshing sleep occurring daily over a period of at least three months**

■ **Cataplexy (sudden loss of muscle tone, most often in association with intense emotion)**

■ **Recurrent intrusion of features of rapid eye movement (REM) sleep into the transition between sleep and wakefulness, as manifested by either hypnopompic/hypnagogic hallucinations or sleep paralysis at the beginning or end of sleep episodes**

■ **The disturbance is not better accounted for by another mental disorder and not due to the direct effects of a substance or a medical condition.**

Adapted from the Diagnostic and Statistical Manual of Mental Disorders, 4th Edition. *Used with permission.*

be a problem for you or someone close to you, these are the questions that should be asked:

- Have you felt overwhelming tiredness during the day?

- Have you had irresistible episodes of falling asleep, regardless of what you were doing at the time?

- Have you suddenly lost muscle control and slumped or fallen?

- When falling asleep or waking up, have you had very vivid dream-like images enter your mind?

- Have you been unable to move for a few moments after waking?

If you answer "yes" to several of these questions, the problem could be narcolepsy. The diagnosis is based on a Multiple Sleep Latency Test, in which a polysomnograph records a series of four or five daytime naps, spaced at two-hour intervals. Typically, people with narcolepsy fall asleep within five minutes of lying down during the day and enter REM very rapidly.

▼

Risks and complications

People with narcolepsy can face an increased risk of automobile and industrial accidents. Some cannot work because of frequent sleep attacks. Those who rely on stimulants to stay alert may develop physiological tolerance and dependence on these drugs. Individuals with narcolepsy have higher than normal rates of major depression, generalized anxiety, and alcohol abuse. It is not known whether these disorders are the consequences of dealing with a chronic and potentially disabling illness or stem from the same causes as narcolepsy itself.

▼
Treating narcolepsy

Scheduled naps throughout the day can help in controlling narcolepsy. For severe cases, physicians may prescribe various medications, including stimulants such as methylphenidate (Ritalin), dextroamphetamine (Dexedrine), and pemoline (Cylert), to overcome daytime sleepiness. Low doses of tricyclic antidepressants that suppress REM sleep or the experimental drug gamma-hydroxybutyrate may be used to prevent cataplexy. Persons are given the lowest dose necessary to control symptoms, interspersed with days without medication to prevent side effects and tolerance. Tranylcypromine (Parnate), a monoamine oxidase (MAO) inhibitor, also may be helpful for cataplexy. Those taking this or any other MAO inhibitor should avoid stimulants and the foods and beverages listed in Chapter 28.

▼
Self-help

Individuals with mild to moderate symptoms of narcolepsy may be able to cope by maintaining good sleep habits, such as regular bedtimes. Sometimes a schedule of regular naps at the same time every day helps dramatically. Local self-help groups sponsored by the American Narcolepsy Association can also be very helpful.

▼
Impact on relationships

Narcolepsy can have a devastating effect on a person's life. Sleep attacks can occur in embarrassing situations and often lead individuals to avoid socializing. Loved ones may interpret the affected individual's chronic tiredness as indifference or rejection. Not surprisingly, narcolepsy often leads to psychological difficulties, and people with this disorder become demoralized and depressed, causing further withdrawal from others. Those who suffer cataplexy may constantly try to control their emotions to prevent attacks, and this lack of normal expressiveness can create difficulties in forming relationships. Individuals with narcolepsy may turn to alcohol as a way of coping, which can exacerbate family tensions. Family members who learn as much as possible about this disorder can offer much-needed empathy, support, and understanding. Meeting with a family therapist can help in identifying and working through issues.

▼
Outlook

Narcolepsy is a lifelong disorder. Stimulants are not always well tolerated, and treatment can be frustrating. Education about the illness as well as psychosocial support are critically important in helping individuals to cope with this chronic and sometimes disabling condition.

Circadian rhythm
sleep disorders

Problems involving sleep-wake schedules are called circadian rhythm disorders because they affect the basic circadian ("about a day") rhythm that influences many biological processes. They include jet lag, shift work disruptions, and advanced or delayed sleep onset.

Most people's personal sleep-wake schedules dovetail with their circadian rhythms and the demands of their environments. They wake when they should to get to work or meet other obligations and fall asleep at a socially appropriate hour. However, there is sometimes a mismatch between sleep-wake patterns and the schedule required by an individual's job, family, or other circumstances. As a result, the person cannot sleep when necessary or remain alert when expected to, although if allowed to follow his or her own schedule this person has no difficulty sleeping well and feeling refreshed afterwards.

For unknown reasons, there is wide individual variation in the ability to tolerate frequently changing sleep-wake schedules. Some people fly over long distances regularly or rotate job shifts for years without any distress. Others are sensitive even to mild changes in schedule. In general, older people have more difficulty adjusting to frequent schedule changes. "Night owls," who feel more energetic in the evening and at night than during the day, tend to adapt better to shift work than "morning larks," who are most energetic early in the day. Individuals whose daily lives are chaotic and whose hours are highly irregular are much more likely to develop a circadian rhythm sleep disorder. People who are struggling to stay alert because of a circadian rhythm disorder are at greater risk for lapses of attention, accidents, and physical ailments, such as ulcers.

In addition to behavioral strategies and good sleep habits, phototherapy—exposure to bright, full-spectrum light for periods ranging from thirty minutes to two hours—has shown promise as an experimental treatment for circadian rhythm disorders, including jet lag and delayed or advanced sleep onset disorder. This approach also has been shown to improve alertness and cognitive performance in night shift workers.

JET LAG

Mental health professionals define jet lag as sleepiness and alertness occurring at inappropriate times during the day, following recent or repeated travel across more than one time zone. Individuals usually adjust more readily to a new time zone after trav-

---

Is it a circadian rhythm sleep disorder?

According to the DSM-IV, *a diagnosis of circadian rhythm sleep disorder should be based on these criteria:*

- ■ **A persistent or recurrent pattern of sleep disruption leading to excessive sleepiness or insomnia that is due to a mismatch between the sleep-wake schedule required by a person's environment and his or her circadian sleep-wake pattern**

- ■ **Significant distress or impairment in social, occupational, or other important areas of functioning as a result of the sleep disturbance**

- ■ **Does not occur exclusively during the course of another sleep disorder or mental disorder**

- ■ **The disturbance is not due to the effects of a substance or medical condition.**

Adapted from the Diagnostic and Statistical Manual of Mental Disorders, 4th Edition. *Used with permission.*

---

eling west rather than east, because it is easier to stay awake and extend the "day" than to try to shorten it by going to sleep at an earlier-than-usual hour.

Jet lag usually improves within two to seven days, depending on individual response, length of trip, and number of time zones crossed. Some people find that they can minimize jet lag if, before their trip, they start shifting their mealtimes and sleep times to coincide with those of their destination. Others find that extra sleep relieves many of the symptoms of jet lag. A short-acting sleeping pill for the first night in the new time zone can help travelers flying from west to east to adapt to the shorter day. Avoiding caffeine and alcohol and immediately switching to the new time zone's schedule can also help to overcome the temporary effects of jet lag.

Individuals who spend one or two weeks a month in a place and time zone far from home may not have fully recovered from the effects of jet lag before they set off on another long trip. The consequences of such repeated long-distance travel include impaired thinking, irritability, and problems in relationships with family members and friends. Nevertheless, many people who travel often on multinational business trips are totally unaware of anything wrong. They may not realize the toll their travel has taken until they take a vacation or stay in one place for a length of time and realize how much better they feel and function.

SHIFT WORK

About 20 percent of Americans have jobs requiring evening or night shifts. On the average, they sleep seven hours a week less than persons with day jobs. A "shift work" circadian rhythm disorder consists of any inability to sleep when one wants to or to stay alert when needed because of frequently changing schedules or night shifts. Rotating shift workers have two to three times the injury rate of co-workers with more stable schedules.

Usually, shift work symptoms are at their worst during the first few days after a change is made. In general, it is easier to adapt to a schedule that shifts from days to evenings to nights than to one that goes from days to nights to evenings. Ideally, work schedules should be changed as infrequently as possible and no more often than once every two weeks. This allows time for the body to adjust. Shift workers who return to a more conventional sleep-wake pattern on weekends or on their days off may never adapt completely to their work shift.

Good sleep habits are critical for shift workers; these include avoiding excessive use of caffeine to enhance alertness or of alcohol to induce drowsiness. In general, people on evening and night shifts should sleep as soon as possible after work for one prolonged sleep period rather than splitting up their sleep times into naps before and after work. Some therapists are experimenting with the use of exposure to bright lights (light therapy) to help shift workers adapt to different schedules.

DELAYED OR ADVANCED SLEEP ONSET

In delayed or advanced sleep onset disorders, a person falls asleep either much later or much earlier than is desired. The most common of these conditions is a problem with delayed sleep, in which individuals—most often young adults—cannot fall asleep until the early hours of the morning. They find it enormously difficult to wake up in the morning to get to work or school. Some drink excessive amounts of coffee or take stimulants to awaken themselves fully; at night they may try sleeping pills to get to sleep. Often they are chronically tired, lack energy, and feel vaguely unhappy and unwell.

In advanced sleep onset, individuals fall asleep much earlier than desired or normal and waken at 3 A.M. or earlier. Older people are more likely to develop this problem, possibly because of age-related changes in the body's biological rhythms. Early morning waking can also be a sign of depression.

Good sleep habits help people with both delayed and advanced sleep onset. Recent studies have shown that morning exposure to bright light can help with delayed sleep phase syndrome. Evening light helps those with advanced sleep phase syndrome to shift to a more normal sleep pattern. These persons can also benefit from sleep restriction, which forces them to limit their time in bed. One tactic is to stay up every night for a certain event, such as the eleven o'clock news; this helps them to sleep later in the morning.

In cases in which delayed sleep onset is causing severe problems and individuals are highly motivated to reset their biological clocks, a very specific treatment called "chronotherapy" can help. People gradually advance their bedtimes by three-hour intervals over a period of several weeks, so that, for example, someone who has not customarily gone to bed until 4 A.M. first moves this to 7 A.M., then to 10 A.M., then to 1 P.M., then to 4 P.M., then to 7 P.M., and then to 10 P.M.—which may ultimately become the person's permanent bedtime. Although often effective, this process is extremely demanding, physically and psychologically, and is highly disruptive during the weeks it is under way. Support and monitoring from a sleep specialist are critically important.

Parasomnias

A parasomnia is any out-of-the-ordinary occurrence that happens during sleep or in the period between wakefulness and sleep. Parasomnias include nightmares, sleep terrors, and sleepwalking episodes. Most of these events occur during the deepest portions (stages 3 and 4) of NREM sleep. These problems are most common in children, who spend more time than adults in very deep sleep and usually do not require treatment. (Chapter 26 discusses sleepwalking, sleep terrors, and bed-wetting in youngsters.)

Anyone suddenly aroused from very deep sleep may be disoriented and later may not remember what happened when awakened, but most people quickly return to normal sleep. This does not usually happen in the parasomnias, which occur more often and are much more distressing.

NIGHTMARES AND NIGHTMARE DISORDER

Individuals with a nightmare disorder repeatedly awaken from REM sleep because of very vivid and frightening dreams, which they recall in great detail. These intense nightmares may occur at almost any time during sleep but usually are more common toward the end of the night, when REM periods are longer. After waking up in a state of extreme anxiety, the person quickly realizes what is happening. Often there is difficulty in returning to sleep, and the memory of the nightmare and of being awakened by it remains the next morning.

▼

**How common are
nightmares?**

Although 4 to 5 percent of all people say that they are troubled by
nightmares, the severe and frequent nightmares characteristic of
nightmare disorder are less common. About two-thirds of all cases
begin before the age of twenty, and many start in childhood.

▼

**What causes
nightmares?**

In about 60 percent of cases, repeated nightmares start after
a major stressful life event, often in childhood or adolescence.
People with frequent physical and mental health problems appear
to be especially vulnerable. Some researchers have found that
individuals who suffer from frequent nightmares show signs of
psychological abnormalities, such as suspiciousness, social and
emotional isolation, alienation, and overanxiety, or have traits
characteristic of schizoid or borderline personality disorders.
Nightmares are common in persons with posttraumatic stress
disorder (PTSD) and may involve reliving of the traumatic events
themselves.

Certain drugs (including reserpine, thioridazine, mesoridazine,
and benzodiazepines) can cause nightmares. Abrupt withdrawal
from substances that suppress REM sleep, such as alcohol and
tricyclic antidepressants, often triggers *REM rebound*—increased
REM periods filled with intense and often frightening dreams.

▼

**How nightmare
disorder feels**

Nightmares are deeply troubling dreams that often contain realistic threats to the person's survival or well-being and themes that
occur again and again. Disturbing dreams typically increase during times of stress or, less often, after extreme physical exertion.
In a few cases, a changed sleep environment may trigger very upsetting dreams.

▼

Seeking help

An occasional nightmare does not require therapy. However, if you
suspect that nightmare disorder may be a problem for you or someone close to you, these are the questions that should be asked:

- Do you repeatedly awaken from sleep or naps because of frightening nightmares?

- Are you able to remember the distressing dream in detail after
  awakening?

- Does the nightmare or subsequent loss of sleep greatly upset you?

If you answer "yes" to these questions, the problem could be
nightmare disorder or another mental disorder, and you may want
to consult a mental health professional.

Is it a nightmare disorder?

According to the DSM-IV, a diagnosis of nightmare disorder should be based on these criteria:

- Repeated awakening from sleep or naps with detailed recall of extended and extremely frightening dreams, usually involving threats to survival, security, or self-esteem; the awakenings usually occur during the second half of the sleep period

- On awakening, rapid orientation and alertness

- The dream experience or the sleep disturbance causes significant distress or impairment in social, occupational, or other important areas of functioning

- The disturbance is not due to the direct effects of a substance or medical condition.

Adapted from the Diagnostic and Statistical Manual of Mental Disorders, 4th Edition. *Used with permission.*

▼

Risks and complications

The nightmares themselves have no major effect on daytime functioning. However, people who experience nightmares may become extremely upset if they recur often and may develop problems in sleeping through the night.

▼

Treating nightmare disorder

In most cases, occasional nightmares do not require therapy. When they occur frequently they may be a sign of too much stress. Relaxation and stress management techniques can help. Psychotherapy can deal with underlying conflicts or difficulties. In some cases, a psychiatrist may prescribe a low-dose benzodiazepine sleeping pill for a short period.

▼

Impact on relationships

Family members can become concerned about the nature of the dreams that are disturbing a loved one's sleep. In young people, nightmares tend to represent the normal conflicts and challenges of growing up. In adults, their causes are more complex, although stress and psychological difficulties or disorders often play a role. The bed partner of someone troubled by nightmares—whose own sleep may be disrupted as a result—may want to probe for explanations or make unwelcome attempts to offer comfort.

▼

Outlook

Nightmares are common throughout childhood, adolescence, and young adulthood, but most people outgrow them. In adults, untreated nightmare disorder can be a chronic problem that recurs as often as three or more times a week for decades. Psychotherapy, relaxation techniques, and low-dose benzodiazepines have all proved effective in helping people troubled by chronic nightmares.

SLEEP TERROR DISORDER

A sleep terror consists of repeated, sudden awakening from deep NREM sleep in the first third of the night, usually accompanied by screams of fright and feelings of agitation that last for up to ten minutes. Although sleep terror episodes may occur once every few days or weeks, some individuals experience them night after night; if these recurrences cause distress or impairment, the condition is sleep terror disorder.

▼

How common is sleep terror disorder?

One to four percent of children between the ages of four and twelve develop sleep terrors, which they usually outgrow. Episodes are less common in adults; the incidence is thought to be less than 1 percent. The frequency of sleep terror disorder in the general population is not known, although data indicate that the usual age of onset in adults is the twenties and thirties; it is rare for it to begin after the age of forty. Sleep terrors occur more often in boys than in girls; there is no gender difference in frequency among adults.

▼

What causes sleep terrors?

High fevers can trigger sleep terrors in children and teenagers. Adults who develop sleep terrors often have symptoms of other mental disorders, such as anxiety. The problem appears to run in families and is much more common among first-degree relatives of a person with sleep terrors than in the population at large. Stress or erratic sleep schedules may increase sleep terrors.

▼

How sleep terror disorder feels

A sleep terror causes profound distress. Individuals scream or yell and may sweat heavily, breathe rapidly, and experience a pounding heart and racing pulse. Nothing anyone says or does can comfort them until time passes and they gradually grow calmer. They may remember waking because of panic and fear, and may recall a few images, but they have no memory of a complete dream. By morning, they may have forgotten the entire episode.

▼

Seeking help

An occasional sleep terror does not require therapy. However, if the episodes recur and you suspect that the problem troubling you or someone close to you may be sleep terror disorder, these are the questions that should be asked:

- Do you repeatedly awaken from sleep screaming or extremely upset?
- At these times, does your heart beat rapidly, do you breathe quickly, sweat profusely, or show other signs of intense anxiety?

<table>
<tr><td>

Is it sleep terror disorder?

According to the DSM-IV, a diagnosis of sleep terror disorder should be based on these criteria:

</td><td>

■ **Recurrent episodes of abrupt awakening from sleep, usually occurring during the first third of the night and beginning with a panicky scream**

■ **Intense anxiety and signs of autonomic nervous system arousal, such as an increased heart rate, rapid breathing, and sweating**

■ **No memory of a detailed dream or, later, of the awakening**

■ **Relative unresponsiveness to efforts to provide comfort**

■ **The disturbance is not due to the direct effects of a medication or substance of abuse or to a general medical condition.**

Adapted from the Diagnostic and Statistical Manual of Mental Disorders, 4th Edition. *Used with permission.*

</td></tr>
</table>

• Do you have no memory of a dream or, later, of waking up in the night?

• Do those who try to comfort you say that you seem unresponsive and inconsolable?

If you answer "yes" to these questions, the problem could be sleep terror disorder. You should consult a mental health professional, who may advise a thorough evaluation to rule out medical problems, such as epilepsy, and evaluate you for other disorders, such as nighttime panic attacks or sleep apnea. An all-night sleep laboratory evaluation may be necessary.

Risks and complications

Occasionally a person suffers an accidental injury (for example, from falling out of bed) during an episode. Embarrassment because of this problem may lead an individual to avoid situations in which others might realize that he or she suffers from sleep terrors, such as sleeping at a friend's house.

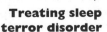

Treating sleep terror disorder

Various forms of psychotherapy have helped people with frequent sleep terrors. Hypnosis can be highly effective in teaching individuals with sleep terrors how to give themselves nightly instructions so they do not suffer an attack. For severe cases, psychiatrists can prescribe low-dose benzodiazepines for a brief period to reduce very deep sleep.

Self-help

Since tension, sleep deprivation, and an erratic sleep schedule increase the risk for night terrors, people who are prone to this problem should try to maintain regular hours for sleeping and should use behavioral techniques, such as relaxation exercises, for dealing with stress.

▼
Impact on relationships

Sleep terrors are very disturbing to parents and partners because their efforts to offer the person reassurance seem futile. They need to recognize that individuals waking from a sleep terror are so agitated and disoriented that they need time to calm themselves.

▼
Outlook

As a rule, sleep terrors in children gradually disappear by early adolescence. Those that begin in adulthood often become a chronic problem. Psychotherapy, relaxation techniques, and hypnosis can help, but little is known about their long-term efficacy.

SLEEPWALKING DISORDER

Individuals with sleepwalking disorder repeatedly leave their beds and walk around without waking up for as long as half an hour; they later have no memory or awareness of these nocturnal excursions. Sleepwalking usually occurs during deep sleep, that is, during stages 3 and 4 of NREM sleep in the first third of the night.

▼
How common is sleepwalking disorder?

One to five percent of children between the ages of six and twelve have sleepwalking disorder; between 10 and 30 percent have had an occasional episode. Childhood sleepwalking tends to peak at around the age of twelve and to cease spontaneously during adolescence. Boys and men are more likely to sleepwalk than girls and women. The incidence of sleepwalking episodes in adulthood is 1 to 7 percent. The disorder is much less common in adults than in children, and in adults tends to be chronic.

▼
What causes sleepwalking disorder?

There appears to be a genetic predisposition to sleepwalking, which is ten times more common in the close relatives of a sleepwalker than in the public at large. Families of sleepwalkers also tend to be deep sleepers, and sleepwalking occurs in the deepest stages of sleep. Certain drugs, such as antipsychotic medications, can induce sleepwalking in individuals prone to this condition.

Children are more likely to sleepwalk when they have high fevers. Adult sleepwalkers, who tend to walk in their sleep when extremely exhausted or under stress, have a higher than usual incidence of other parasomnias, such as sleep terrors, and may have symptoms of other mental disorders, such as personality disorders, or problems in dealing with frustration, failure, or a loss of self-esteem.

▼

**How sleepwalking
disorder feels**

Sleepwalkers are not aware of their actions, but their behavior is evident to others. An episode can begin with a simple movement, such as clutching a blanket; then the sleeper may sit or stand up, get dressed, open doors, eat, or use the bathroom. The faces of sleepwalkers are expressionless; their eyes stare blankly ahead. Although they seem to see objects standing in their way, their co-ordination is poor. Contrary to common assumptions, they can fall, stumble, or be hurt by falls down stairs or through windows. Sleepwalkers are very difficult to awaken and usually do not respond to the efforts of others to communicate with them; if they do talk, they are difficult to understand. In general, sleepwalkers are not dangerous to others, although on rare occasions, especially if they had been using drugs or alcohol, they have assaulted others while at least partially asleep and disoriented.

Often sleepwalkers return to bed or fall asleep elsewhere without waking, and usually have no recollection of ever leaving their bed. Sometimes, however, they awaken while away from their beds and feel confused for several minutes before becoming fully alert.

▼

Seeking help

If you suspect that sleepwalking disorder may be a problem for you or someone close to you, these are the questions that should be asked:

- Do you recall or have others reported that you repeatedly leave your bed and walk about in your sleep?

- Do others report that you seem unaware of where you are and what you are doing and do not respond to their efforts to wake you?

- Do you ever awaken in a place other than where you fell asleep with no memory of how you got there?

- Do you usually have no memory of sleepwalking?

If you answer "yes" to several of these questions, the problem could be a sleepwalking disorder. Adults who sleepwalk often over a period of six months to a year should see their primary physician or a mental health professional. They may be referred to a sleep disorder center for a polysomnogram to rule out physical problems.

▼

**Risks and
complications**

The major danger is accidental injury while sleepwalking. Sleepwalkers may tumble down stairs, fall through windows, burn themselves with irons, or cut themselves with knives.

Treating sleepwalking disorder

Most children outgrow sleepwalking without any treatment. In adults, if stress seems to be the problem, relaxation therapies, such as progressive muscle relaxation, can reduce both daytime tension and nighttime restlessness. Hypnosis has helped some sleepwalkers to stop by teaching them to wake up whenever their feet touch the floor. Psychotherapy can help individuals who have underlying psychological difficulties. In extreme cases of frequent sleepwalking and a serious risk of injury, drugs that reduce deep sleep, such as the benzodiazepines, may be prescribed in the lowest possible doses and for the briefest possible time.

Self-help

Regular hours and afternoon naps (which reduce deep sleep at night) can help. Adults who walk in their sleep or the parents of sleepwalking children should make the environment as safe as possible. That may require putting a gate at the foot and head of stairs, locking windows and doors, and hiding knives, guns, or other dangerous objects.

Impact on relationships

The primary concern of family members is possible danger to the sleepwalker. Taking steps to create a safe sleep environment is crucial. If family members come upon a sleepwalker, they should try not to startle the person and, if possible, should lead him gently back to bed without waking him. If they must arouse a sleepwalker because of imminent danger, they should repeat the person's name in a calm voice, then reassure him or her that everything is all right.

Outlook   Sleepwalking in children and adolescents, whether frequent or not, usually lasts for several years. However, almost all of those affected outgrow the disorder by their twenties. Sleepwalking that begins in adulthood tends to be more chronic. There have been reports of successful treatment with psychotherapy, relaxation training, hypnosis, and the time-limited use of low-dose benzodiazepines.

REM SLEEP BEHAVIOR DISORDER

REM sleep behavior disorder, which is officially categorized as a "parasomnia not otherwise specified" in the *DSM-IV*, has been identified only during the past decade. Its primary characteristic is the occurrence of unusual motor activity during REM sleep, a period when the major muscles are normally paralyzed. In some cases, individuals—chiefly middle-aged or older men—develop bizarre sleep movements, such as pawing at the air or lunging at a bedpost. Many report having nightmares of being chased or attacked while engaging in potentially dangerous activities that are distinctly out of character compared with their tranquil daytime demeanor. One retired grocer dreamed he was a football halfback and tackled his dresser so forcefully that he tore a wide gash in his forehead. Another man woke from a vivid dream, in which he was about to snap a doe's neck, to find his hands poised over his wife's chin.

REM sleep behavior disorder can occur during drug intoxication or withdrawal. Some people with this problem have a neurological condition, such as Alzheimer's disease or stroke. However, most who seek help show no sign of psychiatric problems; the culprit may be aging itself. "Something about the brain may change structurally in older men and interfere with the brain's messages not to move during REM sleep," says psychiatrist Carlos Schenck, M.D., of the Minneapolis Regional Sleep Disorders Center, a leading expert on this problem.

Treatment options include hypnosis, psychotherapy, and medication—primarily clonazepam (Klonopin), a benzodiazepine, and carbamazepine (Tegretol), an anticonvulsant drug. These approaches, particularly drug therapy, greatly reduce episodes of REM sleep behavior disorder.

Is it an impulse control disorder?

Individuals with an impulse control disorder may:

☐ **Be preoccupied with a potentially harmful activity, such as gambling, stealing, hair-pulling, fire-setting, or physically hurting themselves**

☐ **Devote increased time or energy to this activity**

☐ **Feel tense or aroused before giving in to an impulse**

☐ **Find it very hard to resist the impulse**

☐ **Feel immediate pleasure, relief, release, or gratification after giving in to the impulse**

☐ **Forego time for family or work for the sake of this activity**

☐ **Jeopardize personal relationships or jobs**

☐ **Risk serious consequences, such as bankruptcy or imprisonment**

☐ **Become restless or irritable if they do not give in to the impulse**

☐ **Try but fail to control or stop their impulsive behavior**

The more boxes checked, the more reason there is for concern about a possible impulse control disorder. This chapter describes some of the most common impulse-related problems and provides guidance for recognizing their specific symptoms and seeking help.

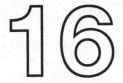

16

Problems of Impulse Control

A bright, successful commodities broker in Manhattan travels to Atlantic City every weekend for some high-stakes "action." A thirtyish woman who could afford practically any luxury steals inexpensive items that she neither wants nor needs. A commercial illustrator plucks so much hair from her scalp that she wears scarves to disguise bald spots. A man sets a fire in an abandoned building, then rushes to help firefighters put it out. A self-described "cutter" uses razor blades, knives, and needles in elaborate rituals of self-mutilation.

Individuals with impulse control disorders such as these repeatedly give in to an urge to perform an act that is harmful to them or to others. Typically, they feel a growing sense of tension or excitement and an urge or temptation that they know they should resist but cannot. Once they act on their impulse, they may feel pleasure, gratification, or relief—responses that for many, if not all, quickly lead to guilt or remorse.

Each of the impulse control disorders in this chapter—pathological gambling, impulsive stealing, irrational spending, hair-pulling, fire-setting, and self-mutilation—serves as a way for the affected person to avoid or relieve painful thoughts or feelings. Individuals with these conditions, unable to acknowledge or express normal emotions, take action instead. When disappointed or frustrated, they may set fires. When a relationship ends, they may go on a spending spree. When they feel abandoned, they may steal something. When overcome by pain or numbness, they may cut or burn themselves. (Another impulse disorder, intermittent explosive disorder, is discussed in Chapter 23.)

With the exception of pathological gambling, the impulse control disorders have not been as extensively researched as other mental disorders, and what we know about treatments and prognosis is often based on relatively few and small studies. Genetic, neurobiological, psychological, developmental, behavioral, and sociological factors may contribute to the development of these conditions. Impulsivity may be related to childhood conduct problems (especially the more serious and less common ones, such as cruelty to animals) and family dynamics. Almost always, impulse control disorders begin or flare up under conditions of stress.

Some mental health professionals believe that at least some of the impulse disorders are addictions that affect individuals in much the same way as alcohol or drug dependence. Pathological gambling, for example, is chronic and, like addictive disorders, worsens over time as individuals wager more money more and more frequently. Other disorders, such as kleptomania, may wax and wane over many years. People who find it hard to control their impulses are more likely to become depressed, to attempt suicide, and to develop other psychiatric problems, including substance abuse. Those who set fires or gamble compulsively often lead risky lives, and their chance of violent death is greater than that of the average person.

Researchers have identified a relationship between impulsivity and levels of serotonin, a key neurotransmitter in the brain. The selective serotonin reuptake inhibitors (SSRIs), such as fluoxetine (Prozac), and clomipramine (Anafranil), a treatment for obsessive-compulsive disorder, have proved effective in treating impulse control disorders. (See Chapter 28 on psychiatric drugs.)

The new understanding of the possible biological roots of impulse control disorders may pave the way to more targeted and effective treatments. Traditional psychotherapy often does not work because it can be very difficult for individuals with impulse control disorders to comprehend their motives or behaviors. Some cannot cope with the turmoil involved in self-exploration. They need empathic, nonjudgmental therapists who can offer support in overcoming problems that many people, including some mental health professionals, view as bizarre and disturbing.

Pathological gambling

Pathological, or compulsive, gambling* is the persistent inability to resist or control the urge to gamble. First officially recognized as a psychiatric disorder in 1980, this invisible illness

---

*The general public and Gamblers Anonymous use the term *compulsive* for gambling that is beyond rational control. In psychiatry, a compulsion brings no enjoyment or satisfaction. Since gamblers enjoy gambling, mental health professionals prefer the term *pathological.*

causes no physical symptoms and may go unrecognized for years. Gambling itself is not the problem. Eighty percent of Americans gamble legally, usually as a recreational activity shared with friends. "Social gamblers" usually plan how much they are willing to wager—and possibly lose—before they head for the bingo hall, racetrack, poker game, or casino. Pathological gamblers, on the other hand, suffer from an addiction, like alcoholism or drug dependence, that they cannot control.

Like other addictions, pathological gambling is progressive. Individuals become increasingly preoccupied with and spend more and more time gambling. As tolerance develops, they bet ever-increasing amounts of money and take greater risks to produce the euphoric, excited "high" that they desire. Often they compare this elation and sense of total well-being to being on cocaine. They may go for hours without eating or days without sleeping. Some report cravings, a "rush" (characterized by sweaty palms, rapid heartbeat, nausea, or queasiness) when they anticipate gambling, and blackouts during or after an intense period of gambling. When they try to cut back or stop, they may suffer classic symptoms of withdrawal, such as restlessness and irritability.

One particular group of gamblers, called *problem gamblers*, are similar to alcohol abusers: They go on periodic binges. This results in some degree of trouble, although not to the extent caused by pathological gambling. Some problem gamblers may develop into pathological gamblers; it is not clear if this is true of all. As with problem drinkers, they can benefit from professional help.

Pathological gamblers may use gambling to escape from or avoid confronting their problems or unhappiness. As long as they have access to any money at all, they gamble. No jackpot is ever big enough; no long shot is ever daring enough. After their biggest win, they cannot wait for their next chance to gamble. When they lose, they are determined to gamble again and win. To them, a loss is a personal setback that makes them feel ashamed and inadequate. As soon as they can, they "chase" their losses, trying to win back their money, even if that means betting recklessly or gambling for double or nothing. They believe that if they can only get back the money, they need not feel guilty about their gambling. If they continue to lose, they feel worthless.

Despite their financial woes, pathological gamblers never make a serious attempt to save or budget money. Their solution to any problem is gambling. When they feel upset or misunderstood, they gamble. When confronted by family, friends, colleagues, or a boss, they lie to conceal their gambling. When their money problems worsen, they may sell their belongings, use family savings, or falsify information to borrow money for gambling. As their debts grow, pathological gamblers consider or resort to criminal means of getting gambling money, including forgery, fraud, theft, and embezzlement. Ultimately they may risk or actually lose their marriages, friendships, jobs, and careers.

▼

How common is pathological gambling?

The *Diagnostic and Statistical Manual of Mental Disorders, Fourth Edition (DSM-IV)* estimates that 1 to 3 percent of American adults are pathological gamblers. The rate is higher among those who abuse alcohol or drugs. Although equal numbers of men and women may gamble, pathological gambling is more common among men.

The age at which individuals seek treatment for gambling has been getting younger, and pathological gambling has become more common among teenagers, who may steal or shoplift to get money and skip school to go gambling.

▼

What causes pathological gambling?

Freud observed that gamblers gamble not for the money but for what today's gamblers call "the action"—the excitement or high that comes from taking risks, placing bets, upping the ante, scoring a big win. Freud was the first to view pathological gambling as an addiction, like alcoholism and drug dependence, and believed that all three stemmed from an underlying addiction to masturbation or fantasies of masturbation.

Other theorists have interpreted pathological gambling as a symptom of low self-esteem, a form of masochism, a way of denying feelings of smallness and dependency, or a rebellion against parents or other authority figures that creates guilt and a desire for self-punishment. According to one view, pathological gambling may be an attempt to "control the uncontrollable" and gives gamblers the illusion of taking charge of their fate.

From a developmental perspective, pathological gambling has been linked with inconsistent, insufficient, or excessively harsh parental discipline in childhood, together with a lack of emphasis on saving, planning, and budgeting. Children whose parents were pathological gamblers or alcoholics are more likely to become pathological gamblers themselves. Other predisposing factors include rejection or neglect by a parent, family emphasis on status and material success, attention-deficit/hyperactivity disorder, and early exposure to gambling as a valued activity.

Women usually begin to gamble at a later age than men, more to relieve depression or to escape loneliness or unhappiness than for excitement. Often they are married to men who drink heavily or spend a great deal of time away from home. Some report having parents or partners who were abusive or had addictive behaviors.

From a behavioral perspective, gamblers, in responding to the stimulation of the racetrack, the roulette wheel, or the high-stakes poker game, may learn certain behaviors that, along with sizable winnings, reinforce their habit. At the track, for example, frequent gamblers are more likely to place their bets during the last two minutes before a race begins, a behavior that heightens the tension and excitement. At least in theory, such learned behaviors can be "unlearned" with behavior therapy.

Pathological gambling may have a biological basis. Several studies have found differences in the brain chemistry of such individuals, including lower than normal levels of brain chemicals such as the endorphins. Gambling may boost these substances, which regulate feelings of excitement and well-being, to normal levels.

▼
How pathological gambling feels

Pathological gamblers tend to be bright, aggressive, successful people whose apparent confidence, optimism, and risk-taking may boost their careers—up to a point. Highly competitive and often overly generous, they strive to impress others. They want almost desperately to be liked, admired, and appreciated. Energetic and hardworking, they are often restless and easily bored. When not gambling, they may work in furious spurts, often waiting until just before a deadline before making an all-out effort to finish.

Many men who become pathological gamblers report being good with numbers and very interested in sports. They may know a great deal about the technical aspects of gambling and often use sophisticated strategies to win. Only when they begin to lose do they become sloppy in their gambling. Women, who gamble more for escape from loneliness than for the thrill of the action, typically choose less competitive forms of gambling. They rely on luck rather than on skill, and are likely to become "hooked" more quickly than men.

Researchers have identified different stages in the course of pathological gambling: winning, losing, desperation, and giving up. In the initial stage of winning, these gamblers win more—often much more, sometimes more than they earn in a year—than they lose, and their winning streak may continue for months or years. Their confidence and pride in their gambling skills swell. They fantasize that they will continue to win big and become wealthy.

When pathological gamblers experience a losing streak or a big loss, they can become obsessed with getting back what they lost. As they chase their money, they gamble recklessly and lose more and more. They may go *on tilt*, a term used by gamblers to describe a loss of control or skill. Their gambling ability may continue to deteriorate because of drinking or drug use, playing while angry or upset, or continuing to play for long periods despite ongoing losses.

Once they start to lose, gamblers often lie about their gambling, may not pay household bills, and may spend all the money they can get, including their families' savings, on gambling. They may gamble during work hours or during time usually spent with their families. Needing more and more money to keep up their habit, they may borrow from friends and family, apply for loans, or spend unemployment or welfare checks.

Eventually, pathological gamblers cannot borrow any more. They may lose their jobs; their families may fall apart. They may promise to cut down or stop gambling in return for a bail-out by a relative or friend. Unfortunately, if they do succeed in obtaining money, they feel more powerful than ever and believe that they can get away with anything.

When they finally reach the desperation phase, pathological gamblers find themselves doing things that they once would have found unthinkable: writing bad checks, embezzling from their companies, forging a relative's signature to get a loan. To rationalize such behavior, they tell themselves these are simply short-term loans, which will be paid back with the big win that will solve all their problems.

At home, pathological gamblers may be irritable, even physically or emotionally abusive. They cannot sleep; they eat poorly. Many fantasize about starting life over, with a new name and identity. Ultimately, they gamble not in pursuit of a high but in fear and despair. They may increasingly think about suicide and may attempt to take their own lives.

When pathological gamblers finally realize that they can never catch up with their losses, they no longer care. Convinced that they will lose, they gamble so carelessly that they don't win even if they have a good hand or sure bet. Long after the thrill is gone, they continue to gamble until they reach the point of exhaustion.

▼

Seeking help If you suspect that you or someone close to you has a problem with pathological gambling, these are the questions that should be asked:

- Do you feel stimulated and intensely alive while gambling?
- Do you think you will get lucky if you keep gambling?
- Do you gamble even though you lose more than you win?
- Have you sold possessions to pay off gambling debts?
- Have you borrowed money to pay off debts?
- Do you try to hide your gambling from friends or relatives?
- Do you have problems sleeping because of worry about debts?
- Have you jeopardized your family's financial security because of gambling debts?
- Are you increasingly anxious and worried about gambling?
- Do you gamble more money in riskier ways to win back your losses?

If the answer to several of these questions is "yes," the gambling may have gotten out of control. If you or the person close to you still believes that there is no problem, the next step is to try to stop gambling for a month. If this proves impossible, it is definitely time to get help.

In evaluating a person for pathological gambling, mental health professionals look for a *pattern* of gambling rather than a one-time or occasional gambling binge. The dramatic swings from the highs of winning to the lows of losing can resemble the mood swings of bipolar illness, but it is gambling alone that dictates the changes in mood. However, other disorders often accompany pathological gambling. These include major depression, alcohol abuse or dependence, bipolar disorder, attention-deficit/hyperactivity disorder, and antisocial, borderline, and narcissistic personality disorders.

▼

Risks and complications

Gambling can lead to financial disaster, including enormous debt, defaulting on debts, loss of credit, and personal bankruptcy. At one treatment center the average debt among individuals who sought help was $54,350; at another it was $92,999. According to the National Council on Compulsive Gambling, at least half of all pathological gamblers eventually turn to illegal means to obtain funds. They face the risk of arrest and imprisonment for embezzlement, theft, bookmaking, con games, fencing stolen goods, loan fraud, tax evasion, pimping, selling drugs, or other crimes.

Pathological gamblers often develop simultaneous addictions to alcohol or drugs; 95 percent of them smoke. Some become compulsive spenders, and others are compulsive eaters. Depression often accompanies pathological gambling, but in some instances it is not clear whether depression is the root of the gambling or whether the gambling leads to depression. In several studies, a high percentage of pathological gamblers had thought of killing themselves, planned or prepared for a gesture or serious attempt, or had actually attempted suicide. In addition, pathological gamblers are more likely to develop stress-related physical illnesses, such as hypertension, cardiac arrhythmias, ulcers, digestive problems, skin conditions, headaches, backaches, muscle spasms, or urological problems.

▼

Treating pathological gambling

Treatments for pathological gambling have included behavioral therapy, cognitive therapy, psychodynamic psychotherapy, and medication. Thus far there have been no scientific studies to compare these approaches. No matter which therapy or therapies are tried, however, the road to recovery is rocky, and relapses are common. Abstinence is the crucial foundation of success.

Is it pathological gambling?

According to the DSM-IV, a diagnosis of pathological gambling should be based on these criteria:

Persistent and recurrent maladaptive gambling behavior, as indicated by at least five of these criteria:

1. Preoccupation with gambling (reliving past gambling experiences, handicapping or planning the next venture, or thinking of ways to obtain money with which to gamble)
2. The need to gamble with increasing amounts of money to achieve the desired excitement
3. Repeated unsuccessful efforts to control, cut back, or stop gambling
4. Restlessness or irritability when attempting to cut down or stop gambling
5. Gambling as a way of escaping from problems or of relieving feelings of helplessness, guilt, anxiety, or depression
6. After losing money gambling, often returns another day to get even ("chasing" one's losses)
7. Lies to family members, therapists, or others to conceal the extent of involvement with gambling
8. Has committed illegal acts, such as forgery, fraud, embezzlement, or theft, to finance gambling
9. Has jeopardized or lost a significant relationship, job, or educational or career opportunity because of gambling
10. Reliance on others to provide money to relieve a desperate financial situation caused by gambling
11. Gambling not caused by a manic episode of bipolar illness

Adapted from the Diagnostic and Statistical Manual of Mental Disorders, 4th Edition. *Used with permission.*

The mainstay of treatment is Gamblers Anonymous (GA), a twelve-step program founded in 1957 and patterned after Alcoholics Anonymous (see Chapter 10). The only requirement for membership is a desire to stop gambling. Members of about one thousand GA groups across the world (seven hundred of them in the United States) attend weekly meetings and talk about gambling and their lives—a process they call giving therapy. Long-time members serve as sponsors who offer support to newcomers and form a *pressure group*, designed to ease stress on an individual by devising a comprehensive plan for handling debts and legal problems, working out family issues, and dealing with work-related difficulties.

Some public and private treatment centers focus specifically on pathological gambling. Most combine several approaches, such as one-on-one counseling, family and group therapy, and attendance at GA meetings. According to case reports, behavioral therapy (described in Chapter 27) helps some pathological gamblers. Individuals at high risk for emotional deterioration or suicide may be hospitalized to undergo intensive and comprehensive treatment.

▼
Impact on relationships

The families of pathological gamblers, like those of alcoholics or drug users, are often dysfunctional and develop codependent behaviors (discussed in depth in Chapter 10). Researchers whose studies have chiefly focused on the wives of male gamblers have identified three distinct stages experienced by the spouses:

Denial. The spouse, although suspicious and worried because the gambler is often away from home, tends to believe that there is no real problem. When the gambler is confronted, he promises to stay home—which he does for a while, then goes back to his old ways. If confronted again, he may get angry. His wife then changes her own expectations and behavior to avoid further confrontation.

The couple falls into a behavior pattern dubbed the *discovery cycle.* She uncovers some evidence of his gambling. He begs for forgiveness and cuts back or stops. Eventually he relapses and hides his gambling until "discovered" again. She, telling herself that things aren't so bad, keeps trying to preserve the marriage.

Stress. This phase typically begins with a major crisis triggered by gambling that causes financial or emotional problems at home. Despite this stressful situation, the wife continues to forgive her husband and to believe that he will quit. The gambler may accuse her of pushing him to gamble because of her nagging and lack of understanding. She, too, may blame herself for the problem.

Exhaustion. The wife can no longer endure the situation. She knows that, however contrite her husband is, however sincere his promises sound, he will return to gambling. She cannot sleep, may drink or use tranquilizers, and may develop physical symptoms, such as severe headaches or digestive problems. Badgered incessantly by the gambler, she may start questioning reality or believe that she is losing her mind. If she does not obtain help for herself, she may develop further medical problems, become depressed, develop an addiction to drugs or alcohol, or attempt to kill herself.

Gam-Anon, closely allied with GA, is a twelve-step program that offers support to families and friends of pathological gamblers. At regular meetings, they learn how to change their own attitudes and behavior rather than trying to change the gambler. Members share feelings, coping methods, and practical strategies.

The children of pathological gamblers inevitably feel the impact of their parents' behavior. Buoyed by a big win, gamblers may shower their youngsters with gifts and attention. Depressed by a loss or anxious about money, they may barely acknowledge their children's existence. Watching a parent swing between these extremes and seeing the tension between their parents build up and explode episodically, children may feel deeply hurt, angry, or confused. As teenagers they may run away from home, turn to drugs, or become depressed. A study of high school students found that those whose parents were pathological gamblers were more likely to overeat, use stimulant drugs, report an unhappy childhood, become entangled in a legal problem, or feel depressed or suicidal. Children of pathological gamblers are more likely to develop gambling problems themselves. Gam-A-Teen, similar to the Alateen program for teenagers with an alcoholic parent, offers meetings and support for young people.

▼

Outlook   Gambling, like other addictions, can be very difficult to overcome, and relapses are common. However, individuals who get help can and do recover. A one-year follow-up of 124 male gamblers found that abstinence rates were highest among those who received professional treatment and who attended GA meetings regularly.

Kleptomania

Kleptomania, or pathological theft, is the repeated failure to resist the impulse to steal. The act of stealing itself—not the specific object stolen—is the goal. Individuals with this problem almost always can afford to pay for what they take. Usually they hide, secretly return, or give away the items they have stolen.

▼

How common is kleptomania?   In the past, true kleptomania was considered rare, but researchers now believe it may be more common than was previously thought. Among arrested shoplifters, less than 5 percent appear to have kleptomania. Shoplifting seems to be more common among females; therefore, although the male-to-female ratio for kleptomania is not known, it is possible that more women than men may have this disorder.

   Recent research has found that women who have depressive, anxiety, or eating disorders may be more likely to develop kleptomania. According to one extensive review of medical reports on kleptomania, the typical individual with this problem is a thirty-five-year-old woman who began stealing at the age of twenty.

▼

What causes kleptomania?   Very young children do not have a clear sense of possession and often take things that appeal to them. As they grow older, youngsters recognize their own right, and eventually the rights of others, to personal property. Children who deliberately steal may feel deprived of a parent's affection or are convinced that a sibling has unfairly received more toys or presents. By taking what they want, they make up for a lack of attention or for any perceived favoritism without having to rely on their parents. However, youngsters usually *want* the object they steal. Unlike a child nabbing a treat and savoring it afterward or a shoplifter pawning stolen jewelry, in kleptomania the act of stealing itself is the key.

Adults with kleptomania do not take something because they desire it but because stealing itself provides some emotional release or comfort. Often the affected individuals have other mental disorders, such as major or chronic depression, bipolar disorder, anxiety disorders, anorexia nervosa, bulimia nervosa, or pyromania (in women). For some persons, stealing may serve as a kind of antidepressant that compensates for an actual or anticipated loss. Sometimes kleptomania begins during times of stress. Occasionally it is a symptom of a brain disorder, such as dementia.

▼

How kleptomania feels   Adults with kleptomania often have serious problems with interpersonal relationships, and their stealing may represent a way to avoid difficult issues or painful feelings. Kleptomania, like many other impulse disorders, occurs most often at times of crisis, loss, or disappointment. People with this problem may impulsively take something that doesn't belong to them so that they can experience a brief sense of pleasure or release from stress. Although they do not consciously consider the consequences of stealing, at the subconscious level they want to get caught and often call attention to themselves. At the same time, they may become depressed, anxious, or guilty about the possibility (or reality) of being caught and the impact that an arrest might have on their reputations and families.

▼

Seeking help   Few people seek treatment for kleptomania until they are caught. However, if you have a problem in resisting the urge to steal, or if you suspect that this is true of someone close to you, these are the questions that should be asked:

- Do you steal repeatedly even though you don't need the items?
- Do you feel mounting tension before, during, or after stealing an object?
- Are you stealing for the eventual pleasure or relief you feel, not because of anger or revenge?

If the answer to these questions is "yes," seek professional help for yourself or the person close to you. Without treatment, problems with the law are almost inevitable. In evaluating individuals

<table>
<tr><td>

Is it kleptomania?

According to the DSM-IV, a diagnosis of kleptomania should be based on these criteria:

</td><td>

- **Recurrent failure to resist impulses to steal objects not needed for personal use or for their monetary value**
- **Increasing sense of tension immediately before committing the theft**
- **Pleasure, gratification, or relief at the time of committing the theft**
- **Stealing not committed to express anger or vengeance, nor in response to a delusion or hallucination**
- **Stealing not better accounted for by a conduct disorder, manic episode of bipolar illness, or antisocial personality disorder**

Adapted from the Diagnostic and Statistical Manual of Mental Disorders, 4th Edition. *Used with permission.*

</td></tr>
</table>

for kleptomania, mental health professionals make sure that the stealing is not a symptom of another psychiatric illness, such as conduct disorder, mania, or antisocial personality disorder.

Risks and complications

The major complications of kleptomania are the legal, social, and personal consequences of being arrested. Family members may feel betrayed and angry. Friends may pull away. Employers or prospective employers may consider the individual a poor job candidate.

Treating kleptomania

Treatments for kleptomania include medication, behavioral therapy, and psychotherapy, although there have been few scientific studies of the effectiveness of these approaches. Recently, mental health professionals have reported improvement after treatment with antidepressant drugs that boost serotonin levels, such as the SSRI fluoxetine (Prozac).

Because the success of insight-oriented psychodynamic psychotherapy depends on the person's motivation, those most likely to be helped by this approach are individuals who feel guilt and shame and want to change. Behavioral therapy, including systematic desensitization, aversive conditioning, and a combination of both, has succeeded even with individuals who did not appear to be strongly motivated. Some therapists use negative conditioning, with images of nausea and vomiting, to help overcome the urge to steal; others use systematic desensitization to reduce the anxiety that builds up prior to stealing.

Impact on relationships

The families of adults with kleptomania may have no awareness of the person's compulsive stealing until he or she is caught. This revelation may cause intense embarrassment and anger. Unable to understand why persons would steal things they can afford or do not want or need, their relatives may be baffled and critical. Family therapy can often help everyone in the family to gain insight into the roots of this problem, to deal directly with sources of stress and conflict in their relationships, and to learn more effective ways of communicating with each other.

▼
Outlook   The urge to steal something may come and go over a long period of time. Persons with this disorder may have bouts of being unable to resist the impulse to steal, followed by weeks or months without feeling tempted. After being caught once, some never steal again, but many are unable to stop without treatment. There are few scientific data about the long-term success of various therapies.

Trichotillomania

Trichotillomania, which can be a chronic and severe condition, is the compulsive plucking or tugging at hair and pulling it out. A French dermatologist first described this disorder in 1889 as "an irresistible urge to pull one's hair . . . [in persons] otherwise sane." Usually the result is a small bald patch on the scalp, although in severe cases individuals may pull out hair from the entire head, including the eyebrows and eyelashes, and from other parts of the body. Some researchers view adult hair-pulling as a form of self-mutilation (discussed later in this chapter).

▼
How common is trichotillomania?   There are no reliable data about the number of people who experience trichotillomania. Because few people have sought treatment for this condition, mental health professionals have considered it rare. However, recent studies question this assumption. In a survey of 2,579 college freshmen, 0.6 to 3.4 percent of women and 0.6 to 1.5 percent of men reported pulling out their hair. In a clinic that specializes in habit disorders, the number of people with trichotillomania was one-fifth the number that sought help for nail-biting. Because about 20 percent of Americans bite their nails, this suggests that the incidence of trichotillomania in the general population may be as high as 4 percent—some 8 million men and women.

During adolescence and adulthood, trichotillomania affects far more females than males. The mean age of onset is thirteen. In a study of sixty hair-pullers at the University of Minnesota Trichotillomania Clinic, the typical patient was a thirty-four-year-old woman who had plucked hair from two or more places on her body for twenty-one years.

Hair-pulling may be a symptom of a depressive or anxiety disorder. Individuals with trichotillomania have a significantly higher than expected rate of close relatives with obsessive-compulsive disorder (OCD); some researchers have argued that trichotillomania may be a form of this illness. However, the consensus among mental health professionals is that it is a distinct problem in itself.

▼
What causes trichotillomania?

Many toddlers and young children simultaneously tug at their hair and suck their fingers or thumbs, especially when they are stressed or tired. This benign habit usually goes away without treatment by the age of six. Some youngsters may continue to do this, however, particularly during a time of stress, such as a hospitalization, the recent loss of someone or something dear to them, or the arrival of a new baby in the family. It then can become a habit that is continued into adolescence and adulthood.

It is possible that there is a biological basis for trichotillomania. Neuroimaging studies have found differences in glucose metabolism in certain regions of the brains of individuals with trichotillomania. The condition may also be more common among close relatives of persons with this problem.

▼
How trichotillomania feels

Like individuals with other impulse control disorders, those with trichotillomania may experience a build-up of tension that is followed by feelings of relief and release once they give in to their impulse. Most, but not all, experience anxiety before they act on the urge to pull. In the University of Minnesota study group, mounting tension was true of 95 percent of the individuals, and 88 percent reported pleasure or relief afterwards.

Most pull hair primarily from the scalp, eyebrows, eyelashes, or beard. Less common sites are the torso, armpits, and pubic area. People with trichotillomania may not experience pain from hair-pulling, although some feel itching and tingling. Many develop specific patterns and rituals for tugging out their hair, such as pulling out tufts or only short or long strands. Some use tweezers as well as their fingers. Many chew, lick, or eat the plucked strands. Adult hair-pullers often report other "nervous" habits, such as nail-biting, nose-picking, thumb-sucking, tongue-chewing, cheek-chewing, lip-biting, or scab-picking.

In severe cases, women may spend three or four hours a day plucking out hair and another hour or two covering up the bald spots. Self-consciousness and shame are common. Many want desperately to stop. In one extreme case, a woman taped her fingers together; then, as a last resort, she cut her fingertips. Never-theless, the impulse to pluck is so compelling that it may be al-most impossible to resist without professional treatment.

▼
Seeking help   As noted above, hair-pulling is common in young children and may simply be a habit, like thumb-sucking or nail-biting, that they use to comfort themselves. Over time, the behavior may become so auto-matic that youngsters return to it whenever they are upset or under stress. As a rule, however, hair-pulling tends to disappear as chil-dren get older. Sometimes simply drawing the child's attention to the behavior and indicating that it is undesirable leads to cessation. Parents who are concerned about the practice should seek the advice of their pediatrician or a child psychiatrist.

Adults tend to deny any psychological basis for their problem, although they are painfully aware of the physical consequences. They usually disguise the hair loss, either by styling their hair to cover bald spots or by applying makeup to eyelashes or eyebrows. Some wear scarves or wigs. People with trichotillomania often seek help from dermatologists rather than mental health professionals.

If you suspect that trichotillomania may be a problem for you or someone close to you, these are the questions that should be asked:

• Do you repeatedly pull out hair from your scalp or body?

• Do you feel mounting tension immediately before plucking hair?

• Do you feel gratification or a sense of relief while or after plucking hair?

If you or the person close to you answers "yes" to these questions, it would be wise to seek professional help. One clue in deciding whether to see a mental health professional or a dermatologist is the state of the fingernails or toenails. Most skin-related conditions affect the nails as well as the hair and scalp; trichotillomania does not.

▼

Risks and complications

The primary complication of trichotillomania is hair loss. Persistent plucking creates patchy areas of partial baldness, usually with short, broken strands mixed with long, normal hairs. In some cases trichotillomania leads to total baldness. Because of their appearance, individuals may become embarrassed or depressed and may avoid social involvement or intimate relationships; may withdraw from pleasurable activities, such as sports, because of concern about disguising their hair loss; and, in extreme cases, may even avoid working for fear of exposure. Those who chew or eat hair may develop medical complications, including nausea, vomiting, abdominal pain, anemia, and obstruction of the bowel by a hairball (particularly in children).

▼

Treating trichotillomania

There is no specific therapy for trichotillomania, but a variety or combination of therapies can help to decrease the practice. Several medications that boost serotonin—including clomipramine (Anafranil), a drug used for obsessive-compulsive disorders, and the SSRIs, especially fluoxetine (Prozac)—have been used to treat trichotillomania, with various degrees of success. Researchers have also reported benefits from the use of lithium, a mood-stabilizing agent, and a combination of an SSRI and pimozide (Orap), which blocks the neurotransmitter dopamine.

Various behavioral techniques may also be helpful. These include self-monitoring to record the time, place, and circumstances when hair-pulling occurs, collecting plucked hairs in an envelope, relaxation training, positive imagery, behavioral contracts, and giving oneself instructions to stop before plucking any hair.

Children who pull their hair often respond well to psychotherapy, and their parents also benefit from counseling or family therapy. Psychotherapy alone has not proved very effective in adolescents and adults, although anecdotal reports indicate that it can be beneficial when used in combination with hypnosis. Hypnosis has been used both alone and together with psychotherapy to provide suggestions to stop plucking hair, to explore any link between hair-pulling and emotional trauma, or to regress individuals to the age at which they began hair-pulling.

A nasty little secret

As far back as she could remember, Alexandra used to twirl a strand of her red hair around her finger and tug at it as she fell asleep. When she got upset during the day, she'd do the same thing. "It's perfectly normal," the pediatrician reassured her mother. "Other kids suck their thumbs. She'll grow out of it."

Alexandra didn't grow out of the habit, although she learned to keep it secret because her mother nagged whenever she caught her doing it. As she got older, Alexandra would do more than tug at her hair; she would pull it out. When she was studying or reading, she'd run her fingers through her hair and feel for a short strand. As she played with it, she'd feel a sort of tension inside. Plucking it out brought a brief but sweet sense of relief.

By the time she was in her twenties, Alexandra had developed bald spots. The first ones were small, and she was able to cover them by switching the part in her hair to the other side. But the impulse to pluck the hairs around the bald spots was irresistible, so the bare patches got bigger. She kept changing her hair styles and creating elaborate ways to cover the patches. If she was in a hurry, though, she had to wrap a scarf around her head or wear a hat she could pull down over her ears. Eventually she had to wear hairpieces or a wig.

One day Alexandra was flipping through a woman's magazine when she saw an article called "Nasty Little Secrets." A quotation across the page in bold type jumped out at her: "I couldn't stop pulling out my hair." As she read the piece, she learned that hair-plucking was a treatable mental disorder with the tongue-twisting name of trichotillomania. One of the psychiatrists quoted in the article lived in the same city as Alexandra. When she went to see her, she carried the magazine with her. "This is me," she said stumblingly. "This is my dirty little secret."

The psychiatrist reassured her that trichotillomania was a secret Alexandra didn't have to hold onto any more. She described psychiatric medications, used in the treatment of obsessive-compulsive disorder, that boost serotonin—including fluoxetine (Prozac)—and suggested that Alexandra try drug treatment along with behavioral techniques.

As instructed, Alexandra began to monitor her behavior carefully, recording every time and place she pulled her hair and collecting all the plucked hair in an envelope. At their next session, she and her therapist reviewed her journal, identified high-risk situations, and worked on relaxation techniques and "thought-stopping" so that she could block the impulse to pull out her hair and learn to relax in other ways.

Within a few months Alexandra's bald patches were filling in. She decided to get a new short haircut that would keep all the hair on her head a uniform length. Particularly during the first year of treatment, she frequently found herself going back to tugging at her hair whenever she felt anxious or upset. However, by conscientiously practicing her relaxation techniques and using her training in thought-stopping, she was able to reduce the power of the impulse and to enhance her power to resist it.

▼

Outlook   Most children outgrow their tendency to tug at their hair, or respond either to suggestions that they stop or to psychotherapy. In adults, untreated trichotillomania may be a more persistent problem, lasting for a decade or longer. Some individuals have frequent flare-ups, followed by remissions. Treatments do help, but there are few data on their long-term efficacy.

Pyromania

Pyromania is the repeated, intentional setting of fires, a behavior sometimes described as "motivationless arson." Individuals with this problem do not start fires as an expression of anger, a means of revenge, a political protest, an attempt at sabotage, or a chance to profit in any way. They set fires because they cannot control their urge to do so.

Fire is intriguing to people of all ages. Children, naturally curious about fire, may experiment with matches and lighters and accidentally set fires. Older individuals may remain intensely interested in fire and different aspects of firefighting. But whereas a fascination with fire is normal, deliberately setting a fire is not.

▼

How common is pyromania?

Pyromania is probably very rare. It can develop from the age of three on into adulthood. Boys and men are far more likely to develop the disorder than girls and women. By some estimates, more than 90 percent of those with pyromania are male. Although pyromania can occur at all socioeconomic levels, it is most frequently found in lower and middle economic groups.

▼

What causes pyromania?

From a classic psychoanalytical viewpoint, pyromania stems from sexual feelings. Freud, who saw fire as a symbol of sexuality, noted that "the warmth that is radiated by fire calls up the same sensation that accompanies a state of sexual excitation." For some, there appears to be a link between fire-setting and sexual arousal.

Adult fire-setters often come from large families that were splintered by divorce. Many report that their fathers were absent when they were growing up. One theory suggests that these individuals may begin setting fires out of a desire to bring a missing father home to extinguish the blaze and rescue them from an unhappy life.

Pyromania usually begins during a period of family or personal stress. Children, in particular, may yearn for more nurturing when a parent is ill or absent. Realizing they will not get the love and attention they crave, they develop what many later describe in therapy as a "sad-lonely" feeling. Because they do not know how to comfort themselves or cope with their distress, their unhappiness intensifies to the point where they cannot bear it. Rage replaces the sadness, and they may fantasize about harming or destroying whoever or whatever caused the initial crisis. Setting a fire displaces and releases their pent-up fury. Usually individuals are not aware of their hidden anger until they start dealing with it in psychotherapy.

Some have theorized that those who set fires are acting out a desire for aggression, power, or prestige. Adolescents and adults with this disorder are more likely to set fires after personal set-backs that make them feel helpless, embarrassed, or inadequate. Starting, reporting, watching, or helping to put out a fire may make them feel proud or powerful and may boost their self-esteem. In some instances they do not act immediately on their urge to set a fire; rather, they fantasize about doing so and spend days on planning and preparation. Some set off false alarms or set fires to summon firefighters into action. They may report the fire and help to bring it under control. Others volunteer or work as firefighters and are eager to demonstrate their courage and skill.

Researchers disagree about a possible correlation between pyromania and physical abuse in childhood. Pyromania is more common in individuals who are mildly retarded, abuse alcohol, suffer sexual dysfunctions, report chronic personal frustration, or have a history of antisocial behaviors, such as stealing, running away, or skipping school. Many people with this problem do poorly at school and have learning disabilities, attention disorders, speech problems, or visual or other physical abnormalities. There is a strong association between fire-setting and cruelty to animals.

Pyromania may also have a biological basis. Individuals with this disorder tend to have low blood sugar levels and decreased levels of metabolites of norepinephrine and serotonin in the fluid surrounding the brain and spinal cord, which may in some way interfere with their ability to control their impulses.

▼

How pyromania feels

Like other individuals who cannot control their impulses, those with pyromania may not be able to recognize and respond to normal feelings, either in themselves or in others. They tend to take things at face value; even as children they show little creativity. For them, setting fires may be the only way they know to express feelings such as frustration, shame, or inadequacy.

Individuals with pyromania feel a fascination with fire and sometimes with the apparatus and excitement involved in firefighting. Typically they are tense or anxious before setting a fire, possibly because of the danger and the possibility of punishment, and feel gratified, excited, or have a sense of release when they set the fire, watch it burn, or observe its consequences. Some become sexually aroused by the fire. Many have no feeling of regret or guilt afterward, or concern about possible harm to life or property; in fact, some feel excitement at the destruction the fire has caused.

▼

Seeking help

Children may accidentally set fires while experimenting with matches or lighters or deliberately start them as an act of defiance or disobedience. Parents should always treat fire-setting in children with utmost seriousness. If the fire clearly was an accident, they should make sure that the child fully understands the serious consequences and dangers of playing with matches or lighters. If fire-setting recurs, or if it is accompanied by other behavioral problems, parents should seek professional help, not to punish the youngster but to prevent future episodes and to deal with possible underlying problems.

Adult fire-setters rarely seek help unless they are arrested and jailed. However, if you suspect that you or someone close to you may have a problem with fire-setting, these are the questions that should be asked:

- Have you deliberately set a fire more than once?
- Did you feel tense or excited beforehand?
- Are you attracted to or fascinated with fire?
- Are you very interested in or curious about the equipment used in fighting fires or other things associated with fires?
- Did you feel pleasure, gratification, or relief when setting fires?
- Did you feel similar emotions while watching the fires or helping to put them out?

If you or a person close to you has deliberately set a fire and answers "yes" to these questions, seek professional help immediately. In addition to pyromania, deliberate fire-setting may be a symptom of other mental disorders, including antisocial and other personality disorders, schizophrenia, mental retardation, or a manic episode.

Risks and complications

Fire-setting may injure or kill the person who starts the blaze as well as others, and can destroy buildings and property. Fire-setters face the risk of arrest and imprisonment.

Treating pyromania

Behavioral approaches, including positive reinforcement and aversive conditioning, are often the first choice of treatment. One particularly effective technique is *graphing*. Working with a therapist, individuals create a line graph of the events, behaviors, and emotions associated with fire-setting. This process helps them to become aware of the cause-and-effect relationship between feelings and behaviors. With the therapist's help, they learn to identify and use the initial feeling as a signal of risk and to substitute more adaptive methods of dealing with their emotions. The therapist also emphasizes that all people have intense feelings and that they

- Deliberate and purposeful fire-setting on more than one occasion

- Tension or emotional arousal before the act

- Fascination with, interest in, curiosity about, or attraction to fire and its associated characteristics (e.g., paraphernalia, uses, consequences)

- Pleasure, gratification, or relief when setting fires or when witnessing or participating in their aftermath

- Fires not set for monetary gain, as an expression of sociopolitical ideology, to conceal criminal activity, to express anger or vengeance, to improve one's living circumstances, or in response to a delusion or hallucination

- Fire-setting is not better accounted for by antisocial personality disorder, conduct disorder, or a manic episode of bipolar illness.

Adapted from the Diagnostic and Statistical Manual of Mental Disorders, 4th Edition. *Used with permission.*

must learn to live with them. Once people can fully grasp these concepts, they are highly likely to stop setting fires.

However, graphing deals only with behavior, not the underlying problems, and many mental health professionals view it as only a first step in helping individuals to develop the capacity to recognize and express their feelings so that they can successfully participate in psychotherapy. Persons with pyromania who lack insight and deny or refuse to take responsibility for their actions do not benefit from psychotherapy.

Some psychiatrists have reported that SSRI antidepressants such as fluoxetine (Prozac) can help in cases of pyromania. "Serotonin seems to play some role in regulating an individual's response to impulses," says psychiatrist Michael Wise, M.D., a clinical professor at Tulane University. "With Prozac, patients say they feel less impulsive."

A few mental health professionals have reported success with crisis-oriented family therapy for young fire-setters and community-based intervention programs that treat any fire-setting (whether accidental or deliberate) very seriously and teach children safety skills, such as using a fire extinguisher and mapping a home escape route. In addition, youngsters who have set several fires spend several hours a week with a firefighter, who helps them rechannel their energy and rebuild their self-esteem.

▼

Impact on relationships

In children, fire-setting may be a cry for attention and help in dealing with family tensions and problems, such as marital discord, an absent parent, or divorce. Families that recognize it as such can begin to deal with the underlying problems.

Family members rarely have any idea that a relative may be setting fires. When the person is caught, the discovery can be enormously shocking and upsetting. Families may need help dealing with a host of unexpected problems, including legal as well as psychological issues.

▼
Outlook

Children who have set fires respond very well to therapy, and fewer than 5 percent continue these acts. Among almost one thousand young fire-setters who went through intervention programs in Texas, fewer than 2 percent continued to set fires.

There is little follow-up information on adults and adolescents with pyromania. Many may set a fire during a crisis and then give up this dangerous behavior without treatment. Others may have little or no motivation to stop setting fires unless they are caught. Those who can express their feelings in words and work through their frustrations in therapy have a better prognosis than those who cannot or suffer from mental retardation or alcoholism.

Repetitive self-mutilation

Repetitive self-mutilation, which is not an officially recognized mental disorder and is not included in the *DSM-IV*, is a pattern of deliberately harming oneself without the intention of committing suicide. The most common types are cutting, burning, or severely scratching one's skin, continuously picking at wounds or scabs, punching or slapping one's face, needle-sticking, bone-breaking, and swallowing glass or other harmful substances. Mental health professionals disagree as to whether such acts are a distinct syndrome or are symptoms of other mental disorders.

Like other problems involving impulse control, repetitive self-mutilation appears to be a means by which some individuals relieve tension. Over time, they may become completely preoccupied with this behavior and harm themselves with increasing frequency and intensity.

▼
How common is repetitive self-mutilation?

Repetitive self-mutilation usually begins in late childhood or the early teen years and appears to be more common among females. It is also a common symptom of borderline personality disorder and of certain schizophrenic disorders.

Repetitive self-mutilation typically begins at times of perceived rejection by a parent, boyfriend, or girlfriend, or in stressful situations in individuals who were physically or sexually abused as children, who underwent surgery or major illness very early in life, whose parents suffered from alcoholism or depression, or who are institutionalized. Among the traits often found in persons who harm themselves are a tendency to perfectionism, to be prone to accidental injury, to be unhappy with the appearance of their bodies or sexual organs, or to be unable to express or deal with emotions. In individuals with this last trait, self-mutilation may be a cry for help from those who cannot express their feelings in other ways.

According to classic psychoanalytical theory, individuals mutilate themselves as a way of avoiding suicide or as a form of symbolic castration. Others explain self-harm as the venting of rage against the self or others, a response to the traumatic loss or death of a loved one, or a way of dealing with sexual fears and conflicts. Some persons may use their self-inflicted injuries to manipulate others into giving them more nurturance.

Psychiatrist Armando Favazza, M.D., of the University of Missouri–Columbia, an expert in this subject, notes that self-mutilators give various reasons for their behavior: It relieves tension, helps them overcome feelings of unreality, makes them feel special or in control, allows them to manipulate others, creates a high or sense of excitement, or helps them express rage.

Often they simply cannot resist the urge to harm themselves. "Cutting, burning and poking needles into my arms is a security for me because I know that if all else fails and leaves me feeling emotionless and empty, the pain and blood will always be there for me," an eighteen-year-old waitress explains. A college teacher, age thirty, says, "Self-mutilation allows me to live on the edge. It is titillating to see just how far I can go and how much real pain I can endure. . . . I can be swept away on a tidal wave of feelings."

Repetitive self-mutilation may have biological roots, and some have speculated that self-mutilation stimulates release of pleasure-inducing endorphins, natural opiate-like substances produced in the brain. There is no conclusive evidence that this occurs, however.

Self-mutilation is common among individuals with multiple personality disorder and may occur in persons with schizophrenia, borderline, histrionic, or antisocial personality disorders, and post-traumatic stress disorder (most often in response to rape, incest, and sexual abuse).

The most extreme forms of self-mutilation, such as amputating a limb or gouging out an eye, occur in cases of schizophrenia, other psychotic disorders, or brain disease, such as encephalitis. Individuals who are mentally retarded or who suffer from neuro-

Is it repetitive self-mutilation? *Although there are no official diagnostic criteria for this problem, mental health professionals usually look for these characteristics:*	■ Repeated self-injury ■ Frequent, intense brooding about hurting oneself, planning self-harm, rubbing or looking at scars, etc. ■ Heightened tension before hurting oneself ■ Feelings of pleasure or release when committing the act ■ No desire to commit suicide and no other psychiatric symptom that might trigger self-mutilation (delusions, hallucinations, transsexual fixed ideas, or serious mental retardation)

logical disorders such as Tourette's syndrome or Lesch-Nyhan disease may engage in "stereotypical" self-mutilation, such as repetitive head-banging or biting of lips or fingertips.

▼

How repetitive self-mutilation feels

Individuals with this disorder often describe themselves as addicted to their acts of self-mutilation. They may use several methods of physical injury, spend hours or days thinking about it, and establish elaborate rituals for hurting themselves. Some drink or save their blood. They may identify themselves—sometimes with shame, sometimes with pride—as "cutters."

Acts of self-mutilation may relieve, at least briefly, psychological distress, including anxiety, tension, rage, racing thoughts, depression, and isolation. In one study, individuals spoke of feelings of anger, fear, self-hatred and, most commonly, numbness—a sense of unreality—leading up to the act of self-mutilation. "When 'it' strikes, self-mutilation is the one thing that provides relief; 'it' being a frantic, desperate, profound sense of alienation from the rest of the world, primarily loved ones," says a twenty-eight-year-old librarian. "Sometimes I think a dose of the good things—loving, hugging—would do it, but it's simpler to reach for a razor blade."

Self-mutilators often report no sensation when they begin injuring themselves. At the point when they see blood or feel pain, they experience relief and a sense of being alive and human again. Afterwards, seeing or rubbing the scar provides a sense of uniqueness, security, and comfort.

As this problem worsens, individuals may harm themselves more often and in more serious ways. Their rituals for self-mutilation, such as carefully laying out the instruments they use, become the center of their thoughts and lives. Because they cannot stop or control this behavior, they may ultimately try to kill themselves.

Seeking help

If you suspect that you or someone close to you may have a problem with repetitive self-mutilation, these are the questions that should be asked:

- Do you repeatedly injure yourself in some way?
- Do you often think about hurting yourself?
- Do you spend time planning ways of hurting yourself?
- Do you touch or look at the scars afterward?
- Do you feel increased tension or anxiety before hurting yourself?
- Do you feel pleasure or release during or after the act?

If the answer to any of these questions is "yes," you or the person close to you should seek professional help.

Risks and complications

Repetitive self-mutilation can create wound infections or disfiguring scars. Some individuals are embarrassed by the way they look and avoid going out in public. About half have had or develop eating disorders; a smaller percentage have had or develop substance abuse problems. The greatest risk is that of suicide, usually by drug overdose or by some means other than wrist-slashing or another form of self-mutilation.

Treating repetitive self-mutilation

Repetitive self-mutilation is one of the most difficult psychiatric problems to understand and treat. Often individuals also suffer from other mental disorders. Treating these problems with psychotherapy, medication, or both may help reduce or eliminate episodes of self-mutilation. Some mental health professionals have reported success with clomipramine (Anafranil), a medication used primarily for OCD that increases serotonin levels in the brain.

A supportive long-term relationship with a mental health professional who helps persons with this disorder to express feelings of anger, sadness, or anxiety may be crucial. Specific coping techniques—such as spending as much time as possible in public places, using earphones and turning up the volume to snap out of the sense of numbness or unreality that often precedes self-mutilation, and wearing rubber or leather gloves during times of extreme tension—also help.

In severe cases, hospitalization may be recommended. Since people almost always self-mutilate only in private, constant supervision in the hospital, which may include one-on-one nursing around the clock, may halt self-harm. After their first experience of not harming themselves for a prolonged time, individuals are sometimes motivated to stop permanently.

▼

Impact on relationships

Self-mutilation is a solitary act that isolates individuals from others. Those with this problem try to keep their cutting or other injuries secret and may lie when questioned about scars or bruises. If family members or friends discover what has been happening, they are likely to be shocked and horrified and can find it very difficult to comprehend how persons they love and value could inflict pain on themselves. Family therapy can help in dealing with long-standing problems of communicating or coping in a family, as well as with the harmful behavior.

▼

Outlook

Without treatment, repetitive self-mutilation may flare up and then ease or it may persist steadily for ten to fifteen years, if not longer. Self-mutilation in individuals who receive treatment for any other mental disorders that may be troubling them may improve after therapy.

Pathological spending

Anyone can splurge or go into debt once in a while. Pathological, or compulsive, spending—a problem that is not an officially recognized mental disorder and is not included in the *DSM-IV*—is the repeated inability to control the impulse to buy much more than a person needs or can afford. It is also a common symptom of bipolar illness (manic depression) and other disorders.

▼

How common is pathological spending?

The number of Americans who cannot resist or control their desire to shop and buy is unknown. Pathological spending occurs in all ages, socioeconomic groups, and genders, although women seem more likely than men to become pathological shoppers. Often their own parents were substance abusers, gamblers, spenders, or borrowers, or were emotionally or physically absent. Some therapists have linked pathological spending with eating disorders and childhood neglect or abuse, especially sexual abuse. Like other impulse control problems, pathological spending tends to increase during times of stress.

▼

What causes pathological spending?

The origins of an irresistible urge to acquire material things may lie in childhood. Some youngsters who do not get adequate attention and approval from a parent may spend excessive amounts of money to make themselves feel more important and valuable. Children who feel that they have never met their parents' expectations or standards (however unrealistic) may want to buy things to give themselves an extra boost in confidence. During a manic episode, individuals with bipolar illness may spend vast amounts of money because of their impaired judgment and grandiose ideas.

▼

How pathological spending feels

"Shopaholics" go on wild buying sprees, which relieve painful feelings of worthlessness, anxiety, or depression and produce excitement and happiness. They rarely buy what they need; instead they purchase luxuries that signify qualities they lack—power, love, self-esteem. Women are most likely to buy clothes, perfume, and other items that make them feel more attractive and feminine. Men tend to buy sporting gear, cars, or exercise equipment.

The act of buying provides a brief moment of immediate gratification or excitement that temporarily alleviates feelings of sadness or inferiority. However, this high is transitory, and quickly fades as shoppers realize that their latest acquisitions have not eliminated their feelings of emptiness.

▼

Seeking help

If you suspect that spending is out of control for you or someone close to you, these are the questions that should be asked:

- Have you been devoting increasing amounts of time, energy, and effort to shopping?

- Do you feel a sense of heightened tension before spending money, followed by feelings of pleasure or relief during or after making a purchase?

- Have you used money set aside for something important, such as tuition or medical care, for an impulsive purchase?

- Do you shop or think about shopping to "feel better"?

- Do you forego important family, social, or work activities in order to shop?

- Have your spending patterns put you in debt or jeopardized your personal relationships?

- Have you written bad checks, shoplifted, or engaged in other illegal activities to obtain money for your purchases?

Is it pathological spending?

Although there are no official diagnostic criteria for pathological spending, mental health professionals usually look for these characteristics:

- Spending patterns that lead to debt or jeopardize personal relationships

- Increasing amounts of time, energy, and effort devoted to shopping

- A sense of heightened tension before shopping, followed by feelings of pleasure or relief during or after making a purchase

- Applying for an increasing number of credit cards and running up significant interest charges on the cards

- Using money set aside for something important, such as tuition or medical care, for the impulsive purchase of an unnecessary item

- Shopping or thinking about shopping to feel better

- Giving up important family, social, or work functions in order to shop

- Writing bad checks, shoplifting, or engaging in other illegal activities to get money for purchases

If you or the person close to you answers "yes" to several of these questions, it may be advisable to discuss these spending habits with a mental health professional. They may indicate problems that could lead to serious consequences.

▼

Risks and complications

Pathological spenders can usually conceal their buying habits long after they have lost control of them. Therefore, the consequences of their actions may become evident only when their spending leads to job loss, bankruptcy, or financial ruin.

▼

Treating pathological spending

Many people do not take pathological buying as seriously as more obviously destructive addictive behaviors and impulse disorders, and few mental health professionals specialize in treating money-related problems. If individuals are spending money as a way to overcome depressed feelings, therapists may provide treatment for the underlying depression. In other cases they may use a behavioral approach, such as having individuals record every purchase. Psychodynamically oriented therapy focuses on the person's childhood in order to deal with feelings of inadequacy or craving for approval.

Since the key to recovery from money addictions is learning new ways of handling money, treatment may include financial counseling. Rather than using money as a way to build self-esteem, persons learn how to become financially responsible, how to manage their spending, and how to pay off old debts.

Self-help Individuals who find themselves spending or buying more than they intend can take steps to change their behavior. Here are some basic guidelines for self-help:

- Keep track of spending "binges." By writing down what happens or how you feel before a shopping spree, you may be able to pinpoint the triggers of your behavior.

- Avoid the places where you usually shop, especially malls in which you may be most tempted to linger and browse.

- Schedule other activities, such as hikes or family outings, during the times you are likely to spend shopping. Develop hobbies or join groups so that you can divert your attention from shopping.

- Destroy all your credit cards or put them where you cannot get at them easily (such as in a friend's safety deposit box or at the home of a relative who lives at a distance).

- Keep money in a savings rather than checking account.

- Make a shopping list before entering a store; limit purchases to the items on the list.

- Give most of your paycheck to a partner, relative, or friend to pay bills and limit spending to a preset "allowance."

- Don't shop by television. You may want to keep the set off or avoid order-by-phone shopping channels when you're bored, upset, and most likely to order something.

- Contact your local chapter of Debtors Anonymous, which was founded in 1976 and has two hundred chapters in the United States, Canada, and abroad, or Spender-Menders, which has a network for people in remote areas that enables them to participate in long-distance calls with counselors and fellow spenders. (See the Resource Directory at the back of the book for listings.)

Impact on relationships Money, one of the most common topics in marital disputes, can become an intense focal point for conflict. Often spouses who buy compulsively try to conceal the amount they've spent. When partners discover that money set aside for a child's tuition, medical bills, or mortgage payments is gone, they feel betrayed and angry. In some cases, pathological spending can be so extensive that it leads to bankruptcy. Family members may lose all trust in the person who has brought them to financial ruin, and may resent what they see as selfish and self-destructive behavior.

Is it schizophrenia or another psychotic disorder?

Individuals with schizophrenia or another psychotic disorder may:

- [ ] **See things, experience sensations, or hear voices and sounds that do not exist (hallucinations)**
- [ ] **Persistently believe in fixed ideas despite proof that they are false (delusions)**
- [ ] **Be unable to think in a logical manner (thought disorder)**
- [ ] **Talk in rambling, disconnected, or incoherent ways**
- [ ] **Make odd or purposeless movements; not talk or move at all**
- [ ] **Repeat others' words or mimic their gestures**
- [ ] **Show few, if any, feelings; respond with inappropriate emotions**
- [ ] **Lack will or motivation to complete a task or accomplish something**
- [ ] **Function at a much lower level than in the past at work, in interpersonal relations, or in taking care of themselves**
- [ ] **Develop symptoms of major depression or of mania (bipolar illness) along with other symptoms on this list**
- [ ] **Have delusions involving real-life situations, such as that they are being followed, poisoned, infected, loved from a distance, or deceived by a spouse**

Family members and close friends are often the first to notice that a loved one with psychotic symptoms is somehow not the same as before. The more of the descriptive boxes above checked, the more reason there is to be concerned about schizophrenia or other psychotic disorders. This chapter can provide information and guidelines for seeking help and available treatments for these illnesses.

17

Schizophrenia and Other Psychotic Disorders

A college student spends his days and nights listening to a CD that, he explains to his roommate, contains secret clues about the second coming of Christ. A cocaine user is sure that an international drug cartel has targeted him for assassination. A depressed young woman hears voices telling her that she is evil and should take her life. A fan of a local newscaster, convinced that they share a special bond, deluges her with love letters and waits outside the studio to follow her home every night.

These individuals share a common characteristic of psychosis: They are unable to distinguish between what is real and what is not. The most common psychotic symptoms are *hallucinations*, sensations involving any of the senses that a person experiences as real even though there is no evidence that they exist; *delusions*, fixed beliefs that a person clings to despite evidence that they are false; and *thought disorders*, disturbances in a person's capacity to reason or think logically.

Many factors, including mental disorders such as major depression and bipolar illness, physical illnesses such as brain tumors or infections, and reactions to drugs or toxic substances, can impair an individual's perceptions, thoughts, and emotional responses. Some psychotic episodes are acute and interfere only briefly with a person's ability to distinguish between the real and the unreal. If such episodes are induced by illness, injury, or substance use, appropriate treatment of the underlying cause can

409

lead to a quick and full recovery. Other forms of psychosis, such as schizophrenia, can be chronic, with symptoms flaring up or persisting for decades.

For those affected and their loved ones, psychosis can be extremely frightening. Psychotic symptoms always require prompt professional evaluation. This chapter presents current beliefs about the diagnosis, treatment, and prognosis for individuals with schizophrenia or other psychotic disorders.

Schizophrenia

Schizophrenia profoundly distorts an individual's sense of external and internal reality. Typically developing in the teens and twenties, this condition strikes young men and women who are at the brink of discovering their possibilities as adults. Considered one of the most intractable mental disorders, schizophrenia can forever change the course of their lives and the lives of their families.

Schizophrenia has existed in every era and every culture; it represents what many people think of when they use terms such as "insanity" and "madness." More prevalent than Alzheimer's disease, insulin-dependent diabetes, multiple sclerosis, or muscular dystrophy, schizophrenia costs the United States some $33 billion annually. Individuals with this illness occupy one-fourth of the nation's hospital beds and account for 40 percent of treatment days at long-term care facilities.

Views of schizophrenia as a hopeless, incurable illness have changed greatly in recent decades. In the 1950s and 1960s, when the first antipsychotic medications enabled hundreds of thousands of hospitalized mental patients to return to the community, there was great optimism that this devastating disorder could be cured. Unfortunately, schizophrenia is a disease with many manifestations, and the new medications provided only partial and limited solutions for the treatment of the illness. Many discharged patients were unable to work or to care for themselves. Some returned to mental health facilities; others joined the ranks of the homeless and, lacking medication, slid back into psychosis, once again becoming desperately out of touch with reality.

Today, years of research have led to what some experts in schizophrenia call "a new era of guarded optimism." Advances in genetics, neuroscience, and neuroimaging have provided new clues about the origins of the disorder. Careful clinical studies have paved the way for more effective treatments, including new approaches in medication and in psychosocial care. But there still is no cure for schizophrenia, and psychiatrists continue to describe it as the most challenging disorder that they treat.

Although some individuals with schizophrenia recover completely, most continue to experience at least some symptoms for decades, even if they make progress and improve with treatment. Many never regain their full ability to function, and their youthful dreams of happiness may never be fulfilled. They are less likely than others of their age to marry. Even with treatment, a significant number cannot complete their schooling, support themselves, or live independently. Nevertheless, given the breakthroughs in the understanding and treatment of schizophrenia, there is reason for the "guarded optimism" that the future may hold brighter promise.

UNDERSTANDING SCHIZOPHRENIA

The Swiss psychiatrist Eugene Bleuler first used the word *schizophrenia* in 1911 to describe a mental illness that shatters meaningful connections between thought, feelings, and behavior. He conceived of schizophrenia as a splitting of the mind's capacities. Some people still think of it, incorrectly, as a disorder involving "split" personalities, or what is now called *dissociative identity disorder* (discussed in Chapter 18). It is not.

As the National Institute of Mental Health (NIMH) puts it, schizophrenia destroys "the inner unity of the mind" and weakens "the will and drive that constitute our essential character." It affects every aspect of psychological functioning, including all the ways in which individuals think, feel, perceive, decide, view themselves, and relate to others.

Every case of schizophrenia is unique. Some people develop only minimal symptoms; others suffer extreme impairment. In a given individual, the symptoms themselves often vary, so that an affected person may appear calm and rational at one time but agitated and incoherent a few hours later.

THE PHASES OF SCHIZOPHRENIA

Schizophrenia typically consists of several stages. The *prodromal phase*, which usually precedes the onset of the illness by about one year, is a period during which behavior gradually changes. Individuals begin to withdraw from social interactions, pay less attention to keeping clean or dressing appropriately, or act in peculiar ways. The length of the prodromal phase is extremely variable, and the prognosis is especially poor if the illness develops insidiously over a period of many years.

During the *acute*, or *active, phase*, medical intervention, including hospitalization, typically is necessary because of "positive symptoms" that reflect abnormal mental activity and cause grossly abnormal behavior. These include:

- Delusions, fixed ideas that a person continues to believe despite all proof that they are false, for example, that their thoughts are being broadcast over the radio or that space aliens have taken control of their bodies

- Hallucinations, in which a person sees things, experiences sensations, or hears voices and sounds that do not exist, such as commands to harm oneself or another person

- Disorders in thought processes, characterized by abnormalities in how a person thinks and what he or she thinks about, such as believing that he or she can read others' minds or has superhuman abilities. Some individuals with schizophrenia report an absence of thoughts or a feeling of emptiness inside their minds.

- Disorganized speaking, such as nonstop talking, rambling on without making any clear point, shifting from one topic to an unrelated subject, or making up words

- Disorganized behavior, such as repeatedly shaking the head or tapping a foot. Some persons assume odd postures or positions.

In the *residual phase* of schizophrenia, positive symptoms subside, and "negative," or deficit, symptoms—signs of a deficiency in certain mental functions and an absence of normal behaviors—develop. Although less dramatic than positive symptoms, negative symptoms such as the following can be very disabling:

- General apathy, flattened emotions, or inappropriate reactions, as, for example, not responding to events, showing no feelings in circumstances that would make others happy, sad, or angry, or reacting in odd ways, such as laughing when someone is hurt

- Lack of will (*avolition*), which interferes with the ability to complete a task at work or school, such as writing a report

- Lack of logic (*alogia*), which is evident in speech and behavior when individuals jump from topic to topic with no seeming order to what they are saying, or shift from one activity to another

- Inability to experience pleasure (*anhedonia*), such as a lack of joy when spending time with friends or in social activities

- Impaired attention, so that individuals cannot focus even on a simple chore, such as preparing a meal

- An impaired capacity for relating to others, which may lead to almost complete withdrawal and avoidance or to extreme over-dependence on parents or other caregivers.

According to the *Diagnostic and Statistical Manual of Mental Disorders, Fourth Edition (DSM-IV)*, schizophrenia is diagnosed if symptoms last for a minimum of six months, including at least one month with a minimum of two positive or negative symptoms, and if deterioration is observed in functioning at work, school, home, or in relationships. If the disturbance lasts for less than six months, the diagnosis is *schizophreniform disorder*. If the disturbance has lasted for less than four weeks and there has been obvious stress or emotional trauma, the diagnosis may be *brief psychotic disorder*. (These disorders are discussed later in this chapter.) Most cases of schizophrenia are chronic, and 20 to 30 percent of affected individuals relapse during their first year of treatment with conventional antipsychotic drugs.

TYPES OF SCHIZOPHRENIA

Mental health professionals use the following classifications as a form of clinical shorthand for describing the way schizophrenia manifests itself in individuals. Primarily descriptive, these categories do not provide clues to the origins of the illness and have limited usefulness in predicting how disabling the disorder will be over the course of a lifetime or how a given individual will respond to specific treatments. Sometimes the symptoms that appear early in the course of schizophrenia lead to a provisional diagnosis of one type; then, over time, other symptoms come to dominate, and the type changes. In many cases, symptoms overlap.

Paranoid (or positive) type, characterized by preoccupation with a delusion or frequent auditory hallucinations related to a single theme, such as being pursued by FBI agents. Although speech and behavior may appear fairly normal, individuals may be anxious, angry, argumentative, even violent, and exhibit a stilted, formal quality or extreme intensity in their interactions with others. This type of schizophrenia can develop somewhat later in life—after the age of thirty—and has a better prognosis, particularly with regard to employment and independent living, than other types.

Disorganized (or hebephrenic) type, in which the dominant symptoms are rambling, incoherent speech, odd or senseless behavior, and a dampened or inappropriate range of feelings. Persons with this type of schizophrenia, who do not have complex delusions or hallucinations, may grimace or giggle inappropriately, behave in a silly or childish way, and withdraw from any social contact. This type usually begins in adolescence or young adulthood and continues throughout a person's life without significant remissions.

Catatonic type, in which persons develop abnormalities affecting their speech, senses, and movements. They may remain in one fixed position, engage in purposeless movements (such as ceaselessly pacing back and forth), maintain a rigid posture against attempts to be moved, not speak, assume bizarre positions, grimace or gesture in odd ways, resist or refuse commands, repeat whatever another person says or does, or lie in a stupor. Sometimes they alternate rapidly between extremes of excitement and stupor and need careful supervision to prevent them from hurting themselves or others or from becoming exhausted and malnourished. This type of schizophrenia has become extremely rare.

Undifferentiated type, in which individuals have various active symptoms but no dominant one.

▼

How common is schizophrenia?

One-half to 1 percent of the world's population—about one in every 150 people—suffers from this disorder, which occurs in every part of the globe. According to the NIMH's epidemiological data, the total lifetime prevalence for schizophrenia in the United States ranges from 1 to 1.9 percent. This means that at least 2.5 million Americans may have schizophrenia at any given time.

Most of those with schizophrenia develop symptoms between the ages of seventeen and twenty-four. Many researchers believe that all types of schizophrenia always develop before age forty-five, but an illness similar in many respects, schizophreniform disorder (described later in this chapter), can occur after age fifty. Schizophrenia affects about as many men as women, but men tend to develop symptoms earlier in life and to suffer more chronic and severe symptoms.

Because of the chronic and disabling nature of this disorder, many affected individuals are unable to live on their own. An estimated 360,000 persons with schizophrenia reside in state hospitals, halfway houses, subsidized hotels, or group homes. Although reported numbers vary greatly, many thousands more—perhaps as many as 200,000—live on the street or in homeless shelters.

▼

What causes schizophrenia?

Schizophrenia is a biological illness characterized by abnormalities in brain structure and chemistry but influenced by environment and stress. Although there is debate over the relative influences of biological and environmental factors, the interaction between the two appears to be more important than either factor alone.

Schizophrenia is definitely more common in certain families. According to various estimates, a child with one schizophrenic parent has a 5 to 12 percent lifetime risk of developing the disorder; if both parents have it, the risk of their child developing schizophrenia is much greater—35 percent. Among susceptible youngsters, those adopted by mentally healthy parents are as likely to develop schizophrenia as those who remain with their biological parents, a finding that underscores the importance of heredity. The lifetime risk for the sibling of someone with schizophrenia is about 10 percent but rises if other family members also have the illness.

The strongest evidence for a genetic factor in schizophrenia comes from studies of identical twins, who share the same genes. According to genetic studies sponsored by NIMH, if one identical twin suffers from schizophrenia, the average risk for the other twin to develop the disorder is 46 percent. Among fraternal twins, the risk is 14 percent. The fact that not all identical twins develop schizophrenia indicates that environmental factors can influence built-in susceptibility. Scientists have not yet been able to identify a specific gene or group of genes that may hold the key to transmission of schizophrenia.

Neuroimaging techniques, such as positron emission tomography (PET), have greatly increased our understanding of schizophrenia. As one of the premier researchers in this area, Daniel Weinberger, M.D., chief of the clinical brain disorders branch of the NIMH, has noted, neuroscientists can now "look at the anatomy, physiology, and chemistry of the living brain" and compare them in healthy individuals and those with schizophrenia. Abnormalities in brain structure observed early in the illness may indicate that the brain suffered some type of injury prior to the development of schizophrenia, possibly before or shortly after birth. There also may be abnormalities in particular brain cells and in blood flow to certain parts of the brain.

Neuroimaging studies comparing pairs of identical twins in which one has the disorder and one has no symptoms have revealed clear anatomic defects and differences. Those with schizophrenia often have slightly larger ventricles (fluid-filled cavities in the center of the brain) and other abnormalities, including smaller brain volumes, especially in the areas involved in thinking, concentration, memory, and perception, and signs of missing, atrophied, or poorly developed brain tissue.

Researchers have identified alterations in brain chemistry in schizophrenia, possibly involving receptors for the neurotransmitter dopamine. It is believed that persons with this illness may have an excessive number of dopamine receptors or excessively active or sensitive receptors, in particular a specific subtype called D_2 receptors. The receptors for the serotonin metabolite 5HT also seem to be involved in the disorder. Other neurotransmitters, including norepinephrine and gamma-aminobutyric acid (GABA), may play still-unknown roles in influencing the symptoms of schizophrenia.

Environmental factors may contribute to the illness in various ways. An unusually high incidence of birth complications and childhood head injuries has been observed in individuals who are later hospitalized for schizophrenia. Viruses have long been suspects. A viral infection during pregnancy or infancy may affect the developing brain of a fetus or newborn, and some studies have found an association between schizophrenia and the incidence of births in late winter or early spring, seasons when viral illnesses are widespread. For unknown reasons—possibly because of genetic programming that heightens susceptibility—a person's immune system sometimes attacks the brain after a viral infection. Scientists have detected abnormal antibodies (immune system cells that normally fight off infection) that target the brain in some individuals with schizophrenia.

Families of people with schizophrenia are at higher risk for psychotic disorders in general and for schizophrenia-like personality disorders (see Chapter 21). Whether diagnosed with a psychotic disorder or not, such family members often share characteristics, such as suspiciousness, poor rapport with other people, social isolation, idiosyncratic use of language, or eccentric behavior.

Families are no longer held responsible for causing schizophrenia, as they once were, nor is there any evidence to support the once-touted psychological theory that traced the disease to problems in an individual's relationship with his or her mother. "People do not cause schizophrenia," psychiatrist E. Fuller Torrey, M.D., a leading figure in schizophrenia research and treatment, has observed. "They merely blame each other for doing so." Social theories that linked schizophrenia to the stress of living in poverty in urban slums have also been discounted. A "drift" downward to poverty and bad living conditions is more likely to be the consequence of schizophrenia than its cause.

▼

How schizophrenia feels

Schizophrenia steals the sense that all is right with the world. For people with this disorder, reality is not a given. They hear, see, or feel things—often frightening and baffling—that they cannot be sure truly exist. A young man may be crossing a busy street and hear a voice telling him to jump in front of a truck. Is the voice in his head? Did a person standing nearby issue the command? Did someone shout from a passing car? He cannot tell. A teenage girl may glance into a baby carriage and see an infant covered with blood. Is the blood real? Is she imagining it? She doesn't know what to make of it or what to do.

Unable to trust their own ears and eyes, those with schizophrenia feel fearful and vulnerable. In a diary, one teenager described feeling as if "someone took a file and sandpaper and scratched off my epidermis. I feel raw and sore and ugly and loathsome.... Something inside me is going through this funny, alien state, a sense of being at the mercy of some strange force, and this pathetic scarecrow figure inside me at the mercy of other forces. My stomach is empty and gnawing and uneasy as if anything could fall in and break the superstructure I hold up with all my strength."

As their suffering intensifies, persons with schizophrenia feel tense, cannot concentrate or sleep, and spend more and more time alone. School or work performance, personal appearance, and relationships deteriorate. Behavior becomes more bizarre, and individuals may talk nonsense or report unusual perceptions or beliefs, such as their conviction that the CIA has masterminded a complex plot to arrest them for "crimes" they cannot specify.

Individuals with active symptoms, such as hallucinations, find it harder and harder to carry out many normal tasks of day-to-day living. All of their energies are directed to warding off the demons within. They are not completely out of touch with reality, yet the lines between reality and unreality blur. When they watch television, they may think that a news reporter is mocking them. They may assume that casual acquaintances know embarrassing details of their sexual histories. Unable to take care of themselves, they may wear dirty or inappropriate clothing and look messy and disheveled. They often move in unusual ways, such as rocking or pacing, or repeat certain gestures again and again. A lack of insight into the oddness or the impact on others of their appearance and behavior is characteristic of this disorder.

Auditory hallucinations, the most common type of hallucinations in schizophrenia, may plague affected persons. At first the voices may issue simple directives, such as "Stand up!" or "Quiet!" Later they may start to ridicule or insult the person or give dangerous commands to jump off a bridge or press a razor blade against a wrist. Although terrified, schizophrenic individuals cannot block out the noises, music, mumbles, or shouts that fill their heads. Some experience tactile hallucinations, such as tingling or burning sensations or a feeling that bugs are crawling under their skin or that internal organs are rotting inside them. Others become extremely sensitive to tastes or smells.

As many as three-quarters of schizophrenic individuals experience delusions. They may believe that someone or something, such as the devil, is putting thoughts into their heads (*thought insertion*); that others can read their thoughts (*thought broadcasting*); that thoughts are being removed from their brain by some external force (*thought withdrawal*); or that their impulses or actions are being controlled by an unknown agent or force (*thought control*). Some believe that they have a rare gift, such as extrasensory perception, or that they are reincarnations of Christ or Napoleon. Others are convinced that their internal organs are changing shape, that they are prostitutes or rapists, or that they are sinners or the devil himself, doomed to burn in hell forever.

Schizophrenia disrupts thinking and talking. Individuals shift from one idea to another as they speak, without any awareness that topics are unconnected. They may start out talking about breakfast and switch to a conversation about favorite colors or start inventing words and rhymes. In severe cases, they may become incomprehensible. Some talk very little. Others seem more verbal, but what they say is so vague, abstract, or repetitive that they convey very little information. (Therapists refer to this as *poverty of speech.*)

Individuals with schizophrenia often lack the normal sense of self that produces feelings of individuality, uniqueness, and self-direction. Some develop other psychiatric symptoms, such as depersonalization (see Chapter 18), in which their bodies or body parts do not feel real to them. In extreme cases they may not be able to distinguish between themselves and other individuals or inanimate objects. If they hear a charismatic speaker or become involved with a religious cult, they may overidentify and become avid followers. The feeling of belonging gives them a yearned-for sense of identity.

Many people with schizophrenia seem distant or remote. They speak in a monotone; their faces show no expression. Others display emotions that are not consistent with what is happening or what seems to be on their minds. They may smile while cursing or laugh uncontrollably when told a beloved grandparent has died. In some cases they may not seem to have any feelings at all. Others may undergo sudden and unpredictable mood changes, including irrational outbursts of anger. Even when they no longer have active symptoms, such as hallucinations, schizophrenic individuals often lack the ability to follow through on a course of action and cannot work toward a goal, however simple. Vulnerable to stress, they deteriorate in circumstances or situations that are too confusing, stimulating, or challenging for them to handle.

Isolated in a bewildering world, people with schizophrenia may develop depressive or anxiety disorders. They may attempt to take their own lives, often in response to a command or impulse. Some become so intensely preoccupied with objects, ideas, or even parts of their bodies that they totally avoid other people. Those with catatonic schizophrenia may seem completely unaware of or uninvolved in their environment and may not speak or move.

▼

Seeking help   Family members and close friends are usually the first to notice the early signs of schizophrenia. If you suspect that someone close to you may be suffering from schizophrenia, these are the questions that should be asked:

- Has the person withdrawn from interactions with others?
- Does the person show signs of delusions, such as believing that he or she knows of a plot to kill the president?
- Has the person mentioned or shown signs of any hallucinations, such as hearing voices, seeing objects that do not exist, or experiencing odd sensations?
- Are the person's thoughts or conversations illogical?
- Is the person behaving in a bizarre, disorganized way?
- Has he or she been neglecting basic hygiene and grooming?
- Does the person move in strange ways or hardly move or speak at all?
- Does the individual's mood or range of emotions appear flat or constricted?
- Does he or she seem incapable of following through on any activity?
- Is the person unable to function at school or work, to relate to others, or to care for him- or herself in the same way as before this disturbance?

If you answer "yes" to several of these questions, seek professional help for your loved one. The problem could be schizophrenia or another psychotic disorder.

There is no definitive biological test for schizophrenia. Psychiatrists base a provisional diagnosis primarily on their assessment of an individual's ability to think clearly and logically and on symptoms, behavior, and history. In making a diagnosis of schizophrenia, they note whether a person is in the prodromal, active, or residual phase and distinguish among the types of schizophrenia described earlier.

▼
Risks and complications

Substance abuse, especially alcohol abuse, is common and can exacerbate symptoms. Schizophrenic individuals, particularly young men, may use drugs or alcohol to relieve anxiety or depression or to help them cope with the symptoms of their illness. As many as 60 percent of those with schizophrenia develop major depression. It is not clear whether schizophrenia itself leads to depression, whether there was a preexisting depression "masked" by psychotic symptoms, or whether antipsychotic drugs used to treat the illness may in some way trigger depression. Sleep disturbances are also common.

People with schizophrenia, particularly those under age fifty-five, have a mortality rate eight times higher than those who do

Is it schizophrenia?

According to the DSM-IV, *a diagnosis of schizophrenia should be based on these criteria:*

■ **Characteristic symptoms.** At least two of the following, occurring for a significant portion of the time during a one-month period (only one if delusions are bizarre or if a voice makes comments about the individual or converses with another voice)

1. Delusions
2. Hallucinations
3. Disorganized speech (incoherence or frequent derailment)
4. Grossly disorganized or catatonic behavior
5. Negative symptoms, such as flattening of emotions and mood, lack of will (*avolition*), or lack of logic (*alogia*)

■ **Social or occupational dysfunction.** Markedly lower functioning at work, in interpersonal relations, or in self-care since the onset of the disturbance, compared with a previous level (in children or adolescents: failure to attain expected levels of interpersonal, academic, or occupational functioning)

■ **Duration.** Persistence of continuous signs of the disturbance for at least six months, including at least one month with the characteristic symptoms described above

■ **Exclusion of other possible diagnoses.** Schizoaffective disorder, medical conditions, and substance-induced problems ruled out by psychiatric evaluation as possible causes of the disturbance

Adapted from the Diagnostic and Statistical Manual of Mental Disorders, 4th Edition. *Used with permission.*

not have it. Suicide is the greatest danger. About one-quarter to one-half of schizophrenic individuals attempt suicide, and one in ten succeeds. Risk factors for suicide include male gender, age under thirty, living alone, unemployment, recurrent relapses, prior depression, a history of substance abuse, and recent discharge from a psychiatric facility. Schizophrenic individuals often do not express their suicidal intent and act impulsively, making prevention very difficult. Violent acts in public by schizophrenic individuals often attract media attention when they are newsworthy, but a far more common problem for parents and other family members is aggressive behavior or violence at home. (This problem is discussed in Chapters 23 and 30.)

A complication of drug treatment for schizophrenia is a condition called *tardive dyskinesia.* According to the American Psychiatric Association Task Force on Tardive Dyskinesia, 15 to 20 percent of individuals receiving long-term treatment with typical antipsychotic drugs exhibit some sign of this problem, which is marked by uncontrollable facial tics, tongue tremors, and jaw movements. The movements are often mild and barely noticeable, but occasionally they become so severe that they interfere with walking or eating. Frequent examinations (every six months) can detect early signs of tardive dyskinesia, such as small, wormlike movements under the surface of the tongue; stopping medication usually reduces these effects.

To prevent this side effect of drug treatment, psychiatrists prescribe the lowest possible dose of antipsychotic medications. The risk for development of this condition increases with age and the length of time the individual receives an antipsychotic drug. Schizophrenic persons who also have bipolar illness or are being treated for psychotic depression are at much greater risk for tardive dyskinesia than are those who do not have a mood disorder. (See Chapter 28 on psychiatric drugs.)

▼

Treating schizophrenia

For centuries, the quest for a cure for this frightening and often tragic disease led to desperate methods of treatment. In the belief that centrifugal force would drive more blood to the head and improve thinking, schizophrenic individuals were strapped onto a board, their heads pointing outward, and rotated rapidly. Theorizing that fear of injury might shock a psychotic individual back to sanity, at one time doctors sprayed a strong stream of water at the spine. In the 1920s, psychiatrists advised pulling out teeth to eliminate hidden toxins that they thought might be causing the disorder. In the 1930s, they tried injections of horse serum; in the 1940s, enemas; in the 1950s, huge doses of vitamins.

Since then, psychiatrists have treated schizophrenia primarily with powerful drugs called antipsychotics or neuroleptics, which reduce confusion, anxiety, delusions, hallucinations, and other symptoms. Current treatment of schizophrenia usually consists of a combination of medication, psychosocial counseling, and rehabilitation, and great progress has been made in helping individuals to improve. However, there still is no cure for this disabling disorder, and many individuals continue to suffer baffling symptoms for decades.

Treatment of acute schizophrenia   An acute episode of schizophrenia almost always requires hospitalization and treatment with antipsychotic drugs. Individuals experiencing an initial psychotic episode may first undergo observation for a day or two, without treatment, in the safe environment provided by a hospital. This allows time for a complete medical examination, standard laboratory tests, including blood chemistries and liver function, and the ruling out of other possible causes, such as cocaine-induced psychosis, which can appear identical to schizophrenia.

A large number of studies have clearly established the efficacy of antipsychotic medications when they are given at the proper doses for an adequate period of time. Some psychiatrists theorize that delays in using them may increase the length of hospitalization and worsen the long-term prognosis for individuals with schizophrenia. It is not known exactly how long is "too long" to withhold medications, but it is generally felt that a day or two is not likely to make a significant difference. However, individuals with recurrences of active symptoms should receive immediate treatment with antipsychotic medications. In most cases, hallucinations and delusions decrease in intensity after one or two weeks of treatment.

Medication   For the vast majority of individuals with schizophrenia, antipsychotic drugs are the foundation of treatment. They make most people with schizophrenia feel more comfortable and in control of themselves, help them to organize chaotic thinking, and reduce or eliminate delusions or hallucinations, allowing fuller participation in normal activities. Even those who do not improve significantly on medication almost invariably do worse without it.

According to studies comparing medication to various forms of psychotherapy in the treatment of schizophrenia, antipsychotic drugs produce much greater improvement. In the long term, the combination of medication with psychosocial and supportive approaches, especially those that emphasize education and counseling, is more effective than drug therapy alone. Family therapy, together with medication and counseling, has been shown to reduce the risk for relapse.

Most of the antipsychotic drugs have a similar mode of action, differing only in dosages, side effects, and cost. Although some may act more quickly than others, almost all are equally effective. Yet certain people, for unknown reasons, may respond better to one drug than to another. In addition, some individuals tend to tolerate certain side effects, such as sedation, better than they do others, such as muscle stiffness. The only way to determine which drug and which dosage will help a person most is by trial and error, and the process of finding the best kind and dosage of medication can be time-consuming.

The side effects of antipsychotic drugs vary in duration and intensity. Dry mouth, blurred vision, constipation, dizziness on standing, and drowsiness are most likely to occur during the first few weeks of therapy, and eventually may disappear. Other side effects include muscle spasms or stiffness in the head or neck, restlessness, sexual dysfunction, or slowing and stiffening of muscle activity in the face, body, arms, and legs. Although uncomfortable, these effects are usually not medically significant and do not cause lasting impairment. The risk for tardive dyskinesia, noted above, is discussed more fully later in this chapter.

Almost one-third of individuals who are given conventional

antipsychotics continue to have residual negative symptoms, such as apathy and withdrawal. In the past, little if anything could be done to relieve these symptoms. A major breakthrough in treatment came with the development of clozapine (Clozaril), a different type of antipsychotic that can help to relieve both positive and negative symptoms in individuals who do not improve with standard antipsychotic medications or who develop intolerable side effects. In one study, 30 percent of those with so-called refractory schizophrenia—that is, who were not helped by other antipsychotics—improved with clozapine. It is believed that clozapine acts not only on dopamine receptors but also on serotonin receptors, and this may enhance its efficacy.

Although clozapine is highly effective and relatively free of side effects and helps to reduce the number and duration of hospital stays, it has one serious drawback. About 1 percent of those who use it may develop agranulocytosis, a potentially fatal reduction in infection-fighting white blood cells. For this reason, individuals taking clozapine must have their blood checked weekly and must stop taking the medication if their white cell counts drop dangerously low. The need for frequent monitoring makes use of this drug very costly: an estimated $5,300 to $9,000 annually. Because of the high price, mental health advocates have argued that only a fraction of those who might benefit from clozapine have been able to afford the drug.

A newer medication, risperidone (Risperdal), which also blocks receptors for serotonin and dopamine, became available in the United States in 1994. Less is known about risperidone than about the older antipsychotics, but clinical trials and reports indicate that it significantly reduces both positive and negative symptoms of schizophrenia, produces fewer side effects than clozapine, and does not require intensive and expensive weekly blood monitoring. According to manufacturer estimates, a year's dose costs about $1,900 to $2,400.

Electroconvulsive therapy (ECT) has been used for schizophrenic individuals who show no improvement after several months of drug therapy and for those with catatonia or depression. Although it relieves depressive symptoms and reverses catatonia, there have been few reports on its long-term effectiveness. (ECT is described in Chapter 28.) The use of other types of medications, including lithium, benzodiazepines, and antidepressants, together with antipsychotics is currently being studied by investigators around the world.

Maintenance therapy   Relapses are common, especially in the first year after an initial episode of active schizophrenia. Most psychiatrists recommend at least one to two years of medication after the first schizophrenic episode, five years of treatment after a second attack, and indefinite, possibly lifelong medication after three or more relapses. Such maintenance treatment can reduce the chance of a relapse by almost fourfold.

A major problem in drug treatment is noncompliance. Sometimes individuals and their families, not recognizing that maintenance therapy is crucial in preventing recurrences, decide not to use medication when symptoms are very mild. Others may not remember or pay adequate attention to their medication schedule. Relapse rates consistently go up when individuals stop taking antipsychotic drugs. In one study, only 10 percent of those who continued taking their medication relapsed, compared with 80 to 90 percent whose illness recurred when they stopped taking their antipsychotic medication.

Psychotherapy In a landmark study that compared psychotherapy alone with a combination of medication and psychotherapy in the treatment of schizophrenia, insight-oriented psychotherapy by itself provided very little benefit. Individuals with this disorder are usually incapable of analyzing their feelings and motivations. However, supportive therapy, which is less demanding, and psychosocial counseling, which may help individuals to obtain vocational training or housing, are very useful. Group therapy may have a positive effect by providing the added benefit of peer support. It is most likely to be beneficial when groups are highly structured and the therapist limits the goals so that they are within the capabilities of the members.

Family therapy Because schizophrenia profoundly affects the person's close relatives over the course of many years, family therapy can be an important factor in the long-term prognosis and can help to reduce the risk for relapse. It is not clear exactly how family therapy lowers relapse rates. Some therapists believe that it may ease daily stress and increase the individual's compliance in taking medication.

The initial focus is on what therapists term *psychoeducation*. Everyone in the family needs to learn that schizophrenia is a chronic disease for which no one is responsible. In addition to providing a full description of the disorder, therapists teach basic principles of communication, social skills, effective problem solving, and behavioral management techniques. These are all important factors in living with a schizophrenic family member.

In regular sessions, family members learn how to communicate with one another clearly and directly, and to function as a team in facing the difficulties the disorder poses. They practice making clear "I" statements about their own feelings, needs or desires ("I feel frustrated—or angry or sad or hurt—when . . . ."); listening actively; expressing feelings, opinions, and requests directly; and clarifying verbal and nonverbal messages (such as saying explicitly that they are upset when the person leaves a room messy, rather than frowning, sighing, and angrily picking up the vacuum cleaner). With the therapist's help, they can identify a few key stressors, come up with suggestions for new solutions, and learn how to negotiate issues of day-to-day living. For example, if one family member does most of the caretaking, the entire family may brainstorm about ways in which others could contribute more. If a parent is upset about the smell from a schizophrenic son's cigarettes, the family may designate smoking and no-smoking areas of the house, or the schizophrenic individual might agree to smoke only outside or in a room with an open window.

Therapists often use cognitive therapy to identify and correct negative thinking by family members. They work with one person at a time, and the others, as they listen, can gain insight into their own behavior. If, for example, a parent tends to generalize and accuses a schizophrenic individual who spills something at dinner of "always" ruining family meals, the therapist might underscore the need to avoid "always" and "never" statements, to keep the focus on the here and now, and to remain calm.

One key factor in the way that different family members respond to schizophrenia is in the expression of emotion. When therapists ask open-ended questions, family members with "high expressed emotion" make more critical remarks and show greater emotional involvement, including being overprotective, intrusive, or self-sacrificing. They talk more or at the same time as others, engage in more heated discussions, make less eye contact, appear less attentive, and are less effective at problem solving. They are more likely to think that the schizophrenic relative is lazy and does not have a real illness, to be critical and intolerant, not to understand the individual's needs for reassurance, and to have unrealistic expectations—for example, that he or she behave like "a normal person."

By comparison, relatives with "low-expressed emotion" talk less and remain calmer, more neutral, positive, and supportive. They accept symptoms as signs of a real illness and provide more reassurance and social support. Family therapy can lower the level of expressed emotion through education and training in more effective ways of coping. In turn, reducing criticism and emotional overinvolvement lowers stress for everyone in the family, including the patient, and helps to prevent relapses.

Many families continue in therapy for a year or longer and rely on informal groups thereafter for ongoing support over the course of many years. This group support can be invaluable. Some groups meet every other week, some monthly. Usually each family describes current issues and its efforts to cope, and other participants comment on the family's strengths and suggest alternative solutions to unsolved problems.

Rehabilitation   Even though antipsychotic medications can relieve symptoms and enable patients to leave hospitals, most cannot begin to rebuild their shattered lives without active rehabilitation. This usually consists of behavioral approaches, social skills training, attention-focusing procedures, and instruction in personal grooming. Structured activities can help to reduce the bizarre behavior of people with chronic schizophrenia. Vocational rehabilitation can provide job-seeking skills as well as apprenticeship and other job-training programs.

As schizophrenic individuals build their competence, confidence, and coping skills, they become less vulnerable to stress and relapse. However, they often require intensive practice sessions, which present them with a variety of situations, to help them apply what they have learned, along with booster sessions to maintain their skills. Simply being instructed in the basics of budgeting, for instance, is not enough. They then need to be taught how to master food shopping within a budget, how to set up a budget for clothing, how to budget for other purchases. They also may need repeated instruction on how to use an automated teller machine (ATM) or balance a checkbook.

Hospitalization   In most cases, people are hospitalized only during the acute stage of schizophrenia, whether an initial episode or a relapse, and are discharged once their symptoms are under control. Hospital stays today, in contrast to several decades ago, rarely last more than a few days or weeks or, on occasion, months. The primary reasons for hospitalization are concern that individuals may be dangerous to themselves or others and a need for observation, evaluation, or treatment. If they refuse hospitalization but are considered in danger or dangerous, a court order must be secured for involuntary hospitalization. Short-term hospitalization for persons diagnosed as having schizophrenia is usually covered by private insurance, disability coverage, or Medicaid.

Inpatient treatment for an acute episode of schizophrenia is fairly standard, whether the institution is a private psychiatric center or a public hospital. The quality and experience of the staff and their ability to work together as an effective team are crucial components of quality care.

Although medication is the mainstay of treatment for active schizophrenia, the design, structure, and organization of a psychiatric unit or ward—its "milieu"—can themselves be therapeutic.

Individuals tend to do best with relatively short stays in small units that have a high staff-to-patient ratio and low staff turnover, a low percentage of actively psychotic patients, and a supportive, practical approach that emphasizes problem solving.

However, some people experience such severe and progressive deterioration that they require long-term institutionalization. Even with antipsychotic medication, their symptoms remain so incapacitating that they cannot function at home or in group living situations. There are not many options for families seeking care for a loved one who needs long-term, skilled, around-the-clock psychiatric care. Hospitalization in the limited number of private mental health facilities in the United States is expensive, and many families do not have the financial resources to afford such care. National advocacy organizations and local support groups can refer families to financial counselors who can help them assess their economic situation.

State mental hospitals provide care for thousands of mentally ill individuals, but often admit only those who are extremely violent or completely incapable of caring for themselves. Many people, although disabled by schizophrenia, do not meet these criteria. Even those who are admitted may be discharged as soon as their condition improves, despite the fact that they still have some disabling symptoms. If such people have nowhere to turn, if family care is not possible, or if they refuse to live with relatives, many of them end up on the street or in homeless shelters.

Residential treatment centers   After treatment for an acute episode, individuals can transfer to a residential treatment center that also provides a therapeutic milieu. As hospital stays have grown shorter, an increasing number of programs have provided partial hospitalization options and special living arrangements that offer the counseling and group support vital to successful treatment. Most of these programs reduce social or environmental stresses, assist individuals in interpreting reality and making decisions requiring judgment, and discourage substance abuse. (Abstinence is an essential step in recovery.) These settings are beneficial, but they are expensive and are not available in all communities. Day treatment centers, which offer the same group support that residential centers provide at much lower cost, also can serve as effective therapeutic settings.

Whether residential or day, treatment centers typically organize programs aimed at helping individuals meet short-term goals. To overcome the apathy that is common in the residual stage of schizophrenia, for instance, they may set up a token economy or credit incentive system in which individuals earn "credits" if they participate in therapy groups, work on conversational and vocational skills, or improve their personal grooming. At day centers, participants may earn credits if they arrive promptly or pitch in with cooking and cleanup. Their credits may entitle them to assorted privileges, such as use of a computer or CD player, a supervised outing, time off from the day center, or a chance to spend time alone with a favorite staff member. Those who earn the most credits each week may win a special reward, such as a movie pass or a trip to a park with a counselor.

Other living arrangements Group homes and halfway houses run by experienced mental health professionals provide excellent options for many individuals with schizophrenia. The environment is structured, the administration of medication is supervised, and opportunities for continuing rehabilitation and education are offered. Many provide an all-important bridge from institutional care to some form of independent living. Often families participate in counseling sessions and in support groups sponsored or overseen by the facility.

Many people with schizophrenia eventually return home to live with their families, at least temporarily. Others move into adult homes that provide greater independence than halfway houses or group homes, along with ready access to mental health care services. Clinical social workers affiliated with private or public mental health institutions can help schizophrenic individuals and their families to sort out options, evaluate their quality, and decide on those that best meet their needs.

Several states, including Wisconsin, Michigan, Delaware, and Rhode Island, have set up Programs for Assertive Community Training (PACT), in which a multidisciplinary team of professionals visits schizophrenic individuals at their homes or job sites, on a daily basis if needed. They provide medication and counseling, teach coping and life management skills (such as shopping and housekeeping), and respond to crises around the clock. The cost per client is estimated to be $5,000 to $10,000 a year, less than full hospitalization or day treatment. Because of the support they receive, PACT clients usually show significant improvements in living skills, are able to live more independently, often work at least part-time, and require fewer hospitalizations than might otherwise be expected.

▼

Impact on relationships The intense suffering that schizophrenia can cause extends beyond those who develop this disorder to all who care about them. "The family is a victim just as much as is the person with schizophrenia," observes Stuart Yudofsky, M.D., chairman of the department of psychiatry and behavioral sciences at Baylor College of

Medicine in Houston. Schizophrenia can disrupt family life for many years and cause emotional, social, and financial difficulties. Family members may feel worried about their relative, anxious about the illness, guilty about being responsible for it in some way, and angry and frustrated if treatment does not bring about a complete recovery. (Chapter 30 discusses the impact of mental illness on relatives.)

"The relations a person with schizophrenia has with his or her family members are usually intense and chaotic," notes Yudofsky. "Overdependence, violent interchanges, dramatic shifts from intimacy and trust to distrust and distress are common." The stress of such conflicts and tensions can make families feel that they are falling apart. Members may blame one another for somehow causing the illness or—consciously or unconsciously—may isolate the schizophrenic individual.

The withdrawal and detachment that commonly occur in schizophrenia can be the most difficult aspect of the disease for family members. They need to understand that this remoteness is not deliberate or defiant. The more that relatives learn about the illness and its treatment, the better they can cope with their loved one's behavior and the demands of helping him or her to improve. They also must come to terms with the fact that schizophrenia may have changed this person forever, that their family routines may never be the same, and that they may have to sacrifice time and energy indefinitely to provide direct care. Families may have to make financial sacrifices as well. The costs of care for schizophrenia can be staggering, and many insurance plans and health care programs provide only limited coverage or a preset "cap" that is quickly reached and exceeded.

For parents, the anguish of watching the torment of a schizophrenic child is intense. One father described it as "a nightmare in broad daylight." Guilt and fear often haunt parents as they struggle toward acceptance of this reality. They continue to love their child but hate the disease that has transformed him or her. They may do everything humanly possible to make sure the young person gets the "best" care and treatment, only to discover that it is not enough, that their son or daughter is still a lonely soul lost in a private hell. Parents of children with schizophrenia have a high rate of marital problems and mental disorders that may be consequences of the stress of dealing with the impact of their youngsters' mental illness.

Brothers and sisters also must deal with painful feelings. Parents may devote so much time, energy, and emotional preoccupation to a child with schizophrenia that siblings feel neglected. As adults, brothers and sisters may feel a burden of responsibility for their schizophrenic sibling, particularly after their parents' deaths.

Danny—'old' and 'new'

Marcia has spent a lot of time poring over old family albums, looking for signs of something "different" about Danny. He was a towheaded all-American kid, smiling with his front teeth missing, proudly wearing his Little League uniform, grinning as he hung up his Christmas stocking. When did the glow fade? In his high school photos, his expression has taken on a certain sullenness. But don't all teens cultivate that look? And maybe he does stand to the side in many of the shots—but isn't that, too, typical of adolescence?

Long before there were any tangible signs, Marcia had sensed something was wrong. Once Danny had tried to explain that sometimes he heard her voice even when she wasn't around. There were other voices he couldn't confide to her, scary ones that told him he was bad, that mocked everything he said and knew about stuff—sexual stuff, thoughts he'd had, things he'd done. Sometimes these voices would tell him to do things he knew he shouldn't, like walk into the middle of a busy street or burn his arm with a cigarette.

Despite the tormenting voices, Danny was able, at least for a while, to keep going through the motions of daily life. His grades fell, his friends slipped away, but his parents kept telling themselves it must be a phase. When he went away to college, they felt that being on his own might help.

But midway through his freshman year, Danny stopped shaving, taking showers, brushing his teeth, washing his hands, changing his clothes. He'd spend hours locked in his room, talking and laughing to himself, the same song blaring night and day. After one of these episodes, Danny finally emerged from his room gaunt and wild-eyed, words rushing out about "The Force" that had taken control of his mind. "It is time now for the sacrifice," he said ominously. His frightened housemates rushed him to the hospital.

Antipsychotic medications drove away the voices and brought Danny back to reality. During his four-week hospitalization he calmed down, participated in group activities, and met regularly with a therapist. When he returned home, his parents were relieved that he seemed less tormented, but crushed to discover that this "new Danny" was very different from the carefree boy whom they had known and loved. The new Danny seemed distant, as if his soul lived in some far-off place. He spoke in a monotone, with almost no expression on his face. Sometimes he'd burst into a rage if they asked him to turn down the TV or not smoke in the house. At dinner he might laugh uncontrollably. Even a simple task like clearing the table seemed too much for him.

Danny's parents enrolled him in a day-treatment program in which he participated in therapy and training groups. He gradually improved to the extent where he could take on some independent responsibilities. One weekend Danny's parents put him on a bus to visit his uncle. He never got there. For several frantic days, his relatives searched for him. Finally, the police found him disheveled and incoherent, wandering the streets of a nearby city.

For two years this pattern continued. Finally the psychiatrists suggested a new medication, clozapine (Clozaril). The results were dramatic—not just in relieving Danny's hallucinations but also his "negative" symptoms, such as his lack of emotion, apathy, and withdrawal. "For the first time, I can see parts of our old Danny again," says Marcia. "But the most wonderful thing is that now he has a chance of finding the good things in life that every parent wishes for a child."

They may feel torn between their sibling's demands and the needs of their own spouses and children.

Even when schizophrenic individuals live more or less independently in some form of community housing, the worries continue. Parents and siblings know that an emergency call could come at any time, reporting that their loved one is not taking his or her medication, has developed acute symptoms, has gotten into trouble on the job or with the law, or has attempted or committed suicide. "You reach the point of thinking, 'Now what?'" says one mother whose daughter has spent twenty years in and out of institutions. "You think, 'I can't take any more,' but somehow you do. You can't close your heart to a child who needs you."

Families who do not have formal or informal sources of support can become emotionally exhausted from the strain of having to cope with crisis after crisis. Counseling and support from groups such as the National Alliance for the Mentally Ill (NAMI) can help families come to terms with their own feelings, develop realistic expectations for their loved ones, and cope with the ongoing stress in their lives.

▼

Outlook   Researchers have described four patterns for the course of schizophrenia: complete recovery; recurrences of the illness but with full recovery each time; repeated recurrences but incomplete recovery, leading to some persistent symptoms; and progressive deterioration. The first two outcomes are less common than the last two, and no one can predict which pattern a particular patient will follow. In general, women appear to have a more favorable prognosis and better social functioning than men.

Overall, about one in every four or five individuals with schizophrenia has a relatively good outcome and improves dramatically within two years of the onset of psychotic symptoms. In general, those most likely to do well over the long term are married and from a high socioeconomic class, have no family history of schizophrenia, develop psychotic symptoms quickly and for a brief duration, had functioned well previously, have had no previous mental disorders, and show signs of confusion or depression during the psychotic episode (which is an indication of some awareness of what is happening).

The great majority of schizophrenic individuals continue to need treatment over a prolonged period of time. Nevertheless, although they suffer remissions and residual negative symptoms, most continue to make slow, fluctuating progress over a period of up to thirty years. With appropriate treatment, they are able to work in some capacity, live with their families or in some form of independent living arrangement, and develop friendships.

<table>
<tr>
<td>

Is it schizophreniform disorder?

According to the DSM-IV, a diagnosis of schizophreniform disorder should be based on these criteria:

</td>
<td>

■ **Characteristic symptoms.** At least two of the following, occurring for a significant portion of the time during a one-month period:

1. Delusions
2. Hallucinations
3. Disorganized speech
4. Grossly disorganized or catatonic behavior
5. Negative symptoms, such as flattening of emotions and mood, lack of will (*avolition*), or lack of logic (*alogia*)

■ **Duration.** An episode lasts at least one month but less than six months.

■ **Exclusion of other possible diagnoses.** Schizoaffective disorder, medical conditions, and substance-induced problems ruled out by psychiatric evaluation as possible causes of the disturbance

Adapted from the Diagnostic and Statistical Manual of Mental Disorders, 4th Edition. *Used with permission.*

</td>
</tr>
</table>

Some studies indicate that after a decade or two, even some of those severely affected by schizophrenia often show remarkable improvement.

NAMI estimates that about 15 percent of people with schizophrenia do not respond to existing treatments and that another 15 percent respond only moderately to medication and require extensive support throughout their lives. The factors linked to a poor outcome include not being married, social isolation, insidious onset and long duration of symptoms, previous psychiatric treatment, low socioeconomic status, poor previous functioning, structural brain abnormalities, assaultiveness, and a history of childhood behavior problems, such as truancy.

Schizophreniform disorder

Schizophreniform disorder is identical to schizophrenia, but briefer in duration. The relationship between the two conditions is unclear. Some researchers believe that this problem is distinct from classic schizophrenia; others do not. By definition, all symptoms of schizophreniform disorder, including those of the prodromal, active, and residual phases, last for less than six months.

Treatment is usually the same as for schizophrenia and consists of medication and psychosocial care. Persons with this disorder have a better prognosis than those with schizophrenia, and a greater percentage recover completely. Those most likely to do so typically develop psychotic symptoms quickly (within four weeks of the first noticeable change in their behavior or functioning), are confused or disoriented during the psychotic episode (which implies some awareness of what is happening to them), had functioned well before the onset of symptoms, and maintain a normal range and display of emotions rather than blunted feelings.

Schizoaffective disorder

Some individuals develop symptoms of both schizophrenia *and* a mood, or "affective," disorder: either major depression or bipolar illness (manic depression). These persons are diagnosed as having schizoaffective disorder. Some develop a depressed mood, as well as other symptoms of major depression, together with psychotic symptoms, such as delusions or hallucinations. A depressed woman, for example, may report hearing babies crying in the night and develop the delusion that someone is stalking the neighborhood and killing children. Others develop mania in combination with psychotic symptoms. In a manic episode that occurs in schizoaffective disorder, a man with bipolar illness may develop the delusion that he is the new Messiah and gather followers to prepare for Judgment Day.

The combination of a psychotic disorder and a depressive disorder is the key element in the diagnosis of schizoaffective disorder. Often clinicians, not immediately aware of the existence of two disorders, may make a diagnosis of major depression and treat the person with antidepressants, only to discover that the psychotic symptoms continue unrelieved. When they prescribe antipsychotics, the patients improve.

Less common than schizophrenia, schizoaffective disorder also develops in late adolescence or early adulthood. In addition to the characteristic symptoms and complications of depression (see Chapter 5) or mania (see Chapter 6), individuals with schizoaffective disorder face a special risk: the combination of a depressive disorder and psychosis greatly increases the danger of suicide.

Treatment, as always, is tailored to the individual. Occasionally symptoms of both major depression and psychosis subside with antidepressant medication alone. If they do not, an antipsychotic agent may be prescribed. In some cases electroconvulsive therapy (ECT) may be advised. For those with mania, a mood-stabilizing medication such as lithium may be combined with an antipsychotic. Although drug treatment is the cornerstone of therapy, psychotherapy may also be beneficial for some individuals.

The long-term outlook for persons with schizoaffective disorder is somewhat better than for those with schizophrenia, most of whom do *not* recover completely. However, it is not as good as for those with a depressive disorder, most of whom *do* resume full functioning. Some individuals improve significantly between episodes of depression or mania. Others suffer chronic residual symptoms and never recover completely or function normally.

Brief psychotic disorder

In this disorder, individuals suddenly develop at least one active or positive symptom of psychosis—delusions, hallucinations, disorganized speech, or catatonic or disorganized behavior—but recover within a period ranging from a few hours to, at most, a month. Psychiatrists may use this designation as a provisional diagnosis for individuals who suddenly develop psychotic symptoms until they can assess their medical and mental condition fully and rule out substances and physical illnesses as causes.

In brief psychotic disorder, psychotic symptoms may appear after an event or series of events that would be extremely stressful to almost anyone in similar circumstances, such as combat, a violent attack, or a loved one's death. This is most likely to occur in adolescence or early adulthood. The average age of onset is the late twenties to early thirties. Those with personality disorders are particularly vulnerable, although anyone caught in a situation involving overwhelming stress can develop psychotic symptoms. (Chapter 12 discusses other disorders that can develop after a

■ **At least one of the following symptoms:**
 1. **Delusions**
 2. **Hallucinations**
 3. **Disorganized speech**
 4. **Grossly disorganized or catatonic behavior**

■ **Duration of at least one day but no more than one month, with eventual full return to the previous level of functioning**

■ **The disturbance is not better accounted for by schizophrenia, or the direct effects of a substance (a drug of abuse or a medication), a mood disorder, or a general medical condition.**

Adapted from the Diagnostic and Statistical Manual of Mental Disorders, 4th Edition. *Used with permission.*

trauma.) In making the diagnosis, psychiatrists note whether psychotic symptoms followed a "marked stressor" or if they occurred within four weeks of childbirth (if so, this may be referred to as *postpartum psychosis*).

Brief psychotic disorder can be extremely frightening for the affected persons and for those around them. Individuals may behave in bizarre ways, screaming or refusing to speak, assuming strange postures, dressing in outlandish fashion. Disoriented and unable to remember recent events, they may repeat nonsense phrases or spout gibberish. The emotions they display may not fit what they are doing or saying. When asked straightforward questions, they may respond with silly or obviously made-up answers. Some become aggressive or suicidal.

The initial treatment recommendation may be close observation in a safe setting. If medical tests reveal the use of a drug, such as cocaine, that triggered the psychotic episode, symptoms disappear within a day or two of treatment with what one psychiatrist sums up as "plain old room air." If an underlying illness, such as a brain tumor or infection, is discovered, appropriate treatment is essential. When tests show that no drug or illness is implicated as a cause, psychotic symptoms sometimes go away on their own, and the individual recovers quickly. If not, antipsychotic medications are prescribed; as soon as the symptoms subside, these agents are tapered. Individuals may then recover fully, although some may be troubled by secondary effects, such as diminished self-esteem and mild depression, for some time.

In other cases, symptoms persist, requiring continuing treatment with antipsychotics. By definition, brief psychotic episodes last no longer than a month; therefore, depending on the duration and severity of the symptoms, the diagnosis may change to schizo-phreniform disorder or schizophrenia. Sometimes the symptoms of a depressive disorder become more prominent as the psychosis improves with medication. It may turn out, for example, that an individual's psychotic symptoms developed as part of a manic episode in bipolar illness. In such cases, psychiatrists focus on treating the underlying mental disorder.

Delusional disorder

Delusions are persistent beliefs that a person holds in spite of all proof that they are false. Individuals with a delusional disorder have an unshakable false belief concerning events that can occur in real-life circumstances. Thus, they may believe that a rock singer is in love with them, that a coworker is spying on them, or that a spouse is unfaithful. In psychiatric terms, their delusions are *well systematized*—that is, they fit into an all-encompassing conceptual scheme that makes sense to the individual—and *encapsulated*—meaning they do not intrude onto most aspects of the person's life. In contrast, the delusions that occur in persons with schizophrenia tend to be bizarre, as in believing, for example, that one has been befriended by Martians or that their internal organs are changing shape.

▼
How common is delusional disorder?

Delusional disorder is relatively uncommon. Although this condition accounts for 1 to 2 percent of all annual admissions to psychiatric hospitals, its actual incidence in the general population is estimated to be only around 0.03 percent. Many cases begin in middle or late adult life, and occur slightly more often in women than in men. The average age of onset is between thirty-five and fifty-five.

▼
What causes delusional disorder?

The causes are not known. Psychosocial factors may lead to persecutory delusions; one form described by mental health professionals is *migration psychosis*, usually persecutory, found in persons migrating from one nation to another. Paranoid, schizoid, or avoidant personality disorders (described in Chapter 21) may increase the likelihood of delusional disorders.

▼
How delusional disorder feels

Most individuals with a delusional disorder look and act more or less normally *unless* they are talking about or acting on their delusion, although many are angry, hostile, or suspicious. Some become reclusive and socially isolated or behave in eccentric ways. Most delusions are classified as persecutory, erotic, grandiose, jealous, or somatic (related to bodily changes or symptoms).

The most common delusions are persecutory. Individuals believe they or their loved ones are being harmed in some way. They are convinced that someone is cheating, maligning, harassing, following, poisoning, or drugging them. As evidence, they may exaggerate a slight or threat and try to take defensive action, either legally by appealing to courts and government agencies, or by resorting to violence against the people they see as dangers or the institutions they feel have betrayed them.

Those with erotic delusions (a condition sometimes called *erotomania*) believe that someone, usually rich or famous, desires them, not just on the basis of a simple sexual attraction, but because of a deep, spiritual, romantic love. They may write, call, send letters and gifts, show up at the person's house, even stalk him or her. The data indicate that most of those who seek treatment for this problem are women, although police or court cases usually involve men. Erotic delusions typically involve former boyfriends, girlfriends, and spouses, but they are focused on celebrities sufficiently often for many public figures to consider the unwanted attention of delusional individuals a major source of harassment.

Those with grandiose delusions may be convinced that they have great power and influence, possess unrecognized ability or talent, or have made a groundbreaking discovery. Occasionally such individuals develop a delusion that they have a special relationship with a prominent person, such as the president, or believe that they actually *are* president. Some people with grandiose delusions, such as being singled out by God, become leaders of religious cults.

Men and women with jealous delusions are convinced that their sexual partner is unfaithful. To prove infidelity, they may search for scraps of evidence (such as lipstick stains or phone callers who hang up without speaking) and then confront the partner. Some try to stop the imagined infidelity through drastic means, such as not letting the partner leave the house alone or secretly following the other "lover." Occasionally, individuals with this disorder physically attack their partner or, more rarely, the suspected lover.

Somatic delusions involve an imagined physical defect or medical condition. Persons may believe that they are giving off a foul odor, that insects have gotten under their skin, that they have an internal parasite, that certain parts of their body are misshapen and ugly, or that certain organs are not functioning. Usually they turn to general medical physicians for treatment of what they believe are purely physical problems. A less common delusional disorder is Capgras' syndrome, in which individuals believe that someone close to them has been replaced by a double and accuse the person of being an impostor.

Seeking help Most individuals with delusional disorder have little or no insight into their problem and refuse to admit that anything is wrong with them. If you suspect that someone close to you may have this problem, these are the questions that should be asked:

- Does the person persistently hold on to a belief despite evidence that it is false?
- Does the delusion involve real-life people and situations?
- Does the person think that others are following, plotting against, or planning to harm him or her?
- Does the person think that someone loves him or her in a special way and wants his or her attention and devotion?
- Does the person believe that he or she has been granted some special power or unique talent?
- Is the person convinced that his or her spouse is having an affair despite a lack of evidence?
- Does the person believe that he or she has a disease or physical abnormality, despite reassurance that nothing is wrong?
- Have the delusions lasted for at least one month?
- Except for the delusion and its ramifications, does the person's behavior seem normal?

If someone close to you answers "yes" to several of these questions, insist that he or she see a mental health professional, or consult one yourself. Diagnosis requires a careful examination to rule out physical causes, such as alcoholism, drug use, dementia, infections, and metabolic or hormonal disorders. Imaging of the brain with computed tomography (CT) or magnetic resonance imaging (MRI) can identify brain abnormalities that may cause delusions.

Risks and complications Sexual problems and depressive symptoms are common complications of delusional disorder. Those whose paranoid delusions lead to legal action against supposed enemies may devote huge amounts of time and money to litigation.

Violence is rare but can occur. In cases of erotomania, "stalkers" who act on their delusions may be hospitalized, legally restrained,

Is it delusional disorder?

According to the DSM-IV, a diagnosis of delusional disorder should be based on these criteria:

- ■ **Non-bizarre delusions (involving real-life situations, such as being followed, poisoned, infected, loved at a distance, having a disease, or being deceived by a spouse or lover) lasting for at least one month**

- ■ **None of the symptoms of schizophrenia for more than a few hours**

- ■ **No impairment of functioning or obviously odd or bizarre behavior, except for the delusion and its ramifications**

- ■ **Brief symptoms of mood disorders, if any**

- ■ **Symptoms not caused by the direct effects of a substance (a drug of abuse or a medication) or a general medical condition**

Adapted from the Diagnostic and Statistical Manual of Mental Disorders, 4th Edition. *Used with permission.*

or jailed; more than twenty state legislatures have passed stalking laws to protect potential victims. Recent research indicates that although violence is a danger in erotomania, the stalker's significant others are more likely to become the targets than the "fantasy love object." However, there have been incidents in which stalkers have assaulted and, in some cases, murdered the persons they had watched and desired from afar.

▼

Treating delusional disorder

Individuals with delusional disorder usually do not admit that they have any problem and do not seek therapy unless forced to by family members or by legal action, as when, for example, they violate a court injunction to stay away from the individual they have been stalking. It is important for persons with this problem to get into treatment and to become aware of the potential benefits of medication and therapy.

Antipsychotic medications, such as pimozide (Orap), decrease delusions and anxiousness, although these symptoms may not disappear completely. Pimozide may relieve somatic delusions, including the belief that some aspect of a person's appearance is ugly; this particular delusion is also responsive to treatment with the selective serotonin reuptake inhibitors (SSRIs). Other psychiatric drugs, such as anti-anxiety medications, may be prescribed for symptoms that accompany these problems, but they have not been systematically tested for delusional disorder per se.

Psychotherapy also can contribute to recovery. If persons with a delusional disorder can establish trust and rapport with a mental health professional, in time they may come to acknowledge that their beliefs may be interfering with their lives.

▼

Impact on relationships

Individuals with this disorder are likely to have difficulty in their friendships and marriages because of their tendency to develop delusions about jealousy or betrayal. They may demand constant reassurance that a partner is loving and faithful and may be suspicious of the spouse's friends and colleagues. Some manage to function well at work, while others develop occupational as well as personal and social difficulties. Those with paranoid delusions may suspect coworkers of trying to sabotage their projects, stealing their ideas, or making critical comments to their bosses. Their accusations may alienate colleagues and lead to lasting resentment and conflict.

▼

Outlook

Unlike those with schizophrenia, many individuals with delusional disorder can function fairly normally in the world, support themselves, and remain employed. However, this is somewhat dependent on both the nature and the intensity of the delusion. It is less likely to be true of those whose delusions involve looking ugly or giving off a foul smell or of those whose delusions come to dominate their lives. In some cases, particularly in jealous delusions, the delusion disappears within a few months; but in most, especially for persecutory delusions (which are the most common type), the condition remains chronic, with the delusion waxing and waning but persisting over time.

Shared psychotic disorder

In this rare disorder, an individual in a close relationship with someone who has psychotic delusions develops a delusion that is similar in content. There is no sign of any prior psychotic disorder. Although as a rule only two people are involved in this disorder—hence, its other name, *folie à deux*—there have been cases in which as many as twelve persons in a family have shared the same delusion.

The shared delusion usually is realistic enough to be possible (although occasionally it is bizarre) and often is based on past experiences the two people have in common. For example, one spouse may convince the other that their food is being poisoned by recalling past incidents in which they did indeed suffer food poisoning. Usually the person who first developed the delusion is the dominant one in the relationship and gradually imposes his or her delusion on the more passive partner.

Although shared psychotic disorder can begin at any age, usually the people who share a delusion have lived together for a long time and may be relatively isolated from contact with other persons. Almost invariably the condition develops when the long-standing relationship is being threatened or altered by external forces, such as one person's desire or need to move or make a change in the relationship.

Usually these individuals are less impaired in their ability to function normally than those with a primary delusional disorder or schizophrenia. If the relationship with the person with the initial delusion ends, the delusional beliefs diminish or disappear. If the relationship endures, the condition is likely to become chronic unless treated.

Individuals rarely seek professional help for shared psychotic disorder. A therapist learns about its existence only if the person who first developed the delusion comes for treatment and reveals that a partner or family members have the condition. There is no specific treatment for this disorder, although therapists may suggest psychotherapy and antipsychotic medications. They work to establish trust and rapport and to ensure that individuals are protected from any harm that might be the result of poor judgment or of acting on the shared delusion.

Is it a dissociative disorder?

Individuals with a dissociative disorder may:

☐ **Develop two or more distinct, unique, enduring identities that repeatedly take control of behavior**

☐ **Be unable to recall certain important personal information**

☐ **Find themselves in strange places or situations, with no memory of how they got there**

☐ **Experience distortions or lapses in time**

☐ **Be unable to remember events or behaviors that others tell them about**

☐ **Discover letters, diaries, or possessions that are supposedly theirs but that they do not recognize or cannot account for**

☐ **Not remember a traumatic or stressful experience or some aspect of it**

☐ **Travel suddenly away from home or work**

☐ **Be confused about personal identity**

☐ **Repeatedly feel detached from the mind or body, as though they are observing themselves**

☐ **Perceive objects as changing size or shape**

☐ **Sense that other people seem dead, fake, or mechanical**

☐ **Experience significant distress or impairment in their usual functioning, activities, or relationships**

The more boxes that you check, the more reason you have to be concerned about a possible dissociative disorder. This chapter provides information on dissociative disorders and guidance for seeking help and obtaining appropriate treatment.

18

Dissociative Disorders: Disorders of Identity and Sense of Self

Each of us has a unique sense of identity, based on our awareness of the present and our memory of the past. This identity is the core of our psychological being. *Dissociation* refers to any altered form of consciousness that alters our sense of identity or self, or our ability to integrate memories and perceptions. In dissociation, events that would normally be connected are separated from one other. Rape victims, for example, may be unable to remember the assault, yet they become increasingly fearful, demoralized, and estranged from friends and family. They cannot integrate the memory of the attack with their present identity. Others may feel detached from their bodies, as if they are observing rather than experiencing ordinary sensations.

Mild dissociative states are common among normal, healthy persons, especially in youth. We become lost in thought or are so caught up in listening to music that we don't register what is happening around us. According to one study, about a third of people report that they have occasionally felt as though they were watching themselves in a movie; a small percentage of this group feel this way fairly often. Among young adults, as many as 70 percent report short periods of feeling that they are not themselves or that the world seems dreamlike.

Given the complex processes involved in perception, memory storage, and information processing, what is remarkable, notes David Spiegel, M.D., a professor of psychiatry and behavioral sciences at Stanford University and a leading expert in dissociation, "is not that dissociative symptoms or disorders occur, but that they do not occur more often."

The problems described in this chapter are not mild dissociative states but rather are dissociative *disorders* that involve profound and disturbing changes in psychological state. Individuals may develop several internal personalities (as in dissociative identity disorder), experience a feeling of unreality (as in depersonalization), or forget important information about themselves (as in amnesia and fugue). The symptoms of dissociative disorders depend on each person's reactions to his or her surroundings, and they exhibit wide variation among cultural settings.

Although these problems are extremely distressing, they also have a definite psychological function: Usually, they serve to shield a person in some way from an overwhelming, intolerable trauma. "Trauma can be understood as the experience of being made into an object, a thing, the victim of someone else's rage, of nature's indifference," notes Spiegel. "It is the ultimate experience of helplessness and loss of control over one's own body." Increasingly, mental health professionals have come to view dissociation as a defense against trauma, an attempt, as Spiegel puts it, "to maintain mental control at the very moment when physical control has been lost."

Dissociative symptoms and disorders are more likely to occur in individuals who have suffered physical or sexual abuse in childhood or in those who have had life-threatening experiences. In studies of the survivors of disasters—such as the firestorm in Oakland, California, in 1991; the Loma Prieta earthquake in the San Francisco Bay area in 1989; the Ash Wednesday bushfire in Australia in 1983; and the Hyatt Regency skywalk collapse in Kansas City in 1981—a quarter to a third of the survivors developed symptoms such as emotional numbing and an inability to feel deeply about anything. Far fewer developed actual disorders.

Because of their dramatic nature, dissociative disorders are often the stuff of which novels and screenplays are made. Much of what the general public knows about what once was called "multiple personality" is based on movies, television shows, and books and is not always correct. In part because of the widespread fascination with these problems, mental health professionals, who long believed that dissociative disorders are very rare, have taken a new look at them. Their research shows that these serious forms of mental illness, although uncommon, occur more often and are much more responsive to treatment than had been believed.

Dissociative identity disorder

Dissociative identity disorder, formerly called *multiple personality disorder* and renamed in the *Diagnostic and Statistical Manual of Mental Disorders, Fourth Edition (DSM-IV)*, is a complex and chronic illness, involving both identity and memory for important personal information. Persons with dissociative personality disorder lack something that others take for granted: a sense, at the very core of their being, of a single identity. Instead, they are splintered into selves, each one distinct rather than merely the embodiment of a particular mood. "The problem is a failure of integration," says Spiegel. "These patients suffer, not from having more than one personality, but from having less than one personality."

In classic cases of dissociative identity disorder, there are at least two personalities or *alters*, although they can number more than one hundred. The more abuse an individual has endured and the younger the age at which it took place, the more personalities typically develop; the more personalities, the more extensive the treatment the person needs. About half of recently reported cases have involved ten or more alters.

▼

How common is dissociative identity disorder?

At one time, mental health professionals believed that in many instances individuals often confused mood swings with distinct personalities or deliberately feigned different identities. During the last decade, however, the number of confirmed cases of dissociative identity disorder has skyrocketed. In 1980, the total of all such cases ever reported was two hundred; the number of *current* cases in the United States was recently estimated to be six thousand. It is now believed that dissociative identity disorder may be far more common than had been thought, largely because child abuse has proved to be much more widespread than many once thought. An estimated 3 percent of individuals hospitalized for psychiatric treatment have this disorder.

Almost invariably the disorder begins in childhood, usually before the age of nine years. Although it is sometimes diagnosed in children, it usually is not correctly identified until the teens or twenties. Typically, there is a delay of more than six years between the time the first symptoms emerge and the time at which the diagnosis is made.

Most individuals with dissociative personality disorder—75 to 90 percent, according to various reports—are women, possibly because females experience more sexual abuse as children. Also, as Spiegel observes, "Men resolve the conflict over impossible helplessness differently, often by turning the abuse on others or using alcohol or drugs." As a result, they are more likely to land in jails than in therapists' offices.

Not all therapists are convinced that dissociative identity disorder is as widespread as now appears to be the case. Although it seems certain that the condition is much more prevalent than had once been thought, there are reasonable grounds for some degree of skepticism. In several well-publicized criminal cases, including the trial of the "Hillside Strangler" in Los Angeles, accused criminals have tried to use dissociative identity disorder as a defense, usually without success. In much less dramatic instances, skillful manipulators may simulate the disorder to avoid blame for their actions. Some skeptics contend that therapists may ask questions about childhood memory lapses in such a way that suggestible individuals come to believe that they have dissociative personalities. Certain people, sometimes unconsciously, sometimes deliberately, state that they have had experiences or behaved in ways like those in media depictions of multiple personalities. It may be very difficult for therapists with limited experience in treating this condition to sort out what is really going on.

▼

What causes dissociative identity disorder?

In the overwhelming majority of cases, intense and repeated physical, sexual, or emotional abuse in childhood leads to the creation of dissociative personalities. The disorder may also develop after other severe emotional traumas in childhood, such as continued neglect, the loss of a loved one, illness and pain, or exposure to brutal accidents or violence.

Whatever the nature of the intolerable circumstances, a terrified, emotionally overwhelmed child, unable to understand and escape, may dissociate as a way of dealing with the trauma. "Dissociative identity disorder is a way of making the unbearable bearable," Spiegel explains. "A child is not as completely vulnerable if she can say, 'It happened to her, not me.'" Betrayed by the persons they love or need most, too little and too powerless to fight or to flee, traumatized youngsters escape in the only way they can—by running away in their minds. Dissociative identity disorder, in this sense, is similar to posttraumatic stress disorder.

Children who develop this disorder "typically endure sustained, chronic abuse over many years," says psychiatrist Richard Kluft, M.D., director of the dissociative disorders program at The Institute of Pennsylvania Hospital in Philadelphia. Often they have been sexually abused, kicked, burned, slashed, locked in closets, trunks, or basements, or sadistically tortured. Children who survive more impersonal traumas, such as internment in concentration camps or wartime bombardments, are less likely to develop dissociative identity disorder than those who suffer sexual, psychological, or physical abuse at the hands of the individuals they trust, love, or need.

The disorder is more common in first-degree biological relatives of people with the same condition than in the general population, and it can occur in several generations and in siblings within families. The reasons are not clear. There may be an inherited susceptibility. It also may be that parents, themselves abused as children, treat their own youngsters in the same way or cannot protect their children from abuse. In other cases, a child may identify with and emulate a parent with dissociative personality disorder.

▼

How dissociative identity disorder feels

The great majority of individuals with this disorder lead lives that, at least on the surface, seem normal. As one psychiatrist puts it, "They are pretty ordinary people who could well be your neighbors or colleagues." One in six earns a graduate degree; some work as social workers, physicians, nurses, managers, teachers. "For years I coped by jumping into work and studying," says a woman physician with dissociative identity disorder. "I wanted to help people even though I didn't know how to help myself."

For a while, having other personalities can be adaptive. The mother of two young children relies on her alters to take care of responsibilities she hates: "Some handle sex. One takes the kids to the doctor because I can't stand to see them getting shots. If it weren't for my alters, I'd be dead or a lot worse off psychologically than I am now."

But sooner or later—most often in young adulthood—the intricate inner world of alters breaks down. Often the trigger is a rape or beating. Even without such trauma, these individuals are prone to develop mental disorders, such as depression and eating disorders, to abuse drugs and alcohol, or to start cutting or burning themselves.

"About 80 percent of the 'hosts' are not aware of having other personalities," says psychiatrist Stephen Buie, M.D., who has extensive experience in treating individuals with dissociative disorders. "When they develop strange symptoms, they are afraid that something is terribly wrong, but they don't tell anybody. And when they first learn the diagnosis, they refuse to believe it."

One of the most common telltale signs is what one woman calls "losing time," when individuals cannot account for minutes, hours, or days and find themselves in unfamiliar, often dangerous places. One woman repeatedly found herself in strangers' cars, with no memory of how she had gotten there. Others find checks or letters in a handwriting they don't recognize, or clothes in their closets that they don't recall buying. "They try to cover up," says Buie. "They grow up in families with lots of secrets, so they're used to hiding."

Individuals with dissociative identity disorder are also used to blaming themselves for whatever happens to them. "All they know is pain, and they think that's what they deserve," says Spiegel. "Often they don't show any anger toward their abusers. They make excuses for a father who beat or raped them, like 'He was just drunk' or 'I provoked him.' They think they did something to deserve what happened, that they're the ones who are bad, that they should be punished."

Such self-loathing often leads to mutilation and suicide attempts. "Dissociative identity disorder is a lethal disease," notes Kluft. "Many patients hear commands from their alters to hurt or kill the host or other alters. Because of their delusion of actual separateness, the alters think of what they're doing as homicide, as killing another person, rather than suicide."

Alters can indeed seem, in some ways, as different as separate persons. Researchers have documented dramatic differences in their handwriting, voice patterns, brain waves, visual acuity, allergic reactions, and medical symptoms. One woman's child alter had the characteristic signs of "lazy eye" that she had had as a youngster; the older alters had outgrown the problem, just as she had. Sometimes one alter develops hives or a rash after eating a particular food or taking a certain drug; the others do not.

Alters typically include at least one scared and traumatized child, along with protectors, persecutors, managers, observers, sometimes even animals. The personalities may see themselves as being of different ages, genders, ethnic backgrounds, and physical types. They may differ in perceptions, values, purposes, memories, ways of dressing, and individual interests. One may be prim and shy, another reckless and promiscuous, and still another macho and tough. They also cope with difficult issues and problems in different ways. For example, one might respond to a physical attack with panic, one might submit passively, one might fight back, one might become seductive. Often they reflect the age of the child at the time of a trauma. Some may be based on characters seen in childhood on television or in the movies.

Usually each alter has a name, but sometimes they are known by descriptive terms: the Protector, the Whore, the Little Girl, the Angry One, the Screamer. Often the personalities exist in groups

Is it dissociative identity disorder?

According to the DSM-IV, a diagnosis of dissociative identity disorder should be based on these criteria:

■ **Presence within a person of two or more distinct identities or personality states (each with its own relatively enduring pattern of perceiving, relating to, and thinking about the environment and self)**

■ **At least two of these personality states recurrently take control of the person's behavior.**

■ **Inability to recall important personal information that is too extensive to be explained by ordinary forgetfulness**

■ **The disturbance is not due to the direct effects of a substance or a general medical condition.**

Adapted from the Diagnostic and Statistical Manual of Mental Disorders, 4th Edition. *Used with permission.*

of two or more, all representing the same period of life, such as adolescence. When this occurs, one may have the role of the protector of the others in the group. In general, no more than six personalities play major roles at any given time. Often the personalities are aware of some or all of the others. Some may experience the others as friends, companions, or enemies; others may threaten or actually harm the "host."

At any given moment, usually only one alter interacts with the external environment. However, any number of the other personalities may actively listen in on or influence all or part of what is going on. In most cases, the switch from one personality to another occurs suddenly, usually within seconds or minutes. The transformations can be startling, with an individual shifting from a sobbing child, to a furious man, to a defiant teenager, to a bewildered woman, within a brief period of time. In daily life, psychosocial stressors, conflict among the alters, or intrapsychic conflicts can trigger a switch to a different personality. In therapy, alters may emerge in response to direct requests or hypnosis.

Most of the alters cannot remember certain experiences or periods of time but may hesitate to admit these lapses for fear of being called liars or considered crazy. Sometimes they make up stories to cover up the missing parts of their lives. A small minority—perhaps 6 to 10 percent—are flamboyant about their condition. Most try desperately to hide it.

▼

Seeking help Although this disorder invariably develops during childhood, most individuals are not diagnosed until their teens or twenties, if not later. Often the personality who seeks help has little or no knowledge of the existence of the others. This personality tends to be depressed, anxious, compulsively good, conscience-stricken, and suffering from headaches, psychosomatic symptoms, and some degree of amnesia, for which he or she seeks relief. If you suspect dissociative identity disorder, these are the questions that should be asked:

- Are you aware of two or more distinct identities or personality states within yourself?

- Do they repeatedly "take control" of your behavior?

- Are you unable to recall certain parts of your life or important information about yourself?

- Have you ever found yourself in a strange place or situation with no memory of how you got there?

- Do you experience distortions or lapses in time?

- Are you unable to remember events or behaviors that others tell you about?

- Have others noticed changes in your personality?

- Have you come across letters, diaries, or possessions that are supposedly yours but that you do not recognize or cannot account for?

- Have you ever heard voices within your head that you perceive as separate and that urge you toward some activity?

If you or the person close to you answers "yes" to several of these questions, the problem may be a dissociative disorder, and you should consult a mental health professional.

Dissociative identity disorder can be difficult to diagnose. Sometimes the alters deliberately collude to pass as a single individual, or years go by during which they are quiet or nonintrusive. In one report, one hundred individuals with this problem averaged 6.8 years between their initial assessment and their ultimate diagnosis. In the meantime, they received an average of 3.6 erroneous diagnoses.

There is no specific physiological or biochemical test that can confirm dissociative identity disorder. In addition to a comprehensive physical examination, psychological testing can be helpful. Psychiatrists also must rule out other mental disorders, including fugue, amnesia, and psychotic disorders. Although some people, including experts in mental health, believe that dissociative identity disorder can be feigned, whether deliberately or not, there is no evidence that individuals can create and sustain for an extended period of time the complex symptoms of this condition.

▼

Risks and complications

There is considerable overlap between dissociative identity disorder and other mental disorders, including depressive disorders, substance abuse, borderline personality disorder, and sexual, eating, and sleep disorders. Self-mutilation is common. Many individuals with this problem attempt suicide at some point in their lives. Other complications include violence (such as child abuse or assault) and criminal activity.

▼

Treating dissociative identity disorder

Long-term psychotherapy is the primary approach to helping people with this condition. Although it has proved effective, the process is intense and demanding for both the affected person and the therapist. Usually, individuals visit therapists at least twice a week over the course of two to five years or longer.

Treatment focuses on bringing the fact of abuse into consciousness and dealing with its emotional and psychological impact. "The only approach that works is compassionate psychotherapy," says Kluft. "These individuals, by and large, have never had the chance to heal their hurts and be soothed and comforted. Sure, you cannot make up for a house that's burned down, but you can create a safe, adequate place to live."

The process is slow and hard. "I don't think you would find a single person with this disorder who would not say that therapy is the most painful thing he or she has ever done," says one woman with dissociative identity disorder. "Maybe that's because, for the first time in our lives, we are actually *feeling*. Our entire self is beginning to thaw after a long, long time of being completely frozen."

Getting to know all the alters and establishing a rapport with them are the first tasks for therapists. As they emerge, alters may vie for attention or become hostile and menacing. Harrowing memories may emerge in the form of hallucinations or nightmares. Because strong self-destructive urges can occur, therapists often develop a contract with the personalities in which they agree not to harm themselves or others and to share any thoughts of harm with all the personalities. Hospitalization may be necessary if self-destructive behavior or suicide attempts are a real danger.

Individuals with dissociative identity disorder are usually highly hypnotizable, and hypnosis can help in communicating with the various personalities, who may simply "come out" or respond to a therapist's request. Sometimes therapists use hypnosis to "age-regress," or take the individual back to a time when another dissociative personality was "out."

As they become aware of each other, the alters themselves start to communicate—sometimes silently in the person's mind, sometimes by taking turns writing in a journal, sometimes by drawing pictures. Often the differences among alters fade over time. Hostile ones become less menacing; passive ones more assertive; adult alters may hold and comfort child alters. If there are conflicts among personalities, the therapist may encourage resolution of their differences.

Recalling traumatic experiences from the perspectives of the different personalities is an important component of the therapeutic process, but it can be an emotionally wrenching one. Usually the affected person goes through a process called *abreaction*, the intense reliving of abuse in the presence of a therapist. Some therapists have individuals visualize memories rather than relive them so that the experience will be less intense. One effective technique involves imagining a screen split in two, with an image of a scene of abuse on one side and an image of what the person did to adapt or protect him- or herself on the other. This can help to make traumatic memories more bearable.

Throughout therapy, individuals try to put remembered traumas into perspective, work through their feelings about them, and share the information among their personalities so that eventually there is less fragmentation. Above all else, they must struggle to understand and accept the fact that they were not "bad" children whose abuse was really well-deserved punishment. As they emerge from years of guilt and shame, they experience every conceivable emotion: severe anxiety, sorrow, grief, depression, fury, anger, embarrassment, apathy, numbness. Only by finding ways to manage such powerful feelings can dissociative personalities come together. However, there can be great resistance to an ultimate integration, which may seem like an attempt to "kill" off parts of the self and can produce great fear and vulnerability. These issues must also be worked through in psychotherapy.

The process of *integrating*, or coming together into one personality, often occurs gradually. "I had expected fireworks, noise, deep insights, and orgasmic feelings when we began to integrate," comments one woman. "That didn't happen. It was and is a very quiet and very personal thing. Having this disorder is like being hungry. Integrating is like becoming less hungry—only in small steps."

As the personalities come together, the individual must develop new coping skills and learn to respond to difficulties within a unified personality. Group and family therapy may be useful during this period. Regular follow-up sessions help individuals to deal with any lingering or new problems or sources of stress. Most continue in therapy for a year or more after integration to learn how to deal with setbacks and stresses as a single personality.

No psychiatric medication has proved beneficial for dissociative

Hannah's secret lives

Beth is a friendly, precocious five-year-old. Tommy is a tough guy who leads a teenage gang. Chatty Felicity gets along with everyone. Abigail, nervous and sad, worries about everything. The Judge doles out harsh punishments to those who reveal family secrets. All are among the fifty-four personalities inhabiting the mind of Hannah, a former executive with dissociative identity disorder.

"When things get quiet, I know they're plotting," Hannah says. "The last time, all I could hear was: 'It doesn't matter what you do or where you go. You won't be safe. We're going to get you anyway.'" Terrified, she checked into a psychiatric hospital. Hours later a nurse found her lying unconscious in a pool of blood; an emergency transfusion saved her life. Two of her violent "alters," or dissociated personalities, had smuggled in razor blades and cut an artery.

Just two years before this harrowing experience, Hannah "had all the things that would make anyone happy: a great job, a house, a fiancé." But none of her friends and coworkers knew about the darker side of her life: the deep depressions, the blackouts, the drug overdoses, the razor blade slashes on her wrists, arms, and soles.

"I could handle any business situation, then I'd go home and cut myself. I wasn't aware of it at the time, but four alters—Miss Socialite, Mr. Logic, Miss Vocabulary, and the Competitive One—actually did various parts of my job. The same must have happened in school. I graduated with honors but have no memories of going to school."

Hannah, now on medical disability, lives by herself, paints and draws (in different styles, depending on which alter is the artist), and does volunteer service in the community. Three times a week she works with her psychiatrist to come to grips with the personalities that live within her imagination and the dreadful, dark secrets that led to their creation.

Hannah's goal is simple: she longs for "less chaos in my life." After more than a year of therapy, she is just beginning the hard work of dealing with memories and feelings that have been buried for decades. "I've gotten some memories back of sexual abuse by neighborhood children, by teachers, by people in our church. I can remember other incidents, but I can't see the face of who's hurting me. What scares little Beth, my five-year-old, is finding out that it was our father who abused me sexually as well as physically.

When I say that now, I don't feel anything; it's as if I were dead inside. But I know that somewhere inside are alters who carry the pain, and that scares me. I picture them standing in a circle, like a football huddle, and I can hear them saying that I'm bad, that I'm the one to blame."

In a recent session, one of Hannah's teenage alters, Celeste, remembered and relived a painful beating by her father. "The Judge felt Celeste had to be punished for telling secrets to the psychiatrist," says Hannah, who ended up with two slashed veins that required ten stitches. "I never learned how to deal with feelings," she says. "I'd rather handle physical pain."

Although she still is haunted by urges to harm herself, Hannah, thirty-one, is making progress. After years of being cut off from memories of the past and uncertain of moments in the present, she has begun to think about the future and to feel some stirrings of hope:

"Until the last few months, given the option to live or die, I'd have chosen to die. Now I want to live. I can see light, some joy, the possibility of something good coming out of my life, and that's what keeps me going. If I can protect one child or prevent one case of abuse, what I've been through will be worth it."

identity disorder, although antidepressants can help individuals who also have major depression.

▼

Impact on relationships

Dissociative identity disorder can create great misunderstanding and conflict. Family members often realize that something is very strange, but they have no explanation for their loved ones' shifting moods, unexplained absences, or different ways of speaking and dressing. Spouses may be convinced that their partners are lying to them about where they have been, what they have done, or how they have behaved. The realization that other personalities exist within their loved one can in itself be profoundly upsetting. In some cases, the affected person uses alters to escape from problems in the relationship. Therapy can help both partners to deal with such issues.

▼

Outlook

The long-term prognosis for persons with dissociative identity disorder who obtain the help they need is excellent. In one group followed for up to fifteen years after integration, 96 percent no longer had dissociated personalities. Without treatment, however, those with this disorder are at high risk for revictimization, that is, for getting into situations in which they are hurt again—by abusive partners, by rapists, by others who betray their trust. In controlled studies of follow-up three to ten years later, individuals who received no treatment other than benign neglect of their separate personalities continued to suffer from this disorder, whereas of those who had been actively treated, only 3 to 6 percent did.

Dissociative amnesia

D issociative amnesia is psychologically caused memory loss. Individuals with this disorder, which usually is not permanent, cannot recall important information about themselves, sometimes including who they are. Most often they cannot remember anything that happened during a certain period of time, usually the time during or after a profoundly disturbing event. One woman had no memory of what happened between the time a fire destroyed her home and neighborhood and the following day. In cases of what is called *selective amnesia*, individuals can recall some but not all of the events that occurred during a certain period. A father who found his two-year-old drowned in the pool, for instance, could remember calling 911 for help but not diving into the pool and bringing the child's body into the house. Unlike am-

---

Is it dissociative amnesia?

According to the DSM-IV, a diagnosis of dissociative amnesia should be based on these criteria:

■ One or more episodes of inability to recall important personal information, usually of a traumatic or stressful nature, to an extent that cannot be explained by ordinary forgetfulness

■ This disturbance does not occur exclusively as a symptom of dissociative identity disorder, dissociative fugue, posttraumatic stress disorder, acute stress disorder, or somatization disorder, and is not due to the direct effects of a substance (e.g., a drug of abuse or a medication), or a neurological or other general medical condition).

■ The symptoms cause significant distress or impair social, occupational, or other important areas of functioning.

Adapted from the Diagnostic and Statistical Manual of Mental Disorders, 4th Edition. *Used with permission.*

---

nesia caused by illness or injury, dissociative amnesia does not interfere with the ability to learn and remember new information.

▼

How common is dissociative amnesia?

People rarely suffer psychological memory loss under normal circumstances, but dissociative amnesia is common in response to overwhelming stress, such as war, rape, violence, fires, or natural disasters such as floods and earthquakes. During wartime, 5 to 20 percent of combat veterans forget some or all of their battlefield experiences. This disorder is most common among individuals in their twenties or thirties. Older men and women rarely develop it.

▼

What causes dissociative amnesia?

The direct cause of dissociative amnesia is overwhelming stress, which creates a situation that a person finds impossible to cope with or tolerate. It may involve the threat of injury or death; fear of not being able to escape; actual or anticipated loss of someone deeply valued; or an unacceptable impulse or act, such as a desire to have an affair with a spouse's friend or to kill a despised enemy. In life-threatening circumstances, such as being caught in a shoot-out on the street, amnesia usually begins abruptly. In cases of inner conflict, it may develop gradually as the result of repeated stress.

▼

How dissociative amnesia feels

Dissociative amnesia typically follows the stress of a major trauma and often develops in two stages. Initially, individuals enter an altered state of consciousness. Disoriented and confused, they can wander about aimlessly and may experience hallucinations. This stage can last for minutes, hours, or days. In the second stage, affected persons become aware that they cannot remember who they are or what has happened before, during, or after an event.

Persons with amnesia may not be able to do simple math. Some seem to have completely blank minds and may not recognize even those closest to them. Nevertheless, although they may not recall certain information or experiences, their behavior reflects what has happened to them. Thus, a rape victim who cannot remember the assault nevertheless suffers the usual symptoms of this trauma, may feel detached and demoralized, and may be incapable of enjoying intimate relationships. A parent with no memory of a car crash in which he was injured and his child died still suffers anguishing grief.

Seeking help   Individuals with dissociative amnesia usually are taken or find their own way to emergency facilities or police stations. Some are enormously upset by their amnesia and are eager to participate in any treatment that might restore their memory. Others show little emotion and may seem indifferent or even cheerful. Still others are sullen and withdrawn or may refuse to cooperate with those who are trying to treat them.

If you suspect that the problem may be dissociative amnesia, these are the questions that should be asked:

- Is the individual unable to recall important personal information: for example, what happened before he or she was injured or found?

- Is the memory loss far more extensive than might be explained by ordinary forgetfulness?

- As far as you can tell, is the memory loss unrelated to other mental disorders, a physically caused state, such as a blackout while intoxicated, or substance use or withdrawal?

If the answers to these questions are "yes," seek medical attention. In evaluating individuals who have suffered memory loss, physicians check for physical causes of amnesia, such as head injury, stroke, medical illness, alcohol intoxication, and epilepsy. (Amnesia due to medical causes is discussed in Chapter 20.)

Risks and   Dissociative amnesia ranges from mild to severe, depending on the
complications   extent of memory loss and its duration. Most cases last for twenty-four hours or less, although occasionally memory loss persists for months or even years. The condition is also associated with other mental disorders, including conversion disorder, bulimia nervosa,

alcohol abuse, and depression, as well as with borderline or histrionic personality disorders.

▼

**Treating
dissociative
amnesia**

Above all else, people with dissociative amnesia need to feel safe
from whatever stress caused their memory loss. Hospitalization,
by providing a secure haven, greatly reduces their anxiety. Once
individuals feel safe, their memories may return spontaneously.
If amnesia persists, hypnosis may help in regaining lost memories
and identifying the life stress that led to the amnesia. They then
may benefit from therapy to help them understand why they developed dissociative amnesia and to deal with the psychological
impact of the trauma or stress they experienced.

▼

Outlook

Most affected individuals spontaneously regain their memories
and recover completely. Usually they experience only one episode,
although recurrences can develop. In rare cases, the condition can
persist indefinitely.

Depersonalization disorder

Depersonalization involves a persistent, strong, disquieting,
and unpleasant sense of unreality about one's self. People
typically find it hard to describe the frightening and bizarre nature
of such an experience. They may simply say they feel they are "going crazy." Some have the feeling that they are made out of wood
or that they have become robots or puppets. Others have the
sense of stepping out of their body and observing themselves,
sometimes from above. Often they also perceive the environment
as unreal or strange, a phenomenon called *derealization.*

Episodes of depersonalization usually occur suddenly, last for
minutes, hours, or days, and then gradually go away. In depueron-
alization disorder, these episodes are persistent or recurrent and
cause significant distress or difficulty in functioning. Some therapists believe that depersonalization occurs far more often as a
symptom of another disorder, such as an anxiety disorder or
schizophrenia, rather than as a separate problem. However, so
little is known and understood about depersonalization disorder
that it is impossible to say this with certainty.

▼

**How common is
depersonalization?**

As many as 70 percent of young adults have reported single brief
episodes of depersonalization. Among individuals receiving psy-

Is it depersonalization disorder?

According to the DSM-IV, a diagnosis of depersonalization disorder should be based on these criteria:

- ■ Persistent or recurrent experiences of feeling detached from, and as if one is an outside observer of, one's mental processes or body (e.g., feeling like one is in a dream)

- ■ During this experience, perception of reality remains intact.

- ■ The depersonalization causes significant impairment in social, occupational, or other areas of functioning, or marked distress.

- ■ The experience does not occur exclusively during the course of another mental disorder, such as schizophrenia, dissociative identity, acute stress, or panic disorder, and is not due to the direct effects of a substance or a general medical condition.

Adapted from the Diagnostic and Statistical Manual of Mental Disorders, 4th Edition. *Used with permission.*

chiatric care, depersonalization symptoms are the third most common group of complaints, after depression and anxiety. The incidence of this disorder, which is more severe and incapacitating, is not known. It is believed to begin in adolescence or early adult life.

▼

What causes depersonalization?

Symptoms of depersonalization often occur in response to life-threatening circumstances (gunfire, a hurricane, a fire) or to sustained trauma, such as combat, and also may emerge in other very stressful situations, such as the breakup of a cherished relationship. Persons who have had near-death experiences frequently report feelings of depersonalization, as do those with anxiety disorders, posttraumatic stress disorder, and schizophrenia. Depersonalization symptoms can be a consequence of alcohol and drug abuse or a side effect of prescription medication.

▼

How depersonalization feels

In depersonalization, individuals feel strange, yet typically find it hard to find words to describe the eeriness of their experience. One person said he "felt fuzzy." Another spoke of feeling as if she were in a dream. Others talk of being "outside" themselves or explain they have a sense of "deadness" in their bodies. Many report a disquieting sense of feeling separated from their thoughts, emotions, or identity. They are aware of events but are not touched by them, and perceive feelings and sensations as somehow not their own. Those who have near-death experiences typically perceive themselves as outside observers of the attempts to bring them back to life.

Because of their detachment from their usual experience of themselves, people feel that they have lost control over their bodies, actions, or utterances—an often terrifying sensation that can make them fear they are losing their minds. Anxiety, depression, and extreme distress are common. Some persons experience altered perceptions, such as numbness or hyperacute hearing. Many have dizzy spells. As they tune in to each and every sensation they are going through, they may become preoccupied with their bodies and try to relieve or cure their symptoms through various means, including substance abuse.

Those who experience derealization perceive objects as different in size or shape from what they really are, or view other people as dead, fake, or mechanical. Their sense of time can become distorted. They may feel that something is wrong with their memories because they have difficulty recalling facts or experiences.

▼
Seeking help If you suspect that depersonalization or derealization may be troubling you or someone close to you, these are the questions that should be asked:

- Are you having repeated experiences of feeling detached from your mind or body?

- Do you see yourself as an outside observer?

- Do objects appear different in size or in shape from what they usually are?

- Do other people seem dead, fake, or mechanical?

- Are you having difficulty recalling facts or experiences?

- Have these experiences upset or worried you?

- Have they interfered with your usual activities or relationships?

If you or someone close to you answers "yes" to these questions, the problem could be depersonalization, derealization, or another mental disorder. A psychiatrist can rule out possible medical and psychiatric causes of depersonalization symptoms. The severity and duration of symptoms determine whether an individual is diagnosed as having depersonalization disorder.

▼
Risks and complications Many individuals with depersonalization disorder continue to function adequately, and their symptoms, although distressing, may cause only slight impairment. However, depersonalization may worsen over time and, uncommonly, may become incapacitat-

ing. Some people are plagued by chronic anxiety about their state of mind and worry about going insane. Others develop hypochondriasis (discussed in Chapter 19) or turn to drugs or alcohol for relief and thus incur a substance abuse disorder.

▼

Treating depersonalization disorder

Episodes of depersonalization are usually temporary. If they do not go away without treatment or if they recur, training in self-hypnosis may help. Individuals can learn to induce a pleasant sense of floating lightness to replace their distressing feelings. Relaxation techniques, such as progressive muscle relaxation and biofeedback, also can help. Psychotherapy that focuses at working through emotional responses to trauma or stress is beneficial for those with the disorder. Some physicians prescribe anti-anxiety medications, which may provide some relief but also pose a risk because depersonalization and derealization can themselves be side effects of these drugs. If depersonalization is a symptom of anxiety or schizophrenia, appropriate treatment for these disorders usually relieves the depersonalization.

▼

Outlook

Depersonalization is a common and usually transient experience. Depersonalization disorder tends to be chronic, recurring during mild anxiety or depression and then abating. In most cases, it gradually disappears over time.

Dissociative fugue

Individuals with dissociative fugue forget who they are, may assume a new identity, and may travel to a new location. When they recover their memories, they often cannot recall what took place during their fugue. Fugues tend to be fairly brief and do not usually recur.

▼

How common is dissociative fugue?

This disorder, believed to be extremely rare, is most likely to occur in wartime or after a natural disaster or overwhelming psychological stress. A soldier, for example, may wander away from the front line and wake up in a strange place with no idea of who he is or how he got there.

▼

What causes dissociative fugue?

A traumatic life experience, such as the extremely distressing breakup of a marriage or close relationship, great financial pres-

<table>
<tr><td>

Is it dissociative fugue?

According to the DSM-IV, a diagnosis of dissociative fugue should be based on these criteria:

</td><td>

■ **The predominant disturbance is sudden, unexpected travel away from home or work, with inability to recall the past.**

■ **Confusion about personal identity or assumption of a partially or completely new identity**

■ **The disturbance does not occur exclusively during the course of a dissociative identity disorder and is not due to the direct effects of a substance or general medical condition.**

■ **Symptoms cause significant distress or impairment in social, occupational, or other areas of functioning.**

Adapted from the Diagnostic and Statistical Manual of Mental Disorders, 4th Edition. *Used with permission.*

</td></tr>
</table>

sures, combat, or a catastrophic earthquake, flood, or fire, can lead to dissociative fugue in susceptible individuals. Mental health professionals have noted that persons who experience fugues are highly suggestible and use massive repression and escape as a coping style. Heavy alcohol use may increase the risk in such people. Therapists disagree about the possible role of childhood abuse or neglect or of prior mental illness. Some individuals who experience fugues have intense suicidal or homicidal impulses. For them, fugue may represent a partial suicide attempt.

Dissociative fugue also may be a symptom of illness involving the central nervous system, such as epilepsy or Alzheimer's disease, traumatic brain injury, or the use of drugs that affect mental functioning.

▼

How dissociative fugue feels

Many fugues begin after an individual wakes from sleep or after a long period without sleep. In most cases the fugue lasts no more than hours or days and consists of little more than brief, apparently purposeful travel, unlike the aimless, confused wandering of someone with amnesia. Usually the amount of traveling is limited.

Often perplexed and disoriented, individuals in a fugue avoid others or have only minimal social contacts. In most cases they lose their sense of identity but do not assume a new one, although they may take a new name and find a new place to live. Occasionally they experience violent outbursts, verbally or physically attacking someone or something. Sexual behavior may be less inhibited than usual, and these persons may engage in other behaviors—sometimes criminal—that would normally be unacceptable to them.

▼
Seeking help

Confusion and disorientation may lead some individuals to seek help. Usually they seek therapy only after the fugue has ended, although in other cases, friends and family members may consult a therapist after the person returns. If dissociative fugue may be the problem, these are the questions that should be asked:

- Did the person suddenly made an unplanned trip away from home or work?

- Has he or she been unable to recall the past?

- Has the individual been confused about his or her identity?

- As far as you can tell, is the individual's behavior unrelated to a substance-induced disorder or to a medical condition such as epilepsy?

If you or the person close to you answers "yes" to these questions, seek help. In evaluating the person, a physician will rule out brain injuries such as head trauma and illnesses such as a stroke or tumor. Assessment may require a complete physical examination, mental status examination, toxicological studies, and an electroencephalogram (EEG). An individual who develops separate identities may actually have dissociative identity disorder. Mental health professionals also may suspect malingering, a deliberate attempt to feign an illness in order to evade obligations or the consequences of an act (see Chapter 19).

▼
Risks and complications

Risks depend on how long the fugue lasts and on its consequent impact on the person and on family and friends. In most cases there is little, if any, lasting damage, although individuals in a fugue state may be harmed, commit a crime, or become violent themselves, and have sometimes ended up in jail.

▼
Treating dissociative fugue

Memory of life before the fugue episode usually returns spontaneously, without any specific treatment. If it does not, psychotherapy, often aided by hypnosis, can help in recovering it. Sometimes a single session restores memory; more often, several are necessary. In therapy, persons are encouraged to talk about what they remember immediately before the onset of the fugue and, by free-associating, to fill in the gaps. Writing automatically, without thinking about content, can also provide clues that trigger memories. Further therapy may be recommended to help the person cope with the impact of any traumatic life experience that may have precipitated the fugue.

▼
**Impact on
relationships**

If the fugue was brief, as most are, there may be little, if any, impact. Family members and friends, who may have feared abduction or other forms of foul play when a loved one disappeared, are immensely relieved by the person's return, although they often find it hard to understand why he or she left without a word. If the fugue continued for a while, however, or if the individual assumed a new identity or became involved in questionable activities, family members and friends may feel confused, angry, or even betrayed, and may have difficulty accepting the fact that their loved one's actions were not deliberate.

▼
Outlook

Dissociative fugues typically end as suddenly as they begin, often when a person wakes from sleep. People vary in how much they can recall of what happened during the fugue. Recovery from a dissociative fugue is usually rapid, and recurrences are rare.

Is a mental disorder affecting your physical well-being?

Individuals with a mental disorder that affects their physical well-being may:

- [ ] **Continually worry about having a serious physical illness, even though medical evaluations show no signs of a problem**

- [ ] **Believe that a part of their body is ugly or grossly abnormal, although others see nothing wrong**

- [ ] **Be extremely self-conscious about a slight physical imperfection, such as a birthmark or mole**

- [ ] **Develop one or more extremely distressing or disabling physical complaints that have no known medical basis**

- [ ] **Have a number of persistent physical complaints that begin before the age of thirty and have no known physical basis**

- [ ] **Develop an unexplained neurological symptom, such as impaired vision, hearing, swallowing, or movement**

- [ ] **Intentionally feign physical or psychological symptoms in themselves or another person**

If you or someone close to you checks any of these boxes, the problem may be a *somatoform* disorder, a mental condition involving physical concerns or symptoms. This chapter provides information on these disorders as well as guidance on seeking help. Chapter 24 discusses psychosomatic disorders, in which psychological factors trigger or exacerbate physical illnesses.

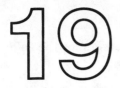

19

Disorders of the Mind that Affect the Body

I t is not unusual for feelings or emotional experiences to affect us physically. A job applicant may be so anxious about an interview that she cannot sleep. An actor opening in a new play may be so nervous that he vomits before the curtain goes up. A widow overwhelmed with sadness may feel that she has a lump in her throat. A man whose father died of a heart attack at an early age may worry that chest pains may indicate a similar fate for him.

Concerns and reactions like these are entirely normal. As with many other problems, distinguishing between these behaviors and those that may indicate a mental disorder depends mainly on two factors: severity and duration. In some cases, physical symptoms and excessive preoccupation with medical illness are due to treatable depressive, anxiety, or adjustment disorders. In others, the less common *somatoform disorders* described in this chapter are responsible.

All of these conditions, including somatization and conversion disorders, which involve physical symptoms with no known physical basis, and hypochondriasis and body dysmorphic disorder, which center on a preoccupation with illness or appearance, produce significant distress and interfere with normal functioning. People with these disorders cannot control what they feel, nor do they consciously produce or feign their symptoms.

In a different illness, factitious disorder, individuals deliberately produce or fake symptoms in themselves or in others for the sake of getting medical attention.

Somatoform disorders

The various somatoform disorders all involve bodily, or *somatic* (from the Greek word *soma*, meaning "body") complaints that occur without any sign of a physical cause. The lives of individuals with these disorders often revolve around their symptoms, which may occur or intensify at times of personal stress or trauma, or around sensations they believe are signs of illness.

Persons with somatoform disorders are at great risk for unnecessary testing, medical procedures, drugs, or surgery. This is especially true of those who "doctor shop," seeking help from physician after physician in the vain quest for someone who can provide relief. These individuals are particularly likely to undergo extensive and unwarranted medical evaluations, spend a great deal of money, and suffer physical complications.

HYPOCHONDRIASIS

The *American Psychiatric Press Textbook of Psychiatry* defines *hypochondriasis* as "an unrealistic preoccupation with fear of having a disease." Individuals with this problem misinterpret sensations in their bodies as abnormal or as signs of illness. They become excessively concerned about their health. Their worry about AIDS, cancer, or another disease may be so intense that even careful, repeated examinations and tests revealing no sign of a problem do not persuade them that they are healthy. They acknowledge that they may be exaggerating their symptoms or that they may not be ill at all, yet their preoccupation persists even when time passes, when many doctors reassure them that they are in good health, and when they do not develop the disease they fear.

▼

How common is hypochondriasis?

According to various surveys, 10 to 20 percent of healthy persons and about 45 percent of those seeing mental health professionals worry about illness from time to time. Most can accept their physicians' reassurance that they are fine, but about 4 to 9 percent do not or cannot believe their doctors and continue to be fearful about their health. Hypochondriasis, which occurs equally in men and women, can develop at any age, although it most often begins in a person's twenties and peaks in middle age.

▼

What causes hypochondriasis?

Over the years, mental health professionals have suggested a variety of theories about the origins of hypochondriasis. Individuals with this disorder have often had experiences that lead them to pay greater than usual attention to bodily symptoms. Some have experienced a serious disease or have had illness in their family during their childhood. Those with a hypersensitivity to normal physical sensations sometimes had a parent who was overly attentive to childhood illnesses or neglectful when the child was not ill. Various psychological and social stressors also can contribute, although usually there is no single trauma that triggers symptoms. Any event that induces fear of disease, such as witnessing death, or any mental disorder that causes anxiety or depression may lead to somatic symptoms.

Because reassurance often does not persuade people with hypochondriasis that there is no illness, they become anxious. The symptoms of their anxiety—a fast-beating heart, for example—further convince them that something is wrong. They *know* that they have distressing symptoms, so they do not believe doctors who tell them they are healthy. They pay increasing attention to their symptoms and focus even more on their bodies. The more anxious they become, the more "symptoms" they notice, and a vicious cycle develops. (Individuals involved in learning about illness, such as medical students, may be especially vulnerable to temporary hypochondriasis.)

▼

How hypochondriasis feels

Individuals with hypochondriasis become preoccupied with bodily functions, such as their heartbeat, sweating, or digestion. They may be quick to sense hunger, easily disturbed by loud, sudden noises, or made very uncomfortable by heat or cold. Minor physical abnormalities, such as a small sore, or transient symptoms, such as a cough, can become signs of disease. The slightest irregularity can trigger apprehension and alarm.

These individuals are quick to notice something odd—for example, a moment of dizziness—and rather than dismissing it as the consequence of sitting or standing up too quickly, they begin to watch for its recurrence. If it does happen again, or they think it might have, they become even more attentive. Over time, their vigilance turns into worry. They may fear illness in general, specific diseases, or a single malady. In *cardiac neurosis*, for example, individuals become convinced that they have heart disease.

Often people with hypochondriasis become dissatisfied with any physician who is unable to detect a medical problem and go from doctor to doctor, "shopping" for one who will give them a diagnosis. Indeed, they may seem more interested in getting a diagnosis than in gaining relief from their symptoms. Typically they feel that they are not receiving good medical care and that they should be given a certain test or prescribed a medication that their doctor will not order.

Some become angry because of their unrelieved distress or their frustration with skeptical, impatient, or hostile doctors. They often exhibit traits associated with obsessive-compulsive personality disorder, such as a need for extreme control and orderliness. They frequently become depressed because they are suffering yet cannot find help.

▼

Seeking help   If you or someone close to you seems excessively concerned about illness, and hypochondriasis may be a possibility, these are the questions that should be asked:

- Do you often think or worry about having a serious disease?

- Do you tend to interpret any unusual physical sensations as signs of illness?

- Has your concern persisted despite reassurances from physicians?

- Is there a treatment or test that you think your doctors should try, even though they tell you that it is unnecessary?

- Have medical tests revealed no physical problems that could account for the sensations you are experiencing or your interpretation of them?

- Has your worry or fear of illness lasted for at least six months?

If you or the person close to you answers "yes" to several of these questions, the problem could be hypochondriasis. Some people are so offended by the suggestion that their fears are unwarranted or that the problem is mental rather than physical that they refuse to see a psychiatrist, or do so only when they have reached the point of living like invalids, often spending most or all of their time in bed. It can be most helpful to bring up the issue with your primary physician, who may advise consulting a mental health professional while still remaining under his or her care.

Hypochondriasis also can exist along with proven medical illness. Any evaluation for this disorder must begin with a thorough investigation of physical symptoms to rule out medical illnesses and conditions. On occasion it can be a symptom of other mental conditions, such as depressive, panic, obsessive-compulsive, or generalized anxiety disorders, but in such cases it usually does not persist unless these disorders remain untreated for an extended time.

▼

Risks and   Ironically, people with hypochondriasis may develop physical
complications   problems and complications as a result of their efforts to get medical attention. Doctors may fail to diagnose a physical illness be-

Is it hypochondriasis?

According to the DSM-IV, a diagnosis of hypochondriasis should be based on these criteria:

- A preoccupation with fears of having, or the idea that one has, a serious disease, based on misinterpretation of bodily symptoms

- Persistent fear and worry despite appropriate medical evaluation and reassurance

- Significant distress or impairment in social, occupational, or other important areas of functioning

- Duration of at least six months

- The disturbance is not part of generalized anxiety, obsessive-compulsive, panic, major depression, separation anxiety, or another somatoform disorder.

Adapted from the Diagnostic and Statistical Manual of Mental Disorders, 4th Edition. *Used with permission.*

cause individuals report so many confusing symptoms. They also face medical risks from repeated, often expensive, and unnecessary diagnostic procedures, such as exploratory surgery, and from medications (including potentially addictive drugs) that may be prescribed to relieve symptoms. Anxiety and depression, which can be severe, are common.

▼
Treating hypochondriasis

Individuals who develop this problem vary widely in personalities, beliefs, and fears, and therapy must always be tailored to their unique situations and needs. However, psychiatric evaluation and treatment are a supplement to, not a replacement for, continuing medical care. Individuals with hypochondriasis should find a single primary doctor whom they can trust, who listens to their concerns about illness, and who is conservative about ordering potentially harmful tests and treatments. They should resist the temptation to seek opinions from new doctors and instead should schedule regular visits with their primary physician to make certain their condition hasn't changed.

In our judgment, a psychiatrist is the best mental health professional to consult in cases of hypochondriasis because of the importance of medical training in working with this disorder. The psychiatrist may want to review previous records and hospital charts and to talk with the person's primary physician. If there is no evidence of any serious physical illness or abnormality, the psychiatrist can explain the findings and provide further reassurance about the person's physical condition. If individuals develop new symptoms or believe that they have a new illness, they may undergo another brief examination, but the focus in therapy should gradually shift away from symptoms to social or personal concerns and the ability to function at work and at home. If symptoms remain the focus, both the individual and the psychiatrist will become dissatisfied, since the symptoms rarely abate for more than a brief time.

Many different psychotherapy approaches have been tried. Some concentrate on education; others encourage individuals to ventilate and talk about their fears and what they believe their symptoms indicate. Frequent sessions, at least once a week, are most helpful because they offer continuing reassurance.

Most people with hypochondriasis have a poor understanding of the relationship between emotions and bodily symptoms. They need information, such as the fact that physical symptoms are extremely common and only a small proportion are caused by disease. They also need to recognize that selective attention to one part of the body makes a person more conscious of sensations in that part than elsewhere. Many people tend to be anxious when they see physicians; this is especially true for those with hypochondriasis, whose apprehensiveness can make it difficult for them to absorb such information. It is important to find a psychiatrist who is willing to repeat explanations and who can offer helpful suggestions, such as teaching distraction, relaxation, and stress management techniques (described in Chapter 29).

Sometimes group sessions or courses can be beneficial. In an innovative program created by psychiatrist Arthur Barsky, M.D., of Harvard Medical School, individuals meet in small groups for eight weeks for a course on "the perception of physical symptoms." First, they learn that paying attention to symptoms intensifies them. They also learn that thinking of minor aches and pains as medical symptoms makes them seem more ominous than they actually are. Participants are taught to use their ability to concentrate on bodily sensations in a more positive way, for example, focusing on the natural flow of their breathing in a meditation exercise. This is helpful because it relaxes them when they find themselves worrying about the sensations they feel.

There is no evidence that drug treatment is beneficial in hypochondriasis unless individuals suffer from another mental disorder, such as depression or panic disorder. In such cases, some therapists do try to break the cycle of fear, symptoms, and more fear with anti-anxiety or antidepressant drugs. These medications can reduce symptoms in persons with these disorders and make it easier for them to avoid paying attention to physical discomfort and to concentrate on other matters. With effective therapy, they usually use the drugs less frequently and eventually stop taking them altogether.

▼

**Impact on
relationships**
A person's constant preoccupation with physical health can strain friendships and family relationships; people often grow weary of listening to a litany of woes. Family members may resent the time, energy, and expense their relative devotes to concern about illness and, once medical tests reveal no physical abnormalities, may dismiss complaints as trivial or "all in your head." Ironically, at the very time that people with hypochondriasis most need support and empathy, their persistent worries may drive others away.

▼

Outlook
People with hypochondriasis cannot become better psychologically until they accept the facts that they have little to fear medically and that their problems do not have medical solutions. Reports concerning those who do receive treatment indicate that many improve or recover completely, finally giving up their fruitless search for such remedies. The prognosis is best for those who undergo evaluation and treatment for hypochondriasis soon after their troubling symptoms and intense concerns begin, rather than pursue extensive medical evaluations and treatments.

BODY DYSMORPHIC DISORDER

Body dysmorphic disorder, often described as "imagined ugliness," involves individuals who look normal but are intensely preoccupied with an imagined defect in their appearance. Whatever its target—and there usually are several over their lifetime—their concern is always extremely upsetting and interferes with their work or relationships. Most often they focus on a part of the face or head: pimples, wrinkles, spots on the skin, swelling, too much or too little hair, the shape of their nose, mouth, jaw, or eyebrows. Some concentrate on the hands, arms, breasts, buttocks, penis, back, hips, legs, or feet.

Although some people simply describe themselves as ugly, many with this disorder can pinpoint very precisely what is wrong; for example, pointed ears or a too-pale complexion. Others have a more general complaint, such as a sagging face or frizzy hair. It is not unusual for these individuals to feel anguish for more than one reason, such as large teeth, a prominent Adam's apple, and splotchy skin.

The complaints of individuals with imagined ugliness may or may not have a basis in reality. When there is an actual but slight imperfection, such as a large mole on the neck or a bald spot, the person is far more self-conscious or concerned than the imperfection warrants. Paradoxically, a real and more noticeable physical abnormality, such as large ears or a bump on the nose, may not cause any concern.

▼

How common is body dysmorphic disorder?

Although many people are not satisfied with their appearance, most do not become so preoccupied with it that they are unable to function because of their less-than-perfect looks. The intense dissatisfaction of body dysmorphic disorder is considered relatively rare. The condition is most likely to begin in the teens through the twenties, and occurs equally in men and women. By some estimates, 2 percent of those who seek cosmetic surgery may have this disorder.

▼

What causes body dysmorphic disorder?

Imagined ugliness is not a new mental disorder spawned by our appearance-conscious age. Freud wrote that one of his patients, known as the Wolf Man, "neglected his daily life and work because he was engrossed to the exclusion of all else in the state of his nose," making painstaking observations of it in a pocket mirror. Little research has been done into the etiology of this disorder, which seems more likely to occur in persons with depressive symptoms or an obsessive-compulsive personality disorder. Members of the families of individuals with body dysmorphic disorder are more prone to develop depressive disorders, substance abuse, and obsessive-compulsive disorder themselves. Some experts have noted similarities between body dysmorphia and obsessive-compulsive disorder.

▼

How body dysmorphic disorder feels

Almost all young people feel self-conscious about some aspect of their appearance, but those with body dysmorphic disorder are genuinely convinced that they are repulsive because of a slight or imagined imperfection. Thus, whereas many teenagers worry about acne, someone with body dysmorphic disorder feels ugly because of a single pimple.

Individuals with this disorder often describe their feelings as devastatingly painful. Often they cannot work, complete important tasks, or engage in normal social activities because of their extreme distress or the time they spend checking, improving, or ruminating about their appearance. They may spend hours staring in the mirror at their "defects" and keep checking their image in store windows, car bumpers, or any reflecting material they encounter. Some use magnifying mirrors or special lights to examine themselves. They devote hours every day to thinking about how they look or trying to hide their appearance with cosmetics or

Is it body dysmorphic disorder?

According to the DSM-IV, a diagnosis of body dysmorphic disorder should be based on these criteria:

- Preoccupation with an imagined defect in appearance; if a slight physical anomaly exists, the concern is clearly excessive

- Significant distress or impairment in social, occupational, or other important areas of functioning

- The preoccupation is not better accounted for by another mental disorder.

Adapted from the Diagnostic and Statistical Manual of Mental Disorders, 4th Edition. *Used with permission.*

clothing. This constant checking and grooming only intensifies their anxiety and preoccupation with their appearance.

Body dysmorphic disorder can also generate the opposite response, in which persons avoid looking at themselves. Some try to camouflage their imagined abnormality—for example, by wearing a hat to disguise hair loss, growing a beard to hide supposed blemishes or scars, or padding their underwear because of too-small breasts or a "shrunken" penis.

Although individuals who believe they are ugly may seek constant reassurance about their appearance, they feel no better when told that they look fine. They may constantly compare their "ugly" body part with the same area in others, and often believe that other people are staring at them, talking about their imagined defect, or even making fun of them. Some report physical sensations, such as tingling or tightness, in the affected area.

▼
Seeking help

Individuals with this problem almost never seek psychiatric help for their imagined ugliness, although they may undergo therapy to deal with other problems, especially depression. Even then, they may be so ashamed of their "disfigurement" that they cannot confide even in their therapists. They are more likely to seek "corrective" treatment for it from a plastic surgeon, dermatologist, or other physician. On occasion, such doctors, who come to recognize individuals whose dissatisfaction with their appearance goes far beyond the normal, will suggest that they seek psychotherapy, but even in these circumstances the individuals may consider consultation with a mental health professional chiefly as a "ticket punch" to the cosmetic procedure they really desire.

The face in the mirror

Marcie never met a mirror she didn't love. That's what her brother used to say when she was a teenager. And Marcie had every reason to like what she saw: blond hair, blue-green eyes, a flawless complexion, pert features. But by the time Marcie reached her mid-twenties, after an early marriage and an ugly divorce, the mirror turned into her enemy.

What bothered her first were the bags under her eyes. "I look like Bette Davis in her declining years," she'd complain. Although friends reassured her that she looked fine, she didn't believe them. Once she used to smile when she caught a reflection of herself in a store window, but now she immediately zeroed in on the pouches she saw under her eyes. She was also concerned about the fine lines that were beginning to spread across her forehead and the arc she saw forming between her nose and her mouth.

"They say blondes age more quickly, and they're right," she would think as she stared into her magnifying mirror at home. "By the time I'm thirty, people will think I'm forty-five."

Marcie, whose make-up once consisted of mascara, blusher, and lipstick, began spending hours experimenting with different cosmetics. If a friend dropped by unexpectedly, she wouldn't even answer the doorbell if she hadn't put on her make-up. When she went out to a club, she'd choose a dim corner where the light seemed more flattering. Once an avid tennis player and swimmer, she swore off spending any time in the sun. She haunted the cosmetics counters at the department store where she worked, always looking for new products that might help with what she called "my problem." She carried a compact with her always and constantly checked and rechecked her face.

Marcie's friends and family began to weary of her constant need for reassurance that she looked fine. "You're still the prettiest of us all," a friend told her. "We're just getting a little character in our faces."

If "character" meant bags and wrinkles, Marcie wanted none of it. On her twenty-eighth birthday she decided to see a plastic surgeon about having the bags under her eyes surgically removed. "We hardly ever do this procedure on someone so young," the first doctor she consulted said. "I don't really think that surgery is needed. Why don't you come back in twenty years?"

Outraged at what she felt was his callous attitude, Marcie visited other surgeons, who also discouraged her from undergoing surgery. Finally a dermatologist told her that a chemical peel might help with some of the fine lines Marcie felt were spreading like a cobweb over her face. The procedure was expensive, painful, and, from a technical standpoint, a complete success. But Marcie thought the results were disastrous. "You've ruined my skin tone," she complained to the doctor. "It's all blotchy. I'm more hideous than ever." When the physician suggested Marcie see a psychiatrist, she was furious. "I am not crazy!" she declared.

Soon afterward, one of Marcie's friends practically dragged her to a lecture a local therapist was giving called "Women Who Hate Their Bodies." So much of what the psychologist said struck home that Marcie made an appointment to see her. The diagnosis of body dysmorphic disorder has been a hard one for Marcie to accept, but in her sessions she is working to redefine what she sees as normal and attractive. "I'm not sure I'll ever love the way I look," she says. "But at least I might be able to look in a mirror without wincing."

If you suspect that body dysmorphic disorder may be a problem for you or someone close to you, these are the questions that should be asked:

- Do you believe that some part of your body or aspect of your appearance is ugly, abnormal, or defective?

- Does this perceived imperfection cause you great concern or embarrassment?

- Do doctors or others you trust tell you that your concern is exaggerated or unrealistic?

- Do you spend a significant amount of time thinking about or trying to disguise what you see as the problem?

- Have you sought medical advice or undergone treatment for it?

- Has your concern about the way you look interfered with your relationships, social activities, or ability to work?

If you or a person close to you answers "yes" to several of these questions, the problem may be body dysmorphic disorder. Mental health professionals can rule out other problems, such as social phobia, in which a person may exaggerate physical defects, or anorexia nervosa, in which a person may feel fat even when severely underweight. They can also diagnose and treat associated psychiatric problems, such as depression and obsessive-compulsive disorder.

▼

Risks and complications

Individuals with body dysmorphic disorder may feel so much shame and distress that they drop out of school, avoid socializing, choose inconspicuous jobs in order to avoid public exposure, or quit working rather than face possible humiliation. They often have few friends, avoid dating, have marital difficulties, or get divorced. Some become extremely isolated, not leaving their houses for months or even years, or leaving only when others will not see them.

Body dysmorphic disorder is linked to depression, social phobia, and obsessive-compulsive disorder. It may lead to repeated hospitalization, unnecessary surgery and its complications, and suicide.

▼

Treating body dysmorphic disorder

Mental health professionals tend to take the same approaches to this condition as those used to treat hypochondriasis, and emphasize reassurance and education about what is normal and what is not. There have been no scientific studies of treatments for body dysmorphic disorder, although various therapists have reported success with behavior therapy and psychodynamic psychotherapy. Antidepressants may help those with symptoms of depression.

The "treatment" many individuals choose on their own is medical, dermatological, dental, or surgical correction of the presumed defect. The results still do not satisfy them, and they often feel worse or develop new preoccupations, which can lead to more unnecessary and unsuccessful treatments. In time, some individuals become, as one psychiatrist put it, "synthetic creations of artificial noses, breasts, ears, and hips."

▼

Impact on relationships

Individuals with body dysmorphic disorder are often so self-conscious that they avoid social situations and are unwilling to become involved in close relationships with co-workers or other acquaintances. Relatives or friends to whom they voice their concerns may not know how to respond, and if they do offer reassurances, these are not likely to be believed. Sometimes friends or family members encourage the person to get medical or surgical treatments simply so he or she will feel better. If, as is often the case, dissatisfaction and preoccupation with appearance persist despite the treatment, those close to the person may become unsympathetic or critical.

▼

Outlook

This problem typically persists for years, although the intensity of the unhappiness can wax and wane. Sometimes the focus of the individual's preoccupation changes, and concerns about a different body part replace old ones. There have been no scientific studies of the long-term prognosis for those who receive treatment.

SOMATIZATION DISORDER

Somatization is a type of somatoform disorder consisting of many different physical complaints that persist for years and lead to medical treatment or changes in lifestyle. This complex chronic illness, once called Briquet's syndrome, usually begins in the teens or twenties. Menstrual difficulties are often one of the earliest complaints, although girls and young women may also report seizures, depressive symptoms, headache, or abdominal pain. Other symptoms typically include the following characteristic patterns:

- Pain that occurs in at least four different parts of the body, such as the head, abdomen, back, joints, arms, legs, chest, or rectum, or during sexual intercourse, menstruation, or urination

- At least two digestive symptoms other than pain, such as nausea, diarrhea, bloating, vomiting, or adverse reactions to several different foods

- At least one sexual or reproductive symptom other than pain, such as sexual indifference, impotence, irregular menstrual periods, excessive menstrual bleeding, or vomiting throughout pregnancy

- At least one neurological problem, such as double vision, blindness, deafness, loss of touch or pain sensation, inability to speak, impaired coordination or balance, paralysis or localized weakness, difficulty in swallowing, urinary retention, seizures, loss of memory, or loss of consciousness other than fainting

- Complaints cannot be explained fully by a medical condition or illness. If there are findings of an abnormality, the symptoms are greatly in excess of what would be expected.

▼

How common is somatization disorder?   The National Institute of Mental Health's (NIMH) Epidemiologic Catchment Area (ECA) study estimated that about one in every one thousand people suffers from somatization disorder; the *DSM-IV* cites ranges of 0.2 percent to 2 percent in women and less than 0.2 percent in men. These individuals use health care often, and one study of the highest 10 percent of medical care users found that 20 percent had somatization disorder. It is diagnosed much more often in women than in men, perhaps because some bodily symptoms, such as menstrual irregularities, are uniquely female, and also because men tend not to report physical symptoms. According to the *American Psychiatric Press Textbook of Psychiatry*, the typical patient with somatization disorder referred to a psychiatrist is a married woman in her twenties.

▼

What causes somatization disorder?   Somatization disorder clearly runs in families. Studies of individuals with this problem, some reared by their birth parents and some by adoptive parents, suggest that both genetic and environmental factors contribute to the problem. As many as 20 percent of the first-degree female relatives (mothers, sisters, daughters) of individuals with somatization disorder develop the same illness. Their male relatives have an increased incidence of antisocial personality disorder and substance abuse.

Experiments using tests of brain chemistry and functioning have found some difficulties with information processing related to attention and memory, and indications of certain brain abnormalities. People with somatization disorder often report a history of abuse or molestation as children, impaired relationships as adults, and high levels of distress over their lifetime. They are

Is it a somatization disorder?

According to the DSM-IV, a diagnosis of somatization disorder should be based on these criteria:

■ A history of many physical complaints beginning before the age of thirty, occurring over a period of several years, and resulting in a search for medical treatment or in significant impairment in social or occupational functioning

■ In the course of the disorder, development of each of the following:

  1. Four pain symptoms related to at least four different body sites or functions, such as pain in the head, abdomen, back, joints, extremities, chest, or rectum, or occurring during sexual intercourse, menstruation, or urination

  2. Two digestive (gastrointestinal) symptoms other than pain, such as nausea, diarrhea, bloating, vomiting other than during pregnancy, or intolerance of several different foods

  3. One sexual or reproductive symptom other than pain, such as sexual indifference, erectile or ejaculatory dysfunction, irregular menses, excessive menstrual bleeding, or vomiting throughout pregnancy

  4. One "pseudoneurologic" symptom (suggesting a neurological disorder) not limited to pain: conversion symptoms such as blindness, double vision, deafness, loss of touch or pain sensation, hallucinations, inability to talk, impaired coordination or balance, paralysis or localized weakness, difficulty swallowing, difficulty breathing, urinary retention, seizures, dissociative symptoms, such as amnesia, or loss of consciousness other than fainting

■ The disturbance is not fully explained by a medical condition, or the resulting complaints or impairment are in excess of what could be expected from the history, physical examination, or laboratory findings.

Adapted from the Diagnostic and Statistical Manual of Mental Disorders, 4th Edition. *Used with permission.*

more likely than the average person to suffer from mental disorders, especially depression, anxiety, and personality disorders.

▼

How somatization disorder feels

Unlike most people, who rarely do anything to relieve minor aches and pains, those with somatization disorder seek medical help, take a prescription medicine, or alter the way they live to accommodate their symptoms. A year in the life of such individuals rarely passes without the pursuit of medical attention for generally ill-defined symptoms or vague medical syndromes. Because of their complicated medical histories and symptoms, they may see themselves as long-suffering and plagued by health problems far more serious than those that actually afflict them.

Persons with this disorder suffer both physically and mentally.

They often are depressed or anxious and encounter problems on the job and in their relationships and marriages. Although they are in touch with reality, they may experience hallucinations, most commonly that of hearing their own name called.

▼

Seeking help   Individuals with somatization disorder seek health care frequently, often from a number of physicians at the same time, yet most resist mental health care because they see their problem as medical, not emotional. In time, however, many eventually turn to mental health professionals because of depression or suicidal thoughts or attempts.

If you suspect that somatization disorder may be a problem for you or someone close to you, these are the questions that should be asked:

- Do you have a number of physical complaints that began before the age of thirty and have persisted over a period of several years?

- Have you undergone medical treatment or altered your lifestyle as a result of these problems?

- Have you experienced the following:
  1. Pain in different parts of your body or during sexual intercourse, menstruation, or urination?
  2. At least two digestive symptoms other than pain, such as nausea, diarrhea, bloating, or vomiting?
  3. Sexual or reproductive complaints, such as sexual indifference, impotence, or irregular periods?
  4. At least one neurological symptom, such as double vision, paralysis or localized weakness, or difficulty swallowing?

- Have medical examinations and tests revealed no physical cause for these complaints, or are the symptoms much greater than would be expected on the basis of the medical findings?

If you or someone close to you answers "yes" to these questions, a somatization disorder is a possibility. You may want to discuss this with your primary physician, who may suggest consulting a psychiatrist. In our judgment, this is a wise course to follow because psychiatrists may be able to provide insight or offer suggestions that other physicians may miss on their own. Although it can be tempting to continue seeking different opinions from different doctors, in the long run it is far better to establish a good relationship with a primary physician, a psychiatrist, or both.

Consulting psychiatrists may want to review old medical charts, talk with the individual's other physicians, or interview the person several times to obtain a complete history and to ensure that there is no medical explanation for the symptoms. They also will determine whether the symptoms might be caused by another mental disorder, such as schizophrenia, depression, early dementia, or panic disorder.

▼

Risks and complications

Because those with somatization disorder are constantly undergoing medical evaluations, they are at increased risk for complications from unnecessary surgery, abuse of or dependence on prescribed medications, long periods of disability, or suicide attempts because of depression. Some also have histrionic or, more rarely, antisocial personality disorders.

▼

Treating somatization disorder

Over the years an eclectic approach, based on re-education, reassurance, and suggestion, has proved helpful. A "therapeutic alliance"—a partnership between an individual and a health professional based on mutual trust and respect—is particularly important. People with somatization disorder should feel that their complaints are taken seriously, that their suffering is recognized as real, and that the clinician, whether a primary physician or a psychiatrist, is committed to understanding and helping them. In one well-designed study, the involvement of a psychiatrist—who urged the primary physicians to see patients regularly (every four to six weeks), to perform an examination at each visit, to use the person's history and physical examination to look for signs of disease rather than taking complaints at face value, and to avoid laboratory tests, diagnostic procedures, and hospitalization unless clearly indicated—cut the costs of health care for these individuals by approximately half.

Education is critical in helping people to understand that somatization disorder is a medically recognized complex illness, that it is not "crazy," and that it does not lead to progressive mental deterioration or other dire consequences. Initially, individuals often need repeated reassurance that they have been thoroughly evaluated and are receiving the best possible type of care. Over time, the focus shifts from symptoms to strategies for helping them to function well and manage their lives effectively. The physician should explain that although stress does not cause somatization disorder, there *is* a relationship between stress and physical complaints, and he or she should suggest stress management or behavioral coping strategies.

Group therapy with others who have somatic complaints may be helpful if the members can go beyond discussion of their symptoms and deal with the underlying stress that may be causing or exacerbating their physical problems. Ideally, individuals should receive as few drugs as possible, assuming that any at all are necessary.

▼

Impact on relationships

People with somatization disorder can strain the tolerance and understanding of friends and relatives. Sometimes symptoms are used to seek attention or manipulate others, but even when this is not the case, the intense focus on symptoms can make the person seem self-absorbed and uninterested in other pursuits or people. Once medical tests have ruled out possible physical causes, or if the impairment is much greater than such problems normally cause, family members may lose sympathy and become resentful of the time, attention, and energy that their relative devotes to his or her body.

Often symptoms worsen during marital or family crises, and separation and divorce are common complications. Family members should consult with the individual's physician or psychiatrist so they can understand the medical and psychological complexities of this disorder. Family therapy may also be useful.

▼

Outlook

Somatization disorder tends to be chronic and fluctuating, improving and worsening over time. However, treatment can help. In a classic study of an approach that emphasized reassurance and education, about half of the individuals showed significant improvement at a three-year follow-up.

CONVERSION DISORDER

Persons with conversion disorder develop one or more symptoms affecting awareness, perception, sensation, or movement that have no apparent physical cause or are out of proportion to the cause. The most common are blindness, double vision, deafness, loss of sensation, inability to speak, impaired coordination or balance, weakness or paralysis, difficulty in swallowing, seizures, loss of consciousness, or what is called "glove-and-stocking anesthesia"—numbness of the hands and feet. Conversion symptoms are not consciously or intentionally produced, nor can they be fully explained by any physical illness or abnormality. Psychological factors, such as stress or conflict, appear to trigger or worsen them.

▼

How common is conversion disorder?

Conversion symptoms typically develop in the teens or early adulthood, usually before the age of thirty-five, although they can also appear for the first time during middle age or even later in life, often after a traumatic event. Those who develop characteristic symptoms later in life are more likely to have some as yet undetected physical disease accounting for the symptom.

Conversion disorder often occurs in soldiers during battle or among hospital patients, primarily those with neurological or orthopedic problems. Various reports have estimated that 1 to 3 percent of outpatients are referred to mental health clinics because of conversion disorder; as many as 20 to 25 percent of all individuals admitted to general hospitals have experienced conversion symptoms at some time during their lives. This disorder is diagnosed more often in women than in men.

▼

What causes conversion disorder?

Usually, conversion symptoms develop suddenly at a time of extreme stress. The traditional explanation has been that individuals unconsciously "convert" emotions they cannot express into physical symptoms that serve as a form of punishment for a forbidden wish, that allow them to escape from a threatening situation, or that enable them to become dependent on others. In some circumstances, conversion symptoms may allow them to avoid something they do not want to do, as when, for example, a soldier who cannot walk or move his fingers cannot be sent into battle. In psychoanalytic theory, conversion symptoms represent a compromise between the unconscious need to express ideas or feelings and the fear of expressing them. Behavioral theorists explain conversion symptoms as learned responses that follow a particular event or psychological state and that are reinforced by certain conditions. Thus, an individual who cannot speak after learning of a tragic death in the family may unconsciously respond to the sympathy and attention of others and experience the same symptom under other stressful circumstances.

As many as half of those with conversion disorders have an underlying neurological disorder, and conversion causes symptoms out of proportion to the severity of this disorder. The high rate of conversion symptoms after head injury or other brain disorders also suggests a biological basis for this problem.

Conversion symptoms appear to be more common in relatives of individuals with this disorder. Previous physical conditions, exposure to people disabled by similar symptoms, and extreme psychosocial stress can also contribute to conversion disorder. About one-third of individuals with conversion disorder also have somatization disorder. Conversion disorder often develops during the course of other mental disorders, such as a major depression, panic disorder, substance abuse, or schizophrenia.

▼

How conversion disorder feels

Individuals with a conversion disorder respond to a traumatic event by developing a physical problem. Someone who witnesses a brutal murder or catastrophe may become blind. After a fierce argument, a man struggling to control his rage might become paralyzed in one arm. Many persons unconsciously model their symptoms on a previous illness or the symptoms suffered by an important figure in their life, such as a parent or grandparent.

Common conversion symptoms include paralysis, abnormal movements, inability to speak, blindness, and deafness. Usually they conform to the person's idea of how the disease affects people rather than to its actual symptoms and typical patterns. Many are deeply upset and concerned about their symptoms, but others, despite often severe impairment, show relatively little concern, an attitude described by the French phrase *la belle indifference.*

▼

Seeking help

If you or someone close to you has developed symptoms such as loss of vision or hearing, muscle weakness, paralysis, or difficulty in swallowing, and the causes are not clear, these are some questions to consider:

- Did the symptoms develop at a time of stress, personal crisis, or conflict?
- Are the symptoms beyond conscious control?
- Have the symptoms caused great distress or interfered with normal relationships, activities, or work?

If the answers to these questions are "yes," you may want to discuss them with your physician, who may find your insight helpful in arriving at an accurate diagnosis and who may suggest consulting a psychiatrist.

It is often difficult for physicians to determine if individuals do indeed have a physical disease, conversion disorder, or both. Thorough physical and psychiatric evaluations are essential, and laboratory and neuroimaging tests are often necessary. If there are few or no physical indications of disease, clinicians may consider a diagnosis of conversion disorder.

Sometimes it is impossible to rule out a physical problem. In follow-up studies, a significant proportion of those diagnosed with conversion disorder are later found to have an illness (usually neurological) that, in retrospect, accounted for their symptoms.

▼

Risks and complications

Individuals with unrecognized conversion disorder may undergo unnecessary diagnostic or therapeutic procedures, including dis-

■ One or more symptoms or deficits affecting voluntary motor or sensory function that suggest a neurological or general medical condition

■ Psychological factors are judged to be associated with the symptom or deficit because its initiation or exacerbation is preceded by conflicts or other stressors.

■ The symptom or deficit is not intentionally produced or feigned.

■ The symptom or deficit cannot, after appropriate investigation, be fully explained by a neurological or general medical condition and is not a culturally sanctioned behavior or experience.

■ The symptom or deficit causes clinically significant distress or impairment in social, occupational, or other important areas of functioning or warrants medical evaluation.

■ The symptom or deficit is not limited to pain or sexual dysfunction, does not occur exclusively during the course of somatization disorder, and is not better accounted for by another mental disorder.

Adapted from the Diagnostic and Statistical Manual of Mental Disorders, 4th Edition. *Used with permission.*

figuring operations, that may cause serious side effects. Prolonged loss of function can produce real and serious complications, such as muscle atrophy in individuals who develop conversion paralysis, and may severely interfere with normal life activities.

▼
Treating conversion disorder

There is no well-established systematic treatment for conversion disorder. In general, the primary physician or consulting psychiatrist provides reassurance and support while trying to deal with the stressful situation that may have triggered the symptoms. Often more direct approaches can also help.

The objectives are threefold: to provide reassurance and support; to demonstrate, if possible, that the change or impairment in physical function caused by the symptoms can be reversed; and to help the person develop some insight into the origin of the symptom. Usually individuals who seek help can be shown that they are capable of doing things with their muscles or senses that they believe are beyond their power, such as reaching out and catching a ball tossed toward them even though they are "blind." Those who have lost their ability to speak may be helped by learning to cough, then to say "ah," then to move on to more varied syllables such as "bah" or "pah," until they resume normal speaking.

Some people develop striking insight into the origin of their symptoms after only one or two therapy sessions. If acute symptoms persist, hypnosis may help them to relive the events that provoked their problem, enabling them to express painful, suppressed emotions. Insight-oriented psychotherapy, which focuses on childhood sexual behavior and other developmental problems, has not proved any more effective than general supportive psychotherapy. Although there is little research on specific therapies, physicians report that the treatments described in this chapter are usually beneficial.

▼

Impact on relationships

Conversion disorder is deeply distressing for individuals and their loved ones. All fear that the person will never be able to see, hear, speak, or walk again. The family may demand aggressive testing and treatment. Once conversion disorder is diagnosed, relatives should talk with the primary physician or consulting psychiatrist so that they can become fully informed about this condition and the best ways to respond to it. Often they are tremendously reassured to learn that many people improve rapidly and without residual adverse effects.

▼

Outlook

Conversion symptoms usually develop quickly and last for only a short time. Even without treatment, most individuals improve and do not suffer lasting complications. However, relapse may occur, and some cases can persist for several years. The prognosis is best when symptoms begin suddenly after a stressful event and when the person was previously in good health and had no physical or psychiatric illness. The nature of the symptom also affects the prognosis. Those who develop blindness, inability to speak, and paralysis tend to do better than those who experience seizures or tremors.

UNDIFFERENTIATED SOMATOFORM DISORDER

In this disorder, individuals develop a single symptom, such as difficulty in swallowing, or, more commonly, several symptoms, such as fatigue, loss of appetite, and digestive complaints, that persist for six months or more and cannot be explained on the basis of any physical findings. The symptoms are most likely to appear at times of depression, anxiety, or stress.

▼

How common is undifferentiated somatoform disorder?

Somatic symptoms with no physical basis are extremely common. It is believed that in any given week, as many as 60 to 80 percent of all men and women develop some complaint that has no biological cause. What is uncommon is becoming so preoccupied or concerned that it is impossible for the person to function normally. There has been little research on this problem and its incidence in the general population.

▼

What causes undifferentiated somatoform disorder?

According to traditional psychodynamic thinking, this disorder may have its roots in early childhood. In normal development, children gradually learn to identify feelings, initially by expressing them in physical ways—crying, smiling, clapping, kicking—and then, as they learn to speak, by putting them into words. It is theorized that youngsters who have difficulty doing this may be prone to development of somatoform disorder.

People vary widely in their perceptions of "the sick role." Some with somatoform disorder may unconsciously seek release from normal obligations, such as work and school. Others may welcome the special privileges that come with being sick: being cared for and being allowed to depend on others. But individuals with somatoform disorder are not aware of such desires and do not intentionally produce symptoms for the sake of such benefits.

Family and cultural influences can play a major role. Parents who are most loving, nurturing, and attentive at times when a child is ill may, consciously or unconsciously, encourage their youngsters to rely on sickness as a way of obtaining attention and love. In other cases, parents punish children when they express emotions such as anger or fear, thereby conveying the message that it is bad, wrong, or simply not wise to show feelings. The only acceptable way for their youngsters to get attention may be by developing physical complaints. In cultures and settings that discourage the expression of emotion, physical complaints may be a legitimate and effective way of dealing with feelings. In general, somatization is more common among rural, religious, ethnic, and lower socioeconomic groups.

▼

How undifferentiated somatoform disorder feels

Individuals with this disorder do not think in emotional terms. They do not see themselves as depressed, anxious, frustrated, angry, or worried. They may not be capable of expressing feelings openly or of acknowledging psychological problems. Instead, they develop symptoms that cause them considerable distress.

▼

Seeking help

Typically, men and women with troublesome symptoms turn to their primary physicians or to specialists, such as neurologists and cardiologists, for help. When possible physical causes are ruled out, they resist any suggestion of seeing a mental health professional. If you or someone close to you develops an inexpli-

Is it undifferentiated somatoform disorder?

According to the DSM-IV, a diagnosis of undifferentiated somatoform disorder should be based on these criteria:

- One or more physical complaints (e.g., fatigue, loss of appetite, digestive or urinary problems)

- EITHER:
  1. After appropriate investigation, the symptoms cannot be explained by a general medical condition or the effects of injury, medications, or alcohol or drugs of abuse.

  OR

  2. When there is a medical condition, the physical complaints and social or occupational impairment grossly exceed what would be expected.

- Significant distress or impairment in social, occupational, or other important areas of functioning

- The disturbance persists for at least six months.

- The disturbance is not better accounted for by another mental disorder, such as another somatoform disorder, sexual dysfunction, mood disorder, anxiety disorder, sleep disorder, or psychotic disorder.

Adapted from the Diagnostic and Statistical Manual of Mental Disorders, *4th Edition. Used with permission.*

cable physical symptom, these are the questions that should be considered:

- Do you have one or more distressing physical symptoms, such as constant fatigue, loss of appetite, or digestive problems?

- Did they start or do they flare up at a time of stress, conflict, or personal crisis?

- Have medical examinations and tests found no physical cause for what you are experiencing?

- If there is a confirmed physical problem, is your distress or inability to work and function much greater than what would be expected on the basis of the problem?

- Have the symptoms persisted for at least six months?

If you or a person close to you answers "yes" to these questions, the source of the physical symptoms could be undifferentiated somatoform disorder. You may want to discuss this possibility with your physician, who may advise consulting a psychiatrist.

▼

Risks and complications   Repeated medical tests or unnecessary surgery to attempt to discover the source of the symptoms may lead to serious physical complications and side effects.

▼

**Treating
undifferentiated
somatoform
disorder**

There is no carefully studied, systematic treatment for this disorder. People appear to benefit most when they develop an empathic, accepting relationship with a single physician. Often the doctor will schedule regular appointments every few weeks or months so that the person does not feel that he or she needs to develop new symptoms in order to obtain medical attention.

In the past, individuals with somatic complaints were viewed as less likely to benefit from psychotherapy than those who had only psychological symptoms. However, recent controlled studies suggest that psychotherapy is as—or even more—effective for people with undifferentiated somatoform disorder as for those with some other mental disorders.

In general, medications offer little benefit for bodily symptoms that have no identifiable physical basis. Some psychiatrists prescribe antidepressants for individuals who also suffer from depression. These medications can also reduce unexplained bodily symptoms in people who have chronic pain and panic disorder in addition to a somatoform disorder. Those with an anxiety disorder may benefit from the short-term use of a benzodiazepine (see Chapter 28), although because of their potential for abuse, it is important that the use of these drugs be viewed as only a temporary measure.

▼

**Impact on
relationships**

Sometimes illness or symptoms serve a hidden purpose in families who cannot acknowledge psychological problems. The person's condition may serve as a diversion from difficulties the family finds too threatening to discuss and resolve openly. Family therapy can help work out these problems.

▼

Outlook

Some individuals experience only a single episode of a somatoform disorder; others have recurrent problems. Many people with somatic symptoms improve or recover simply with a physician's explanation and reassurance. However, often individuals are eventually diagnosed with a general medical condition or another mental disorder.

Feigned illness

Most people fake illness on occasion. A child who does not want to go to school may claim to have an upset stomach. An employee hoping to get an extension on a deadline may complain of a headache. Individuals may pretend to be suffering for the sake of getting out of jury duty, qualifying for disability benefits, or winning a legal judgment. All these behaviors are examples of malingering, discussed later in this chapter. Far more baffling are instances in which individuals produce symptoms, often painful ones, for no obvious or tangible reason. This condition is called *factitious disorder.*

FACTITIOUS DISORDER

Factitious means "artificial," and people with factitious disorder deliberately produce or pretend to have physical or psychological symptoms. They consciously try to deceive health care professionals and simulate illness in ways that are not likely to be discovered. However, even though their actions are deliberate, these individuals cannot explain or control what they are doing. This disorder stems from an irresistible psychological need to assume the sick role.

There is a broad spectrum of factitious behaviors, ranging from feigning illness under stress to becoming a "hospital hobo" and devoting all one's time and energy to a quest for medical care. Persons with factitious disorder may induce psychological symptoms, physical symptoms, or, as is most common, a combination of both. Physicians have reported cases of factitious AIDS, anemia, diabetes, leukemia, kidney stones, hysteria, posttraumatic stress disorder, seizures, and psychosis. Factitious disorder is usually chronic, although occasionally it consists of a few brief episodes.

About 10 percent of individuals with factitious disorder develop the extreme form called *Munchausen syndrome,* named for the nineteenth-century Baron von Munchausen, who was known for his tall tales and fanciful exaggeration. People with Munchausen syndrome lie pathologically about their symptoms and illness, often devoting their entire lives to trying to get admitted to or remain in hospitals.

Although those with factitious disorder often discuss their condition in vivid, melodramatic terms, their descriptions lack detail and consistency. Because they know a great deal about medical terminology and hospital routine, they can lie convincingly about their past histories and present symptoms. Once hospitalized, they are demanding, difficult patients who want constant attention; they break hospital rules and request specific medications or treatments. If tests fail to reveal a physical cause for their initial symptoms, they complain of new ones.

▼

How common is factitious disorder?   No one knows how common this disorder is. Rarely reported, it may not be recognized, especially in milder forms. One study of fevers of unknown origin found that up to 10 percent of the fevers were factitious. Usually factitious disorder begins in early adulthood, often with hospitalization for actual illness. Most cases are not severe. Young women are more likely to develop mild forms, while men with a history of substance abuse and psychopathological or criminal behavior fit the profile of "classic" Munchausen patients.

▼
What causes factitious disorder?

A variety of factors may underlie factitious disorder. True physical disorders, extensive medical treatment, or hospitalization during childhood or adolescence may set the stage for development of the condition. According to one theory, some individuals have a personal history of emotional deprivation. Children who were neglected or were physically or sexually abused at home may have been treated well when hospitalized, so they conclude that being sick is a way of being loved and cared for. As adults, they may seek to re-create this early nurturing by health care providers.

Some individuals have had a significant relationship with a physician in the past (for example, a family member or lover may have been a doctor). Conversely, others may harbor a grudge against the medical profession, perhaps because they feel they received poor care in the past, and may feign illness for the sake of feeling a sense of mastery as they thwart the doctors who cannot cure them.

Nurses, laboratory technicians, and other medical paraprofessionals are more likely to develop factitious disorder than the population at large. One study found that the majority of individuals with factitious illnesses had worked in medically related occupations. Factitious disorder has been linked with personality disorders, particularly borderline or antisocial personality. Some persons with this disorder have masochistic traits.

In one study of thirty-two individuals with Munchausen syndrome, testing revealed subtle abnormalities in brain functioning. On the basis of these findings, some researchers have theorized that the almost desperate quest for medical treatment and the pathological lying that are characteristic of factitious disorder may in fact be an individual's way of coping with problems created by brain dysfunction.

▼
How factitious disorder feels

Although they consciously produce the signs or symptoms of illness, people with factitious disorder typically do not know why they do so and cannot stop or control the behaviors that make them sick (or seem sick), even when these behaviors jeopardize their health. Their actions seem "voluntary" in the sense that they are deliberate and intentional, but their behavior is driven by a compulsive need that they neither understand nor recognize.

Some individuals with factitious disorder simply claim to be suffering pain when they are not, or falsify thermometer readings or other test results. Others inflict symptoms on themselves in varied ways. They may cause infection by injecting themselves with feces or other toxic material, take too much or too little of a prescription medicine for an actual illness, deliberately consume substances that bring on vomiting or diarrhea, hit themselves to cause bruises. They may also worsen actual medical problems, as by purposely picking at a wound so it becomes infected. Some move from doctor to doctor and hospital to hospital simulating illness. Typical complaints include severe abdominal pain, nausea and vomiting, dizziness, rashes, abscesses, fevers, bleeding, and lupus-like symptoms. As one physician notes, their symptoms may be limited only by their "medical knowledge, sophistication, and imagination."

Those with classic Munchausen syndrome often become knowledgeable about the ins and outs of the health care system. They seek care in emergency rooms on evenings and weekends when less experienced physicians in training are likely to be on duty, and provide a plausible history for a medical illness. They use sophisticated medical terminology and make specific requests for diagnostic tests and painkillers. Much of the time, however, they have one symptom of an illness, such as an elevated temperature indicating infection, but not the others that would accompany a real infection (such as sweating, flushing, and increased pulse rate). They also may show physical signs of previous treatments. Some have undergone so many exploratory operations to look for the source of their symptoms that they are left with a "gridiron" pattern of surgical scars on the abdomen. Indeed, they may require further invasive treatment for legitimate complications of these procedures.

Those who feign mental illness may behave in a bizarre manner or report depression, delusions, auditory hallucinations, and other psychiatric symptoms. When they are aware of being watched, they typically become much worse. Their descriptions fit their idea of mental illness, not the typical clinical signs. If a therapist mentions other symptoms, these individuals may report having them as well. If they undergo standardized psychological tests, their responses are usually not characteristic of any mental disorder; rather, they conform to the person's concept of the disorder.

When challenged or confronted by physicians, people with factitious disorder deny the allegations or rapidly discharge themselves

Is it factitious disorder?

According to the DSM-IV, *a diagnosis of factitious disorder should be based on these criteria:*

- ■ Intentional production or feigning of physical or psychological signs or symptoms

- ■ The motivation for the behavior is to assume the sick role.

- ■ No external incentives for the behavior (e.g., economic gain, avoiding legal responsibility, or improving physical well-being)

- ■ The disturbance is not better accounted for by another mental disorder.

Adapted from the Diagnostic and Statistical Manual of Mental Disorders, 4th Edition. *Used with permission.*

from the hospital against medical advice. Often they seek admission at another hospital the same day. Some travel to different cities, states, even different countries and continents, so that they can continue to get the medical attention they crave.

▼

Seeking help

Individuals with factitious disorder are always seeking medical help yet resist any suggestion that they should see a mental-health professional. However, if you suspect that this might be a problem for someone close to you, you may want to discuss this possibility with the physicians who provide the person with care.

Physicians evaluating people whom they suspect may have factitious disorder look for tip-offs, such as a long, complicated medical history that does not fit the person's apparent state of health, a description of symptoms that too closely resembles the textbook definition of an illness, sophisticated medical vocabulary, demands for specific medications or treatments, and a history of many operations. A consulting psychiatrist may gather previous hospital charts and talk to doctors who have treated the individual and to family members or friends who may be able to provide information. If the person refuses to permit these relatives or friends to talk to the consulting physician or claims that records have been lost, this can itself be a clue.

▼

Risks and complications

Individuals with factitious disorder face risks of complications from unnecessary surgery and adverse drug reactions. Some use medications to produce symptoms, such as stimulants that make them agitated or sedatives that induce lethargy. Substance abuse, especially of painkillers and sedatives, is common in people with this disorder. Their attempts to produce symptoms may actually lead to illness—for example, serious infection after injections with toxic material. Those with the most severe form of this disorder often cannot work or develop normal relationships because they spend so much time in the hospital.

▼

Treating factitious disorder

Individuals with this disorder usually do not seek help on their own, and it is not known what percentage ever undergo therapy. On the basis of the person's history and complaints, the primary physician may become suspicious and consult a psychiatrist to determine how to proceed. Then, assuming that the person is willing to see a psychiatrist, it is best for both doctors—the primary physician and the psychiatrist—to talk with the individual together in a nonthreatening, matter-of-fact manner. Responding to the condition as a cry for help, they offer reassurance that they can and will provide the medical and psychiatric care the person needs. The most important point is to ensure that the person does not undergo more unnecessary and possibly dangerous tests or treatments.

Psychiatrists disagree as to whether and when people should be confronted with evidence that they are faking their symptoms. Some believe that the first step should be for the psychiatrist to develop a trusting, supportive relationship with the person and learn what psychological function the disorder serves, with confrontation coming later. Others recommend immediate confrontation to force the issue into the open.

There are no controlled studies indicating which types of treatment are best. Several reports suggest that psychotherapy may be helpful. Because individuals with factitious disorder may have no one in their lives to offer empathy, supportive psychotherapy may be more beneficial, at least initially, than insight-oriented treatment. There is no evidence that psychiatric drugs help individuals with factitious illness.

In one case report, therapists used biofeedback to "treat" factitious seizures. This served as a face-saving way for the person to reduce the number of seizures without revealing the true nature of her disorder and risking the scorn of her family. By the end of nine months of weekly treatments, she was free of seizures.

▼

Impact on relationships

Many individuals with milder forms of factitious illness have stable relationships, but severe forms of the disorder, such as Munchausen syndrome, are extremely incapacitating and make lasting relationships or normal family ties all but impossible.

Friends and relatives, who may initially find it hard to accept the diagnosis, can help by encouraging psychiatric treatment and discouraging further testing or medical treatments.

Outlook Psychotherapy, biofeedback, and behavior modification have all had limited success. However, there has been little follow-up research on the long-term prognosis for people with factitious disorder, which is often chronic.

FACTITIOUS DISORDER BY PROXY

In this rare disorder, one individual deliberately produces symptoms in a person under his or her care. The great majority of victims are children. Typically, a parent or caregiver artificially creates physical symptoms in a child; for example, by giving the child medications that induce diarrhea or vomiting. Little is known about factitious disorder by proxy (also called Munchausen syndrome by proxy), which has been recognized only in the last two decades. There have been reports, not always substantiated, of several hundred cases in the United States; some have been the subject of intense media coverage.

In the majority of cases involving children, the mother proved to be the person responsible for the youngsters' ailments; in others it was a foster mother or other care provider. Often these women suffered from depression or a personality disorder, although some had no other mental illness. Many worked in health care positions. Economic gain or other external motivations are not involved. The women, mental health professionals theorize, do not want to inflict pain and suffering on a child but to indirectly assume the sick role, to become the focus of attention from pediatricians and other health care workers, and to receive sympathy and support from others. One psychiatrist describes these persons as "so narcissistic and needful of approval" that they do not see a child as a separate individual but as an almost inanimate object. In one review of cases, the death rate for youngsters in whom symptoms were deliberately induced was 8.5 percent.

MALINGERING

Malingering, which is not a psychiatric disorder, is the intentional production of false or grossly exaggerated symptoms for a specific purpose, such as avoiding work or military service, obtaining money, evading criminal prosecution, securing drugs, or gaining better living conditions. Unlike with factitious disorder, external incentives such as these are the motive for producing or feigning symptoms. Under special circumstances malingering may be

adaptive, such as faking illness while a hostage in order to win release, but usually the motivations are less benign. Malingering is
most likely to occur when a person is seeking medical evaluation
as part of a legal action or disability claim. Individuals with antisocial personality disorder (discussed in Chapter 21) are especially
prone to malingering for these reasons. There is no physical or
psychological test that clearly identifies malingering, and mental
health professionals tend to rely on their experience, expertise,
and instincts in spotting signs of deception and determining the
truth of a situation.

Is it a cognitive disorder?

Individuals with a cognitive disorder, such as delirium, dementia, or amnesia, may:

☐ **Not be fully aware of their surroundings**

☐ **Find it difficult to focus, concentrate, or shift attention**

☐ **Become disoriented about time, day, date, or location**

☐ **Show fluctuations in alertness and awareness over the course of a day**

☐ **Not be able to learn new material or to remember information about the past**

☐ **Speak in rambling, disorganized ways**

☐ **Not be capable of performing simple tasks, even though comprehension and motor skills seem fine**

☐ **Not be able to recognize and identify everyday objects**

☐ **Find it difficult to plan, organize, put things into sequence, or comprehend abstract concepts**

☐ **No longer function normally**

Because cognitive disorders interfere with the ability to think and to perceive what is happening, the persons affected may not be able to recognize symptoms in themselves. If you have checked several boxes that describe troubling changes you have observed in someone close to you, there may be reason to be concerned about cognitive impairment. This chapter provides information on the most common disorders that affect thinking and memory, including guidelines on seeking help and appropriate treatments.

20 Cognitive Disorders

Flu or fever can make it hard for anyone to concentrate. Nervousness may temporarily push the names of familiar people or objects out of memory. Pain can make us irritable or distracted. But whereas many physical and psychological circumstances can temporarily interfere with our mental abilities, the conditions discussed in this chapter—delirium, dementia, and amnesia—profoundly impair the ability to think, reason, or remember.

Cognitive disorders may stem from an illness (mental or physical), an injury, or substance use or withdrawal. They often develop in people who have never before had any mental disorder or serious psychological problem, and they can affect emotions, behaviors, and motivations as well as thoughts and perceptions. Often it is impossible to tell whether the psychological symptoms associated with these problems are the result of direct damage to the brain or a reaction to the often devastating effects of the disorders themselves.

Cognitive impairment may occur at any age. The very young and the very old are most vulnerable to delirium, whereas dementia is most common in the elderly. Sometimes these problems develop suddenly, most often as a result of illness or injury. In other cases the early symptoms are so insidious that neither the person nor close relatives may realize that something is wrong for several years. Depending on the underlying cause, these disorders may be temporary or may progressively worsen.

Once they become aware of a problem, individuals who suffer cognitive impairment are often extremely upset by their diminished abilities. They may become anxious, depressed, ashamed, or irritable. Some try to cope by imposing strict control and orderliness in their lives, keeping things in exactly the same places, making detailed notes to compensate for forgetfulness, and avoiding situations that might reveal their mental difficulties. Others try to conceal memory gaps by rambling on about details or making up plausible explanations. Those who are habitually suspicious may become paranoid, accusing others of taking their possessions or trying to trick them, and becoming intensely angry or aggressive. A few show inappropriate emotions, such as euphoria or complete indifference.

Cognitive disorders can interfere with impulse control and social judgment. As a result, people may behave in ways that they never have before: making sexual advances, exposing themselves, assaulting others (verbally or physically). Unless they understand that these are not conscious or malicious acts, family and friends may think their loved one is deliberately provoking them. This kind of inappropriate behavior can force affected persons to withdraw or may cause others to pull away from them, yet social isolation only worsens cognitive disability and psychological symptoms.

With early diagnosis and appropriate treatment, individuals with cognitive impairment disorders can often improve. Some completely recover their mental abilities, and even for those with permanent brain damage, the quality of daily living can be greatly enhanced.

Delirium

Delirium is a state of disorganized thinking and diminished ability to focus and shift attention, characterized by fluctuations in a person's mental state from day to day, hour to hour, or even minute to minute. "It is the equivalent of acute brain failure," says psychiatrist Michael Wise, M.D., a clinical professor at Tulane University in New Orleans. In general, delirium develops suddenly and affects all thinking processes, especially alertness, attention, perception, and sense of person, place, and time. The individual quite simply seems "out of it." While delirious, people don't understand what's going on, see or hear things that do not exist, and frequently are paranoid, believing that their doctors are trying to harm or poison them or that a family member is in collusion with someone who intends to do so. Delirium usually lasts only a few hours to a few days, and most people recover completely; however, it can be extremely alarming while it is going on.

Many conditions can lead to delirium, although in some instances the cause of delirium is never identified. These include medical problems, high fever, substance abuse, medications, mental disorders, sensory deprivation, or an unfamiliar environment. Sometimes several factors in combination, such as a serious illness along with the disorienting effects of being hospitalized, may contribute to it. When the person has another illness, delirium greatly increases the likelihood of complications and a longer hospital stay. Some health care experts have estimated that prompt and effective treatment to reduce the hospital stay of each delirious patient by a single day would save the U.S. economy $1 billion to $2 billion annually.

Those at highest risk for developing delirium are the elderly, persons who have undergone major heart surgery, burn patients, those who have suffered previous brain damage (from a stroke, for instance), and people with AIDS. Men and women over the age of sixty are most susceptible for a variety of reasons, including severe medical illness, impaired physical health, chronic brain disease, and multiple medications. The likelihood of delirium after heart surgery depends on several factors, including the duration and complexity of the operation.

▼

How common is delirium?

Delirium is the most common mental disorder caused directly by a disease, drug, or trauma. Although it can occur at any age, men and women over the age of sixty may be most vulnerable. In those over age sixty-five hospitalized for a general medical condition, about 10 percent show signs of delirium on admission. Another 10 to 15 percent may develop delirium in the hospital.

▼

What causes delirium?

The most common medical causes of delirium are fever, hypoxia (lack of oxygen), ischemia (lack of blood flow to the brain), brain infections such as meningitis or encephalitis, liver or kidney disease, thiamine (vitamin B_1) deficiency, hypoglycemia, intracranial bleeding, and hypertensive encephalopathy (spasms of the central nervous system arteries caused by high blood pressure). Delirium can also follow a seizure or a traumatic brain injury.

Many medications, illegal drugs, and alcohol, used either in combination or in excess, may induce delirium directly or, if stopped abruptly after prolonged use, may lead to delirium during withdrawal. Alcoholics who stop drinking may develop delirium tremens (DTs), a particularly agitated form. Use of steroids can trigger delirium characterized by euphoria as well as disorientation. In the elderly, even standard dosages of common medications, such as digoxin (Lanoxin), may result in delirium. Some psychiatric medications, especially sedating antipsychotic, or neuroleptic, drugs such as chlorpromazine (Thorazine) and thioridazine (Mellaril), antidepressants, and lithium, can cause mild cases of delirium. So can withdrawal from benzodiazepines. Certain pesticides and solvents can also be responsible for delirium.

Although the environment alone rarely causes delirium, it can exacerbate it. This is why individuals in hospitals or nursing homes, upset by an unfamiliar, intimidating setting such as an intensive care unit, often become confused. They may be particularly vulnerable in the evening, when there is less environmental stimulation and interaction with other people; this phenomenon is sometimes called *sundowning*.

▼
How delirium feels

Delirium usually develops over a relatively short period of time. It can occur quite abruptly after head injury or a seizure, although if an illness or physical condition is the cause, individuals typically experience a prodromal period of several hours or days, during which they develop restlessness, difficulty in thinking clearly, hypersensitivity to sights and sounds, insomnia, daytime sleepiness, and vivid dreams and nightmares.

Persons with delirium cannot concentrate. Easily distracted, they have difficulty in sustaining a coherent stream of thought. In mild cases, their thoughts may seem sped up or slowed down. In severe cases, their thinking is completely disorganized, and they may be unable to name objects, tell time, or write their own names. Because their attention wanders, they may not be able to follow a normal conversation; questions must be repeated several times. They cannot reason or work toward a goal. When they talk, their speech seems fragmented and disjointed. They may ramble, make irrelevant comments, and switch from subject to subject.

Delirious patients usually know who they are but typically are confused about time, place, and situation. They invariably have problems in remembering, especially recent events. Their emotional distress can take many forms: anxiety, fear, depression, irritability, and anger. Some swing rapidly and unpredictably from one emotional state to another. Fear is very common, sometimes because of threatening hallucinations or delusions, and individuals may try to flee from or attack a supposed assailant. Because they often cannot perceive things clearly, they may mistake the slamming of a door for a pistol shot or think that a crumpled blanket is a ghost. In severe delirium, misperceptions may go beyond brief illusions and develop into hallucinations or delusions. The intravenous tubing can become a snake; strange odors are transformed into toxic gases; itching feels like insects crawling under the skin.

Affected persons are usually most lucid in the morning. As evening approaches they may become more confused. Symptoms typically worsen in the dark, when they may cry, call for help, curse, mutter, or moan.

Some individuals reverse their customary hours of sleep and wakefulness. Many become restless and agitated, groping at bed-clothes, trying to get out of bed, striking out at nonexistent objects, changing position abruptly. At other times they may be sluggish and almost catatonic, or may swing from one extreme to another. Tremors (shaking of the extremities) are common in delirious patients; heart rates speed up, they sweat more, and they also may develop a flushed face and dilated pupils.

▼

Seeking help   Friends and family members visiting a sick relative in the hospital may be the first ones to notice changes in the person's thinking and perceptions that could be early signs of delirium. In considering this possibility, these are the questions that should be asked:

- Does the person seem unaware or confused about where he or she is?
- Does he or she know the time, the day, the date, or what is happening around him or her?
- Does the person's attention wander? Does he or she seem to have difficulty concentrating?
- Does the person seem to have forgotten past events or information recently given him or her?
- Is the person's speech incoherent or rambling?
- Have these changes occurred over a fairly brief period of several hours or a day?
- Does the person seem more alert or aware at certain times of day?

If you answer "yes" to several of these questions, speak to the doctors caring for your loved one. Delirium tends to be underdiagnosed and undertreated. Physicians, who usually examine hospitalized patients in the morning, when they are most likely to be relatively calm, may not spot any indications of delirium, yet in the evening these same patients may become confused, anxious, and agitated.

Once alerted to the problem, the primary physician may call in a psychiatrist for a consultation. Delirium is in many ways similar to dementia, discussed later in this chapter. In differentiating between them, the psychiatrist looks for a recent, abrupt change in behavior, thinking, or arousal, especially when individuals have

SIGNS OF DELIRIUM

- ☐ **Fluctuations in awareness, attention, and consciousness**
- ☐ **Disorientation**
- ☐ **Hallucinations, illusions, and other distorted perceptions**
- ☐ **Incoherent speech**
- ☐ **Increased or decreased movements**
- ☐ **Impaired memory (if testable)**

not had any previous psychiatric problems. By comparison, dementia tends to be chronic and impairs mainly higher intellectual functions and memory.

One of the most common quick assessments of mental status is the Mini-Mental Status Questionnaire, which consists of ten questions, including inquiries about the month, year, and day; the patient's location; age, month, and year of birth; and the names of the current president of the United States and the previous president. More extensive tests can help in evaluating orientation, attention, recall, language, and memory. Additional medical tests, such as blood chemistry, urinalysis, electrocardiogram (ECG), electroencephalogram (EEG), chest x-ray, brain imaging scans, screening for drugs, and checks of vitamin levels and blood gases, may be needed to identify the underlying cause of delirium. Because drugs are often a factor, it is important for a consulting psychiatrist to review all medications the patient has been taking.

Risks and complications

Individuals with delirium can suffer injuries from falling out of bed or attempting to run from frightening hallucinations. If inadequately or belatedly treated, delirium may lead to dementia or lasting brain damage, and in some cases may progress to coma, from which the patient may or may not emerge.

Delirium is linked with an increased risk for death. About one-fourth of hospital patients who develop delirium die within three or four months of its onset. This high mortality rate is due in part to the illnesses that cause delirium; other contributing factors include the delirium itself, particularly if untreated, and the individual's age and general condition.

Treating delirium

Ideally, a team of physicians in different specialties—a psychiatrist, internist, and neurologist, for example—work together to identify and treat the underlying cause of the delirium. In severe cases, emergency treatments, such as administration of oxygen or thiamine or lowering of body temperature in cases of high fever,

SIGNS OF DEMENTIA

- ☐ **Decline in intellectual capacity so severe that the person can no longer function normally**

- ☐ **Fewer hour-to-hour fluctuations in awareness and attention than in delirium**

- ☐ **Inability to remember words, concepts, or skills**

- ☐ **Impaired memory, particularly in the short-term memory**

- ☐ **Change in personality**

may be necessary to prevent brain damage. Because delirium is unpredictable, hospitalized patients require close monitoring, which may mean one-on-one nursing or video observation. Agitated and restless individuals are often fearful and paranoid and may be belligerent, combative, or assaultive, possibly injuring themselves or others. Those in danger of falling from bed are sometimes placed on a mattress on the floor. Physical restraints should be avoided, if possible, because they may worsen agitation and cause painful bruises as patients struggle against them.

Once the medical team has determined the reason for the delirium, they can treat the underlying medical problem. Physicians may prescribe various medications to help individuals sleep, to calm them during the day, or to alleviate psychotic symptoms. Antipsychotic medications, such as haloperidol (Haldol), help to reduce the psychosis-like symptoms of delirium. Lorazepam (Ativan) is often given in combination with haloperidol to ease anxiety; this allows physicians to use much lower doses of the antipsychotic drug and thus minimize its side effects. Once symptoms are controlled, the physician should re-evaluate the need for continuing medication.

Because the environment can contribute to an individual's disorientation, it often helps to leave a light on at night, provide calendars and clocks, and use a radio or television to help with orientation and stimulation. Family members can help by putting photographs or cherished objects near the person's bed, staying with him or her, telling the day and date, making sure the room is well-lit, and explaining, clearly and simply, what is happening—for example, that a nurse or physician has come into the room. Reading the daily newspaper or talking about radio or television news can help patients focus on the here and now.

▼

Impact on relationships

Delirium can be frightening to witness, and family members are often shocked and fearful. It is important that they receive clear information from the doctors and other health care professionals. The more they understand about the nature of delirium, the better

The boy in the old man's body

At sixty-eight, Charlie always had a twinkle in his eye, a quip on his lips, and a compliment for the ladies. "I'm a boy in an old man's body," he'd say with a sly wink. His health had always been fairly good. He had suffered a mild heart attack in his early sixties, wore a hearing aid, complained about his legs aching after a walk, and had had a cataract removed. Living at home with his wife, Eileen, Charlie remained active. But lately he had been having a lot of chest pain, not just when he was up and about but even when he was taking it easy and lying down. After extensive tests, his doctor recommended coronary bypass surgery.

Charlie sailed through the operation without any problems, and the next day, in the cardiac intensive care unit, he seemed to be recovering well. But then he developed problems concentrating. He was easily distracted, and his thoughts seemed slowed down. He would try to ask for some water but could not come up with the word he needed. He didn't seem to be paying attention to questions. "Are you cold?" Eileen repeated several times. "The car," he responded. "You've got to park the car." At times Charlie didn't seem to know where he was or why.

"Something's wrong with Charlie's mind," Eileen told his doctor when he came to evaluate him. "What is it?"

"I'm not sure," he replied. "I'm calling in a consultation psychiatrist." The psychiatrist administered some tests to assess Charlie's mental status. His diagnosis: delirium, a not uncommon occurrence after heart surgery. Since Charlie was becoming more agitated and combative, he prescribed a combination of haloperidol (Haldol), an antipsychotic medication, and a short-acting benzo-diazepine called lorazepam (Ativan).

Because the room air that Charlie was breathing might not have been providing him with sufficient oxygen, his doctors inserted a nasal tube to ensure an adequate supply. To help with his orientation, they asked Eileen to bring in a bedside clock and a calendar, along with some family photos. She took up a position at his side, talking to him about where he was, what was happening, what each nurse or doctor was doing. She made a point of reading the newspaper to him every morning and watching the evening news with him on television.

Within a few days, Charlie's mental confusion had cleared. He was making jokes with the staff, complaining about the food, and asking to go home. "For a while there, you were sounding like an old man," Eileen teased him. "I'm glad to see that the boy in you is back."

they can respond to the person's needs and provide both reassurance and help with orientation.

▼
Outlook   Delirium is usually brief, lasting from a day to a week, although rare cases persist for more than a month, and individuals who have been deprived of oxygen for a long period—for example, for several minutes after a cardiac arrest—may experience confusion for weeks or months. Depending on their age, the duration of the delirium, and its cause, with early diagnosis and appropriate treatment most people recover completely, although they may not remember all or parts of the experience. In cases where the delirium does not improve, the individual may gradually develop another brain disorder, such as dementia. Especially for the elderly,

delirium is associated with a high incidence of death in the
months after discharge from the hospital.

Dementia

Dementia consists of persistent, multiple cognitive impairments that affect memory, language, thinking, emotion, and
personality. Its effects are severe enough to interfere significantly
with a person's work, usual social activities, or relationships. The
cognitive changes characteristic of dementia are not an aspect
of normal aging or the result of congenital brain deficits; rather,
they are consequences of one or more medical conditions, other
malfunctions, or reactions to medications or substance abuse.
(Chapter 25 discusses the effects of aging on the mind and brain.)

As the population ages, dementia, primarily a disorder of the
elderly, is becoming a major health challenge. According to the
U.S. Congress Office of Technology Assessment, if the ranks of
older Americans grow as projected, the number with severe
dementia may increase by 60 percent by the year 2000 and by
100 percent by 2020.

Individuals with dementia show less hour-to-hour variation in
their thinking than those with delirium. As a rule, dementia is
more chronic and difficult to treat than delirium, although this
is not always the case. In fact, individuals with chronic dementia
are more susceptible to developing delirium.

In the past many people believed that dementia was progressive,
always worsened, and could not be reversed. Medical science still
has not pinpointed specific causes and treatments for many forms of
dementia, but there has been great progress in relieving the suffering
and improving the functioning of even severely impaired individuals.
Whether dementia is chronic, progressive, or reversible depends on
what has caused it and, to some degree, on timely treatment.

▼

**How common is
dementia?**

According to government estimates, 4 million Americans suffer
from severe dementia, and 1 to 5 million may have mild to moderate dementia. Two to 4 percent of those over age sixty-five have
Alzheimer's disease; other dementias are less common. The likelihood of dementia increases with age; it is most prevalent among
individuals over the age of eighty-five.

▼

**What causes
dementia?**

There are more than seventy possible causes of dementia. Some,
like Alzheimer's disease, affect the cerebral cortex, the cap of
deeply grooved tissue in which the brain's higher powers are located; they mainly impair memory, speech, and other aspects of

cortical functioning. Others, such as dementia caused by HIV infection, affect the deep gray and white matter structures in the subcortical region of the brain; they interfere most with normal arousal, attention, motivation, and information processing.

Alzheimer's disease, formally referred to as *dementia of the Alzheimer type*, accounts for 50 to 60 percent of all cases in the elderly and claims 100,000 lives a year in the United States. Scientists have recently discovered a gene associated with a high risk for Alzheimer's disease. Widespread research is seeking the causes of this devastating disease; it is believed that a virus, pathological changes in the brain, or a combination of factors may contribute to the progressive brain degeneration (especially in the cortex and basal forebrain) that characterizes Alzheimer's disease. (Chapter 25 discusses this illness in greater detail.) Recent studies have shown that taking estrogen after menopause appears to reduce a woman's risk for Alzheimer's disease and to lessen the severity of symptoms in women who do develop it.

Pick's disease, a progressive, degenerative disorder of the frontal and temporal lobes of the brain, produces very different changes in the brain than does Alzheimer's disease, but its symptoms and course are similar.

Vascular dementia, much less common than Alzheimer's disease (although it may occur along with it), is the result of cerebrovascular disease; that is, of problems within the blood vessels of the brain. As a result of clots or bleeding within the brain—what physicians sometimes refer to as "mini-" or "silent" strokes—part of the brain is deprived of blood, which causes neurons to die. Whereas "major" strokes, or cerebrovascular accidents, may cause a loss of movement in an arm or leg or interfere with speech and comprehension, these mini-strokes cause subtle changes in the brain's higher intellectual capacities (such as memory).

Individuals over the age of sixty are most likely to suffer vascular dementia; this condition is more common in men than in women. The risk factors are the same as for major strokes: high blood pressure, heart disease, cigarette smoking, diabetes, excessive alcohol consumption (more than three drinks a day), and high cholesterol levels.

A tremendous variety of effects can develop in vascular dementia, depending on the location and extent of the brain damage. Usually the initial incident of cognitive impairment occurs abruptly and is followed by a gradual recovery, seemingly to a plateau of normal functioning. Then the person suffers another mini-stroke and shows sudden, significant losses in cognitive ability and functioning. The plateau that ensues after this second incident is at a new and lower level. Individuals with vascular dementia are more aware of their impairments, and more distressed by them, than are those with Alzheimer's disease.

Other causes of dementia include traumatic brain injury; metabolic disorders (pernicious anemia, folic acid deficiency, hypothyroidism); neurological diseases (Huntington's disease, multiple sclerosis, Parkinson's disease); severe hypoglycemia; and infectious diseases (including syphilis and HIV). (Chapter 24 discusses the effects of HIV on the brain and mind.)

Certain substances, including alcohol, inhalants, and sedative-hypnotic or anti-anxiety drugs, can cause brain damage and lead to dementia, which may develop during their use or within six weeks of stopping them. Dementia can also result from a combination of causes, such as concurrent medical conditions (for example, Alzheimer's and cerebrovascular disease) or a medical condition accompanied by chronic substance abuse. In some cases there is no identifiable cause.

When major depression interferes with memory and thought processes, it can create what mental health professionals call a *pseudodementia*. However, as psychiatrist Michael Wise, M.D., notes, "There is nothing 'pseudo' about the cognitive impairment in some depressed patients." When the depression is treated, memory and cognitive functioning usually improve.

▼

How dementia feels

There is no such thing as a typical case of dementia. Its signs and symptoms vary greatly, depending on the cause, course, and severity of the underlying disease or problem, the region of the brain most affected, and the individual's personality before the dementia.

Memory impairment is the most prominent characteristic of dementia. In mild cases there is moderate memory loss, especially for recent events, names, telephone numbers, directions, conversations, and events of the day. In more severe cases, individuals may not be able to finish tasks because they forget to return to them after an interruption. They may leave water running in the sink or not turn off the stove. Eventually they may forget the names of their close relatives, their own occupations, their birthdays, occasionally even their own names. Unable to make even simple decisions, they may not discard the most useless objects, such as empty bottles or old newspapers.

In an effort to cope with decreasing mental abilities, people with dementia may establish a rigid pattern for daily life and avoid any departure from the routine, such as traveling, socializing, or trying unfamiliar tasks. Some try to conceal or compensate for memory gaps by relating events in minute detail. They may become increasingly paranoid, accusing others of thefts, betrayal, or plotting against them. Increasingly fearful, they may add more locks to their doors and spend more time behind them.

As cognitive impairment worsens, it becomes impossible to maintain the facade of normality, especially during illness or under stress. Nevertheless, the erratic behaviors associated with dementia are not necessarily related to the degree of impairment. Persons with relatively mild dementia can show extreme emotional and behavioral changes, whereas severe dementia may produce apathy, lethargy, diminished activity, sleepiness, or an emotional numbing.

The personalities of individuals with dementia often change. Sometimes characteristic personality traits, such as impulsiveness or stubbornness, intensify and become more rigid, so that the person seems exactly the same as always—only more so. Others may become markedly different in their usual behaviors, as when a fastidious person turns slovenly or an easygoing one tense, irritable, and cantankerous. Inhibitions often loosen, and individuals may disregard social norms, urinating outdoors, using vulgar language, telling smutty jokes. A cautious businessman may start betting on long shots at the track; an affluent widow may shoplift; a kindly grandfather may expose himself.

Initially people with dementia, especially that induced by vascular problems, may realize to some extent that their mental powers are deteriorating and react by becoming depressed or anxious. When a health professional examines them and confronts them with evidence of their memory loss, some feel deep anguish. Physical and psychosocial stressors, such as the death of a spouse or friend, minor surgery, or retirement, can make their intellectual and emotional difficulties worse.

In Alzheimer's disease, individuals typically have little, if any, awareness of their growing inability to think clearly or to remember directions, keep appointments, or pay bills. Over time they experience more difficulty with daily activities. Eventually they become so impaired that they may no longer be capable of any self-care at all, such as bathing or using the toilet. They may wear the same clothes day after day or put one layer of clothing on top of another. Many develop delusions about relatives plotting against them or a spouse having an affair. As their confusion intensifies, they may cling to family members, pace constantly, finger buttons and clothing, wrap and unwrap bits of string. In time they may not even recognize their own faces in the mirror. In the final stages of Alzheimer's disease, which is ultimately fatal, they can no longer speak and are unable to sit up or walk.

▼

Seeking help The early signs of dementia—memory loss, insomnia, irritability, sensitivity to alcohol and other drugs, decreased energy, and intolerance of frustration—are usually subtle and insidious. Friends and family may suspect a problem but often act only when the person's behavior becomes so erratic, irresponsible, or dangerous that they cannot put it off any longer. Sometimes dementia is diagnosed only when a person becomes ill, needs to be hospitalized, and is observed by a physician to have serious memory loss.

If you suspect that someone close to you may be suffering from dementia, these are the questions that should be asked:

- Is the individual forgetful or unable to learn new information?
- Is the person having difficulty remembering things he or she once knew?
- Does he or she have difficulty speaking?
- Is he or she unable to perform simple tasks even though comprehension and motor skills seem normal?
- Is the person unable to recognize and identify objects?
- Does he or she have difficulty planning, organizing, putting things into sequence, or comprehending abstract ideas?
- Have problems in thinking greatly interfered with the individual's usual social or occupational functioning?

If you answer "yes" to several of these questions, the problem could be dementia, and you should discuss it with your loved one's primary physician or a consulting psychiatrist.

Physicians diagnose dementia on the basis of a comprehensive assessment of an individual's medical history, physical health, and mental status. They try to find out whether symptoms developed suddenly or gradually, which medications and drugs the person may have taken, whether there has been a stressful or traumatic experience, such as the illness of a spouse, and whether there is a history of chronic alcohol abuse. They also distinguish among the symptoms produced by various types of dementia, including Alzheimer's, vascular dementia, and dementias caused by certain other medical conditions or substances.

In diagnosing Alzheimer's disease, psychiatrists must determine that no other condition or cause is responsible for the symptoms. To confirm this, they may perform a combination of physical, psychiatric, and neurological examinations, including brain scans. Until recently this diagnosis was difficult to pinpoint, but new tests hold greater promise of precision, which is crucial because many conditions, including brain tumors, infections, abnormal thyroid function, vitamin and nutritional deficiencies, alcoholism, and a series of small strokes, can mimic Alzheimer's disease. A diagnosis of vascular dementia is based on the same symptoms of cognitive disturbance, along with characteristic findings from neurological testing (such as abnormal reflexes), signs of lesions in computed tomography (CT) or magnetic resonance imaging (MRI) brain scans, and abnormalities on EEG or ECG tests.

▼

Risks and complications

Individuals with dementia can be so disoriented and irrational that they put themselves in danger. They may wander and become lost, attack others, or develop delirium. They are more susceptible than others to accidents and potentially fatal infectious diseases, such as pneumonia.

▼

Treating dementia

The earlier and more accurately that dementia is detected, the greater the hope of preserving healthy brain tissue and halting or slowing the degeneration of neurons. Treatment depends on the type of dementia diagnosed. For dementia caused by substance abuse, withdrawal from alcohol and/or drugs would be the first step. Dementias caused by infections, thyroid malfunction, or vitamin deficiencies improve with appropriate treatment of those conditions. When dementia is caused by blood vessel disease in the brain, low-dose aspirin can help to prevent blood clots and further damage caused by blockage of blood flow. Antihypertension medication can also reduce such risks.

The environment is a key component of treatment because cognitively impaired individuals are highly sensitive to too much or too little stimulation. They do best in consistent, familiar surroundings, with structured daily routines, prominently displayed clocks and calendars, night-lights, checklists, and diaries. Even those hospitalized or institutionalized with severe dementia benefit from adequate rest, exercise, balanced and regular meals, elimination of nonessential drugs, photographs and other familiar objects from home, frequent family visits, and updates on current events through newspapers, radio, or television.

As many as 30 percent of those with dementia also suffer from depression. Persons who are aware of their cognitive impairment may benefit from therapy that helps them to grieve for their losses, accept their disability, and make the most of their remaining abilities and skills. There are few data on whether antidepressants help in treating those who have both depression and dementia.

Treatments for Alzheimer's disease focus on controlling abnormal behavior associated with this type of dementia and trying to enhance or restore as much cognitive ability as possible. Low doses of antipsychotic medications are often used for agitation, wandering, suspiciousness, hallucinations, and hostility.

The first specific medication for Alzheimer's disease is tacrine (Cognex). By inhibiting the enzyme cholinesterase, this drug increases levels of acetylcholine, a neurotransmitter important for memory that is deficient in Alzheimer's disease. Tacrine has produced modest cognitive improvement for about one-third of those who try it; other compounds similar to it are expected to become available soon. Side effects, some of which may make it necessary to discontinue the drug temporarily or permanently, include elevation of liver enzymes, nausea, vomiting, abdominal pain, and diarrhea.

Impact on relationships

Dementia can take an enormous toll on relatives. In severe cases they must watch helplessly as a loved one slowly becomes a stranger to them, and vice versa. It can be devastating when a demented parent shows no hint of kinship and no longer recognizes an adult child. Education and counseling can help the family understand why this has happened and what is causing the emotional swings and loss of inhibitions they are witnessing—behaviors that uninformed relatives may not realize are beyond the person's control.

Family members providing care for individuals with dementia need psychological support as they deal with feelings of anger, guilt, shame, frustration, and helplessness, and with the strain of providing constant care. If a parent or spouse is the patient, some caregivers may also need to deal with unresolved issues and conflicts in those relationships.

Counseling on how to help and what to expect is very useful. Health care professionals should work closely with family members caring for persons with dementia at home so they can anticipate and prevent problems. For example, caregivers need to understand that it may be best to avoid rushing or pushing patients to do things beyond their ability. Even well-intentioned attempts to assist them in getting dressed or taking a bath can trigger angry, even aggressive outbursts. It is easy for caregivers to interpret these reactions as rejection or ingratitude, but such episodes may not be deliberate or conscious. Often the demented individual switches mood and forgets the entire incident within minutes.

In severe cases of dementia, when families must confront the difficult decision of whether to seek nursing home care, mental health professionals can be very helpful in letting family members explore their feelings. Group therapy can provide both educational and emotional support. The Alzheimer's Disease and Related Disorders Association (ADRDA), a national organization of family members, has local chapters throughout the country (see the Resource Directory at the back of the book).

Outlook

The outlook for dementia varies greatly. About 20 percent of dementias are reversible, including those caused by depression and hypothyroidism, heavy metal poisoning (as with lead), medications (a common problem in nursing home residents), and chronic alcohol abuse. In about 30 percent of dementias, treatment can help to maintain current functioning but cannot reverse previous deterioration. In about half of cases nothing can be done, and the dementia slowly progresses, in a generally deteriorating course over a period of several years, until it culminates in death. In such cases, health professionals try to make individuals as comfortable as possible while dealing with problems such as nighttime wandering, incontinence, and violent behavior.

Amnesia

Amnesia is an impairment of short- and long-term memory caused by a disease, drug, or injury. (Loss of memory for psychological reasons is discussed in Chapter 18.) Persons with amnesia cannot learn new material or recall recent events, although they may remember events of the remote past. Thus, someone might recall in vivid detail a hospital stay of a decade before but not realize that he or she is currently hospitalized. Usually people with amnesia know who they are and answer to their names, but may not know where they are or what the date is. Some make up imaginary events to fill in memory gaps; this is called *confabulation*. Most are not aware of their memory deficits and may deny that anything is wrong. Others acknowledge a problem but appear unconcerned.

Amnesia is common in head injury. Trauma to the brain can stretch and twist neuronal axons, the long fibers crucial for conveying messages between neurons. As the result of this damage, individuals may suffer *posttraumatic amnesia*, consisting of unconsciousness; *retrograde amnesia*, the inability to recall events in the past, which can range from a few minutes before the injury to a few years; and *anteretrograde amnesia*, ongoing problems remembering new information. These trauma-induced memory problems can last from a few hours to months after the injury.

Chronic, heavy alcohol use can lead to thiamine (vitamin B_1) deficiency and the development of Korsakoff's syndrome, a complete inability to learn new material. Individuals with this problem can usually still recall information from the past. If they abstain from alcohol, many show cognitive improvement, but there may be some remaining impairment.

Other causes of amnesia include stroke, brain tumors, repeated or severe hypoglycemia in people with poorly controlled diabetes, current or recent substance use (especially of sedative-hypnotic or anti-anxiety drugs), damage to certain structures in the brain caused by surgery, insufficient oxygen, a cutoff of blood flow, or infection.

Some people, most often men between the ages of fifty and eighty, experience *transient global amnesia* and are unable to recall events in the past or to learn new information for a period of several hours. The causes of this temporary amnesia are unknown, although conditions such as epilepsy, cerebrovascular disease, migraine, and drug overdose have come under suspicion. It is not clear whether physical or emotional stress may trigger such episodes. Usually memory returns without treatment, and recurrences are rare.

A psychiatric interview and assessment can reveal the extent of memory loss. According to the *DSM-IV*, the key diagnostic criteria for amnesia are:

- Memory impairment as manifested by the inability to learn new information or to recall previously learned information
- Significant occupational or social impairment or decline from previous level of functioning because of the memory disturbance
- The memory disturbance does not occur only during course of delirium or dementia or intoxication with or withdrawal from a substance
- Evidence that the memory disturbance is a consequence of a medical condition or substance use.

The primary medical focus is treating the underlying cause. Thus, large doses of thiamine may be given to individuals with chronic alcoholism and a thiamine deficiency; in other cases, the infection or injury is treated.

Is it a personality disorder?

Individuals with a personality disorder may:

☐ **Have persistent difficulties in various aspects of their lives**

☐ **Be unable to get along with others or to form and maintain relationships**

☐ **Tend to blame others, luck, or circumstances for whatever goes wrong**

☐ **Repeatedly lie, try to manipulate others, or violate the law or social norms, with no remorse or guilt**

☐ **Have poor control of their emotions and impulses, get involved in intense, stormy relationships, and behave self-destructively**

☐ **Crave constant attention and be extremely emotional and concerned with their appearance**

☐ **Have a grandiose sense of self-importance and entitlement and need admiration**

☐ **Desperately fear being alone, have an excessive need to be taken care of, and be submissive and clinging**

☐ **Feel uncomfortable around other people, have low self-esteem, and be hypersensitive to possible criticism or rejection**

☐ **Be perfectionistic, preoccupied with details and orderliness, and concerned with control**

☐ **Distrust others, be extremely suspicious, and question the loyalty or trustworthiness of friends and associates without reason**

☐ **Not enjoy or lack interest in social relationships and have a restricted range of emotional expression**

☐ **Be acutely uncomfortable with close relationships, have distorted thoughts or perceptions, and behave in odd or eccentric ways**

If you or someone close to you checks several of these boxes, you may want to learn more about specific personality disorders. This chapter provides information on recognizing and understanding these common problems, and guidance on obtaining appropriate treatment.

21

Personality Disorders

A woman finds herself falling in and out of love with a series of men, each of whom initially seems perfect yet turns out to be anything but. A young man yearns for close relationships but is so fearful of rejection that he barely speaks to other people. Brooding over past injustices, a manager is on constant lookout for signs of sabotage or betrayal. Consumed with getting the details absolutely perfect, a bright, hard-working graduate student consistently misses project deadlines and gets poor grades.

These individuals do not believe that they have a problem. In fact, they don't see anything at all wrong with their own behavior. Even though their lives are filled with disappointment and difficulty, they blame everyone and everything else for these outcomes. Like others with personality disorders, they do not realize, even when it is obvious to everyone around them, that their characteristic ways of dealing with other people and with the world lead to the problems they encounter.

Many of the other mental disorders discussed in this book cause acute symptoms for a period of time. They generally improve or go into remission, although some, such as schizophrenia, obsessive-compulsive disorder, and major depression, are often chronic. The personality disorders are different: They are not difficulties that people *have* but fundamental problems about who they *are*—how they feel, how they see themselves, how they cope, how they interact with and relate to others. These disorders begin early in life and continue for years or for decades.

Personality traits—the characteristic ways that we all have of dealing with others and of facing the demands, stresses, and strains of daily living—are neither good nor bad in themselves. Suspiciousness, for instance, can help in potentially dangerous situations, such as living or working in a high-crime neighborhood. However, in some people, distrust of specific situations or individuals may develop into paranoia, the belief that everyone is out to get them. Those with a paranoid personality disorder assume that every situation, every co-worker or acquaintance, is a potential trap or threat. Locked into this rigid, unbending view, they respond with wariness to every new set of circumstances, even when such reactions are inappropriate.

The borders between healthy and unhealthy personality traits and between normal patterns of behavior and personality disorders are not clearly defined. It can be very difficult to say precisely when normal suspiciousness becomes paranoia or a vigorous sense of self-importance becomes so grandiose that it is a sign of a narcissistic personality disorder. However, only a chronic personality problem that causes great distress, interferes with an individual's ability to function or relate to others, affects many aspects of daily living, and endures for an extended period of time warrants diagnosis as a personality disorder. As with other disorders, personality disorders range from mild to severe.

Although there has been an explosion of research into these disorders since 1980, when they were recognized as a distinct category in the American Psychiatric Association's *Diagnostic and Statistical Manual of Mental Disorders (DSM)*, many questions remain unanswered. For example, there are few data on the long-term success of treatment, although many mental health professionals feel that therapy can and does help individuals with personality disorders to develop more adaptive ways of dealing with the world around them.

Types of personality disorders

The *DSM-IV* groups the ten officially recognized personality disorders into three clusters, based on the dominant characteristics they share. Each disorder is described separately later in this chapter.

Dramatic, Emotional, or Erratic

- *Antisocial personality disorder,* a pattern of irresponsible and often illegal behavior reflecting a lack of concern for the rights of others

- *Borderline personality disorder,* characterized by instability in relationships, impulsivity, and poor emotional control
- *Histrionic personality disorder,* in which individuals constantly seek attention and are extremely emotional
- *Narcissistic personality disorder,* characterized by a grandiose sense of self-worth and entitlement and a need for excessive admiration

Anxious or Fearful

- *Avoidant personality disorder,* a combination of feelings of inadequacy, social awkwardness, and extreme sensitivity to rejection or disapproval
- *Dependent personality disorder,* characterized by an enormous need to have others take charge and make decisions, submissiveness, and great fear of being left to take care of oneself
- *Obsessive-compulsive personality disorder,* characterized by perfectionism, excessive attention to details and devotion to work, and a desire for control

Odd or Eccentric

- *Paranoid personality disorder,* a pattern of unwarranted distrust and suspiciousness and doubts about others' loyalty and trustworthiness
- *Schizoid personality disorder,* characterized by a complete lack of interest in close relationships and very limited emotional expressiveness
- *Schizotypal personality disorder,* in which individuals are extremely uncomfortable in close relationships and have odd ways of thinking, talking, and acting

These clusters are what researchers call "fuzzy sets," with borders that often overlap. Most people with one personality disorder have features of others. Thus, someone with a narcissistic personality disorder may also have obsessive-compulsive and avoidant behaviors. In addition, individuals may have both a personality disorder and another mental illness, most often major depression.

▼
How common are personality disorders?   Personality disorders are common, affecting 10 to 15 percent of the population. As many as 30 to 50 percent of men and women who seek mental health care may have a personality disorder, often in addition to another psychiatric problem.

Personality disorders usually develop in childhood or adolescence and become apparent by young adulthood. Personality changes that begin later in life are likely to be the result of a major mental disorder, such as schizophrenia, or a physical illness, such as a brain tumor, and differ in kind, treatment, and prognosis.

Some disorders, such as schizotypal personality disorder, affect men and women equally. Others, among them antisocial, schizoid, and obsessive-compulsive personality disorders, are more common in men. Women are more likely to be diagnosed as having dependent or histrionic personality disorders. There has been considerable debate over whether gender bias may influence the diagnosis of specific personality disorders—for example, therapists may interpret certain behaviors in women, such as wearing revealing clothes or acting flirtatiously, as a histrionic disorder when these behaviors may simply reflect societal or cultural norms.

▼

What causes personality disorders?

The exact causes of personality disorders are not known. A variety of factors affects the way an individual's personality develops: genetic predisposition, biological differences, parental nurturance, and early childhood experiences. Nevertheless, neither nature nor nurture alone can account for personality or for personality disorders. What appears to be most crucial is the complex interaction between biological and environmental influences.

Genetic factors appear to contribute to at least some personality disorders. In an investigation of fifteen thousand pairs of twins, both twins in the identical pairs were several times more likely to develop personality disorders than were the fraternal twins. The genetic link seems to be strongest in antisocial personality disorder, a pattern of socially irresponsible behavior that is five times more common among close relatives of antisocial men than among the general population. Some individuals with a genetic predisposition to alcoholism seem to be predisposed to antisocial personality disorder as well.

Histrionic personality disorder, characterized by intense emotionality and a craving for attention, is also more common among close relatives of people with this disorder than in the population at large. There may be a genetic predisposition among close relatives of schizophrenic men and women that leads to schizotypal personality disorder, which involves odd ways of thinking, talking, and acting. There is also evidence that certain personality traits associated with various personality disorders may be inherited. An example is introversion, which can be a characteristic of schizoid, schizotypal, and avoidant personalities.

Biological differences from the norm may be found in people with certain personality disorders. In some types of schizotypal personality disorder, for example, there are irregularities similar to those observed in schizophrenia, such as abnormal eye movements that occur with the administration of certain tests, and differences in brain volume.

There are various theories about the psychological origins of personality disorders. According to Freud, certain personality types form when individuals become *fixated* or stuck at different stages of psychosexual development. For instance, fixation at the oral stage would result in a personality characterized by demanding and clinging behavior, as in dependent personality disorder. Fixation at the anal stage would lead to personalities distinguished by rigidity and emotional aloofness, as in obsessive-compulsive personality disorder, while fixation at the phallic stage would lead to shallowness and an inability to engage in intimate relationships, as in histrionic personality disorder. There is little real evidence to support Freud's hypothesis that fixation at certain stages actually leads to specific personality patterns. However, psychodynamic theory has offered insight into possible developmental origins of these disorders.

Narcissistic personality disorder, with its characteristically inflated sense of self-worth and need for admiration, for example, may arise between the ages of eighteen months and three years, when a child's sense of having an independent self emerges. If parents need children to be perfect, as often happens when parents themselves are narcissistic, youngsters who do not live up to parental expectations may be criticized, punished, or ignored. Fearing that no one could ever love them just as they are, these youngsters may develop a deep-rooted sense of being somehow repulsive or disgusting. To protect themselves from such deeply disturbing feelings, narcissistic individuals create a facade of grandiosity, self-importance, and invulnerability that masks an overwhelming sense of failure.

Environmental influences, particularly a troubled childhood, may play a major part in personality disorders. Antisocial personality disorder, for example, has been linked to a lack of consistent parental discipline, childhood abuse, and failure to develop a close attachment to parents. In borderline personality disorder there may be a history of early abandonment, physical and sexual abuse, sustained neglect, or a lack of stability that makes it difficult for individuals to maintain a firm sense of themselves or others later in life. A combination of inborn temperament and early rejection—by parents, peers, or both—may contribute to avoidant personality disorder. Children whose early relationships are cold or abusive may conclude that relationships are not worth pursuing or that they themselves are somehow deserving of abuse, factors that could lead to the lack of interest and of enjoyment of relationships that is typical of schizoid personality disorder.

Social learning and conditioning also can contribute. For example, some people with avoidant personality disorder may have been rejected or humiliated early in life; as a result, they remain excessively concerned about being watched and evaluated. Histrionic personality disorder may stem, at least in part, from a misjudgment of what is appealing and appropriate. One theory suggests that little girls who rely on their fathers as the primary source of love may conclude that the way to get men to care for them is by being coy and enticing.

External factors can also be influential. Chronic illnesses, both mental and physical, especially in children and teenagers, may foster excessive reliance on and submission to others and contribute to the development of dependent personality disorder. A disfiguring injury can contribute to avoidant personality disorder. Our fast-moving, high-stress society, with its increased mobility, high divorce rate, and constant change, may increase the risk for borderline personality disorder in susceptible individuals.

▼

How personality disorders feel

Individuals with personality disorders often do not know exactly how or what they feel, although almost all are plagued by a sense of inadequacy. Because of low self-esteem, many do not see themselves as worthy of love, admiration, or success, so they turn to other people for reassurance that they are worthwhile human beings. Without such validation they may become depressed or anxious, but because of their disorder its effects are transient, and their problems with self-esteem soon recur.

Difficulty in acknowledging, expressing, or dealing with emotions is common in personality disorders. Some people view their own emotions as not really belonging to them. Others find it hard to tolerate intense feelings or are unable to express them. Afraid of being overwhelmed by strong emotions, such as anger, sadness, or fear, they may try to avoid feeling anything at all. In other cases, persons may fluctuate between periods of emotional emptiness and sudden outbursts of extreme rage or jealousy. Once their powerful feelings are unleashed, they may find it hard to calm down, and afterwards they typically blame someone or something for "making" them feel that way. Unable to control their emotions, lives, or relationships, they feel that things are always happening *to* them and cannot see how their behavior or responses can have any impact or allow them any control.

Paranoid individuals may cope with their own feelings of hostility and resentment by projecting these emotions onto their presumed enemies. Those with borderline personalities sometimes express their unconscious wishes or conflicts by acting out, often through self-destructive behaviors like fighting or promiscuity.

The problem, as some therapists explain, is that individuals with personality disorders live within *character armor*, a system of internal defense mechanisms on which they rely to avoid or overcome feelings. Although these protective attitudes and behaviors can create great difficulty in their lives, they cling to them as the only way they know of dealing with problems. Indeed, some people with personality disorders regard feelings themselves with suspicion or contempt. Those with antisocial personality disorder may think that the fact that they don't feel guilty indicates that they haven't done anything truly wrong. Those with obsessive-compulsive personality disorder may feel morally superior to "emotional" people who lose control of their feelings.

But living in a world without feelings can be desperately lonely. Individuals with personality disorders may never really connect in a meaningful way with other people. Even when they are with others, they may feel alone. Many are exquisitely sensitive to any form of rejection, criticism, disapproval, or abandonment. Any separation or loss can be a great psychological blow.

Sometimes sex becomes a way of compensating for a lack of emotional closeness. Some people seek out sexual experiences as a way of making some intimate connection; all too often, such encounters turn out to be meaningless or unsatisfying. Some use sex to obtain the admiration and attention they crave rather than as a means of sharing tenderness. Those with avoidant, schizoid, or schizotypal personality disorders typically avoid sex because they fear any intimate contact.

The lack of feeling that can characterize many personality disorders may be physical as well as psychological. Indeed, some individuals, particularly those with borderline personality disorder, may cut, burn, or otherwise mutilate themselves, yet they literally feel no pain and may not fully recognize what they have done. For others, such acts may be a way of releasing emotions that they do not know how to express in other ways.

In severe personality disorders, individuals often have no cohesive sense of themselves. Because they lack a continuous identity, they may not have a stable sense of people close to them. When they are angry, for example, they may not be able to recall what it was that they once loved or valued in another person.

▼
Seeking help   Only about a fifth of those with personality disorders seek professional help. They go through life unintentionally making their worst expectations come true by creating difficult situations, provoking or alienating others, and making poor decisions and choices. However unhappy they may be, however frustrating or irritating others may find them, many individuals see no reason or

need to change, or are unaware that their behavior is maladaptive. Even those who do realize their personality problems may feel that there is nothing to be done about them.

If you suspect that you or someone close to you may have a personality disorder, these are the general questions that should be asked:

- Have you had long-term difficulties in various aspects of life?
- Do you have problems getting along with others or in forming and maintaining relationships?
- Do you tend to blame others or external circumstances or forces for whatever goes wrong in your life?
- Do you find yourself repeatedly deceiving or manipulating others or violating laws or social norms? Do you feel an absence of guilt about these actions?
- Do you find it difficult to control your emotions and impulses? Does your life consist of dramatic highs and lows, volatile relationships, and/or self-destructive behavior?
- Are you extremely emotional? Do you want to be noticed more by others? Do you constantly seek attention by dressing or behaving in a dramatic way?
- Do you feel uniquely gifted and deserving of special treatment and admiration? At the same time, do you have doubts about your basic worthiness?
- Are you so fearful of abandonment and separation that you cling to those around you and want them to take care of you?
- Are you uncomfortable in social situations and overly sensitive to any hint of rejection or criticism?
- Are you a perfectionist who prizes control and orderliness? Do you find it hard to be open in expressing your feelings?
- Are you mistrustful and suspicious of others? Do you doubt the loyalty and honesty of your friends and co-workers, even though you have no reason to do so?
- Do you lack interest in and fail to get enjoyment from relationships? Are you aware of feeling only a limited range of emotions?
- Are you extremely uncomfortable in close relationships? Are you aware of any distortions in the way you think or perceive things around you?
- Have you been feeling great distress or been unable to keep up your usual relationships and activities because of problems in dealing with others?

If you or someone close to you answers "yes" to several of these questions, the problem could be a personality disorder. Typically, individuals with these disorders do not recognize their problem, and seek help for other difficulties, such as depression, substance abuse, or marital conflict. In fact, such difficulties may stem from an underlying personality disorder, and both may require treatment.

The diagnosis of a personality disorder is based on a comprehensive psychiatric interview that may include a detailed history and description of troubling symptoms, the therapist's clinical experience and judgment, and professionally administered assessments or inventories of behaviors. A thorough physical examination can rule out medical and neurological changes that mimic personality disorders. In making their evaluation, mental health professionals have to ascertain that the source of maladaptive traits, such as withdrawal or low self-esteem, is a personality disorder rather than another psychiatric problem, such as depression.

▼

Risks and complications

Although most individuals with personality disorders are able to get jobs without much difficulty, they may find it hard to keep them. They often get into conflicts with co-workers or supervisors or become increasingly frustrated by the demands or limitations of their work. Feeling exploited or unrecognized, they may quit impulsively or be fired. Many who are bright and talented never find jobs that match their abilities and move from one type of work to another fairly often.

Individuals with personality disorders have chronic problems in many other aspects of their lives. They have higher than usual rates of separation, divorce, child custody disputes, accidents, criminal activity, and emergency room visits, and are at increased risk for developing major mental disorders, particularly depression, substance abuse, and alcoholism. Men and women with borderline personality disorder are at risk for dysthymia (chronic mild depression), self-mutilation, and psychotic disorders, such as brief reactive psychosis, and some 5 to 10 percent take their own lives. Antisocial personality disorder increases the risk for substance abuse, alcoholism, vagrancy, suicide, and violent death, including fatal car accidents.

▼

Treating personality disorders

Personality disorders consist of deeply ingrained attitudes and behaviors that cannot be changed quickly. For this reason, mental health professionals used to be pessimistic about treating these problems. This is changing, however, because of recent reports indicating that several forms of psychotherapy can be effective. Treatment of specific disorders is discussed later in this chapter.

The best-established treatment for all these disorders is psychodynamic psychotherapy, which helps people learn better ways

Is it a personality disorder?

According to the DSM-IV, *these are the general diagnostic features for a personality disorder:*

- An enduring pattern of inner experience and behavior that deviates markedly from the expectations of the individual's culture and that occurs in at least two of the following areas:
  1. Cognition (ways of perceiving and interpreting self, other people, and events)
  2. Affectivity (the range, intensity, lability, and appropriateness of emotional responses)
  3. Interpersonal functioning
  4. Impulse control

- The pattern is inflexible and pervasive across a broad range of personal and social situations.

- Significant distress or impairment in social, occupational, or other important areas of functioning as a consequence of the pattern

- The pattern is stable and of long duration, with an onset that can be traced back at least to adolescence or early adulthood.

- The pattern is not better accounted for as a sign or consequence of another mental disorder.

- The pattern is not due to the direct effects of a substance (either a medication or drug of abuse) or medical condition (e.g., head trauma).

Adapted from the Diagnostic and Statistical Manual of Mental Disorders, 4th Edition. *Used with permission.*

of coping, improve everyday functioning, and develop gratifying relationships. The interaction between the therapist and the person seeking help is of the greatest importance because it serves as a model that enables individuals to learn relationship skills they may never have mastered before.

Supportive psychotherapy helps people with personality disorders through periods of stress. Cognitive-behavioral strategies typically work toward reducing impulsivity or increasing assertiveness, often by means of role-playing or relaxation exercises. Cognitive therapy focuses on irrational and distorted thinking styles, which are common in personality disorders. Behavioral therapies can alleviate specific symptoms, such as difficulty in voicing opinions. Interpersonal therapy is effective because personality disorders always involve problems in relating to others. Group therapy can help individuals recognize inappropriate or irritating behaviors and their effects on others. Marital therapy can enable couples to find more healthful ways of relating to each other and to the outside world.

Researchers are exploring a possible role for psychiatric medications in certain of these conditions. Long used to treat accompanying disorders, such as anxiety or depression, these medications also may have a direct effect on the characteristic symptoms of some personality disorders. For example, serotonin-boosting drugs, such as the selective serotonin reuptake inhibitors (SSRIs) and other antidepressants, seem to help in controlling impulsivity, aggression, and mood swings.

Because personality disorders can involve severe depression or anxiety, episodes of self-destructiveness, and an increased risk for suicide, often along with drug and alcohol abuse, some people may require hospitalization to prevent them from harming themselves or others. Usually such hospital stays are brief, and psychotherapy continues both during and after them.

▼
Impact on relationships
Men and women with personality disorders are often viewed as difficult human beings who cannot get along with others, whether at home, at work, or socially. Some do indeed have undesirable or unpleasant traits, such as being paranoid, overdramatic, or manipulative, but many, if not most, are simply lonely, isolated, anxious, or dependent. What they have in common with those with more irritating traits is consistent difficulty in forming healthy, satisfying relationships.

The behavior of individuals with personality disorders can be hard for anyone to understand. Because they tend to think in all-or-nothing terms, they look at another person as either perfect in every way or hopelessly flawed. They expect (and give) unconditional love or none at all. Their swings back and forth from one extreme to another, from idealization to contempt, can leave friends and family members confused, hurt, and in a constant state of tension, never knowing what to expect and feeling helpless about improving matters. Family therapy often is critical if relatives are to understand more about personality disorders and to work to change unhealthy patterns of relating.

Specific personality disorders may have differing effects on relationships. Antisocial individuals usually cannot sustain lasting, close, warm, and responsible relationships with anyone. Because they cannot tolerate being alone, borderline individuals may frantically seek companionship or become very dependent on the few close friends they do have. Histrionic individuals, who also hate to be alone, often use their flirtatious, seductive behavior to attract friends or would-be sexual partners, but because what they are really seeking is attention or reassurance, their intimate relationships tend to be ungratifying. The relationships of narcissistic persons are almost always troubled. They tend to exploit others and take advantage of friends to meet their special needs.

Avoidant men and women often live in the protected environments their families create. Those who are faced with the opportunity to enter into a relationship may become angry, anxious, or depressed. A secure, protective relationship is so important to some dependent individuals that they endure mistreatment because they fear abandonment. Others become so needy and clinging that they drive away partners.

Paranoid, schizoid, and schizotypal individuals often avoid any intimate relationships at all, which can be extremely distressing to family members who try to connect with their loved ones. Those with obsessive-compulsive personality disorder may place a higher value on work than on other people, and their difficulty in expressing cordiality toward others makes them seem aloof, cold, or indifferent.

Specific personality disorders

Following are descriptions of the ten personality disorders officially recognized in the *DSM-IV*, grouped according to the clusters in which they fit.

ANTISOCIAL PERSONALITY DISORDER

Individuals who, although capable of reasoning, violated society's moral code were once described as "morally insane." The term used today, *antisocial personality disorder*, refers to a pattern of behavior that is socially irresponsible, disregards or violates the rights of others, exploits and possibly harms others, and provokes no remorse in the perpetrator. This disorder poses a difficult dilemma for mental health professionals: On the one hand it should not serve as an excuse for antisocial acts, yet on the other it is a long-recognized form of true psychic impairment.

Sociopaths, as persons with this disorder are sometimes called, seem born to be bad. From early childhood they are incapable of following rules. As youngsters, they skip school, bully, steal, torment animals, run away from home, and are likely to develop attention-deficit/hyperactivity disorder (AD/HD) or a conduct disorder (see Chapter 26). As adults they habitually lie, and they cannot hold down a job for long or maintain a close relationship. Although they can seem charming in superficial social interactions, they repeatedly hurt, anger, and exploit others, and may cheat, rob, harass, or injure them. Yet whatever laws they break, whomever they hurt, whatever trouble they get into, they feel no guilt. Even when punished, they show no regret. In fact, they often feel that their behavior, however cruel or selfish, is justified.

An individual with antisocial personality disorder may:

- Be glib or superficial

- Have a grandiose self-image

- Be deceitful or manipulative

- Lack remorse

- Lack empathy

- Be impulsive

- Be irresponsible

- Be easily angered or frustrated

- Have had serious behavior problems as a child and teenager

- Show callous unconcern for others' feelings

- Disregard social norms or the rights of other people

- Be unable to maintain enduring relationships

- Be incapable of experiencing guilt

- Blame others or offer rationalizations for antisocial behavior

- Be constantly irritable.

▼

Understanding antisocial personality disorder

Antisocial individuals stir little sympathy because they hurt others without apparent compunction. Yet although others look at them as tough and resilient, they often are extremely fragile psychologically. Beneath what one psychiatrist has called their "mask of sanity" are tension, hostility, irritability, and rage. Mental health professionals who have worked closely with antisocial individuals report an emptiness, as well as a sadness, at the core of their personality.

Antisocial individuals are defiant and contemptuous of standards for accepted conduct. At an unusually early age, even for their peer group, they often use tobacco, alcohol, or other drugs, and become sexually active. Irritable and aggressive, they tend to get into fights. Paying little heed to their personal safety, they live recklessly and regularly take dangerous risks. They lie easily, can be skillful con artists, often do not repay debts, and squander whatever money they get. Many are drifters who never settle down for any period of time. Traveling aimlessly, they may look for work haphazardly or do whatever they "have to" to get by, including stealing, dealing in drugs, or engaging in other forms of criminal activity. They are indifferent to those they harm or mistreat and may rationalize their behavior by saying the victim "had it coming to him" or using another glib excuse. They are "watching out for number one" and feel that everyone else is doing the same.

Crime is, in fact, closely linked with this disorder. Some estimates suggest that antisocial personality disorder is found in as

Is it antisocial personality disorder?

According to the DSM-IV, a diagnosis of antisocial personality disorder should be based on these features:

■ **A pervasive pattern of disregard for and violation of the rights of others, occurring since age fifteen, as indicated by at least three of the following:**

1. **Failure to conform to social norms for lawful behavior, as indicated by repeatedly performing illegal acts that are grounds for arrest**

2. **Deceitfulness, as indicated by repeated lying, use of aliases, or conning others for personal profit or pleasure**

3. **Impulsivity or failure to plan ahead**

4. **Irritability and aggressiveness, as indicated by repeated physical fights or assaults**

5. **Reckless disregard for safety of self or others**

6. **Consistent irresponsibility, as indicated by repeated failure to keep a job or honor financial obligations**

7. **Lack of remorse, as indicated by indifference or rationalizations for having hurt, mistreated, or stolen from others**

■ **Eighteen years of age or older**

■ **Evidence of a conduct disorder that began before age fifteen**

■ **Antisocial behavior does not occur only during the course of schizophrenia or a manic episode of bipolar illness.**

Adapted from the Diagnostic and Statistical Manual of Mental Disorders, 4th Edition. *Used with permission.*

many as 75 percent of those in prison. Alcohol abuse may be both a contributing cause and a consequence of antisocial behavior, and those who are both antisocial and alcoholic seem particularly prone to violent crimes.

Not everyone with antisocial personality disorder becomes a criminal, but even those who remain law-abiding may act in exploitative, irresponsible, or deceptive ways. They typically are promiscuous, rarely remaining in a monogamous relationship for more than a year. As spouses they tend to be glib, superficial, manipulative, dishonest, abusive, and unfaithful, and those who have children may neglect them or fail to keep them safe. Although they show no remorse about mistreating or hurting others, they frequently report their conviction (often correct) that others are hostile toward them.

In community surveys, 3 percent of men and 1 percent of women have antisocial personality disorder. This diagnosis, which is not used for individuals under age eighteen, peaks between the ages of twenty-four and forty-four, then drops sharply thereafter. After the age of thirty, behaviors such as fighting and criminality diminish, although the disorder can persist into the sixties and seventies. Although older individuals are less likely to get into trouble with the law, they continue to have problems, such as unstable relationships, substance abuse, impulsiveness, poor temper control, and failure to honor financial obligations.

▼

Treating antisocial personality disorder

Antisocial personality disorder can be extremely difficult to treat, although it does tend to remit or become less obvious as individuals enter their thirties. Those who are pressed (or forced) into psychotherapy by family members, employers, or the law may have no desire to change and can find it hard to tolerate the intimacy required in psychotherapy. Mental health professionals experienced in working with antisocial individuals focus on enhancing an individual's strengths, channeling sensation-seeking actions into more positive, socially responsible behaviors, and teaching practical ways of handling the frustrations of daily living.

Medications are not usually recommended. In some instances, however, drugs can help in diminishing violent episodes. Because individuals with antisocial personality disorder may also have AD/HD, some therapists have tried treatment with stimulants, such as Ritalin (see Chapter 14), but there have been no systematic, long-term studies of this approach. Stimulants should not be prescribed unless the individual has been specifically diagnosed with AD/HD and has not responded to alternative medications. Because these drugs can be abused, their use should be carefully monitored.

For those convicted of crimes, "treatment" often consists of incarceration. Some residential facilities, which certain criminal offenders may be able to choose in lieu of time in conventional prisons, provide intensive counseling, but drop-out rates are high. Another alternative to jail time for adolescents with a pattern of delinquent behavior who get in trouble with the law is specially designed wilderness programs, somewhat similar in rigorousness to Outward Bound, which provide difficult, even dangerous challenges. Their efficacy has been debated, and their long-term success in turning around antisocial behavior is not clear.

BORDERLINE PERSONALITY DISORDER

Individuals with borderline personality disorder (BPD) live on a psychological edge. Nothing in their lives—their sense of identity, their moods, their relationships—seems stable. The key factors in this disorder are instability in mood and in relationships, impulsivity, and a greatly impaired capacity for attachment. One therapist describes this condition as a form of "emotional hemophilia," in which individuals lack the clotting mechanisms that control spurts of feelings in normal persons. They are incapable of a *little* sadness, a *little* anger, a *little* worry. Every reaction is extreme, including their occasional feelings that they do not exist at all.

Confused about who they are and what they want, borderline individuals don't know which job to take, which interests to pursue, which friends or lovers to choose. They may swing suddenly and swiftly from one intense emotion to another, begging for help one moment and righteously seeking revenge the next. They may gamble, abuse drugs, binge on foods, mutilate themselves, or attempt suicide. All these behaviors are desperate attempts to deal with their frightening, uncontrollable emotions and the terrible emptiness within, yet they often have no idea why they feel and act the way they do.

Borderline is the most widely studied personality disorder as well as the most common one. Like other personality disorders, it develops in late adolescence or early adulthood. BPD occurs in about 2 percent of the population and in every culture, and may be present in at least 10 percent of individuals seeking mental health care. Yet diagnosis is often difficult, largely because of the overlap with other disorders, and much about this disorder remains unknown. It is about five times more common among those with close biological relatives with this disorder than in the general population.

An individual with borderline personality disorder may:

- Be unable to control emotions or impulses
- Rush into intense, stormy relationships
- Always try to avoid being alone or abandoned
- Think in black-or-white, good-or-bad, all-or-nothing terms
- Experience constant ups and downs in daily living
- Impulsively spend money, abuse drugs or alcohol, shoplift, be promiscuous, go on eating binges, or drive recklessly
- Engage in self-mutilating acts
- Threaten or attempt suicide
- Swing from one extreme mood to another
- Chronically feel empty inside
- Become intensely angry and lose control
- Get involved in frequent physical fights
- Experience temporary feelings of unreality.

▼

Understanding borderline personality disorder   The characteristics associated with borderline personality disorder include intense and chaotic relationships, fluctuating and extreme attitudes toward others, impulsivity, self-destructive behaviors,

Is it borderline personality disorder?

According to the DSM-IV, a diagnosis of borderline personality disorder should be based on these features:

A pervasive pattern of instability of interpersonal relationships, self-image, emotions, and control over impulses, beginning by early adulthood and present in various contexts, as indicated by at least five of the following:

1. Frantic efforts to avoid real or imagined abandonment
2. A pattern of unstable, intense relationships in which the individual first idealizes another person as perfect in every way and then completely devalues him or her
3. A markedly unstable self-image or sense of self
4. Impulsivity in at least two potentially self-damaging areas (e.g., spending, sex, substance abuse, reckless driving, or binge eating)
5. Repeated suicidal threats, gestures, or behaviors, or self-mutilating behavior
6. Frequent mood changes, with intense emotionality, such as episodes of extreme unhappiness, irritability, or anxiety lasting from a few hours to a few days
7. Chronic feelings of emptiness
8. Inappropriate, intense anger or difficulty controlling anger (e.g., frequent displays of temper, physical fights, etc.)
9. Temporary stress-related paranoid ideas or severe dissociative symptoms

Adapted from the Diagnostic and Statistical Manual of Mental Disorders, 4th Edition. *Used with permission.*

and lack of a clear sense of identity. Women with borderline personality disorder outnumber men by a ratio of about 3 to 1. The reasons for this gender discrepancy, like the causes of borderline personality disorder themselves, are not known. Some researchers speculate that women are more vulnerable because they are more likely to be victims of physical and sexual abuse in childhood and because they have more confusing role and identity options to consider in adulthood. It is possible, however, that borderline men may be undercounted because certain behaviors, such as aggression and violent outbursts, lead to imprisonment rather than diagnosis and therapy, or because they may be misdiagnosed as having antisocial personality disorder.

Borderline individuals think in absolutes: They are either ecstatic or miserable. Either they love or they hate. Someone is either perfect or worthless. They may worship a lover or friend one day, but when this perfect person does something disappointing or hurtful, they turn on him and revile him. This tendency to think in absolutes is a psychological defense mechanism called *splitting*, which inevitably leads to great pain.

Unable to tolerate contradictory or inconsistent feelings, borderline individuals tend to have very brief and highly intense romantic relationships but appear to be incapable of true intimacy. Because they fear abandonment, they cling. Because they fear engulfment, they push away. They wind up manipulating those they want to be close to, which ultimately leads to rejection.

For those with borderline personalities, life is an unending emotional roller coaster of highs and lows. Some are productive and successful at work, although they may be easily angered or hypersensitive to criticism and have poor relationships with their co-workers. They describe themselves as depressed, angry, fearful, or sad. Even though they do not get along well with others, they hate to be alone. Their most common feeling is emptiness, and many never develop an abiding sense of self. Lacking this stabilizing sense of identity, they experience dizzying, dramatic mood changes from joy to depression to anger, sometimes in a matter of minutes, sometimes hours. Unable either to understand or control these mood changes, they may come to despise themselves.

When times get rough or when under the influence of drugs or alcohol, borderline individuals may not be capable of thinking or perceiving normally and may lose touch with reality for a period of hours or even days. Because of their intense anger, a desire to manipulate others, or the need simply to prove that they are alive, they often act in impulsive or self-destructive ways, taking drugs, going on sexual binges, gambling, shopping, gorging and purging, mutilating themselves, or attempting suicide.

People with borderline personality disorder also may have histrionic, dependent, antisocial, and schizotypal traits. There is a high incidence of major depression among those with this condition. Men are usually more aggressive and have higher suicide rates than women, but women attempt self-injury and suicide more often. Overall, more than 5 percent of borderline individuals, especially those who also have major depression or substance abuse, eventually kill themselves.

▼
Treating borderline personality disorder

Although the best approaches to treating borderline individuals remain a subject of debate, mental health professionals generally agree that what seems most important is the development of a stable, trusting relationship with a therapist who does not respond punitively to provocative acts, who actively participates in therapy to provide assurance of his or her interest and concern, and who emphasizes the harmful effects of self-destructive behaviors, such as drug abuse, promiscuity, or rage. The goals of therapy are to lessen or eliminate these behaviors and improve adaptation. Therapists may combine cognitive and behavioral approaches to help individuals acquire skills for coping with daily life. Follow-up research indicates that a supportive, problem-oriented approach can bring about the same basic changes in personality as more intensive psychodynamic treatment.

Group therapy provides many benefits that supplement individual therapy. It helps people to identify manipulative or dependent behaviors and enables them to communicate their feelings and personal problems without fear of repercussions. It also may enable individuals to develop new and better relationships, both within and outside the group.

No psychiatric drugs address the underlying problems in borderline personality disorder but, when appropriately prescribed, some can improve the individual's mood or behavior. Psychiatrists are studying the use of anti-anxiety drugs, antidepressants, and antipsychotics to diminish specific problems such as impulsivity, depression, and cognitive and perceptual impairment.

Individuals with severe symptoms, particularly those who abuse alcohol or drugs or attempt suicide, may require brief hospitalization. Halfway houses and day centers can be good alternatives to hospitalization; they provide a safe environment, provide social relations with peers, and offer active rehabilitation programs.

The symptoms of borderline personality disorder and the risk of suicide are greatest in young adulthood. They tend to diminish with age; most people with this disorder achieve some stability—personally and professionally—in their thirties or forties.

HISTRIONIC PERSONALITY DISORDER

Many individuals have a flair for the dramatic. Those with histrionic personality disorder go beyond mere flamboyance. Gregarious and intensely emotional, they crave attention and live as if they were always on center stage. Their speech, dress, and mannerisms are theatrical. They never stop performing in the roles they have chosen for themselves, and in times of stress they may be unable to tell where fantasy ends and reality begins. As in other personality disorders, there is a wide continuum of histrionic behaviors, some of which are considered adaptive in our society and some of which are maladaptive.

Histrionic personality disorder affects about 2 to 3 percent of the general population and about 10 to 15 percent of those seen by mental health professionals. Although it can and does occur in men, it is diagnosed much more frequently in women. This may be because women, living in a world dominated by men, have had to adopt a male-defined concept of femininity, which emphasizes physical attractiveness and seductive behavior. As with other personality disorders, individuals develop histrionic behaviors by early adulthood.

An individual with histrionic personality disorder may:

- Be colorful and dramatic
- Crave attention
- Be extroverted
- Act in flamboyant ways
- Dress or behave seductively
- Be superficial, vain, and self-absorbed
- Be overly trusting and gullible.

Understanding histrionic personality disorder

Histrionic individuals have a weak psychological "core" or sense of self. Some describe them as chameleons, who change their emotional coloring to suit the environment. Persons with this disorder are overly concerned with making themselves attractive. Their desire for attention may lead to other flamboyant acts or self-dramatizing behavior, such as being unusually effusive and demonstrative. They have difficulty in focusing their attention on specifics and speak in vague, highly exaggerated terms. Although often creative and imaginative, they do not apply their intelligence in analytic ways, relying on "gut" feelings rather than facts in making decisions or assessing a situation.

People with histrionic personality disorder pay little heed to the past or the future. Rather, they are trapped in the present, consumed with getting whatever they want at the exact moment they want it. Although they seem eager to please, their needs always take precedence over those of all others. They can be extremely dependent and demanding, as well as manipulative and deceitful, using tears, temper tantrums, or emotional outbursts in the effort to get their way. What they really want is reassurance that they are attractive to the other sex, yet despite their sexual provocativeness and frequent promiscuity they may actually have little interest in sex. Sexual dysfunctions, usually impotence in men and inability to achieve orgasm in women, are not uncommon.

Treating histrionic personality disorder

Individual psychotherapy is the primary form of treatment. No single technique or method has proved most effective in helping histrionic individuals, and many mental health professionals use a combination of approaches.

For those with severe histrionic personality disorder, a long-term, analytic approach may be best. For less severe cases, brief psychotherapy may be effective. This can involve a supportive, problem-solving approach, cognitive techniques to overcome distorted thinking, and interpersonal therapy to focus on difficulties in forming a stable, meaningful relationship. (These therapies are described in Chapter 27.) In therapy, people examine the methods they employ in trying to secure satisfaction from others, such as seductiveness or little-girl cuteness, and their motivations for these actions. Eventually they work toward more independent ways of living and of achieving satisfaction on their own, as opposed to—as one woman put it—"always needing to suck sustenance from a man."

Because histrionic individuals often have poorly developed analytic skills, cognitive techniques can be very helpful in teaching them to pay attention to details, evaluate nonverbal clues, and consider their own motives and those of others. Some therapists videotape sessions to illustrate how the person's behavior looks to others. Group therapy, often used in combination with individual therapy, provides another opportunity for feedback.

Medication is not a recommended treatment except for those with a co-existing disorder such as depression. Occasionally hospitalization is necessary because of suicidal thoughts or behavior.

NARCISSISTIC PERSONALITY DISORDER

"Healthy" narcissism, which many define as strong self-esteem, makes people feel good about themselves without repeated reassurance from others. Narcissism becomes unhealthy when individuals crave constant praise and adulation, feel entitled to special treatment, lack empathy, and put others down in order to feel good about themselves.

Individuals with narcissistic personality disorder develop a grandiose sense of themselves as special or superior and need constant reassurance of their immense and unique value. Brash and self-assured, they are often successful at what they do, but beneath the aura of confidence are feelings of inadequacy that create a constant need to keep inflating their sense of themselves. Indeed, they may be so unsure of themselves that they do not know whether they are worthwhile unless someone else tells them so, yet such reassurances prove to be transient. Narcissists need the trappings of success, such as expensive automobiles or lavish houses, to proclaim their worth to the world. If they cannot get the praise and reassurance they need, they become angry or depressed, convinced that life is empty and they are inconsequential.

Less than 1 percent of the general population suffers from narcissistic personality disorder, which is more common (2 to 16 percent) among those seeking mental health care. It may be somewhat more common in men. It always begins by early adulthood.

An individual with narcissistic personality disorder may:

- Have grandiose feelings of being unique or special
- Feel superior to others
- Crave admiration and adulation
- Need constant bolstering from others
- Respond to criticism with lingering rage
- Feel ashamed and worthless after any failure
- Become deeply depressed or enraged after rejection or injury
- Feel entitled to special treatment
- Be insensitive to others' feelings or needs
- Be ambitious and fantasize about fame and fortune
- Be incapable of empathy.

▼

Understanding narcissistic personality disorder

People with a narcissistic personality disorder are often charming, friendly, and adept at ingratiating themselves with others, but their only concern is with themselves and their greatly inflated view of their accomplishments and talents. Regardless of their actual achievements, they expect to be noticed as "special." Being so special, they believe they can be understood and appreciated only by other special people.

These persons do not work for success per se but for admiration and acclaim. When they do focus on achievement, it is likely to be a pleasureless pursuit. Some choose careers in entertainment or politics, where they can bask in actual applause. Others seek frequent, quieter praise, such as a boss's positive words

Is it narcissistic personality disorder?

According to the DSM-IV, a diagnosis of narcissistic personality disorder should be based on these features:

A pervasive pattern of grandiosity (in fantasy or behavior), need for admiration, and lack of empathy, beginning by early adulthood and present in various contexts, as indicated by at least five of the following:

1. **A grandiose sense of self-importance (exaggerates achievements and talents, expects to be recognized as superior without any basis in achievement)**
2. **Preoccupation with fantasies of unlimited success, power, brilliance, beauty, or ideal love**
3. **Belief that he or she is special and unique and can only be understood by, and should associate with, other special or high-status people (or institutions)**
4. **A need for excessive admiration**
5. **A sense of entitlement, that is, unreasonable expectation of especially favorable treatment**
6. **Taking advantage of others to achieve his or her own ends**
7. **Lack of empathy and unwillingness to recognize or identify with the feelings and needs of others**
8. **Frequent envy of others or belief that others are envious**
9. **Arrogant, haughty behaviors or attitudes**

Adapted from the Diagnostic and Statistical Manual of Mental Disorders, 4th Edition. *Used with permission.*

about their hard work. In business, narcissistic individuals may surround themselves with "yes men" or flattering subordinates. As management analysts have noted, they may try to recreate their childhood in their own businesses so they can be at the center of an admiring world.

Because people with narcissistic personality disorder look outward for gratification, they are exceptionally vulnerable to what others think and say. They pander for compliments with great skill and charm. The slightest hint of criticism can trigger feelings of rage, shame, or humiliation, which they may release explosively or try to mask with indifference. Jealousy of anyone who achieves greater success, makes more money, or simply seems happier or more satisfied with life gnaws at them.

Although they may seem genuinely empathic, individuals with this disorder often have no sense of how others feel. If a friend is upset or tired, they don't see why *their* plans have to be changed or cancelled. Their "narcissistic entitlement" leads them to expect special treatment simply because they don't feel they should have to follow rules, wait their turn, or put up with drudgery. If there is a long line at a ticket counter, they see no reason why they should have to go to the end rather than cutting in front. They view every-

The special child

Charm could have been Ken's middle name. Even as a small boy, he was always so friendly and outgoing that he ingratiated himself with everyone who came to visit his parents. "Yes, he is a darling," his mother would coo. "He's such a special child."

Of course, not everyone could recognize and appreciate Ken's specialness, especially at school. He hated having to listen to the other kids stumble through a lesson when he was a far better reader. Whenever he had to work with a partner or team, Ken would try to get the others to do as much of the preparation as possible while he volunteered to do the presentation. He loved recognition in any form. When he started appearing in high school plays, he felt that he was meant to be on stage. Applause was the loveliest sound he had ever heard.

In college, Ken came into his own. He regularly played the leading male roles in the theater department productions. His good looks and gracious manners made him popular with girls. So many fraternities pursued him that he felt he was doing the house he selected a tremendous favor by agreeing to join. He surrounded himself with others who had what he thought of as a "special something"—in looks, intelligence, talent—and they treated the campus like their private playground.

Ken did get into his share of trouble, mainly because he didn't feel that any rules applied to him. He'd park his car in the faculty lot if it was more convenient and never pay the parking fines. He'd steal reference books from the library so he could read them in the comfort of his room, even though other students needed the same materials. He'd sweet-talk the fraternity cook into setting aside some food so he wouldn't have to wake up early for breakfast.

After graduation Ken headed for Los Angeles, charmed his way into the offices of the top agents, passed out glossy headshots wherever he went, and went on "go-sees" for every commercial, sitcom or movie he heard about. Even though he had to supplement his income with stints as a waiter, Ken managed to get a few national commercials and bit parts on television series. He lived for a director's "Nice job!" or a fellow actor's recognition. But any hint of criticism—a call for several retakes, a suggestion that his handling of a role might not be on target—devastated him. Sometimes he would explode in a tirade and stalk off a set in self-righteous indignation. And whenever he'd see someone else get a role he wanted, he'd feel consumed by jealousy.

When his spirits slumped, Ken expected his friends to cheer him up, yet he found it hard to listen to

their problems. The women he got involved with seemed perfect as long as they were always available and attentive to his needs, but as soon as he slipped from being their top priority, he'd say they were "too wrapped up in themselves" and drop them.

By the time he turned forty, Ken was a regular on a daytime soap opera, but he yearned to break into the movies. He'd pester his agent to get him a tryout for a hot movie, only to be told that he no longer qualified for boyish-charm roles. It wasn't even easy for him to get dates anymore or to find friends who would listen in sympathy and offer support. He felt unappreciated and old.

Ken went to see a psychiatrist in part because several actors had told him how Prozac had kindled their creative energies. But the psychiatrist felt that Ken's difficulties stemmed not from depression or a midlife crisis but from "narcissistic personality disorder." Though this was startling to hear, what the therapist said about living for others' praise rang true. And so Ken began the long and often difficult process of coming to know and understand himself. "I've seen too many actors almost destroyed by narcissism as they get older, doing anything just for a few seconds in the limelight," he says. "They seem pathetic to me, and I don't want to end up like that."

thing and everyone in terms of their impact on their own needs and desires.

Although many narcissistic individuals are successful, some pursue unrealistic goals or run into difficulty in getting along with others. If they fail to achieve the success and win the unconditional love and admiration they yearn for, they suffer. As middle age approaches and tarnishes their grandiose visions, some individuals may become preoccupied with aging and devote great energy, time, and effort to looking youthful.

▼

Treating narcissistic personality disorder

Although there have been no scientific studies of which approaches are most effective in treating narcissistic personality disorder, the general perception is that individual psychotherapy or psychoanalysis can help individuals with this problem.

Some therapists advocate traditional psychoanalysis for narcissistic individuals. They may be more likely to benefit from this approach than those with other personality disorders, but there is no proof that a psychoanalytic approach is more effective than insight-oriented psychotherapy. Both processes usually take several years because the goal is significant personality change, not simply improvement of functioning. Short-term psychotherapy, which can lead to permanent personality change in certain other disorders, has not been shown to have the same effect with narcissistic individuals, although it may boost self-esteem and thereby provide the motivation for individuals to pursue long-term psychotherapy.

As with other personality disorders, the relationship with a mental health professional is crucial. Some therapists primarily empathize with the individual's sensitivities and disappointments and encourage development of new skills. Others are more direct, making interpretations and confronting individuals so that they become aware of their grandiosity and its consequences.

AVOIDANT PERSONALITY DISORDER

Avoidant individuals, extremely self-conscious and fearful of embarrassment, shun closeness or contact with others even though they strongly desire intimate relationships. Uncomfortable in all social situations, they fear being ridiculed, criticized, rejected, or humiliated. They desperately want to be liked and to enjoy social interactions, but their low self-esteem, hypersensitivity, and fear of rejection keep them from reaching out to others. Although most people care about how others view them, avoidant men and women are devastated if anyone even *seems* to dislike them. They may avoid all new activities for fear of humiliating themselves.

Social discomfort, fear of being judged negatively, and lack of self-confidence usually begin by early adulthood and affect all aspects of the person's life. An estimated 0.5 to 1 percent of the general population has avoidant personality disorder, which is equally common in men and women. Avoidant individuals have extremely low self-esteem, which seriously impedes their ability to form relationships. Some also suffer from social phobia, depression, or anxiety.

An individual with avoidant personality disorder may:

- Be extremely shy and timid
- Be introverted
- Feel anxious around others
- Have low self-esteem
- Be extremely sensitive to rejection
- Feel apprehensive about meeting people or trying new experiences
- Mistrust people
- Feel uncomfortable in social situations
- Feel extremely self-conscious
- Fear embarrassment or acting foolishly
- Be troubled by an exaggerated sense of the dangers of daily living.

▼

Understanding avoidant personality disorder

Individuals with avoidant personality disorder yearn for and fantasize about affection and acceptance yet cannot relate comfortably to others. Even before meeting someone new, they want reassurance that they will be liked. When they do form a relationship, they are very clinging and fearful that it may end.

Timid in almost any social situation, avoidant individuals are wary of anything new or different. Because they are afraid of saying something that might sound silly or inappropriate, they may not say anything at all. They are easily hurt by criticism or disapproval, and they worry about being embarrassed in public by blushing, stammering, or showing other visible signs of anxiety.

Avoidant men and women cling to a structured routine. Because they fear doing anything outside this routine, they often exaggerate the potential risks of any change. Thus, they may turn down a promotion if it means that they might have to travel or attend more social functions, although they give their supervisors another reason, such as family obligations.

▼

Treating avoidant personality disorder

Initially avoidant individuals may be able to tolerate only supportive techniques, but with encouragement and empathy they may

<table>
<tr><td>

Is it avoidant personality disorder?

According to the DSM-IV, a diagnosis of avoidant personality disorder should be based on these features:

</td><td>

A pervasive pattern of social inhibition, feelings of inadequacy, and hypersensitivity to negative evaluation, beginning by early adulthood and present in various contexts, as indicated by at least four of the following:

1. Avoidance of occupational activities that involve significant interpersonal contact because of fears of criticism, disapproval, or rejection
2. Unwillingness to get involved with people unless certain of being liked
3. Restraint within intimate relationships for fear of being shamed or ridiculed
4. Preoccupation with being criticized or rejected in social situations
5. Inhibited behavior in new situations because of feelings of inadequacy
6. View of oneself as socially inept, personally unappealing, or inferior to others
7. Unusual reluctance to take personal risks or engage in any new activities because they may prove embarrassing

Adapted from the Diagnostic and Statistical Manual of Mental Disorders, 4th Edition. *Used with permission.*

</td></tr>
</table>

later benefit from other types of psychotherapy. Insight-oriented psychotherapy—brief, long-term, or psychoanalytic, depending chiefly on the persons's goals and preference—is often helpful, either alone or in combination with behavioral techniques. Interpersonal psychotherapy concentrates on relationship difficulties. Sometimes family members or close friends participate in the sessions so that individuals can try out new behaviors with them.

Although there are few data, the behavioral techniques that work extremely well for shyness and social anxiety—assertiveness and social skills training through role-playing, instruction, modeling, graded exposure, flooding, and systematic desensitization—may boost the confidence of avoidant individuals and increase their willingness to take chances in social situations. One specific technique that can be very effective in reducing fear of humiliation and rejection is *paradoxical intention*. The therapist may "prescribe" that an individual seek rejection, for example, be turned down twice when asking for dates. If not rejected, the person goes on the date but must still continue asking other people until being rejected. The rejection becomes less feared because it is a way of winning the therapist's approval.

Cognitive therapy, which challenges incorrect assumptions and self-statements, may be particularly useful in boosting self-confidence. Although they may initially be fearful of participation, individuals also find supportive group therapy very helpful in overcoming social anxiety and in developing trust and rapport. As individuals get older, avoidant personality disorder may remit or become less obvious.

The medications prescribed for social anxiety (discussed in Chapter 7) usually are not necessary in treating this disorder, although some therapists may prescribe them for a person's first attempts to enter situations he or she has long avoided. Indeed, simply having a prescription or pills available can be so reassuring that individuals may never actually use them.

DEPENDENT PERSONALITY DISORDER

Although we all rely on others in many different ways, those with dependent personality disorder go beyond any normal degree of interdependence and reliance. Unable to function independently, they allow others to take over responsibility for major areas of life and subordinate themselves to the persons on whom they depend.

Individuals with dependent personality disorder feel an overpowering desire for support and nurturance. From early adulthood they cling to others out of a profound fear of being abandoned and left to care for themselves. They avoid all disagreements for fear of provoking anger or rejection and the possible loss of care and support.

Although the *DSM-IV* describes dependent personality disorder as among the most frequently reported disorders in mental health clinics, there are no reliable estimates of its prevalence. It seems to occur about equally among men and women, always beginning by early adulthood.

Individuals with dependent personality disorder may:

- Feel an extreme need to be taken care of

- Feel incapable of getting along on their own

- Need constant reassurance from others

- Want others to assume responsibility for major decisions

- Not disagree with others for fear that they will disapprove

- Find it hard to initiate projects or to do things on their own

- Go to any lengths to obtain nurturance and support from others

- Voluntarily do unpleasant things to please another person

- Feel helpless when alone

- Search frantically for another person to turn to when a close relationship ends

- Have unrealistic fears about being left to take care of themselves.

Is it dependent personality disorder?

According to the DSM-IV, a diagnosis of dependent personality disorder should be based on these features:

A pervasive and excessive need to be taken care of that leads to submissive and clinging behavior and fears of separation, beginning by early adulthood and present in various contexts, as indicated by at least five of the following:

1. Difficulty making everyday decisions without excessive advice or reassurance from others

2. A need for others to assume responsibility for most major areas of life

3. Difficulty in expressing disagreement because of fear of loss of support or approval

4. Difficulty in initiating projects or doing things on one's own (because of a lack of self-confidence in judgment or abilities, not from a lack of motivation or energy)

5. Going to excessive lengths to obtain nurturance and support from others to the point of volunteering to do unpleasant things

6. Feeling uncomfortable or helpless when alone because of exaggerated fears of being unable to care for oneself

7. Urgent searching for another relationship as a source of care and support when a close relationship ends

8. Unrealistic preoccupation with fears of being left to take care of oneself

Adapted from the Diagnostic and Statistical Manual of Mental Disorders, 4th Edition. *Used with permission.*

▼

Understanding dependent personality disorder

Dependent individuals live in a prison of need. Invariably lacking self-confidence, they belittle their abilities and may describe themselves as stupid or dumb. They cannot assert themselves and fear expressing their true opinions because of the possibility of criticism or disapproval. They are unable to make simple everyday decisions without turning to others for advice and reassurance. When major decisions must be made, they often allow others to decide for them, such as letting a spouse decide which house to purchase or whether or not the couple should have a child.

Convinced that they cannot do anything on their own, dependent individuals have great difficulty starting a project, not because they lack motivation or energy but because they see themselves as incompetent. Dependent persons feel uncomfortable by themselves and go to great lengths to avoid being alone. They want desperately to be liked, and any hint of disapproval or criticism wounds them. To win people's affections, they may agree with them even when they believe the others are wrong, or do unpleasant or demeaning things just to please their friends or partners. The prospect of having to be on their own is more terrifying and painful than actual abandonment. When a relationship does end, they quickly replace it with another.

Often dependent men and women have another personality disorder, such as histrionic, schizotypal, narcissistic, or avoidant personality, and are at increased risk for developing dysthymia, major depression, and anxiety disorders.

▼

Treating dependent personality disorder

Psychotherapy is the primary treatment for this problem. Much of the "work" in therapy sessions centers on assertiveness, decision-making, and developing increased independence. Assured of the therapist's support, dependent individuals learn to express their genuine feelings, make their own decisions, and deal with episodes of anxiety. They come to identify with and act like the therapist, which boosts their self-esteem. This encourages them to try new behaviors at work or home, and their self-confidence grows. Group and cognitive-behavioral therapy, often along with assertiveness and social skills training, can also be helpful.

OBSESSIVE-COMPULSIVE PERSONALITY DISORDER

Conscientiousness, discipline, punctuality, precision, attention to detail, and reliability—traits considered not only normal but desirable—are common among successful men and women. When taken to extremes, however, such compulsive behaviors can create problems. Some people with these characteristics turn into hard-driving "Type As," at greater risk for heart disease because of their chronic hostility and intense competitiveness. Others strive for perfection but concentrate so intensely on details that they see only the trees, never the forest. They are rigid, critical of themselves and others, stingy with their emotions and with their money or goods. If these compulsive behaviors dominate their lives and interfere with the way they feel, act, and relate to others, they may have obsessive-compulsive personality disorder, sometimes shortened to *compulsive personality disorder.*

Whenever obsessive-compulsive behaviors begin to interfere with normal relationships and performance, they should be considered warning signs. The difference between the irritating ways of an uptight fussbudget and the more serious behaviors associated with obsessive-compulsive personality disorder is more than one of degree. Obsessive-compulsive individuals may want to change their thoughts, feelings, ideas or behavioral impulses, but they cannot. They act the way they do because they are trapped in this inflexible characterological pattern.

Obsessive-compulsive personality disorder always involves a

long-term and pervasive pattern of preoccupation with orderliness, perfectionism, and mental and interpersonal control. Obsessive-compulsive disorder (OCD), discussed in Chapter 8, is a distinctive biochemical disorder characterized by obsessions and rituals. Some, but far from all, individuals with an obsessive-compulsive personality disorder also develop the powerful obsessions— thoughts, images, words, or wishes that intrude into awareness against their will and that they cannot block—and the compulsive ritualistic behaviors that are characteristic of OCD.

About 1 percent of the general population and 3 to 10 percent of those seeking mental health care have obsessive-compulsive personality disorder. This problem, which always develops by early adulthood, is diagnosed about twice as often in men as in women.

Individuals with obsessive-compulsive personality disorder may:

- Be preoccupied with perfectionism
- Prize mental and emotional control
- Insist on orderliness
- Pay excessive attention to details, rules, lists, schedules, etc.
- Be unable to complete a task because every detail must be perfect
- Be so devoted to work that they have no time for leisure or friendships
- Be over-conscientious and inflexible about ethical matters
- Be unable to express warm emotions
- Hang onto worthless or worn-out objects with no sentimental value
- Not delegate work unless it is done in a particular way
- Hoard money rather than spend it
- Be rigid and stubborn.

▼

Understanding obsessive-compulsive personality disorder

Individuals with obsessive-compulsive personality disorder are intensely ambitious, extremely time-conscious, obstinate, meticulous, overly conscientious, and inflexible in their ethical views. Some characterize them as "living machines." They demand certainty, order, and discipline, and are unwilling to settle for imperfection. As one mental health professional observes, their most characteristic thought is "I should"— a reflection of their high standards, drivenness, excessive conscientiousness, perfectionism, rigidity, and devotion to work and duties.

Intellectualizing what they see, do, and experience, these persons think rather than feel. They try to control every aspect of their lives, beginning with their own extremely disciplined behav-

Is it obsessive-compulsive personality disorder?

According to the DSM-IV, a diagnosis of obsessive-compulsive personality disorder should be based on these features:

A pervasive pattern of preoccupation with orderliness, perfectionism, and mental and interpersonal control, at the expense of flexibility, openness, and efficiency, beginning by early adulthood and present in various contexts, as indicated by at least four of the following:

1. Preoccupation with details, rules, lists, order, organization, or schedules to the extent that the major point of the activity is lost

2. Perfectionism that interferes with task completion (e.g., unable to complete a project because one's overly strict standards are not met)

3. Excessive devotion to work and productivity to the exclusion of leisure activities and friendships

4. Over-conscientiousness, scrupulousness, and inflexibility about matters of morality, ethics, or values

5. Inability to discard worn-out or worthless objects even when they have no sentimental value

6. Reluctance to delegate tasks or to work with others unless co-workers submit exactly to one's own way of doing things

7. A miserly spending style toward self and others; money viewed as something to be hoarded for future catastrophes

8. Rigidity and stubbornness

Adapted from the Diagnostic and Statistical Manual of Mental Disorders, 4th Edition. *Used with permission.*

ior, but they are so focused on doing things perfectly that they may never accomplish what they set out to do.

Work and productivity take precedence over pleasure or leisure. Extreme workaholics, these individuals rarely spend time relaxing or take vacations. But despite their dedication and long hours, obsessive-compulsive persons often do not enjoy their work or achieve their full potential. Preoccupied with regulations, details, procedures, or forms, they cannot differentiate between what matters and what doesn't. Often they leave the most important tasks until the last moment or miss a deadline because they spend so much time ruminating about what to do first. Fearful of making a mistake, they may avoid or agonize over decisions. They may not delegate tasks or work unless others do things exactly their way; even then, it is not likely to be up to their standards. And no matter how much they accomplish, much of the time it does not seem good enough to them.

Obsessive-compulsive individuals are excessively moralistic and judgmental, quick to condemn the behavior or decisions of others. They typically find it hard to spend money on themselves or others, and save or invest to provide for unknown future catastrophes. Many are unable to part with anything that might later prove useful and become "pack rats" who save even the most useless items, such as old newspapers and broken dishware.

Control is all-important. If this control is endangered, they may react with irritation and anger, which they usually do not express directly. The emotions they find hardest to show are tenderness, love, and compassion—feelings they equate with weakness and vulnerability. In their interactions with others they are characteristically stiff and formal. Often plagued by self-doubt, they are extremely sensitive to criticism, especially from those with status or authority.

For obsessive-compulsive persons, change is seen as a potential source of danger that may leave them even more vulnerable and uncertain. They resist anything new and different and refuse to accept the fact that there are no guarantees in living and that they cannot control the future—or even the present.

Obsessive-compulsive men and women are prone to depression, especially as they grow older and realize that they have not been as successful as they had hoped, that they are not as close to their children or spouses as they would like, or that the hard work they poured into their careers has not justified their sacrifices in personal relationships.

▼
Treating obsessive-compulsive personality disorder

The cornerstone of treatment for obsessive-compulsive personality disorder is individual psychotherapy, often in conjunction with behavior modification to reduce anxiety and teach new patterns of behavior. The goal is to help persons recognize that anxiety is inevitable in all lives and to abandon their attempts at perfection so they can accept themselves and their limitations.

Various forms of therapy can supplement each other and reinforce the potential for change. Reducing depression or anxiety through medications may enhance the benefits of psychotherapy. Obsessive-compulsive individuals who have been diagnosed with OCD may benefit from treatment with drugs such as clomipramine (Anafranil) or an SSRI like fluoxetine (Prozac), which reduce compulsive behavior.

Symptoms such as undue perfectionism, self-doubt, procrastination, and indecisiveness are best dealt with in psychotherapy. Increasingly, short-term therapy has become the preferred approach, although this may be the result of financial restrictions, and many mental health professionals feel that longer-term therapy is more effective. Cognitive techniques can be especially productive because they directly address illogical or rigid beliefs and suit these individuals' tendency to intellectualize their feelings.

PARANOID PERSONALITY DISORDER

Individuals with paranoid personality disorder are more than cautious or suspicious: they are highly distrustful, always on the lookout for signs and clues of danger or deceit. Everyone is a potential threat or enemy. Without any reason, they may question the loyalty or trustworthiness of friends or associates. Often pathologically jealous, they may doubt the fidelity of a spouse or sexual partner, even when they lack the slightest justification for their suspicions. They are extremely secretive, keeping their thoughts and ideas to themselves and not divulging them to even their closest friends.

Bigots, perpetrators of hate crimes, and litigious individuals who file frequent lawsuits may have paranoid personalities. Expecting to be exploited or harmed, they may constantly look for proof that someone—a racial, ethnic, or religious group, a neighbor, or an employer—is out to get them. They often find such evidence by misinterpreting benign occurrences, like someone cutting in front of them on the freeway, as a threat or deliberate provocation. They overreact to real or perceived threats by becoming excessively angry. Unable to forgive and forget, they may take legal actions against purported enemies or betrayers.

The primary characteristics of paranoid personality disorder—hypervigilance, hypersensitivity, suspiciousness, and guardedness—may not be readily apparent, but individuals with this disorder usually have one telltale trait: They blame others, bad luck, or fate for whatever goes wrong in their lives.

On the surface, these persons may not seem to have serious problems at work or home, but this is usually not the case. In work situations they often have difficulty with authority figures. Since they tend to be incapable of meaningful emotional involvement, their lives may be lived in social isolation.

Paranoid personality disorder is different from paranoid schizophrenia and paranoid delusional disorder. People with these psychotic disorders, discussed in Chapter 17, develop persistent delusions that are completely out of touch with reality and cannot be shaken by any evidence to the contrary. Paranoid schizophrenia also involves hallucinations and other characteristic symptoms of a psychotic disorder.

Paranoid personality disorder occurs in about 0.5 to 2.5 percent of the general population, 10 to 30 percent of psychiatric inpatients, and 2 to 10 percent of those seen as mental health outpatients. It appears to be more common in men and always develops by early adulthood.

An individual with paranoid personality disorder may:

- Expect to be exploited or harmed by others

- Constantly question the loyalty or trustworthiness of friends and associates

- Not want to confide in others

- Read hidden insults or threats into innocent remarks or events

- Bear grudges

- Refuse to forgive insults or slights

- Think that their character or reputation is being attacked

- Respond to any possible slight with anger or a counterattack

- Doubt the fidelity of a spouse without justification.

▼

Understanding paranoid personality disorder

Paranoid individuals spend a great deal of energy looking for sinister motives behind the behavior of others. Confronted with a new situation, they read hidden meanings into innocent remarks or events. If someone bumps into them, they assume it was an attack, not an accident. If there is an error on a bill, they are sure it was a deliberate attempt to cheat them.

These persons show a limited range of emotions, often appearing cold and humorless. They may pride themselves on always being objective, rational, businesslike, and unemotional, although they are not. They are egocentric and lack sentimental and tender feelings.

Easily slighted, they are quick to react with anger or verbal assault. They may bear grudges for a long time and never forgive slights, insults, or injuries. Because they rigidly refuse to compromise, they can make others feel defensive and uneasy. Often fiercely argumentative, they exaggerate difficulties and counterattack when they perceive any threat. Although critical of others, they find it very difficult to accept criticism themselves. Some are quiet and hostile; others are combative. Most have difficulties getting along with co-workers and neighbors.

Paranoid individuals attribute to others their own unacceptable feelings and impulses, a behavior called *projection*. In new situations they do not look at the total context. Instead, they search for confirmation that supports their suspicions or prejudgments and ignore all evidence to the contrary. Some, especially those who are moralistic or grandiose, may become leaders of cults and other fringe groups.

Usually these persons have an overriding need to be self-sufficient, and they shun intimacy except with those very few, if any, whom they trust. During extreme stress their paranoia may transiently become psychotic; that is, they may not be able to distinguish between what is real and what is a delusion.

Is it paranoid personality disorder?

According to the DSM-IV, a diagnosis of paranoid personality disorder should be based on these features:

■ **A pervasive distrust and suspiciousness of others such that their motives are interpreted as malevolent, beginning by early adulthood and present in various contexts, as indicated by at least four of the following:**

1. **Suspicions, without sufficient basis, that others are exploiting, harming or deceiving oneself**
2. **Preoccupation with unjustified doubts about the loyalty or trustworthiness of friends or associates**
3. **Reluctance to confide in others because of unwarranted fear that the information will be used maliciously against oneself**
4. **Reading hidden demeaning or threatening meanings into benign remarks or events**
5. **Persistent bearing of grudges, i.e., not forgiving insults, injuries, or slights**
6. **Perception of attacks on one's character or reputation that are not apparent to others, quickly reacting with anger or counterattacking**
7. **Recurrent suspicions, without justification, regarding fidelity of spouse or sexual partner**

■ **Does not occur exclusively during the course of schizophrenia, depression with psychotic features, or another psychotic disorder, and is not due to the direct physiological effects of a general medical condition**

Adapted from the Diagnostic and Statistical Manual of Mental Disorders, 4th Edition. *Used with permission.*

▼

Treating paranoid personality disorder

There have been few studies of treatments of paranoid personality disorder. These individuals do not usually seek help because they do not see themselves as impaired. Those who do make their way into treatment, usually for anxiety or depression, are often so suspicious that they drop out. Supportive psychotherapy is considered the best initial approach, and individuals who persist with therapy can benefit.

Most people with paranoid personalities have deeply embedded and enduring problems that require intensive treatment over a considerable period of time. As is so often the case, the key to success is development of an honest, supportive relationship between the individual and the therapist. This requires trust, something that is very difficult for paranoid individuals to grant. Once they reach the point of being able to confide in a therapist, they can begin to deal with the feelings of insecurity, vulnerability, weakness, inadequacy, or inferiority that may underlie their paranoia. As they improve, group therapy may help in managing anxiety and developing social skills.

SCHIZOID PERSONALITY DISORDER

Individuals with schizoid personality disorder are the ultimate loners. They do not appear to have warm, tender feelings or form close friendships, and they seem not to care about what others say to praise or criticize them. This detachment from the world of people usually begins in early adulthood and characterizes all aspects of their lives.

Schizoid personality disorder occurs in persons with a profound defect in their ability to form personal relationships and respond to others in a meaningful way. Schizoid individuals have no close relationships, except perhaps with family members, choose solitary activities, rarely experience strong emotions, and have little, if any, desire for sex with another person. Unlike those with avoidant personalities, who crave relationships but cannot develop them because they fear rejection, schizoid individuals have no interest in such relationships.

This disorder, which is uncommon in mental health care settings, is diagnosed somewhat more often in men and may cause more impairment for them than for women.

An individual with schizoid personality disorder may:

- Not get involved with others
- Show only a limited range of emotions
- Not desire or enjoy close relationships
- Consistently prefer solitary pursuits
- Have little, if any, interest in sexual experiences with another person
- Enjoy few, if any, activities
- Have no or almost no close friends or confidants
- Seem indifferent to what others say.

▼

Understanding schizoid personality disorder

Individuals with schizoid personality disorder prefer a solitary life with few or no close friends or confidants. They choose solitary recreations, such as playing video or computer games. Their sexual life may be limited to fantasy. Because they lack social skills or a desire for sex, men with this problem usually do not date and rarely marry. Women may passively accede to courtship and marriage, but remain aloof.

Schizoid individuals live in an emotionally constricted world. They do not lose touch with reality, but the praise and criticism of others mean nothing to them. They rarely experience or express strong feelings, such as anger and joy. Some have unusual speech patterns and talk in a flat tone that gives their voices a robot-like

Is it schizoid personality disorder?

According to the DSM-IV, a diagnosis of schizoid person-ality disorder should be based on these features:

■ A pervasive pattern of detachment from social relationships and a restricted range of expression of emotions in interpersonal settings, beginning by early adulthood and present in various contexts, as indicated by at least four of the following:

1. No desire for or enjoyment of close relationships, including being part of a family

2. Almost always, a preference for solitary activities

3. Little, if any, interest in sexual experiences with another person

4. Pleasure from few, if any, activities

5. Lack of close friends or confidants other than first-degree relatives

6. Apparent indifference to the praise and criticisms of others

7. Emotional coldness, detachment, or flattened emotions

■ Does not occur only during the course of schizophrenia, a mood disorder with psychotic features, another psychotic disorder, or a pervasive developmental disorder, and is not due to the direct physiological effects of a medical condition

Adapted from the Diagnostic and Statistical Manual of Mental Disorders, 4th Edition. *Used with permission.*

quality and makes them seem cold and distant. Because they are unable to express aggressiveness or hostility, they can seem self-absorbed, indecisive, and absent-minded.

Many with schizoid disorder choose jobs that involve little or no contact with others, such as night work, and may do well at them. Some are very creative and talented, and for them painting, draw-ing, or sculpture may take the place of relationships. Some form strong attachments to animals or become engrossed in nutrition and health regimens.

▼

Treating schizoid personality disorder

The primary method of treatment is individual psychotherapy. This prospect may seem overwhelmingly frightening at first, and a gentle, cautious approach can minimize anxiety. Writing, music, and drawing may serve as ways of establishing initial rapport. Over time, persons with this disorder may come to understand more about others' feelings, learn ways of handling social situa-tions, develop confidence in their own opinions, and become less self-conscious, all of which can help them to make the most of solitary pleasures, such as traveling or artistic pursuits, and to interact more with others. Family therapy can be valuable because young men and women with this disorder are less likely to marry or become self-supporting than others and may remain at home much longer than their peers.

Behavioral techniques, such as gradual exposure to specific

tasks, can also help to build social confidence. For example, a therapist may encourage a person to attend a concert, then to join a group tour of a museum, then to participate in a hike. Each activity is a step toward greater socialization. Assertiveness training may help those who feel ill at ease socially and lack confidence in their own opinions.

Some, but not all, schizoid individuals benefit from participating in group, as well as individual, therapy. The group provides a built-in system of social contacts and an accepting environment in which schizoid individuals may open up and hone their newly acquired social skills. Most people with this disorder, however, remain loners, preferring solitary pursuits over social ones.

SCHIZOTYPAL PERSONALITY DISORDER

Individuals with schizotypal personality disorder think, perceive, communicate, and act in eccentric ways. Characteristic symptoms include distorted thoughts and perceptions, such as believing that others are talking about them or hearing a voice calling their name, and peculiarities in behavior, such as odd ways of speaking and dressing. Like those with schizoid personality disorder, they are extremely uncomfortable in and have a reduced capacity for close relationships. They often are suspicious of others and may have paranoid fears that others want to harm or embarrass them. Their strange ways of talking, social awkwardness, and limited emotional range interfere with establishment of friendships or intimate relationships.

First designated an official psychiatric disorder in 1980, this diagnosis remains controversial. Some therapists believe that because schizotypal individuals may think, perceive, and act in ways resembling those associated with schizophrenia, schizotypal personality should be classified as a schizophrenic disorder (see Chapter 17). Others view it as a personality disorder involving symptoms that range from withdrawal and insecurity in unfamiliar social situations to paranoid ideas, suspiciousness, or odd beliefs such as clairvoyance, telepathy, or a sixth sense. In extreme cases, persons may experience brief psychotic episodes during which they cannot distinguish reality from their delusions or hallucinations, yet their symptoms are not severe enough to be termed schizophrenia.

About 3 percent of the population may have this disorder, which may be slightly more common in men and always develops by early adulthood.

Individuals with schizotypal personality disorder may:

- Feel extremely uncomfortable in any close relationship
- Think that passersby are talking about them

- Believe in clairvoyance, telepathy, or a sixth sense

- Experience unusual bodily symptoms, such as pain in the blood or bones

- Think or talk in odd ways

- Be excessively suspicious

- Seem cold and aloof

- Look odd, eccentric, or peculiar

- Have no friends or confidants, or one at most.

▼
Understanding schizotypal personality disorder

Schizotypal men and women feel little, if any, joy in living or in relationships with others. They often describe their lives as gray and empty and themselves as lacking in enthusiasm and motivation. They have little or no sense of humor, which may stem from their tendency to take everything literally or may be rooted in an inner joylessness.

These persons have a very limited emotional range and do not pick up on the subtle cues that take place in normal interactions. Some misinterpret the people and events around them. Often they become increasingly tense and suspicious of others' motives. They have one close friend or confidant at most and often none at all, and become extremely anxious in social situations involving unfamiliar people. Even when given opportunities to form friendships, they may shy away from them. They cannot connect with other people in gratifying, pleasurable ways. If they do form a relationship, they tend to remain distant, or else they terminate it because of their anxiety or paranoia.

Schizotypal individuals may choose jobs that seem beneath their ability because they neither require nor want much interaction with others. Some have difficulty generalizing from one situation to another similar one; each encounter is a brand new experience.

To others, schizotypal individuals seem peculiar. They may talk to themselves in public, gesture meaninglessly, or laugh in a silly manner while discussing problems. Although they remain coherent and comprehensible, they often speak in odd ways, rambling, using unusual phrases and words, and rarely looking others in the eye. They seem incapable of chit-chat, lighthearted teasing, or other forms of conversational give and take, and are stiff or out of place in such exchanges. Their choice of clothing may be eccentric by any standard.

These individuals often have problems with what mental health professionals refer to as ego boundaries, and have a distorted sense of their own identity. They tend to be hypochondriacal, often

Is it schizotypal personality disorder?

According to the DSM-IV, a diagnosis of schizotypal personality disorder should be based on these features:

■ **A pervasive pattern of social and interpersonal deficits marked by acute discomfort with, and reduced capacity for, close relationships as well as by cognitive or perceptual distortions and eccentricities of behavior, beginning by early adulthood and present in various circumstances, as indicated by at least five of the following:**

1. **Ideas of reference (perceiving personal references in others' conversations)**
2. **Odd beliefs or magical thinking that influences behavior and is inconsistent with subcultural norms**
3. **Unusual perceptual experiences, including bodily illusions**
4. **Odd thinking and speech (vague, metaphorical, over-elaborate, etc.)**
5. **Suspiciousness or paranoid ideas**
6. **Inappropriate or constricted emotions**
7. **Behavior or appearance that is odd, eccentric, or peculiar**
8. **Lack of close friends or confidants other than first-degree relatives**
9. **Excessive social anxiety that does not diminish with familiarity and tends to involve paranoid fears rather than negative self-judgments**

■ **Does not occur only during the course of schizophrenia, another psychotic disorder, a mood disorder with psychotic features, or a pervasive developmental disorder**

Adapted from the Diagnostic and Statistical Manual of Mental Disorders, 4th Edition. *Used with permission.*

in bizarre ways. For example, they may feel pain in parts of the body that do not normally produce conscious sensations, such as the blood or bones, or report grotesque symptoms, such as the conviction that something they ate is eating their insides. They may also exaggerate a symptom, such as assuming that they have heart disease if they feel a twinge of chest pain. Typically, the less comfortable these persons are with other people, the more physical discomfort they experience.

Schizotypal individuals may experience various mixtures of anxiety, depression, and other distressing moods. It is estimated that about 30 to 50 percent of those diagnosed as schizotypal also suffer from a depressive disorder; more than half have had previous depressions. Occasionally they develop strong suicidal tendencies and may attempt suicide or actually kill themselves.

▼

Treating schizotypal personality disorder

Individuals with this disorder usually do not seek treatment unless they develop depression or a psychotic episode, or come to a therapist at the urging of a family member. Most cannot tolerate the demands of insight-oriented psychotherapy, although they can benefit from a supportive relationship that aims to overcome distorted thinking and odd behavior. Sometimes simply forming a secure, trusting relationship with a mental health professional helps them to cope better.

Often therapists come to serve as "reality organs," helping individuals to interpret a situation or event and focusing on feelings of alienation, isolation, or suspiciousness. Through therapy, they may realize that they have a choice: They can remain isolated in their lonely, joyless world, or they can reach out to participate more fully in life. Even though they may still find intimacy too threatening to form relationships, they can enrich the quality of their existence through the arts, music, travel, or a craft or hobby.

Cognitive-behavioral techniques, with an emphasis on social skills and risk-taking in social situations, may be useful. Those with peculiar mannerisms or odd ways of talking and dressing can benefit from behavior modification to help them fit in better with other people. Very practical forms of instruction—speech therapy to make their communication clearer and more effective, help in choosing clothing, a diary to record interactions with other people, videotapes that allow them to observe and modify awkward mannerisms—can be extremely helpful.

Low-dose antipsychotic drugs may help to alleviate anxiety and psychosis-like features that develop under stress, particularly in those who experience short-term psychotic breaks. Suicidal individuals may require hospitalization. Those with a severe degree of social impairment may require care in day hospitals or halfway houses, where treatment may focus on encouraging them to make more social contacts within the community, while vocational training prepares them for jobs that do not demand much interaction.

Some individuals with this problem improve significantly with treatment, whereas others make only modest gains. A small number of schizotypal individuals eventually develop schizophrenia.

PART III

Special Issues

Is suicide a risk?

An individual at risk for attempting suicide may:

- [ ] **Feel intense hopelessness**
- [ ] **Have very low self-esteem**
- [ ] **Feel sad and depressed, and may lose interest in favorite activities**
- [ ] **Drink more than usual or take drugs**
- [ ] **Have recently lost or broken up with someone important**
- [ ] **Dramatically change eating, drinking, and sleep patterns**
- [ ] **Become very moody**
- [ ] **Suddenly seem calm or peaceful**
- [ ] **Talk about suicide**
- [ ] **Be preoccupied with death**
- [ ] **Not function as well as usual at school or on the job**
- [ ] **Withdraw from friends**
- [ ] **Withdraw from usual activities**
- [ ] **Neglect personal appearance**
- [ ] **Find it difficult to concentrate**
- [ ] **Develop physical symptoms, such as headache or fatigue**
- [ ] **Feel overwhelming guilt or shame**
- [ ] **Become violent, hostile, or rebellious (especially in young people)**
- [ ] **Have recently been discharged from a hospital for psychiatric treatment**

The more boxes that you check, the more reason you have to be concerned about the threat of suicide. If there is immediate danger, contact a mental health professional as soon as possible. This chapter provides information on suicide and guidance on seeking help.

22

Suicidal Behavior

Every year thirty thousand Americans—among them many who seem to have "everything to live for"—commit suicide. Ten times as many attempt to take their own lives. Why? This question haunts parents, relatives, and friends, yet there is never an adequate explanation for what happened. Usually suicide is a desperate cry for help, a last attempt to communicate from a private hell. To people who take their own lives, death seems the best, if not the only, solution—not only for themselves but for their families and friends.

Suicide, the most absolute of conscious actions, leaves no chance for second thoughts or regrets. It is the end. Suicide is not in itself a mental disorder, but it can be the tragic result of psychiatric disorders and of emotional and psychological problems. Many of those who kill themselves suffer from mental disorders. Some cannot cope any more, cannot think rationally, or feel ashamed, lonely, or helpless. For others, particularly young people, trying to take their own lives may be an impulse, an unthinking reaction to yet another frustration or disappointment. (Chapter 26 discusses youth suicide.) Those with debilitating or terminal diseases may think of suicide as a welcome end to their struggle with infirmity and pain. Older individuals, who are faced with the loss of their own good health, of the people they love most, or of the activities that gave them decades of satisfaction, may view suicide as a sensible solution to their difficulties.

But suicide is not inevitable. If those at high risk are identified, rapid intervention and appropriate treatment can literally be life-saving. The more that people learn about suicide and its warning signals, the greater the hope of more tomorrows for more people.

▼

**How common
is suicide?**

Almost 1 percent of all Americans die as a result of suicide, which has become the eighth leading cause of death in this country. The overall rate of suicide has remained the same: 11 to 12 per 100,000. During the last thirty years, however, reported suicides among young adults between the ages of fifteen and twenty-four have tripled, and suicide is second only to accidents as the leading killer of American youth. Nevertheless, suicide is still most common among the elderly, and eighty-year-olds are more likely to take their own lives than teenagers. The suicide rate for white men at age eighty-five or older is 50 per 100,000.

At all ages, men are three times as likely to commit suicide as women, but women attempt suicide much more frequently than men. Elderly men are ten times more likely to take their own lives than elderly women; the incidence of suicide among teenaged boys is twice as high as among girls. The suicide rate is usually higher for whites than for other races. However, it is rising among young blacks in inner city neighborhoods; their incidence of suicide is twice that of white men of the same age. Native Americans have a suicide rate five times higher than that of the general population.

Suicide rates are lowest among married men and women and highest among the separated, divorced, or widowed. In general, people who live alone are at higher risk. College students commit suicide at about half the rate of young people their age who are not in school. Professionals, especially lawyers and physicians (with women physicians at even greater risk), are more likely to kill themselves than blue-collar workers. Suicide occurs more often in times of economic hardship. The unemployed are at higher risk than those with any type of job.

Suicidal thoughts
and actions

Thinking about taking one's life is not unusual, and the vast majority of people who contemplate suicide never follow through. Suicidal thoughts, however, can range from a fleeting reflection that death might be a welcome form of escape to a more focused wish to die. When thinking begins to take the form of planning, there is serious danger. Those who have thought through a plan for killing themselves may be more likely to act on it impulsively in a moment of desperation.

Suicidal gestures are attempts at suicide that are designed to fail, such as taking an overdose of aspirin or other over-the-counter drugs. More serious attempts, such as taking potentially lethal pills, are clearly motivated by a desire or a willingness to die. Most attempts are impulsive rather than deliberate, and nine out of ten fail. Usually the attempt itself is emotionally cathartic. Afterwards, individuals may be deeply ashamed and regret what they have done. Some may admit that they wanted to gain attention, hurt a loved one, or win back a former lover. Typically, they are grateful to those who saved or helped them.

Two-thirds of those who try but fail at a suicide attempt are women, who are most likely to try to kill themselves by overdosing on medications. In contrast, those who complete suicide are more often men suffering from alcoholism or depression, who shoot or hang themselves.

Suicide attempts are more common in those under age thirty-five. Like the act of suicide, they occur more frequently among those who are divorced, unmarried, and living alone without confidants or friends, and among those who suffer from a mental disorder (usually depression, substance abuse, or a personality disorder). Substance abuse plays a greater role in suicide attempts by teenagers than by older men and women.

A suicide attempt should always be taken very seriously, even when the individual deeply regrets the action. If nothing changes afterward—if the person does not get professional help, if the world seems just as bleak—he or she is likely to try again, and this time may choose a deadlier method. Each year, 1 to 2 percent of those who have attempted suicide finally succeed in killing themselves. Ultimately, more than 10 percent of those who attempted suicide in the past take their own lives.

What leads to suicide?

Researchers have looked for explanations for suicide by studying everything from the phases of the moon to the seasons (suicides peak in the spring) to birth order in the family. They have found no conclusive answers. A constellation of influences (mental disorders, personality traits, biological and genetic vulnerability, medical illness, and psychosocial stressors) may combine in ways that lower an individual's threshold of vulnerability. No single factor in itself may ever explain fully why a person chooses death.

MENTAL ILLNESS

As many as 95 percent of those who commit suicide have a mental disorder. Two of these in particular, depression and alcoholism, account for two-thirds of all suicides. Suicide is also a risk for those with other disorders, including anxiety disorders, schizophrenia, and personality disorders.

The depressive disorders, including major depression and bipolar illness (manic depression), are most closely linked with suicide. The risk for suicide in depression may be particularly high early in the course of the illness, when recovery may seem all but impossible, and again after a person begins treatment and starts to recover. At this point, physical symptoms, such as a lack of energy, are improving, but psychological symptoms, such as hopelessness, have not yet lifted. Because this partial recovery gives them the energy to carry out a plan, depressed individuals may follow through on a suicide attempt they had been considering for some time. The risk also increases during the period after release from a hospital or residential facility following treatment, and after any setbacks in recovery that trigger a return of feelings of despair.

SUBSTANCE ABUSE

Dependence on alcohol or drugs increases a person's suicide risk fivefold. Individuals who abuse several substances are at greatest risk. In addition, many of those who commit suicide drink beforehand, and their use of alcohol may lower their inhibitions. Since alcohol itself is a depressant, it can intensify the despondency that suicidal individuals are already experiencing.

Alcoholics who attempt suicide often have other risk factors, including major depression, poor social support, serious medical illness, and unemployment. Among men hospitalized for alcoholism, the risk for suicide during the first five years after hospitalization is seventy-five times greater than that of the general population. Drugs of abuse can also alter thinking and lower inhibitions against suicide. In recent years, the incidence of cocaine-related suicide has increased significantly.

HOPELESSNESS

A sense of utter hopelessness and helplessness may be the most common contributing factors in suicide. When hope dies, people view every experience in negative terms and come to expect the worst possible outcomes for their problems. Given this way of thinking, suicide often appears to be a reasonable escape from a life that they characterize as not worth living. Hopelessness can occur in many mental disorders, including depression, anxiety disorders, and schizophrenia. Guilt and despair increase the risk of suicide.

FAMILY HISTORY

One in every four people who attempt suicide has a family member who also tried to commit suicide, according to a study of 2,304 Los Angeles residents sponsored by the National Institute of Mental Health (NIMH). Although a family history of suicide is not in itself a predictor of suicide, two mental illnesses that can lead to suicide, depression and bipolar disorder, do run in families. Unmarried women with a family history of suicide are more likely to attempt suicide than men or married women with similar backgrounds.

PHYSICAL ILLNESS

Many people who commit suicide are physically ill or believe they are. More than 80 percent have seen a physician about a medical complaint within the six months preceding suicide. About 5 percent actually have a serious physical disorder, such as a traumatic brain injury, epilepsy, multiple sclerosis, Huntington's chorea, Parkinson's disease, AIDS, or cancer. In various reports, the suicide rate among individuals with HIV infection and AIDS has been from thirty to almost sixty times that of the general population. Among persons undergoing kidney dialysis, it is up to four hundred times higher. Often an undiagnosed, untreated depression is responsible for suicide attempts by the medically ill. Although suicide may seem like a decision rationally arrived at, this may not be the case. Depression, not uncommon in serious illness, can skew judgment. When the depression is treated, the person may no longer have suicidal intentions.

BRAIN CHEMISTRY

Investigators have found abnormalities in the brain chemistry of persons who complete suicide, particularly in low levels of a metabolite of the neurotransmitter serotonin, 5-hydroxyindoleacetic acid or 5-HIAA, in cerebrospinal fluid. As noted in Chapter 2, serotonin is involved in the control of impulses, particularly of impulses toward violent or self-destructive acts. There are indications that individuals with a deficiency of this substance may be at as much as ten times greater risk for committing suicide than those with higher levels.

Also at risk are those who exhibit abnormal responses to the dexamethasone suppression test, which is sometimes used to diagnose depression (see Chapter 5). Like those who are depressed, suicidal individuals may have enlarged adrenal glands and high levels of urinary metabolites of the adrenal steroid hormone cortisol It is not clear whether these markers specifically indicate an increased risk for suicide or merely confirm the diagnosis of depression.

Can suicide be rational?

An elderly widow suffering from advanced cancer takes a lethal overdose of sleeping pills. A young man with several AIDS-related illnesses shoots himself. A woman in her fifties, diagnosed as having Alzheimer's disease, asks a doctor to help her end her life. Are these suicides "rational" because these individuals used logical reasoning in deciding to end their lives?

The question is intensely controversial. Advocates of the right to "self-deliverance" argue that persons in great pain or faced with the prospect of a debilitating, hopeless battle against an incurable disease can and should be able to decide to end their lives. As legislatures and the legal system tackle the thorny ques-tion of an individual's right to die, mental health professionals worry that, even in those with fatal diseases, suicidal wishes often stem from undiagnosed depression.

In one classic study of forty-four terminally ill individuals, thirty-four had never been suicidal or wished for death. The remaining ten— seven who desired early death and three who had specifically considered suicide—all had severe depression. Their despair and preoccupation with dying may well have contributed to their willingness to consider suicide. A large number of studies have indicated that most patients with painful, progressive, or terminal illnesses do not want to kill themselves. The percentage of those who report thinking about suicide ranges from 5 to 20 percent; most of these persons have major depressions. "What makes patients suicidal is depression, not their physical condition," says one psychiatrist.

Because depression may indeed warp the ability to make a rational decision about suicide, mental health professionals urge physicians and family members to make sure that individuals with chronic or fatal illnesses are evaluated for depression and given medication, psychotherapy, or both. It is also important for everyone to allow enough time—an average of three to eight weeks—to see if treatment for depression will make a difference in their desire to continue living.

GENERATIONAL ISSUES

Suicide rates have almost tripled among adolescents and young adults in the last thirty years, especially among white males. No single theory can explain why. Factors such as the mobility and instability of modern life, divorce, economic woes, sexual dangers, and substance abuse all may add to the stress felt by teenagers. Although more than half of teens who attempt suicide suffer from depression, many who have never shown any signs of the disorder also kill themselves, sometimes under the influence of drugs or alcohol, sometimes in an impulsive burst of rage or frustration. Some may feel so overwhelmed or trapped by a long string of setbacks, failures, fights with their families, and losses, particularly the end of a close relationship with a boyfriend or girlfriend, that they see no other way out of their difficulties.

Elderly Americans have the highest suicide rates in our society, with an estimated 8,500 to 9,000 taking their own lives every year. Those at highest risk are men, often recently bereaved. An underlying depression, which often is not recognized, is a common cause. Social isolation and anxiety about finances increase the risk. More than 70 percent of the depressed elderly improve dramatically with treatment, which usually consists of a combination of psycho-therapy and medication. (See Chapter 25 on mental health in the elderly.)

OTHER FACTORS

In the tangle of a complicated life, it is often impossible to sort out which experiences or difficulties may have led a person to suicide. People who kill themselves have often gone through many major life crises—job changes, births, financial reversals, divorce, retirement—in the preceding six months. Long-standing, intense conflict with family members or other important people may add to the danger. In some cases, suicide may be an act of revenge that offers the person a sense of control, however temporary or illusory, such as when a husband whose wife has had an affair gets back at her—and has the final word—by killing himself. Others may feel that by rejecting life they are rejecting a partner or parent who abandoned or betrayed them.

For individuals who are already faced with a combination of pre-disposing factors, access to a means of committing suicide, particu-larly to guns, can add to the risk. The rate of suicide by use of a firearm has soared over recent decades, especially among teenagers and young adults. Unlike other methods of suicide, guns allow very little margin for error. States with strict gun-control laws have much lower rates of suicides than states that lack them.

▼

Seeking help It can be especially hard for relatives and friends to admit to themselves or others that someone they cherish might be consi-dering suicide. Difficult though this is, the danger is too great to ignore warning signals (see table on page 567). If there is any reason to suspect that suicide could be a danger for someone close to you, these are the questions that should be asked:

- Has the person attempted suicide in the past?
- Does he or she have a potentially deadly disease, such as AIDS or cancer?
- Does the person have a chronic debilitating medical illness, such as severe heart disease or arthritis?
- Has he or she made dramatic changes in eating, drinking, and sleep patterns?
- Has he or she seemed more moody, down, or sad?
- Has the individual talked about death or suicide?
- Does he or she seem to have a plan for committing suicide?
- Does he or she make comments such as "What's the use?" or "It doesn't matter any more"?

- Does the person seem preoccupied with death?

- Has he or she given away prized possessions?

- Has he or she taken steps to tie up loose ends, such as organizing personal papers or straightening up a perpetually messy office?

- Has performance at work or school declined?

- Has drug or alcohol use increased?

- Has a close romantic relationship recently ended?

- Has the individual withdrawn from normal activities?

- Has he or she expressed feelings of worthlessness or discouragement?

- Has he or she pulled away from friends and family?

- Is the person neglecting personal appearance?

- Does the person complain about physical symptoms, such as headache or fatigue?

- Has he or she suddenly become cheerful or calm after a period of despondency?

- Has the behavior of an adolescent or young adult become violent, hostile, or rebellious? Has he or she run away?

The more "yes" answers given, the more reason there may be for concern. A suicide threat or attempt is a medical emergency requiring professional help. Special suicide hotlines listed in the front of the phone directory can put you in touch with trained personnel. You also might call a mental health crisis center, your physician, or a therapist. If time is crucial, call 911 rather than flipping through the phone book, and explain the circumstances to the dispatcher. If you call a mental health hotline, describe the situation briefly and clearly. Allow the health workers to ask for details. If you cannot stay on the phone, say where you are and specify the kind of help you, your friend, or your family member needs.

Treating suicidal behavior

Professional assessment and treatment are essential. Therapy can help those who feel overwhelmed by problems to realize that they can work toward solutions. Individuals with an underlying mental disorder need appropriate treatment. In every case, the goal is to restore the person's hope of obtaining effective help and finding positive options for dealing with his or her life.

Initially, treatment serves primarily as a way of buying time for therapy and medication, usually antidepressants, to have an effect. To minimize the risk of overdosage with certain antidepressant drugs, psychiatrists often restrict their use or prescribe only

WARNING SIGNALS

Often a person considering suicide says or does something that should serve as a warning signal. The most obvious clue is a previous attempt. Other indications of danger include:

☐ **Increased moodiness, seeming down or sad**

☐ **Feelings of worthlessness or discouragement**

☐ **A withdrawal from friends, family, and normal activities**

☐ **Changes in eating, sleeping, or sexual habits**

☐ **Specific suicide threats**

☐ **Letters, poems, or essays revealing a preoccupation with death**

☐ **Persistent boredom**

☐ **A decline in performance at work or school**

☐ **In young people, violent, hostile, or rebellious behavior, including running away**

☐ **Breaking off of close relationships**

☐ **Increased drug and alcohol use**

☐ **A failed love relationship**

☐ **Unusual neglect of personal appearance**

☐ **Difficulty in concentrating**

☐ **Radical personality change**

☐ **Complaints about physical symptoms, such as headache or fatigue**

☐ **Statements such as "It's no use" or "Nothing matters anymore"**

☐ **Giving away of possessions, putting affairs in order**

---

enough for a few days at a time, or choose antidepressants, such as the selective serotonin reuptake inhibitors (SSRIs), which have a lower risk of death from overdoses. Electroconvulsive therapy (ECT) may be recommended for suicidal depressed individuals because it relieves acute depression more quickly than drugs (see Chapters 5 and 28).

Many mental health professionals have individuals sign a contract agreeing not to kill themselves before their next appointment and promising to contact the therapist if they should feel any suicidal impulses. Both the person and the family should be able to reach the therapist or another mental health professional at any time of day or night.

Those who have attempted suicide or who have carefully designed plans for suicide and the means of carrying them out require surveillance, usually in a hospital with a locked psychiatric unit. If they refuse to consent to the admission, the treating psychiatrist may fill out the forms necessary for involuntary commitment, a legal process used when individuals are considered dangerous to themselves or others. Hospitalization is most likely to be necessary for those have attempted suicide in the past, are preoccupied with death, have shown serious intent to carry out a suicide plan, abuse drugs or alcohol, have a chronic medical or psychotic illness, have experienced a recent loss, express hopelessness, or have poor social supports. In a safe setting, treatment for an underlying illness such as depression, bipolar illness, or schizophrenia can begin or be continued. During hospitalization, individuals are carefully watched and are kept away from sharp objects, belts, and other items they might use to harm themselves.

Suicide continues to be a major risk after hospitalization, which is only a temporary means of prevention. Patients often attempt to kill themselves again within days or weeks of discharge. Families must be aware of this risk so they can watch for warning signals of danger. The person should undergo follow-up treatment, which can include medication, supportive or insight-oriented therapy, and treatment for drug or alcohol abuse, if this is a problem. Family therapy may help in dealing with underlying conflicts as well as with an actual or threatened suicide attempt. Several studies indicate that the combination of medication with other forms of therapy, including psychotherapy and drug treatment, may produce the greatest benefit for depressed suicidal individuals.

For individuals with bipolar disorder, the best approach may be lithium combined with psychotherapy. Those who do not improve with lithium may be given other antimania drugs to augment lithium therapy. (These treatments are discussed in detail in Chapter 6.)

For suicidal individuals with schizophrenia, therapists provide supportive therapy. Those who show signs of depression may benefit from antidepressant drugs. Education of family members, who must realize the importance of not criticizing or berating the individual, can be very important. Although no one who is suicidal should abuse drugs or alcohol, schizophrenic individuals are especially susceptible to the effects of these substances and should avoid them completely. It is also essential that they comply with their schedule for taking antipsychotic medication. (Chapter 17 discusses psychotic disorders.)

If someone you love may be considering suicide

Individuals who are suicidal need to know that friends and family care and understand. They usually feel they are so worthless that no one can or should be concerned about them. Above all else, relatives should not criticize. Parents must be especially careful about not judging teenagers or dismissing their feelings as "stupid" or "silly."

Remember that you cannot tackle this problem alone and that professional help is essential. Just as love and understanding cannot protect people from all the dangers in the world, the same is true for suicide. However, you may be able to make a difference by following these suggestions:

Encourage the individual to talk. Ask concerned questions. Listen attentively. Show that you take the person's feelings seriously and truly care.

Don't criticize the person for feeling suicidal or offer reassurances that he or she will feel better in the morning or next week. If you do, he may withdraw from you and keep his bleak thoughts and plans to himself.

Don't offer trite counsel or list reasons to go on living. Suicidal individuals can be so consumed with their emotional pain that they are unable to appreciate the good things in their lives or focus on the feelings of those who love them.

Don't analyze the person's motives or try to challenge them. Telling individuals who are considering suicide to go ahead will not shock them into rational thinking and may push them closer to the edge.

Suggest solutions or alternatives to problems. Make plans. Encourage positive action.

Don't be afraid to ask directly whether your loved one or friend has considered suicide. The opportunity to talk about thoughts of suicide may be an enormous relief and, contrary to a long-standing myth, will not fix the idea of suicide more firmly in a person's mind.

If your loved one admits to having considered suicide, ask gentle questions, such as how or why. If he or she has a definite plan, ask for specifics. If the person plans to take pills, ask what kind or whether they have been bought yet. Find out if the person has access to a gun. The degree to which the person has formulated actual plans is a measure of how great the risk is of acting on suicidal feelings.

Express your own feelings. If you feel frightened or sad, say so.

If you start thinking about suicide

At some point, the thought of ending it all—all the disappointments, all the problems, all the bad feelings—may cross your mind. This experience isn't unusual for anyone. But if the idea of taking your life persists or intensifies, if you find yourself thinking of how you might go about it or cannot stop thinking about it, seek professional help. Suicidal thoughts are signs of treatable illnesses, and you should respond to them as you would other warnings of potential threats to your health.

The National Depressive and Manic-Depressive Association (DMDA) offers the following recommendations from doctors experienced in treating depressive disorders and individuals "who know what it feels like when depression digs in, but who have survived and want to share their thoughts on how and why":

☐ **Talk to a mental health professional.** Suicidal thoughts indicate more than ever before that you need their help. Keep your doctor's phone number with you; also have a back-up number, such as a suicide hotline.

☐ **Find someone you can trust and talk with honestly about what you're feeling.** Develop a list of friends or family members who can provide support when you may feel suicidal. Educate them about your condition so they are prepared if you call and tell them you're considering suicide.

☐ **Recognize symptoms for what they are.** With your doctor, identify the symptoms you are likely to experience when depression is at its worst. Write them down to help you keep them in perspective during a suicidal episode.

☐ **Write down your daily thoughts.** A simple record of your hopes for the future and the people you value in your life can remind you of why your own life is worth continuing.

☐ **Avoid drugs and alcohol.** Most suicides are the results of sudden, uncontrolled impulses, and drugs and alcohol can make it harder for you to resist these destructive urges.

☐ **Recognize the earliest warning signs of a suicidal episode.** Often your body will give you signals of an episode coming on. Over time you can learn to be sensitive to these danger signs and take action fast.

☐ **Know when it is best to go to the hospital.** Hospitalization can sometimes be the best way to protect your health and safety. Make sure your doctor knows which hospital you prefer and has your most recent medical records. Know the extent of your insurance coverage, and keep relevant health care information in a convenient and accessible place.

☐ **Develop a formal "plan for life" similar to the one on the opposite page.** If you start thinking about taking your own life, all you have to do is follow it.

Adapted from Suicide and Depressive Illness, *National Depressive and Manic-Depressive Association. Used with permission.*

Remove all guns from your home. Anyone who has given the slightest hint of suicidal intentions should not have access to any type of firearms.

Don't think that people who talk about killing themselves never carry out their threats. Many of those who commit suicide give definite indications of their intent to die.

If the person makes a point of saying good-bye or giving you a treasured possession, be especially suspicious. Assure him or her that suicidal impulses are temporary, and that all problems, however big, can be solved.

A plan for life

Doctor's name/phone number: _____

If doctor is not available call other medical professionals: _____
_____

If I start to think about suicide, I will contact these trusted friends (in order of priority):

NAME   PHONE

1 _____   _____

2 _____   _____

3 _____   _____

I know that I am entering a depressed phase of my illness when I experience the following warning signs:

1 _____

2 _____

3 _____

If someone I cared about were considering suicide, this is what I would say to him/her: _____
_____
_____

Preferred hospital if necessary: _____

My health insurance carrier is: _____

Amount of hospitalization insurance coverage: _____

Policy number: _____

Activity checklist

☐ Contact doctor

☐ Contact friends or family

☐ Read diary entries

☐ Notify employer (if I think I will need time off)

☐ Throw away alcohol and unnecessary medications

☐ Prepare for possible hospitalization (if doctor advises)

☐ Identify stressors that may have led to this crisis

_____
Adapted from Suicide and Depressive Illness, *National Depressive and Manic-Depressive Association. Used with permission.*

If you feel that you aren't making any headway, suggest that both you and the individual talk to a mental health professional together. Even if you seem to be having an impact, professional help remains crucial.

Follow your instincts. If you suspect that your friend or family member may act soon on an impulse, stay with him or her and call a suicide hotline.

If you must leave the person alone, negotiate. Have your friend promise that he or she won't do anything to harm himself or herself without first calling you. If your friend does call, get to him or her as quickly as possible. Call for help immediately.

Even if you feel that you have talked someone out of committing suicide, contact a mental health professional. A calm or improved mood does not mean the danger is over.

Impact on relationships

Any suicide attempt can shake a family to its core. Family members may feel enormously guilty as they try to understand why a loved one tried to take his or her life and may wonder what they could or should have done. At the same time, they may be angry at the person for causing such great anguish, although they may be afraid to acknowledge or express this feeling openly. Relieved and grateful that their relative is still alive and that there will be a second chance for a better tomorrow, family members must also face and live with the fear that there may be another attempt and that it might be fatal.

A "successful" suicide attempt ends one life and shatters many others. Its effects are devastating for the individual's family and friends. As partners, parents, siblings, spouses, friends, and colleagues mourn, they are often haunted by regrets, questions, and "if onlys." Survivors are frequently angry at themselves for not somehow saving the person they loved. Guilt over not having given the person enough support and love can linger longer after a suicide than after a death caused by illness or injury. An important part of the healing process is coming to terms with guilt.

Although survivors may want desperately to find out exactly why a loved one committed suicide, almost always it is impossible to know the precise reasons. Even notes, which only about a third of all those who kill themselves leave behind, are likely to provide only partial answers and insights. This troubling sense of not knowing is another issue the survivors must confront and work through.

Some mental health professionals have described the trauma of losing a loved one to suicide, particularly if there has been no forewarning, as so intense that it can induce a reaction similar to posttraumatic stress disorder. Like those with PTSD, survivors of a suicide may suffer distressing nightmares, avoid experiences that might remind them of the loss, lose interest in activities they once enjoyed, or feel incapable of tender emotions.

Grief after a suicide may be especially intense or prolonged, and mourning family members are at risk for depression and even suicide themselves. Anger, a normal response to any death, may be especially persistent, and survivors typically are most angry at themselves for not having recognized clues to the victim's plans.

"I think the anger pulls you through," observes comedian Joan Rivers in her comments on her husband's suicide in *On the Edge of Darkness.* "You get through the guilt by saying to yourself, which I truly believe, that you can't take a splinter out in depression; people have got to cure themselves. You can't do it for them, there's no way. If a friend has cancer, you can't take the cancer out of them. It's the same thing. If they're lucky, they're going to come out of it." An additional burden for family members is apprehension arising from fears that suicide "runs" in families. Young people are particularly fearful that they, too, will feel an irresistible urge to take their own lives. As Joan Rivers notes, suicide seems like "a viable option" for children with a parent who committed suicide: "After it becomes a reality in your family, it's a definite way out."

Psychotherapy is of great help in enabling the families of suicide victims to understand and deal with the serious emotional and practical crises that they experience. Support groups made up of those who have undergone similar losses can also be valuable, and are particularly helpful if families have not obtained social support from others because of religious and cultural taboos against suicide.

In time, the emotionally draining and difficult process of grieving may enable survivors to achieve a sense of peace and acceptance. Although the pain of their loss stays with them always, the day usually comes when they can face the future and get on with their lives. But one thing never changes. As a mother whose fourteen-year-old son hanged himself put it, "There's an empty place in your heart forever."

▼

Outlook   As many as 70 to 80 percent of those at risk for suicide can be helped with appropriate treatment. The challenge is identifying these individuals and making sure that they receive needed help as promptly as possible. Early recognition and treatment for depressive disorders, including "hidden" depression in those with medical illnesses, could help to save thousands of lives each year.

Is it aggressive or violent behavior?

Individuals with aggressive symptoms requiring treatment may:

- ☐ **Frequently shout in anger or make loud noises**
- ☐ **Yell personal insults**
- ☐ **Use foul language or curse viciously**
- ☐ **Threaten violence toward themselves or others**
- ☐ **Slam doors, deliberately throw clothing on the floor**
- ☐ **Throw objects or kick furniture or walls**
- ☐ **Break objects or smash windows**
- ☐ **Set fires or destroy property in other ways**
- ☐ **Pick or scratch at their skin, pull their hair, hit themselves**
- ☐ **Bang their heads, throw themselves onto the floor, slam their fists into objects**
- ☐ **Mutilate themselves with cuts, bites, or burns**
- ☐ **Swing at people or physically threaten them**
- ☐ **Strike, kick, or push others**
- ☐ **Attack others, causing mild to severe injury**

Even checking a single box may indicate a possible problem requiring evaluation. The more boxes that you check, the more reason you may have to be concerned. This chapter describes common problems involving aggression and violence, both personal and social, and provides guidance on seeking help and appropriate treatment.

23

Aggressive and Violent Behavior

A man carrying an assault weapon charges into a high-rise office building and mows down everyone in sight. A passenger in a speeding car fires at other vehicles on the freeway. An elderly widow breaks her hip when her schizophrenic son knocks her down in a sudden rage. A businessman is brutally beaten during a car-jacking. A college student is raped at a fraternity party.

Such incidents are far from uncommon. Violence in our culture has become both a social and a personal concern. As citizens of a violent society, none of us is completely safe. The murder rate for Americans is the highest in the world, more than seven times that of Great Britain or Japan. The incidence of other violent crimes has soared in recent years. According to the FBI, 218 violent crimes are committed every hour in the United States. For individuals who become victims of violence, such statistics cannot begin to describe the horror and outrage they feel. Assault, mugging, battering, rape, and abuse are attacks on body and mind that leave lasting scars.

For those with severe mental disorders and their families, violent behavior poses special problems. Some individuals with severe mental illnesses can become aggressive and violent, and the ones they are most likely to harm are those providing their care. In a study of fifty-five families caring for mentally ill relatives, more than half named aggressive behavior as the most serious problem they faced. (See Chapter 30, When Someone You Love Has a Mental Disorder.)

For years, mental health professionals have been exploring both the causes and the consequences of violence at a social and personal level. This chapter presents what we currently know about the roots of aggression and violence, the options for treatment, the forms violent behaviors take in modern society, and their impact on victims.

Causes of aggression and violent behavior

Whereas anger is considered a normal, sometimes inevitable emotion, aggression—behavior with the intent to control or dominate—is a threat to individuals and to society. Angry people may want to push or punch someone; aggressive people carry through on such impulses and become violent. Why? The reasons are complex, and a full discussion of the sociological, economic, and psychological forces that give rise to aggression and violence is beyond the scope of this chapter. However, scientists are increasingly coming to realize the importance of biological factors, especially damage to the brain and developmental experiences, in creating a predisposition to violent behavior.

BIOLOGICAL FACTORS

Traumatic brain injury may play a major role in violent behavior. For still unexplained reasons, individuals who suffer head trauma often tend to react to a trivial event with overwhelming fury. As many as 70 percent of those who suffer head injuries report some degree of irritability or explosive rage. Those who were drinking or using drugs at the time of an injury or who use these substances afterward are especially likely to behave aggressively or violently. In one study of fifteen death-row prison inmates who had committed brutal murders, all had histories of severe brain injuries, and twelve had neurological problems, such as blackouts or amnesia.

Head injury can cause lesions, or scars, in the brain that impair the function of the frontal or temporal lobes, areas that control reason, judgment, and primitive emotions such as rage. Aggressive behavior was first linked with this region of the brain because of the tendency of some epileptic individuals with partial complex seizures, which involve the temporal lobe, to become violent. However, the connection between epilepsy and violence is controversial, and large-scale studies have found that violence is actually rare among those with seizure disorders.

In searching for other biological abnormalities that may be

BIOLOGICAL CAUSES OF AGGRESSIVE BEHAVIOR

ILLNESSES

☐ **Alzheimer's disease**

☐ **Brain injury**

☐ **Brain tumors**

☐ **Delirium**

☐ **Hormonal disorders (such as hyperthyroidism)**

☐ **Infectious illnesses**

☐ **Multiple sclerosis**

☐ **Parkinson's, Huntington's, or Wilson's disease**

☐ **Seizure disorders**

☐ **Stroke and other neurological disease**

☐ **Systemic lupus erythematosus**

☐ **Vitamin deficiencies**

SUBSTANCES

☐ **Alcohol**

☐ **Anti-anxiety agents (barbiturates, benzodiazepines)**

☐ **Antidepressants**

☐ **Over-the-counter sedatives (which may produce delirium)**

☐ **Painkillers (opiates and other narcotics)**

☐ **Steroids**

linked with violence, neuroscientists have noted low levels of 5-hydroxyindoleacetic acid or 5-HIAA, a metabolite of the neurotransmitter serotonin, in the cerebrospinal fluid of men convicted of homicide. As noted in Chapter 2, serotonin is involved in the control of impulses, particularly those directed toward violent or self-destructive acts. Low levels of 5-HIAA have also been associated with suicide and with impulse control disorders such as pyromania, and may be a marker for general problems with impulsivity. Other neurotransmitters, including norepinephrine, dopamine, acetylcholine, and gamma-amino butyric acid (GABA), may also play important roles in aggression, and the relations among these chemicals ultimately may prove more critical than the levels of any single one of them.

Sex chromosome abnormalities have been investigated but do not seem to cause a greater tendency toward violence in, for example, men with an extra Y chromosome. Researchers have also explored the role of the male sex hormone testosterone. The highly competitive men most likely to dominate a situation or group—whether a seminar or a street gang—tend to have higher testosterone levels than other men. But testosterone in itself does not make men aggressive. At most, as scientists explain, it is only one of many contributing factors.

Physical illnesses and some medications that affect the brain can also lead to aggressive behavior. However, the theoretical link with certain other disorders that have been said to play a part in such behavior, such as hypoglycemia (low blood sugar) and premenstrual syndrome, is unproven and extremely controversial. Also controversial and so unexpected that it has piqued scientific and general interest, is a possible association between aggressiveness and levels of cholesterol, the fat found in the blood that can increase the risk of heart disease. In experimental studies, lowering cholesterol through medication and diet resulted in fewer deaths from heart problems but increased mortality from accidents, homicides, and suicide. In theory, this may be the result of greater aggressiveness, although this has yet to be proven.

MENTAL ILLNESS

Recent research suggests that individuals with serious mental disorders may be more violent than the general population. In an analysis of epidemiological data from the NIMH landmark Epidemiologic Catchment Area (ECA) survey, psychiatrist and researcher E. Fuller Torrey, M.D., found that individuals with a serious mental illness living in the community, particularly those who also had drug or alcohol disorders, report having been violent much more often than those with no mental disorder. However, the incidence of reported violence is even higher in people with a substance abuse problem but no other mental disorder. In other words, alcohol and drug users are, as a group, more violent than individuals with serious mental illnesses.

When researchers do not include those with substance abuse disorders, the risk for assaultive behavior in the mentally ill has been calculated at 7 percent, compared with 2 percent in the general population. "People with major psychiatric disorders are not the 'powder keg' that the media has portrayed," observes Agnes Hatfield, Ph.D., family education specialist for the National Alliance for the Mentally Ill (NAMI). "But they are a little more likely to be violent than the population at large."

Aggression as a symptom   Whereas the majority of people with mental disorders never become violent, those with severe illnesses such as schizophrenia and bipolar disorder may episodically become aggressive or violent. Some schizophrenic individuals become violent because of a delusion that people are threatening or trying to harm them. Others may have low tolerance for frustration or be incapable of delaying the gratification of an impulse. Those who are in a manic episode of bipolar disorder may experience greatly increased irritability and sudden violent outbursts.

Diseases that directly affect the brain, such as dementia, can also lead to aggression or violence. About half of those who have

Alzheimer's disease periodically become agitated or violent. In the mentally retarded, violence is associated with frustration and anger over the inability to express feelings or achieve goals.

Certain personality disorders increase the risk for violence. Persons with a borderline disorder usually direct violence at themselves through self-mutilation. Antisocial personalities are more likely to assault others. Those with paranoid, narcissistic, or histrionic personality disorders sometimes respond to stress with outbursts of aggression or violence.

Alcohol abuse, which lowers inhibitions against violent behavior and interferes with judgment, is strongly linked with aggression. Violence can also occur in users of cocaine (especially crack and intravenously injected cocaine), hallucinogens, PCP, and certain other drugs of abuse. One-third of men who are murdered die in drug-related homicides.

Intermittent explosive disorder   Although aggression and violent behaviors can be symptoms that occur in certain mental illnesses, there is only one mental disorder specifically confined to such behaviors. This is *intermittent explosive disorder* (violent outbursts), recently recognized as an official psychiatric diagnosis in the *Diagnostic and Statistical Manual of Mental Disorders, Fourth Edition (DSM-IV)*. This impulse control disorder is characterized by intense episodes of anger or aggression grossly out of proportion to the cause of the rage that result in personal assaults or property damage. This pattern of periodic physical violence is extremely dangerous and can lead to serious injury and murder.

Intermittent explosive disorder may develop suddenly at any stage of life, but occurs most often in young people in their teens and twenties. Men with this disorder outnumber women by four to one. Some have a history of unusual reactions to drugs or alcohol. Many have abnormal brain functioning, as indicated by neurological tests and brain imaging. Some have a family history of violence, and there is evidence for familial transmission of temper outbursts.

Individuals who explode into violence often describe their outbursts as "spells" or "attacks" that start suddenly and stop almost as quickly. Some report a feeling of tension or arousal before the attack, which is followed by an immediate sense of relief. Afterwards, they may be astounded and embarrassed by their behavior, deeply regret any harm they have done, and reproach themselves for not being able to control themselves.

According to the *DSM-IV*, a diagnosis of this seemingly rare disorder should be based on the following:

- Several discrete episodes of failure to resist aggressive impulses resulting in serious assaultive acts or destruction of property

- Aggressiveness grossly out of proportion to precipitating stressors

- Not better accounted for by antisocial or borderline personality disorder, a psychotic disorder, a manic episode in those with bipolar illness, conduct disorder, attention-deficit/hyperactivity disorder, or the direct effects of a medication, drug of abuse, or general medical condition, such as head trauma or Alzheimer's disease.

Treatment may include medication, psychotherapy, behavioral therapy, and family therapy. Some individuals with intermittent explosive disorder suffer from complex partial seizures; anticonvulsant medication to control the seizures may eliminate the violent behavior. Anticonvulsants also have proven helpful in controlling this disorder in persons without any physical signs of disease. Other drugs used to treat intermittent explosive disorder include beta-blockers, lithium, benzodiazepines, and antipsychotic drugs. Although there are few scientific studies of treatments for this condition, clinicians have reported improvement with drug therapy.

DEVELOPMENTAL FACTORS

A recent report by the American Psychological Association's Committee on Violence and Youth implicated many developmental factors—childrearing practices, parental discipline, relations to peers, sex role socialization, economic inequality, lack of opportunity, and media influences—as contributing to violence. Parents who reject their youngsters, who are physically abusive, or who have a criminal history or antisocial personality disorder (described in Chapter 21) are most likely to have children who show early signs of aggressive behavior. Clearly, brutalized children often learn to become brutal themselves.

Harsh discipline also increases aggressive or violent behavior, which is likely to be demonstrated with playmates rather than at home. Exposure to community violence may also have an effect. In a study of almost 150 grade schoolers, NIMH researchers found that 14 percent of first- and second-graders had seen someone shot, stabbed, or raped; 30 percent had seen a mugging or someone being chased by a gang. Among these young witnesses to crime, about 30 percent developed behavioral problems or signs of depression and fear.

In other cases, for a variety of reasons, children never seem to learn effective ways of handling frustration. Instead, they lash out violently, which can lead to punishment by adults and rejection by peers. Doing poorly at school or feeling ostracized as "dumb" increases the likelihood of aggression.

EXPOSURE TO VIOLENCE IN THE MEDIA

According to the American Psychiatric Association (APA), there are five to six violent acts per hour on television during prime time and twenty to twenty-five per hour on Saturday morning children's programs. Far more graphic violence is available on uncut commercial films in the 60 percent of all households with cable TV or VCRs. The effects of exposure to violence in movies and on television are complex and long-lasting. According to several major studies, viewing violence contributes to an increased acceptance of aggressive attitudes and behavior. It also desensitizes individuals to the terrible consequences of violence.

The impact on children may be particularly damaging. Studies in the United States and other countries have found that more aggressive children watch more television, prefer violent programs, and identify with TV characters more than less aggressive youngsters. In one twenty-two-year longitudinal study, psychologists documented a strong relationship between the violent TV programs children watched, how aggressive they were in school, and aggressive and criminal behavior in adulthood. The more frequently boys watched television at age eight, the more aggressive they were at age nineteen. At thirty, they were more likely to have been convicted of serious crimes, to be more aggressive under the influence of alcohol, and to punish their own children harshly, possibly perpetuating a cycle of abuse and violence.

SOCIAL FACTORS

Extreme poverty, deprivation, unemployment, prejudice, discrimination, involvement with gangs, and repeated exposure to actual violence all contribute to aggressive and violent behavior. The risk for violence increases for those who can find few, if any, economic and social opportunities in mainstream society. Violence is most common among the poor, regardless of race. Most minority individuals, including those who grow up with poverty, discrimination, and family disruptions, do not engage in violence and are, in fact, more likely to be victims of violent crime than white Americans.

The availability of guns has added to the danger. According to the National Rifle Association, 40 to 50 percent of American homes have guns. The National Education Association estimates that 100,000 students carry guns to school. Ease of access to guns has consistently been found to increase homicide rates since, with a gun at hand, an assault or fight may well culminate in murder. About two-thirds of homicides in the United States are committed with firearms. In inner cities, gunshot wounds are the leading cause of death in teenage boys, who often carry weapons to school. Gang membership multiplies the danger, and gang mem-

AGGRESSIVE BEHAVIOR CHECKLIST

Verbal aggression

☐ **Makes loud noises, shouts angrily**

☐ **Yells mild personal insults, e.g., "You're stupid!"**

☐ **Curses viciously, uses foul language in anger, makes moderate threats to others or self**

☐ **Makes clear threats of violence toward others or self ("I'm going to kill you.") or requests help to control self**

Physical aggression against objects

☐ **Slams door, scatters clothing, makes a mess**

☐ **Throws objects down, kicks furniture without breaking it, marks the wall**

☐ **Breaks objects, smashes windows**

☐ **Sets fires, throws objects dangerously**

Physical aggression against self

☐ **Picks or scratches skin, pulls hair (with no or minor injury only)**

☐ **Bangs head, hits fist into objects, throws self onto floor or into objects (hurts self without serious injury)**

☐ **Small cuts or bruises, minor burns**

☐ **Mutilates self, makes deep cuts, bites that bleed, internal injury, fracture, loss of consciousness, loss of teeth**

Physical aggression against others

☐ **Makes threatening gestures, swings at people, grabs at clothes**

☐ **Strikes, kicks, pushes, pulls hair (without injury to them)**

☐ **Attacks others, causing mild-moderate physical injury (bruises, sprain, welts)**

☐ **Attacks others, causing severe physical injury (broken bones, deep lacerations, internal injury)**

Adapted from "Overt Aggression Scale" (OAS), developed by Stuart Yudofsky, M.D., Jonathan Silver, M.D., Wynn Jackson, M.D., and Jean Endicott, Ph.D. Used with permission.

bers are three times more likely to commit aggravated assault or murder than those who are not in gangs.

Treating aggression and violence

Many people have problems controlling their temper. They may fly off the handle, curse, shout, punch a hole in the wall, throw a dish across the room. Drawing the line between such outbursts and aggression, between temper and threat, can be difficult. The intensity of such episodes makes any objective assessment of their nature and seriousness very difficult. Hotheaded individuals may feel embarrassed and minimize what they said or did. Family members may cover up or try to justify an upsetting incident as the result of stress or too much alcohol. Yet because of the potential dangers of violence, people who find themselves erupting into rages or struggling with aggressive urges—or those close to them—should never hesitate to seek professional help.

If individuals and their families can be persuaded to seek help (which may not happen unless there are repeated incidents or actual physical danger), a psychiatrist may use, and suggest that family members use, the Overt Aggression Scale, developed by neuropsychiatrist Stuart Yudofsky, M.D., of Baylor College of Medicine and his colleagues, to get a clear picture of aggressive behavior. This scale divides aggressive behaviors into four categories: verbal aggression, physical aggression against objects, physical aggression against self, and physical aggression against others. Family members or health care providers make note of specific behaviors, such as vicious cursing, clear threats of violence, breaking objects, hitting fists into objects, making threatening gestures, or attacking others, and also record their own responses or intervention. Often this detailed record helps the psychiatrist to determine how serious a problem is and which responses seem most effective.

In addition, a complete medical examination, including neurological tests such as an EEG, CT scan, or MRI to evaluate brain function, is essential. As they take a history and perform a psychiatric evaluation, psychiatrists check for personality disorders, substance abuse, or evidence of a brain injury. They note previous mental disorders, episodes of violence, impulsive behavior (such as reckless driving or fire-setting), and the use of medications or drugs of abuse. They may also talk with family members, teachers, colleagues, and others to get an overall impression of the scope and severity of the aggressive behaviors.

Therapists cannot reliably predict whether individuals who have been violent in the past will become a danger to themselves or others in the future, but they must act if there is good reason to suspect such danger. In a landmark ruling (*Tarasoff* v. *Regents of the University of California*) in 1976, the California Supreme Court held that mental health professionals have a duty to protect third parties from imminent threats of serious harm made by individuals in their care. Some states have "duty to warn" statutes that define the actions mental health professionals must take. These may include voluntary or involuntary hospitalization, warning the intended victim of the threat, notifying the police, adjusting medication, or providing closer supervision of the patient. Therapists cannot refrain from taking these steps on the basis of doctor-patient confidentiality.

Treatment of aggressive or violent individuals almost always requires a multifaceted approach that combines medication, psychotherapy, behavioral treatments, and family therapy.

CRISIS INTERVENTION

A confrontation with an angry individual wielding a weapon or threatening violence is a clear emergency and should be treated as one. The primary concern is safety. Police, trained to handle the threat of violence, are often the first to intervene. Sometimes violent individuals are brought directly to hospitals or psychiatric facilities. Psychiatrists may be able to calm them down simply by talking with them, but if the threat of violence escalates, sedating medications such as benzodiazepines or antipsychotics may be used. If patients refuse such treatment or remain dangerously aggressive, seclusion and restraints, usually for several hours, may be necessary. Such controls are a means of preventing harm to the patient as well as to staff members and others; they should never be thought of or used as a punishment. Once calm has been restored, the psychiatrist can perform a thorough assessment and decide on a course of treatment.

MEDICATION

Sedating drugs, particularly benzodiazepines and antipsychotics, have often been used—or, more accurately, misused—as a "treatment" for aggressive behavior. Although these medications are useful for acute agitation and aggression, long-term use can mask the underlying causes of aggressive behavior and cause serious and disabling side effects. Unfortunately, they are still sometimes used as a routine method of "calming" (that is, controlling) patients in nursing homes and other facilities. The only time antipsychotic medications should be used, except for crises, is to treat aggres-

DRUG THERAPY FOR CHRONIC AGGRESSION

MEDICATION	REASON FOR ITS USE
Antipsychotics	**Psychotic symptoms, such as delusions**
Benzodiazepines	**Acute agitation**
Beta-blockers	**Chronic or recurrent aggression**
Buspirone	**Persistent, underlying anxiety and/or depression**
Carbamazepine	**Seizure disorders**
Lithium	**Mania or bipolar illness**
Valproic acid	**Aggressive behavior**

sion stemming from psychosis, as when, for example, a person under the delusion of being attacked by aliens assaults someone.

In individuals with an underlying mental illness, such as schizophrenia or mania, treatment with appropriate medications can reduce aggression. If, for example, violence occurs as a result of a manic outburst in someone with bipolar disorder, lithium would be the drug of choice. For aggression that develops in Alzheimer's disease or after a traumatic head injury, the antihypertensive beta-blocker propranolol (Inderal) can be beneficial. Most psychiatrists consider it their first choice, although even with high doses it may require six to eight weeks to take effect.

Certain drugs designed to treat particular physical and mental disorders can successfully reduce violence in people who do not actually have these disorders. Among these are the beta-blockers, anticonvulsants, and lithium. These medications can be effective against aggression and violence, although they should be used in combination with other treatments, such as psychotherapy and stress reduction training.

Buspirone (BuSpar), an anti-anxiety agent, has been reported to lessen both aggression and anxiety in developmentally disabled individuals and to help in managing aggression in individuals with depression, anxiety, traumatic brain injury, or dementia. There have been reports that clonazepam (Klonopin), a benzodiazepine, may help in some cases of chronic aggression. Selective serotonin reuptake inhibitors (SSRIs) such as fluoxetine (Prozac) may be useful in aggression associated with brain lesions.

PSYCHOTHERAPY

The goals of psychotherapy are to help violent individuals develop self-control, gain awareness of the early warning signals of anger, and recognize the circumstances most likely to provoke aggression. In therapy, those whose violence stems from developmental factors, abuse, and certain mental conditions, such as a personality disorder, can come to grips with the weakness and helplessness that are usually the core of their identity and can learn to recognize and appreciate the consequences of their behavior. Because violent people often have difficulty verbally expressing needs and conflicts, psychotherapy can provide encouragement and support for talking rather than acting and using words rather than weapons to express feelings, wants, and needs.

Therapists usually choose group or family therapy for violent individuals, because most violence occurs within families or social groups. Not only is group therapy less threatening to these persons than individual therapy, it also allows them to see others struggling with their tempers or low self-esteem.

Violence in society

The United States has the highest rate of interpersonal violence of any industrialized nation. More than twenty-five thousand Americans are murdered every year, and homicide has become the tenth leading killer in the nation. Among African-American youth, homicide is the most common cause of death. "Fatal and nonfatal injuries resulting from interpersonal violence have become one of the most important public health problems facing our country," says the head of the Division of Injury Control of the federal Centers for Disease Control (CDC) in Atlanta. In addition to murders, there has been a surge in other violent crimes, including carjackings, drive-by shootings, and gang warfare. Both the perpetrators and the victims are likely to be young and male.

The best approach to criminal violence, as to other public health problems, is prevention. National authorities have declared violence a public health emergency. As an initial step, the CDC has called upon parents to prevent unsupervised access to guns by their children and has developed pilot community programs for youngsters in high-crime areas. The American Medical Association has proposed greater restrictions on gun ownership, including strict registration and licensing. The Public Health Service is advocating a reduction in weapon carrying by adolescents. The American Psychological Association (APA) has called for decreased violence in the media.

All these steps could make a difference. According to the APA's recent report on violence and youth, violence is not "random, uncontrollable, or inevitable" and can be prevented. Early intervention is critical because aggression in childhood typically escalates into violence and other harmful behaviors in adulthood. Ideally, programs should teach young children skills for managing anger, solving problems, thinking of alternative solutions, and seeing another person's perspective. Equally important are programs that enhance positive interactions between children and adults. Such relationships may act as protective factors that can lower the risk of aggressive and violent behavior. "Violence is learned," emphasizes Ronald Slaby, Ph.D., a psychologist at Harvard University who served on the APA committee. "We can teach children alternatives." In the process, we can create a safer society for all.

DOMESTIC VIOLENCE

Violence doesn't stop on the streets. According to the FBI, the most common and least-reported violent crimes in the United States are attacks in which the victim and the perpetrator knew each other at the time of or before the incident. One-third of all murders occur within families.

Partner abuse   The FBI estimates that a woman—either a wife or a girlfriend—is physically abused every fifteen seconds, and that women have a 50 percent chance of being hit at least once by their husbands or lovers. Battering appears to be the single most common cause of injury to women, more common than car accidents, muggings, and rapes combined. Battered women (who outnumber battered men ten to one) are victims of severe, deliberate, and repeated physical assaults, often accompanied by psychological abuse and threats against their lives. As many as a third of women who visit hospital emergency rooms seek help for symptoms related to ongoing abuse, yet only 5 percent are identified as victims of domestic violence by the physicians who treat them.

The primary factors contributing to physical abuse are the degree of frustration and stress a man is under, his use of alcohol (involved in up to 60 percent of battering cases), and whether he was raised in an abusive home. Only one in twenty men who beat their partners are violent outside the home; nine in ten refuse to admit that they have a problem. In homes where a wife is beaten, children also may be abused.

According to the American College of Obstetricians and Gynecologists, abusers tend to fit a general profile. Typically they:

- Have low self-esteem
- Use threats, force, or violence to solve problems or control their partners
- Often have an alcohol or drug problem

- Are jealous of the relationships their partners form with other people
- Blame the partner for their violence.

Abused wives and children are often trapped in terror. Wives may stay with abusive husbands because of love, financial dependence, shame, guilt, fear of being pursued, harmed, or killed if they leave, or a sense of responsibility to their children. The incidence of alcoholism, substance abuse, depression, and suicide attempts is higher in battered women than others.

Child abuse   Severe child abuse occurs an estimated 1,700,000 times each year and claims the lives of as many as five thousand children. Although parents in every economic, social, educational, religious, and racial group abuse children, poverty is a significant factor in abuse. Mistreatment is seven times more likely in families with incomes under $15,000.

Abuse can take many forms: physical, psychological, or sexual. Physical abuse often leaves visible marks. However, emotional abuse—rejection, verbal cruelty such as constant berating and belittling, serious threats of harm, frequent tension in the home, violent arguments among parents—can be just as devastating to a child.

Many factors play a role in abuse: ignorance about child rearing, the absence of role models, teenage parenthood, the lack of a partner or supportive family network, the stress of poverty. Abusing parents are not necessarily sick; only 10 percent have mental disorders. However, most abusive parents share a similar psychological history and, as youngsters, felt misunderstood, unrewarded, and criticized. In many respects they were denied the right to behave like children. Sometimes they were abused themselves—if not physically harmed, then psychologically—growing up feeling so worthless and unlovable that as adults they continue to search for mothering and love. Often these individuals marry persons with problems similar to their own. When the new relationship cannot meet their psychological needs, they feel rejected. Their children may seem their last resort in obtaining the love they crave, and children who do not live up to these unrealistic expectations become the victims of abuse in turn.

Among the psychological traits most often associated with child abusers are immaturity and dependency, extremely low self-esteem, a sense of incompetence, difficulty in seeking pleasure and finding satisfaction in the adult world, social isolation and a reluctance to seek help, fear of "spoiling" the children, a strong belief in the value of punishment, false expectations of children, and a complete lack of empathy with the child's condition and needs. When they cannot cope with daily stress or a crisis occurs, such parents are likely to feel pushed beyond their ability to cope and end up abusing their children.

Sexual abuse of children involves *any* sexual contact, whether it is sexually suggestive conversation, prolonged kissing, petting, oral sex, or intercourse, between an adult and child. Because children are not intellectually or emotionally mature enough to consent to sexual involvement, any such action is an illegal violation of a child's rights.

Pedophilia, or child molestation, refers to abuse by individuals—for example, teachers, baby-sitters, or neighbors—who are not related to the child. Incest is sexual contact between two people who are closely related, including siblings as well as children and parents (or step-parents), grandparents, uncles, and aunts.

Researchers have found it difficult to make accurate estimates about the prevalence of incest and child molestation. In a telephone survey of 2,626 randomly selected men and women, about one in four of the women and one in seven of the men said they had been sexually victimized as children. Many victims of childhood sexual abuse are under the age of seven and may not realize that an adult's behavior is improper or may not know how to distinguish between affection and sexual contact. Older children, when molested by a family member or friend, may feel ashamed or somehow responsible for what happened and may not confide in their parents for fear of being punished. Even parents who are informed may not be able to handle the emotional trauma of finding out that someone close to them would "do that."

Abuse, whether emotional, physical, or sexual, can affect every aspect of a child's life. Youngsters may develop physical symptoms such as headaches, stomachaches, and sleep problems, and may run into academic and social difficulties in school. Since children often blame themselves for whatever happened and assume that they are responsible, they may develop a sense of hopelessness, shame, and pessimism. Some become clinically depressed or develop other mental or emotional problems that may continue into adolescence and adulthood, including headaches, depression, insomnia, obesity, and fatigue.

Sexual abuse in childhood can be emotionally devastating, and survivors suffer deep psychological wounds, including a profound sense of betrayal and loss. As adults, many of them find it hard to form intimate relationships and experience sexual difficulties. Other common problems include depression, feelings of guilt or shame, inability to trust, drug and alcohol abuse, and vulnerability to other forms of victimization.

SEXUAL VIOLENCE

At a bar on a weekend night, a group of intoxicated young men grab a woman and squeeze her breasts as she struggles to get free. At a party, a man offers his date drugs and alcohol to lower her resistance to his sexual overtures. Although some people do not realize it, such actions are forms of sexual coercion: forced sexual activity. It is very common. In one survey of 190 college men, 61 percent said that they had fondled women against their will, and 15 percent had forced a woman to have intercourse.

Although sexual victimization can take many forms, *rape* refers to sexual intercourse with an unconsenting partner, male or female, under actual or threatened force. Sexual intercourse between a male, usually over the age of sixteen, and a female under the "age of consent," which differs from state to state and ranges from twelve to twenty-one, is called *statutory rape.* In *acquaintance rape*, the victim knows the rapist, who may be a classmate, neighbor, co-worker, or date.

Both stranger and acquaintance rape are serious crimes that can have a devastating impact on their victims. Because many people never report rape, especially if they know the rapist, it is hard to know exactly how widespread this violent crime is. In several recent surveys, 19 to 25 percent of women reported that they had been raped. There are no limits on who may become a victim of rape. Boys, men, infant girls, old women, pregnant women, and nuns have all been attacked.

For many years the victims of rape were blamed for behaving in some way that brought on the attack. Researchers have since shown that women are raped because they encounter sexually aggressive men, not because they look or act in a certain way. Nevertheless, although no woman is immune to attack, women who were sexually abused as children are at greater risk than others. Scientists are now exploring the reasons for this vulnerability.

Although rape has long been viewed as an act of violence and domination, recent studies indicate that not all rapists share the same motives or characteristics. Those who attack strangers often have problems in establishing intimate relationships, have poor self-esteem, feel inadequate, and may have been sexually abused as children. Some rapists report a long history of fantasizing about rape and violence, usually while masturbating. Others rape out of anger that they cannot express toward a wife or girlfriend. The more sexually aggressive men have been, the more likely they are to view such aggression and violence as normal and to believe myths about rape, such as that it is impossible to rape a woman who doesn't really want sex. Alcohol also plays a major role on both sides. Many rapists drink before an assault, and a victim's drinking may interfere with her ability to avoid danger or resist attack.

Within the broad category of rape, researchers have identified several distinct types, which are not mutually exclusive:

Anger rape. An unplanned violent physical attack, usually on a total stranger, motivated by hatred and a desire for revenge for the rejection the rapist feels he has suffered from women. Anger rapists often harbor long-standing hostility toward women, use far more physical violence than is needed for submission, and usually do not find the rape to be sexually gratifying.

Power rape. Usually a premeditated attack motivated by a desire to dominate and control another person. Power rapists, unable to deal with stress and their sense of failure, may rape to regain some sense of having power. They use only as much force as is needed to make their victims submit and may find the rape sexually gratifying, even though that is not their primary motive.

Sadistic rape. A premeditated assault that often involves bondage, torture, and sexual abuse. Sadistic rapists find power and anger sexually arousing and may subject victims to rituals of humiliation or torture. They are often preoccupied with violent pornography; their motives are more complex and difficult to understand than those found in other types of rape.

Sexual gratification rape. An attack, usually impulsive, by someone willing to use physical coercion for the sake of sex. In general, these rapists use no more force than needed to get a partner to submit and may stop the attack if it becomes clear that they will have to use extreme violence to overcome resistance. Many acquaintance rapes fit into this category.

Gang rapes. These involve three or more rapists. Men in close groups, such as fraternities or athletic teams, with their own housing, unsupervised partying, and drinking, are more likely to participate in such assaults. The reasons may go beyond aggression and sexual gratification to the excitement and camaraderie the men may feel during the experience.

In recent years, there have been more frequent reports of male rape by other men and by women. There have been reports of men being forced by women to participate in sexual intercourse, although there is no consensus on how common this may be.

Researchers estimate that about 10 percent of acquaintance rape cases involve men. These "hidden victims" often keep silent because of embarrassment, shame or humiliation, and their own feelings and fears about homosexuality. However, although there is a widespread assumption that men who rape other men are always homosexuals, most rapists who choose male victims consider themselves to be heterosexual. Contrary to a common assumption, young boys are not the only subjects of rape. The average age of male victims is twenty-four. Rape is a serious problem in prisons, where men may experience brutal assaults by other men who usually resume sexual relations with women once they are released.

The impact of violence

As their numbers have grown and their anguish has been recognized, the victims of violence have received greater attention. In the last decade, hundreds of shelters for battered women and their children have been set up around the country. They offer physical and psychological treatment, and a haven where women can begin to rebuild their shattered self-esteem as well as their daily lives. Rape counseling and crisis centers on college campuses and in the community provide various forms of assistance to victims of rape. In many cities the telephone directory lists hotlines and resources. More than four hundred victims' advocacy groups have been established across the country to advise those hurt by crime. Support organizations help many survivors to deal with the emotional aftermath of their experiences. (See the Resource Directory at the back of the book for listings.)

Any form of violence—a street mugging, sexual assault, or battering at home—is deeply traumatic. Victims of rape and other forms of sexual violence often suffer long-term effects. The American Psychiatric Association has identified sexual victimization as "a significant risk factor" in the development of depression in women. Sexual assault also has been linked with eating disorders, self-mutilation, and other mental disorders. Many victims develop chronic symptoms, such as headaches, backaches, high blood pressure, sleep disorders, pelvic pain, and sexual or fertility problems. The psychological scars take a particularly long time to heal. Mental health professionals have linked sexual victimization with hopelessness, low self-esteem, and destructive relationships.

Rape victims, men as well as women, may develop a *rape trauma syndrome*, a form of posttraumatic stress disorder (described in Chapter 12), in which they experience deeply upsetting flashbacks and "relive" the rape. Acquaintance rape sometimes causes particularly intense psychological torment. Often too ashamed to tell anyone what happened, its victims may suffer alone, without skilled therapists or sympathetic friends to reassure them. They tend to blame themselves more, question their own judgment, and have higher levels of psychological distress than those raped by strangers. Nightmares, anxiety, and flashbacks are common. Years afterward, rape victims who do not obtain professional help may still be struggling with rage against men and with problems in establishing trusting relationships.

HELPING VICTIMS OF VIOLENCE

Sometimes well-intentioned friends and relatives make victims of violence feel worse. Here are suggestions for offering comfort without unintentionally implying criticism:

Don't blame the victim. Even when no one doubts that he or she is completely innocent, the victim may be plagued by regrets and self-accusation: Why didn't he lock the windows? Why did she park on that dark street? What did she do to make her spouse so angry? Any second-guessing, any implied criticism of the person's actions, adds to the burden of blame and shame.

Don't try to deny that it happened. Although it may be hard to talk about—or even listen to—the reality of the event, it must not be ignored. Ignoring it is a form of denial, and denial makes victims doubt their own experience, and question themselves at a time when they crave reassurance.

Don't pressure the victim to talk—or not to talk. Some people need to go over every detail of what happened, again and again, until they work out their feelings of outrage and become ready to get on with their lives. Others find going into details too humiliating. Let the victim set the tone and limits for disclosure. Don't pry or prod.

Don't try to rush the victim to leave the past behind and get on with his or her life. Recovery from any traumatic event takes time, and only the victim knows the appropriate pace. Chapter 12 on stress-related disorders may provide useful insight into what the person is going through. If months pass, however, without any lessening of symptoms or improvement in day-to-day functioning, family members and friends should not hesitate to recommend that their loved one see a mental health professional.

24

Problems that Affect Body and Mind

"**E**veryone who is born holds dual citizenship, in the king-dom of the well and in the kingdom of the sick," Susan Sontag wrote in *Illness as Metaphor*, noting that "al-though we all prefer to use only the good passport, sooner or later each of us is obliged, at least for a spell, to identify ourselves as citizens of that other place."

Many complex forces—heredity, biology, childhood develop-ment, environment, nutrition, exercise, even luck—influence whether we remain in the kingdom of the well or enter the domain of the ill. Sometimes we crash across the border, as when a car careens out of control or a flu virus knocks us off our feet. More often, we simply lose our way and find ourselves in hostile terri-tory. The reasons why may involve intangible psychological factors that do not in themselves cause physical diseases yet can trigger, worsen, or prolong symptoms.

In some conditions, traditionally called *psychosomatic illnesses,* emotional factors are not simply present but are dominant. This does not mean that these problems, and the distress they cause, are imaginary or faked. It does mean that they may begin at a time of crisis in a person's life, flare up during stressful situations, and improve when circumstances change for the better or the per-son learns to adapt.

Almost every illness of the body affects the mind. As many as 65 percent of all hospitalized patients develop mental disorders, primarily anxiety disorders, depression, and disorientation, that may require treatment. About a third of those with medical illnesses develop a clinical depression. Anxiety disorders are almost as common.

Few people with both physical and psychological difficulties ever see a consultation psychiatrist (one who specializes in problems related to medical illness and treatment) or a therapist of any kind. Patients, families, or physicians are often reluctant to suggest or agree to a psychiatric evaluation. They may assume, mistakenly, that it is normal for people with serious diseases to be depressed, anxious, or disoriented, or that psychiatric care won't help. Yet, as research has clearly and carefully shown, hospitalized patients who receive needed psychiatric care develop fewer complications, have shorter hospital stays, incur lower medical costs, and have lower mortality rates. Treating the mind is good for the body as well.

Psychological factors that affect physical health

Psychological factors can influence the course of a physical problem by triggering or intensifying symptoms, interfering with recovery, or making it more difficult for an individual to adapt to a chronic illness. In some cases, because of depression or denial that they are indeed ill, individuals refuse to take medication or follow their physicians' recommendations. Others ignore risk factors that may jeopardize their health, such as drinking too much or eating high-fat foods. Among the ailments most strongly linked to psychological influences are diabetes, skin conditions, digestive disorders, cardiovascular disease, respiratory problems, and connective tissue disorders.

Depression and anxiety have the greatest impact on physical conditions. High rates of depression are associated with strokes and certain skin conditions, such as acne and psoriasis. Depression can also be an early sign of some illnesses, among them multiple sclerosis or Parkinson's disease. Depression complicates many physical conditions and can interfere with treatment and recovery from asthma, stroke, heart disease, cancer, epilepsy, kidney failure, multiple sclerosis, and Parkinson's disease. In a recent Canadian study, heart attack survivors who developed major depression had a three- to fourfold greater risk for dying within six months than those who were not depressed.

Anxiety disorders also affect many physical conditions. They can lead to or intensify asthmatic reactions, skin conditions such as acne, eczema, atopic dermatitis, and itching, and digestive disorders such as indigestion, irritable bowel syndrome, and Crohn's disease. Stress can play a role in hypertension, heart attacks, cardiac arrhythmias, and sudden cardiac death. Inability to cope with an illness, often because the sick person feels overwhelmed by stress, can complicate recovery.

Various traits characteristic of personality disorders occur more often in individuals with certain medical conditions, including peptic ulcers, asthma, rheumatoid arthritis, inflammatory bowel disease, and skin problems. However, there is no strong evidence that any specific personality traits actually cause disease. More often, and more directly, personality disorders interfere with the ability of individuals to get along with health care personnel or with family members who are caring for them.

Psychological and emotional factors can have beneficial as well as negative effects. One of the most potent appears to be faith. Herbert Benson, M.D., a professor of cardiology at Harvard Medical School and a pioneer in behavioral medicine, has long noted that belief—what he calls "the faith factor"—is the hidden ingredient in Western medicine and every traditional system of "healing."

It isn't what individuals believe but the fact that they *do* believe that matters. As Benson observes, the faith factor is not limited to any one religious or philosophical system: "The same basic approach—which has a quantifiable, scientifically measurable effect—can be applied in a variety of specific circumstances and faith contexts," he says.

Perhaps just as important is hope. Psychologist Shlomo Breznitz, Ph.D., director of the Center for the Study of Psychological Stress at the University of Haifa in Israel, defines it more scientifically as the ability "to look at the situation, no matter how negative, to seek the few remaining positive elements and build on them. . . . The healthiest attitude is hope that is based on a realistic evaluation of the situation. Mature hope dwells on what is positive about life, but also what's realistic."

Psychosomatic disorders

Psychosomatic disorders involve physical and psychological vulnerability in combination. People with these problems must have a biological predisposition to a particular condition, caused by heredity, injury, previous disease, exposure to toxic substances, or harmful habits such as smoking or overeating. Thus, a man with a family history of heart disease may be overweight, get little exercise, and be chronically hostile and angry.

Over time, this combination of physical and emotional factors might lead to high blood pressure (hypertension) or heart disease.

CARDIOVASCULAR DISEASE

Heart disease is the nation's number one killer. More than 63 million Americans suffer some form of cardiovascular illness. These facts alone can cause anxiety, especially in those who have cardiovascular risk factors or symptoms. Anxiety itself prompts 10 to 15 percent of patient visits to cardiologists.

The Type A theory and heart attacks   In the 1970s, cardiologists Meyer Friedman, M.D., and Ray Rosenman, M.D., compared their heart attack patients to attack-free people of the same age and developed two general categories of personality: Type A and Type B. Hardworking, aggressive, and competitive, Type As never had time for all they wanted to accomplish, even though they habitually tried to do several tasks at once. Type Bs were more relaxed, though not necessarily less ambitious or successful. Friedman and Rosenman's research found that Type A behavior was the major contributing factor in the early development of heart disease.

The actual impact of Type A behavior remains controversial, and various scientists have criticized the initial research. According to a twenty-two-year follow-up study of three thousand middle-aged men by researchers at the University of California, Berkeley, smoking and hypertension are much greater threats than Type A behavior in terms of heart attack risk. Nevertheless, anger, hostility, cynicism, and aggression do seem to be clear dangers. They can send epinephrine and other stress hormones into the bloodstream and drive up cholesterol levels and blood pressure. In one study, people who scored high on a hostility scale as teenagers were much more likely than their more easygoing age mates to develop high cholesterol levels as adults. The intense arousal triggered by anger may also harm the coronary arteries directly and wear out heart muscle fibers.

Type As can change their heart-damaging ways by learning stress management and relaxation techniques. A report on 1,012 volunteers by Stanford University's Recurrent Coronary Prevention Project found that treatment to reduce Type A behavior helps heart attack survivors to live longer, prevents a second heart attack, and also reduces deaths from other causes. In the study, men who received behavioral counseling to change aggressive, hostile behavior experienced 44 percent fewer heart attacks eight years after their first attack than those given only standard medical care.

The emotions that affect the odds for subsequent heart attacks appear to be different in men and women. For women who have had a heart attack, anxiety and fearfulness, rather than anger, are more likely to lead to a second attack. Nevertheless, like men, women who undergo behavioral treatment after a heart attack are less vulnerable to a second heart attack. The single psychological factor that predicts which men and women are most likely to die after a heart attack is severe depression. Psychiatrists now recommend routine screening of cardiac patients for depression and immediate treatment when indicated.

Hypertension Some 58 million Americans have high blood pressure that requires monitoring or treatment; 30 million do not have their blood pressure under adequate control. The likelihood of developing blood pressure problems may depend on how individuals respond to everyday sources of stress. According to data from the longitudinal Framingham Heart Study, anxiety levels in middle-aged men, but not in women, may be predictive of later incidence of hypertension. Anxiety and anger may trigger the classic "stress response," which releases excessive amounts of adrenal hormones that increase heart rate and blood pressure. Behavioral therapy, such as biofeedback and relaxation training, and psychotherapy may be helpful.

Mitral valve prolapse Mitral valve prolapse (MVP), an abnormality in a heart valve that affects the flow of blood through the heart, occurs in as many as one in ten Americans, more often in women than men. Although this condition is usually benign, there is a risk for irregular heart beats—arrhythmias—that can be fatal.

MVP can cause palpitations and dizziness. About 20 percent of individuals with panic attacks also have MVP; the reason for this is not known (see Chapter 7). Some medications used to treat this condition can cause depression. Ideally, cardiologists and psychiatrists should work together to find the most effective drug or drugs for an individual's physical and psychological symptoms.

RESPIRATORY PROBLEMS

Emotions often affect breathing. We sigh when sad or take shallow, hurried breaths when fearful. Because breathing is essential to life, problems that interfere with it can trigger great anxiety.

Hyperventilation Hyperventilation (very rapid breathing) causes a loss of carbon dioxide from the blood that may lead to light-headedness, dizziness, tingling in the fingers and toes, or other disturbing sensations. Individuals with this problem may be unable to catch their breath, may be extremely anxious, and may believe they are having a heart attack. In some people, hyperventilation may trigger or occur during a panic attack. This problem runs in families, an indication of genetic susceptibility.

Individuals with anxiety disorders often hyperventilate but may not realize that they have changed the rhythm or rate of their breathing. Stressful situations, such as a wedding, an examination, or job interview, can trigger hyperventilation. Breathing into a paper bag, which allows the exhaled carbon dioxide to be reinhaled, usually relieves the symptoms and enables the person to breathe normally again. Those with an underlying anxiety disorder should obtain appropriate treatment.

Asthma Asthma is characterized by periodic attacks of wheezing, difficulty in breathing, shortness of breath, and coughing. About 10 million Americans, 4 million of them children, have asthma. There is a familial element in some cases. Three main factors can trigger an attack in a person prone to asthma: allergy to external irritants, such as dust or pollen, respiratory infections, and stress. During an attack the bronchioles, small tubes inside the lungs, contract as a result of a spasm or constriction, mucous blockage, or a swelling of their linings. Attacks range from mild to so severe that immediate medical treatment is needed to prevent death. Between attacks, patients are relatively free of symptoms. Although there is no actual cure, treatment with medications such as anti-inflammatory drugs and bronchodilators, which widen the airways in the lungs, can keep asthma under control.

Eliminating allergens or treating an infection can prevent attacks. If emotional stress seems to be the primary cause of the attacks, relaxation methods can be effective. Many individuals with asthma are most likely to have a stress-induced attack when other factors, such as an allergy or respiratory infection, have already increased their susceptibility.

DIGESTIVE DISORDERS

Emotions often affect the digestive system, causing symptoms that range from a loss of appetite to "butterflies" in the stomach. More serious problems are also common. According to the National Digestive Diseases Advisory Board, almost half of the U.S. population will suffer a digestive illness at some time. Some conditions, including irritable bowel syndrome and inflammatory bowel disease, are closely linked to psychological factors.

Ulcers For years, psychological factors were considered a major cause of peptic or gastrointestinal ulcers, which afflict about one in ten Americans. But recent research has led to a revolution in the way physicians think of ulcer disease. "We've come to recognize it as an infectious, transmissible disease, just like pneumonia or a urinary tract infection, that can be permanently cured in a matter of weeks," says David Graham, M.D., chief of gastroenterology at the Houston Veterans Association Medical Center.

Scientists have identified a particular type of bacteria, called *Helicobacter pylori (H. pylori)*, as the cause of the vast majority of peptic ulcers. In 1994 a National Institutes of Health consensus conference recommended that antibiotics become a standard part of therapy for patients with recurrent ulcers. The discovery of *H. pylori* and the proven effectiveness of antibiotic treatment have lifted the burden of self-blame long carried by ulcer patients.

Does stress play any role? "There is no conclusive evidence that it does," says gastroenterologist Martin Brotman, M.D., chairman of the Department of Medicine at California Pacific Medical Center in San Francisco. "During the blitz in World War II, Londoners—who certainly were under extreme stress—didn't show a higher incidence of ulcer disease."

Irritable bowel syndrome Irritable bowel syndrome (also called irritable colon or spastic colon) is a common problem caused by intestinal spasms. The muscular contractions that move waste material through the intestines become irregular and uncoordinated, causing a frequent need to defecate, nausea, cramping, pain, gas, and a sensation that the rectum is never emptied.

A flare-up of this problem can be triggered by stress, certain foods, or alcohol. About 25 percent of individuals with this problem may also have dysthymia, major depression, or an attention-deficit disorder, problems that can exacerbate digestive symptoms if not treated. Many people benefit from education about their illness and stress management training.

Inflammatory bowel disease As many as 2 million Americans, including some children and many in the prime of life, suffer from one of the two forms of inflammatory bowel disease (IBD): Crohn's disease, which causes inflammation anywhere in the digestive tract, and ulcerative colitis, which creates severe ulcers or holes in the inner lining of the colon and rectum. Both illnesses can trigger frequent and intense diarrhea, abdominal pain, gas, fever, and rectal bleeding. Without treatment, IBD can cause potentially fatal complications such as blockages, perforations, and hemorrhages. Although there is no cure, many people who receive appropriate therapy go into remissions that can last for years or decades.

Twenty percent of cases involve a genetic or familial predisposition. Although emotional factors do not cause IBD, as once was thought, they can affect its course. IBD tends to flare up at times of stress, and as many as 40 percent of IBD patients develop serious depression that requires treatment with psychiatric drugs or psychotherapy. Others become extremely anxious.

For nine in ten individuals, both adults and children, treatment of IBD consists of medications to control symptoms and prevent more serious complications. Sometimes dietary changes, such as eating a low-fiber diet and avoiding spicy foods, not smoking, and getting regular rest and exercise can help to prevent flare-ups. Persons with more severe symptoms may require treatment with prednisone, a powerful corticosteroid (a synthetic hormone) that reduces inflammation but can cause a wide range of side effects, from weight gain to muscle aches to bone thinning. Newer agents "dampen" the body's immune system to reduce symptoms; their side effects include nausea, headache, dizziness, rashes, and blood abnormalities.

Patients with Crohn's disease who do not improve on medication or who develop life-threatening complications, such as a severe intestinal blockage, may need to undergo surgery to remove or bypass the diseased part of the intestine and reconnect two healthy segments. Those with severe ulcerative colitis may have part or all of their colon and rectum removed. Crohn's disease often recurs in another part of the intestinal tract, but for those with ulcerative colitis, removal of the entire colon brings an end to troubling symptoms.

IMMUNITY

Research into the relationship between the mind, the central nervous system, and the immune system has spawned a new scientific field: psychoneuroimmunology. Studies in both animals and humans have confirmed that the powerful chemicals triggered by stress can dampen or suppress the body's immune system, a network of organs, tissues, and white blood cells that defends against disease.

Infectious illness Traumatic stress, such as losing a loved one through death or divorce, impairs immunity for as long as a year. Even minor hassles take a toll. Under examination stress, students experience a dip in immune function and a higher incidence of infections. Ohio State University researchers found a significant drop in the immune cells that normally ward off infection in medical students during exam periods.

Personal stress management techniques can boost the immune system's ability to fight infectious illnesses. In one study, herpes sufferers who learned relaxation, visualization, and stress management techniques experienced only half as many outbreaks as others who simply attended support groups concerned with the sexual and emotional difficulties of having herpes. When herpes did recur, the episodes in those who had learned stress management techniques were less severe and ended several days sooner.

Autoimmune disorders   The common thread in problems such as systemic lupus erythematosus, rheumatoid arthritis, Sjögren's syndrome, Hashimoto's thyroiditis, Graves' disease, myasthenia gravis, and scleroderma is the body's production of antibodies— biochemical substances in the blood that normally protect it from infection by attacking foreign matter—that instead target healthy tissues. Possible causes include an inherited predisposition, sex hormones (estrogen in particular may greatly influence the immune system), a noninfectious retrovirus (a very small virus that becomes part of the genetic material within healthy cells), and exposure to chemicals and other toxins. Treatments vary according to the specific disorder but may include aspirin, taken more often and in higher doses than for minor aches and pains; nonsteroidal anti-inflammatory drugs, or NSAIDs, such as ibuprofen (Motrin), sulindac (Clinoril), and indomethacin (Indocin); drugs that dampen the immune system; and corticosteroids, synthetic hormones such as prednisone, which if used in high doses or for long periods can produce troubling physical and emotional side effects (lower or alternate-day doses minimize such risks).

Stress has been suspected as a culprit in initiating or worsening these diseases, but the connection is not clear. Some psychological symptoms associated with certain autoimmune disorders may be direct consequences of the illness. In lupus, for example, antibodies may attack the brain, causing learning and concentration problems, seizures, mood swings, depression, and irritability.

SKIN DISORDERS

Because the skin is the most visible (as well as the largest) organ of the body, none of its problems is likely to seem trivial. Emotional upheavals and anxiety can lead to or aggravate certain skin diseases, including acne and eczema.

The most common complaint of people who see dermatologists is itching (pruritus), which may be mild or intense, localized or all over the body. Occasional itching is normal, although it can provoke psychological as well as physical distress. In some cases, anxiety and severe emotional stress can lead to an outbreak of hives (urticaria), although this problem is more commonly caused by allergies or excessive sun exposure. Medications can provide relief for the discomfort of urticaria or other itching problems.

In psoriasis, the rate of epidermal cell production is speeded up. As these skin cells pile up faster than they can be shed, they produce unsightly, deep-pink, raised patches on the skin. Psoriasis may run in families and can be chronic. Emotional stress and life changes can trigger flare-ups. Physicians usually prescribe ointments, creams, or pastes, including some steroidal preparations, or ultraviolet treatment.

Fear, rage, and anxiety can increase perspiration (hyperhidrosis). Emotion-induced sweat appears mainly on the palms, soles, and armpits. The prime areas of heat-induced sweat are the forehead, neck, torso, and backs of the hands and arms. In prolonged stress, excessive sweating can cause rashes, blisters, and infections that require treatment with appropriate medications.

PAIN DISORDER

For a few brief, blissful moments after she awoke every morning, a middle-aged woman would think that maybe, just maybe, the doctors were right, maybe nothing was wrong with her, maybe the pain that had tormented her for months really was all in her head. Then she would get up. "It was a nightmare," she recalls. "Pain would shoot down my back and thighs. I could barely walk. I couldn't sit." Yet despite her agony she could not convince her physicians that her pain was real. Again and again they dismissed her complaints.

All too frequently, people with disabling pain encounter similar rebuffs. Their complaints often baffle and frustrate physicians who cannot find any physical abnormality or malady to account for the existence or intensity of the pain. Yet pain isn't simply in a person's head *or* body, but in both.

The most common causes of chronic pain among persons treated in pain clinics are back problems, neurological disease, and headache. Chronic pain, which deprives a person of daily pleasure, can be so demoralizing that it produces personality changes and psychological symptoms such as depression, irritability, and anger—symptoms that were once considered the cause, rather than the consequence, of pain.

Pain disorder—persistent, intense pain that is related to psychological factors, causes great distress, and interferes with a person's ability to function normally—is an officially recognized but controversial psychiatric diagnosis. Its key characteristics are pain that is associated with a physical condition but is much greater than might be expected, and pain with no identifiable cause.

According to the *Diagnostic and Statistical Manual of Mental Disorders, Fourth Edition (DSM-IV)*, a diagnosis of pain disorder should be based on these criteria:

- Pain in one or more areas of the body, so severe that it requires medical attention

- Significant distress or interference with a person's usual ability to function as a result of the pain

- Psychological factors playing an important role in the onset, severity, worsening, or continuation of the pain

- Pain not intentionally produced or feigned

- Pain not better accounted for by a mood, anxiety, or psychotic disorder.

Psychiatrists distinguish between pain disorders in which psychological factors play the major role and those in which both psychological factors and a medical condition seem to be equally responsible for the pain. Pain caused mainly by an injury or illness is not considered a mental disorder.

Pain disorders, considered common in general medical practice, can occur at any age, from childhood to old age. The most frequent age of onset is the thirties or forties. Possibly because of sexual stereotyping, these conditions are diagnosed almost twice as frequently in women as in men. An acute pain disorder lasts less than six months; a chronic pain disorder lasts longer.

▼

What causes pain disorder?   According to psychoanalytic theories, individuals who develop unexplained pain may not be able to experience and express feelings verbally, a condition therapists refer to as *alexithymia*. As a result, they may translate psychologically stressful events into pain rather than emotions.

Sometimes pain is the only acceptable way people can receive nurturance and support. For others, it may relieve an unconscious difficulty, help in avoiding a conflict or problem, or provide tangible benefits, such as disability pay.

Unexplained pain often occurs with mental disorders such as schizophrenia, somatization disorders, or major depression. In one study, 60 percent of depressed individuals complained of pain. Does depression make individuals more sensitive to pain, or does chronic pain cause depression? It may be difficult to tell which form of misery came first, but treating the depression can help to relieve the physical discomfort.

Pain disorder may also develop immediately after a physical injury, the onset of a disease, or surgery, or in association with migraine, angina, sickle cell disease, or rheumatoid arthritis. Although these conditions are painful in themselves, those with pain disorder experience much greater pain than might be expected, and their pain often begins or worsens at times of stress.

▼
Living with pain

Pain becomes the central focus in the lives of people with pain disorder. They see physicians often in their quest for relief, take larger and larger amounts of painkilling medications in a fruitless effort to relieve their pain, request surgery or elaborate treatments, and ultimately assume the lifestyle of an invalid. Because their suffering is so great, they may not even consider the possible role of psychological factors in contributing to their pain.

Although persons with pain disorder seek medical attention promptly, they may not be referred to a psychotherapist, or may refuse to see one, for many years, even when the pain has clear symbolic significance, such as chest pain in a person whose father recently died of heart disease. Often they fear that a psychiatrist will tell them that their pain is not real. Yet, as one psychiatric textbook reminds clinicians, "Pain occurring in unicorns, griffins, or jabberwocks is always imaginary pain, since these are imaginary animals; patients, on the other hand, are real, and so they always have real pain."

Many individuals with pain disorder also develop other symptoms, such as muscle spasms or numbness in some part of their bodies. Insomnia is common, as are symptoms of depression, especially a lack of pleasure in daily living.

Families have great influence on how persons perceive and cope with pain. Some families are overly solicitous and, consciously or unconsciously, discourage the person from trying to master or cope with the pain. Spouses or partners should always obtain as much information as possible about their loved one's condition and about the impact of their own behavior on the person.

Often individuals who have chronic pain become trapped in a vicious cycle. Because of their pain, they become inactive and their muscles atrophy; this leads to fatigue and a lack of stamina, which discourages activity even further and thus worsens the pain. Physical therapy, using a progressive, stepwise plan, can help individuals to gradually become more active. Specialists in pain control usually offer a variety of options, including various forms of stimulation (massage, heat, cold, vibration, acupuncture, electrical stimulation).

▼
Treating pain disorder

The first step is a thorough evaluation, including a medical history and a review of symptoms and physical findings, to enable the mental health professional to understand the individual's anguish and establish a trusting relationship. The therapist may consult with the person's physician to make sure that there is no physical cause for the pain or for such an extreme level of pain. Many therapists administer psychological tests, including personality assessments and more specific evaluations designed to measure the effects of chronic pain. They also must rule out other psychiatric problems, such as somatization or depressive disorders.

Pain, which is one of the most complex and subjective of symptoms, almost always improves most with a combination of treatments rather than any single approach. The goal of treatment is to relieve suffering and to provide the person with new skills and coping strategies. In time, those with pain disorder are usually able to shift from searching for a cure to finding ways to cope with their symptoms so that they can lead more satisfying lives despite their pain. Psychiatric drugs, primarily antidepressants, may ease pain in some individuals, possibly by reducing anxiety and relieving depression. One review of 40 studies found tricyclic antidepressants especially effective for pain related to neuropathy, headache (including migraines), fibrositis, and arthritis.

Cognitive-behavioral approaches have become the most widely used form of therapy for pain disorders. Although there have been few studies of their effectiveness, they seem to work best for pain of mild to moderate severity. Their goal is to make individuals more aware of the factors that either exacerbate or relieve their pain so that they can modify their behavior accordingly. Those who may have become accustomed to controlling or avoiding situations by complaining of pain or being sick, which is not uncommon in pain disorder, can benefit from training in assertiveness and communication skills, which helps them learn to express their needs more directly.

People often find it helpful to identify exactly what their pain prevents them from doing and then to develop strategies to accomplish specific goals. One strategy, for example, is learning to distance themselves from pain, so that they can say, "It isn't really me who's suffering." Specific coping skills include *imaginative inattention* (thinking of a pleasant day at the beach), *imaginative transformation of the pain* (the sensations are really contractions, not pain), *imaginative transformation of the context* (it hurts but it's like being the hero in an Arnold Schwarzenegger film), *diversion of attention* (counting ceiling tiles, doing mental arithmetic), and *focusing on the pain but analyzing the experience* (as if for a report in a biology class).

Relaxation, deep-breathing exercises, and biofeedback teach individuals to relax and may also have direct effects on muscles and blood vessels. Generalized relaxation training, in various controlled studies, has proved simpler, less expensive, and as effective as biofeedback for relieving pain caused by tension and migraine headaches. Hypnosis and posthypnotic suggestion can help individuals learn to employ dissociative strategies or evoke images and metaphors that distract from or reinterpret pain sensations, so that, for example, they perceive them as tingling rather than pain. Other approaches include physical therapy, acupuncture, and transcutaneous electrical nerve stimulation (TENS).

Keeping a daily behavioral diary can help individuals to note flare-ups of pain, relate them to stressful events, and keep track of drugs taken. They also can record alternative strategies and how well they work in relieving pain. Support groups for individuals with chronic pain can be very helpful.

▼

Outlook   Because of the difficulty of objectively evaluating the effects of specific treatments, health care professionals do not know exactly which forms of treatment are most effective. Nevertheless, both the art and the science of pain control have made great progress during recent years. The short-term outcome for people with chronic pain who are treated at pain centers is excellent; in the long term, pain usually is not completely eliminated, but individuals report improved functioning.

Medical conditions that cause psychiatric symptoms

L earning that you have a serious health problem is upsetting for anyone. However, although it is normal to feel disheartened, worried, or fearful, it is *not* normal to become so upset or to remain upset for so long that you cannot function more or less the way you used to. In such instances, the problem may be a mental disorder. Major depression and anxiety disorders affect 20 to 30 percent of medically ill individuals. In some cases, treating the underlying problem eases or eliminates the psychological symptoms. In others, it has little or no effect, and treatment with psychotherapy or psychiatric medications is necessary.

CANCER

Individuals with cancer struggle with changing issues and concerns during the course of their illness. The initial diagnosis often brings shock, denial, anger, and fear. At the same time, they face difficult decisions about treatment; more and more commonly, oncologists (cancer specialists) present several options but leave the final choice to the individual. Overwhelmed with medical data that can be hard to absorb and understand, worried about which decision is best, patients may develop generalized anxiety, panic attacks, fear of going outside their homes (agoraphobia), or obsessive-compulsive disorder. Major depression tends to occur in the six to ten weeks after initial cancer therapy.

Appropriate medications for depression, panic attacks, or other disorders and psychotherapy are very beneficial. A variety of therapies—cognitive, crisis intervention, supportive, progressive relaxation training, psychodynamic, hypnosis, group—have proved helpful in reducing distress, improving quality of life, and promoting a greater sense of well-being in cancer patients.

Treating the mind can affect not only the quality of life for cancer patients but its duration as well. In one landmark study that followed advanced breast cancer patients for ten years, supportive group therapy *doubled* survival times. The women in the study, all of whom had metastatic breast cancer, received standard cancer care. About 60 percent were assigned to two weekly support groups that dealt with the psychological impact of their disease, doctor-patient issues, and pain control. At the end of a year this treatment group reported less depression, anxiety, fatigue, and pain, and greater self-esteem, than the controls.

"We clearly showed that psychosocial interventions can improve psychological functioning, but we never thought about extending survival," says psychiatrist David Spiegel, M.D., a professor at Stanford University, who initially found the startling results of his ten-year follow-up hard to believe. "I nearly fell out of my chair when I saw the differences in survival. We're not talking weeks, but an average of a year and a half."

The support groups, which were led by a therapist and a counselor who herself had breast cancer in remission, used no visualization or positive thinking techniques. The emphasis was on facing often grim realities. "Even though certain things about dying are frightening, the nothingness of death was less terrifying to the women than pain and physical helplessness at the end of their lives," says Spiegel. "They learned that there were things they could do, that they could keep making choices even as their disease advanced. Watching and reaching out to members whose condition deteriorated helped the women see the process of dying as something endurable rather than overwhelming."

The women also gained a greater sense of control over the time they had left. "They had to give up and grieve for the things they couldn't do, but they learned to focus on life projects that were do-able," says Spiegel. A frustrated writer published two small books of poetry before her death. Another woman devoted herself to imparting her life values to her young children. An unhappy wife decided to write off a bad relationship with a spouse rather than waste more energy on it. "The women emerged with a wisdom in living," Spiegel notes.

In their ninety-minute sessions, the women provided encouragement and shared strategies for better communication and relationships with their physicians. Group members also phoned one another, sent cards and letters, and visited those who had to be hospitalized. "They all felt that their relationships with friends and family had changed, and the group may have provided replacements for bonds that had been broken," says Spiegel. "They came to care deeply about one another."

Within four years of the study's inception, all the women in the control group were dead, whereas 30 percent of group participants were still alive. Average survival time for group members was 36.6 months, compared to 18.9 months for the controls. "There's no magic here; we didn't make the cancer go away," says Spiegel. "But something happened. We don't know what. Maybe the women's general health improved because they had less pain and fatigue and could be more active. Maybe their doctors perceived they were ready to fight and treated them more aggressively. Maybe there were changes in their immune systems. Whatever happened, it was remarkable." Other studies, with patients with malignant melanoma as well as metastatic breast cancer, have also found longer survival and increased immunologic functioning in those who receive psychological as well as medical treatments.

Cancer is a crisis for families as well as individuals. At the same time that they have to deal with their own feelings and fears, the parents, spouses, or adult children of cancer patients must often assume responsibility for direct patient care. During the course of the illness, each member faces a change in family dynamics, disruptions in familiar routines, and the financial consequences of extensive and expensive treatments. Family counseling, with an emphasis on education, emotional support, and acknowledgment of each member's right to personal needs and negative feelings, can be very helpful.

Because of the increasing success of treatments, ever-growing numbers of Americans—by the year 2000 the figure will be 10 million—survive cancer. Yet, just as the disease can lead to long-term physical consequences, survivors may experience unsettling and persistent psychological effects. Some find the transition from the sick to the well role difficult. Many experience a form of anxiety termed the Damocles syndrome, a heightened sense of the fragility of life combined with continuing concerns about illness and death. These worries can undermine self-confidence and the ability to form close relationships and plan for the future. Psychotherapy and self-help groups can help survivors to work through these lingering concerns.

HIV INFECTION AND AIDS

Not very many years ago, no one knew what the human immuno-deficiency virus (HIV) was or had ever heard of acquired immune deficiency syndrome (AIDS). Today, HIV is the most feared infectious agent in the world, and AIDS has become one of the most challenging medical and social issues of our time. As with no other disease of this century, AIDS provokes enormous emotional reactions, not only in those infected with HIV but in the general population. The reason may be that AIDS, a fatal disease that chiefly strikes young, healthy people, forces all of us to confront our own vulnerability. Because it is sexually transmitted, it also may tap into deep feelings about sexuality, particularly homosexuality.

Although there is no cure for this illness, a great deal can be done to enhance the quality of psychological and physical life for those with HIV and AIDS. In studying reactions to HIV infection, researchers have identified a characteristic four-stage progression: shock and a period of crisis that usually lasts for three or four months; a transitional phase marked by anxiety, depression, and internal turmoil; acceptance of physical status; and, finally (often after a period of many years), a stage of preparation for death.

Similar responses have been described with other severe illnesses, such as cancer, but there is a difference. Almost always a diagnosis of cancer leads to treatment, which may be extremely arduous but which has a definite goal; in an ever-increasing number of cancer cases, the prognosis ranges from fair to very good. Individuals who learn that they are HIV-positive may have no symptoms. The only "treatment" may consist of drugs given in the hope of warding off or delaying the development of AIDS. Infected persons do not and cannot know if or when they will develop signs of the disease. There is only one virtual certainty: AIDS is fatal.

As noted, the most common response to a positive HIV antibody test is shock. Depending on their perceptions and understanding of the disease, individuals may feel overwhelmed by fears of dying, disability, a long and painful illness, the loss of work, money, and support from family and friends. They want to know if they are contagious, how long they'll live, whether their partners or children are at risk, if they can have sex again, and a hundred other urgent facts about the future they face.

Newly diagnosed individuals may not be able to sleep; they may monitor themselves vigilantly for any sign of disease or turn constantly to health care providers for reassurance. Most feel a range of dark emotions, including fear, depression, anger, grief over their losses (including the loss of their self-image as a healthy person, their sexual freedom, perhaps the hope of having a child), and guilt over past behaviors that may have led to infection. Some react with strong feelings of denial and continue to practice behaviors that put their well-being in danger (such as not seeking medical care) or that jeopardize others (such as unsafe sex). Counseling before and after HIV antibody testing can make an enormous difference in helping people to understand and come to terms with the diagnosis. With such help, they find it easier to learn what to do to protect themselves and others, to arrange for medical follow-up, and to adapt to the psychological realities of living with HIV.

Despite the stress of being diagnosed with HIV, most people do learn to cope, and to cope well. In some large-scale research studies, rates of depression were lower in HIV-positive individuals than in control groups. Psychotherapy, whether for a few sessions or over a longer period, can make a great difference in providing hope, dealing with stress, and working through psychological issues. Self-help groups and support programs can also play an important role.

Learning that a loved one is HIV-positive affects family members, partners, and friends. They, too, must go through stages of adaptation and may swing back and forth between overwhelming sadness or fear and acceptance. Parents may first learn that their teen or adult children are homosexual or bisexual, or abuse intravenous drugs, at the same time that they find out that they have HIV. Old conflicts may erupt, and everyone may feel guilt or regret.

Partners of individuals with HIV must deal with the prospect of losing a cherished lover and companion and with fears for their own well-being. A spouse may worry about the couple's children or finances. A gay lover may be concerned about the reaction of his partner's family and the prospect of being left alone after the partner's death. A few sessions with a therapist can often help partners and families to deal with such concerns and to focus on making the most of the time they have left with their loved ones.

Psychiatric complications Depression and anxiety can develop or intensify when symptoms worsen or a treatment fails. Individuals who have had previous depressions or a history of drug abuse are most likely to develop serious psychiatric disorders. There also is increased danger of suicide.

Major depression can be difficult to recognize because the fatigue and lethargy caused by the infection can also diminish energy and interest in favored activities. In addition to psychotherapy (often using a combination of behavioral, cognitive, and supportive approaches), treatment with antidepressants, stimulants, or alprazolam (Xanax) has proved effective. The choice of a specific medication depends on the person's mental and physical condition.

Anxiety is common among individuals with HIV infection as they face the stress of repeated tests, diagnoses, treatments, and the inevitable progression of their disease. Those who have had chronic anxiety disorders are most likely to experience severe anxiety. Reassurance and support from friends, loved ones, and caregivers are tremendously important. In cases of intolerable fear or when intense anxiety interferes with a person's ability to understand and cooperate with medical treatment, physicians may prescribe anti-anxiety medications.

Hospitalized patients with AIDS may become delirious as a result of metabolic imbalances, infections, cancers, or a drop in oxygen or blood sugar secondary to the disease. Prompt treatment, usually with haloperidol (Haldol), perhaps combined with other medications, can relieve symptoms and prevent permanent brain damage and potentially fatal complications.

HIV encephalopathy and dementia   HIV can directly affect the brain, spinal cord, and nervous system. Infection of the brain can cause a combination of cognitive, emotional, and behavioral changes referred to by several different terms, including *HIV encephalopathy, subacute encephalitis,* and *AIDS dementia.* Secondary infections of the central nervous system, such as cryptococcal meningitis and toxoplasmosis, also affect thinking and emotional state. A small percentage of patients (4 to 10 percent) develop lymphomas (malignant tumors) in the brain, which can cause confusion, impaired thinking, headaches, seizures, and personality changes. HIV-infected individuals are also at greatly increased risk for stroke.

Usually individuals with HIV infection of the brain first develop subtle symptoms, such as forgetfulness and problems in concentrating or paying attention. They may have difficulty reading a book or following a conversation. Over time it can become harder to do more complex tasks, such as grocery shopping or cooking. Many report symptoms of depression, including disturbed sleep and loss of appetite and energy. Some develop weakness, particularly in their lower legs and feet, problems with fine motor skills such as handwriting, and difficulty in walking or climbing stairs. Friends and family may notice personality changes, such as increased irritability or greater anxiety when faced with any change. Occasionally individuals experience psychotic symptoms, including hallucinations, mania, and paranoid ideas.

The course of this condition varies greatly. Many people suffer minimal impairment and develop effective coping strategies, such as writing reminder notes or keeping a pocket calendar. Those whose physical well-being is also deteriorating may need to rely on others for help with daily tasks. In some cases, individuals become so confused and disoriented that they no longer can make decisions about their treatment or daily life.

HIV encephalopathy can be diagnosed in a variety of ways. Brain imaging techniques, including computed tomography (CT) or positron emission tomography (PET) scans, may reveal atrophy (wasting away) of brain tissue and other signs of deterioration. Abnormalities can also be revealed by testing of cerebrospinal fluid and assessments of attention, abstraction, information processing, and other skills.

Treatment with AZT (azidothymidine, or zidovudine) can improve the symptoms of HIV encephalopathy, including memory and general cognitive ability. Stimulants such as methylphenidate (Ritalin) or dextroamphetamine can also bring about significant improvement in functioning, self-sufficiency, and self-esteem.

CRITICAL ILLNESS OR INJURIES

As noted in the discussions of cancer, HIV infection, and AIDS, potentially fatal diseases or injuries can cause a variety of psychiatric symptoms, including anxiety disorders, major depression, and delirium (extreme confusion). In severe cases, individuals may be hospitalized in critical care units. Although they can and do save lives, by their very nature intensive care units (ICUs) and coronary care units (CCUs) are extremely stressful places to be. The lights are always on. There is little or no privacy and a great deal of noise and activity. Crises are common, and it is not unusual for patients to witness cardiac arrests, other medical emergencies, and deaths.

Most patients who are alert to their surroundings when admitted to such specialized units initially respond with fear and anxiety. By the second or third day, some enter a period of denial and, convinced that nothing is seriously wrong with them and that their doctors are overreacting, may try to sign themselves out of the unit or refuse treatment. In another day or two, when they can no longer deny the seriousness of their condition, they may feel demoralized and depressed. This bout with pessimism usually passes fairly quickly, and most patients manage to rally their internal resources in a fight for recovery.

Nevertheless, because anxiety speeds up or stimulates many physiological processes, it can be dangerous for critically ill patients, especially those with cardiovascular problems. It is extremely important that anxiety be treated promptly. The usual approach is the use of anti-anxiety agents such as a benzodiazepine or buspirone (BuSpar). In addition, ICU and CCU patients often feel much calmer if they can have some control over their environment, even if only to dim the lights near their beds or to sit in a particular chair.

Depression can be difficult to diagnose in many seriously ill patients because symptoms such as lack of appetite, problems in sleeping, or fatigue may be caused by their physical condition or medication rather than by a depressive disorder. Psychiatrists experienced in treating medically ill patients are skilled in sorting out these factors. In some cases a change in medication can eliminate the problem. In others, psychiatric treatment, usually with antidepressant medications, can help. (See Chapter 5 for more information on medically caused depression.)

Many critically ill patients become confused. Those at highest risk of delirium are the elderly, individuals dependent on drugs or alcohol, severe burn patients, those with HIV-related disorders, and those who have suffered previous brain injury. Possible causes of delirium include infections, fever, drug withdrawal, metabolic imbalances, trauma, neurological disorders, vitamin deficiencies, hormonal abnormalities, insufficient oxygen, and reactions to drugs or toxins. Very ill patients often suffer from several of these problems simultaneously. Their doctors, working with a consultation psychiatrist, will try to reverse as many abnormalities as possible. Medication is often necessary for patients who are agitated, combative, or paranoid; the usual choice is the anti-psychotic drug haloperidol (Haldol), sometimes in combination with other sedating drugs.

Family members can play a helpful role by remaining with delirious patients, providing reassurance, helping to keep them aware of time and place, and preventing falls or other mishaps. Placement of familiar objects, as well as a clock and a calendar, near the bed can help to improve their orientation.

Critically ill patients, whether or not they suffer from delirium, may become angry or hostile. Often such emotions stem from the frustration they feel about their condition or from a sense of vulnerability or fear. Some patients refuse medical treatment as a way of asserting control or rebelling against the dependency forced on them by their illness. A consultation psychiatrist often provides valuable insight and help to both patients and their families.

HORMONAL DISORDERS

Before birth, hormones sculpt bodies and brains. In childhood, they stimulate growth and development. Beginning at puberty, they usher in the intricate changes of sexual maturation, menstruation, pregnancy, and menopause. At every age and every stage, hormones influence metabolism and mood, appetite and arousal, energy and well-being, directing the intricate, delicate balance of the human body and brain and affecting the myriad ways in which people think, look, feel, and act.

A mere twenty years ago researchers had identified only about twenty hormones; now we know that there are more than two hundred of these powerful chemicals in the body. The primary hormone-producing, or *endocrine*, glands are the thyroid, parathyroids, pituitary, pancreas, pineal body, adrenals, thymus, and gonads or sex organs (ovaries in women, testes in men).

All the hormones produced by the body are interdependent and work together so closely and in such complex ways that scientists still do not understand exactly how they overlap or complement one another. Because of these interconnections, an imbalance of any single hormone can affect many parts of the body and many emotional states. Thus, when the thyroid gland churns out an excess of thyroid hormones (hyperthyroidism), individuals can develop anxiety, depression, irritability, and nervousness. When thyroid hormone levels fall below normal, body processes slow down, causing depression and problems in concentrating or thinking. Some hypothyroid individuals develop delusional, paranoid, or belligerent behavior, a form of dementia called *myxedema madness* that is sometimes mistaken for schizophrenia.

Excessive or insufficient amounts of other hormones, including adrenal, pituitary, and parathyroid hormones, can also cause psychiatric symptoms, which often develop slowly and insidiously. Diagnosis usually is straightforward and is based on physical symptoms and standard screening tests that can detect most hormonal imbalances. In most cases, treatment, which may involve replacement hormones, medications, or other therapies (such as radiation to destroy an overactive thyroid), can ease or eliminate psychological symptoms.

KIDNEY DISEASE

The kidneys perform the essential function of removing metabolic waste products from the blood. A number of diseases can lead to kidney failure, a life-threatening condition. Acute kidney failure, usually caused by shock, infection, toxins, or drugs, is usually reversible if treated promptly. Chronic kidney failure is not curable, and a mechanical process of clearing wastes from the body, called *dialysis*, is necessary on an ongoing basis. Approximately 100,000 Americans receive dialysis every year. About 50 to 60 percent are able to live fairly normal lives, depending on many factors, including cognitive side effects. Continuous ambulatory peritoneal dialysis, which can be done at home, has a lesser impact on daily functioning than hemodialysis, the conventional form of blood cleansing performed at a dialysis center.

Dialysis patients often feel psychological distress as they come to terms with an incurable disease, their dependence on technology and medical care, and the limitations their disease places on their life. Depressive symptoms (although not major depression) are common. They may be the result of these factors, the kidney disease itself, or medications. Many individuals report sexual dysfunction. Suicide can be a risk.

Self-help groups for dialysis patients can provide a new social network and enhance feelings of self-esteem and self-mastery. Brief problem-oriented psychotherapy, sometimes combined with antidepressants, can help patients who are having problems in adjusting to their disease or to dialysis.

Various degrees of impaired thinking and atrophy of the brain are common in chronic dialysis patients, although there is no correlation between these problems and the duration of dialysis or kidney failure. Some patients who have been on dialysis for many years develop a rare, progressive condition called *dialysis dementia*, which can cause personality change, loss of memory, disorientation, seizures, mutism, and death, usually within a year. The cause may be aluminum toxicity caused by agents used in dialysis; chelating (blood cleansing) medications sometimes help relieve symptoms, although they do not restore kidney function.

NEUROLOGICAL PROBLEMS

Injuries and illnesses involving the brain often affect the mind. As many as half of those with neurological problems, whether they are hospitalized or outpatients, may develop psychiatric disorders; treating them is critical for recovery. For depression, psychiatrists generally try antidepressant medications, usually those least likely to be sedating or to lower blood pressure and affect other vital functions. Patients who do not improve or who develop serious side effects from medication may benefit from electroconvulsive therapy (ECT). For panic attacks, antidepressant drugs can be as effective as benzodiazepines and cause fewer side effects.

Individuals who have suffered any form of brain damage should be extremely cautious about using drugs. Even over-the-counter sleep or cold preparations can cause unexpected negative reactions. Alcohol is equally risky for such persons.

HEAD INJURY

Two million men, women, and children in the United States suffer head injuries annually; half a million are serious enough to require hospitalization. Head trauma is the number one cause of death and disability among Americans under the age of forty-four and of medically induced mental disorders at any age. Neuropsychiatrists have come to the realization that even "mild" injuries that do not involve a loss of consciousness can cause persistent symptoms and cognitive difficulties.

Postconcussion syndrome   Concussion is injury to the brain caused by a blow or other shock to the head. Persons who lose consciousness only briefly (usually for less than twenty minutes) may not require hospitalization. However, even minor brain injury may lead to a complication, referred to as *postconcussion syndrome* or *postconcussion disorder*, which is characterized by the following symptoms:

- *Physical:* Headache, dizziness, fatigue, insomnia
- *Cognitive:* Impaired concentration, memory problems
- *Perceptual:* Ringing in the ears, sensitivity to noise or light
- *Emotional:* Depression, anxiety, irritability.

These symptoms often improve greatly within three months, although some, particularly headaches, may persist for a longer time. Ten to twenty percent of persons with concussion suffer some symptoms for six months or longer, and a much smaller percentage experience some residual symptoms for a year or more. Treatments similar to those used in traumatic brain injury— medication combined with behavioral approaches—may help.

Traumatic brain injury   More serious brain injuries can cause physical disability, including general weakness and paralysis. Equally traumatic are the invisible wounds, including problems in reading and thinking, memory, finding the right word, speaking, and personality changes. Psychiatric problems—depression, anxiety, and uncontrollable mood swings—are common. Their likelihood and seriousness depend on the type, severity, and location of the injury itself and the severity of the "invisible wounds," as well as the person's behavior, intelligence, and psychological well-being before the injury. About 70 percent of head trauma patients, or their families, report significant irritability or aggression.

To date, the greatest success in remedying brain damage has come with intense rehabilitation, beginning as soon as possible after the accident and continuing for months or years. New drugs may limit or halt the chemical interactions responsible for much of the damage to the brain that follows a blow or fall.

Improvement of physical and emotional symptoms occurs gradually over eighteen months or so as swelling lessens and the brain heals. Medications can control some symptoms, such as violent outbursts. In general, behavioral approaches—rewards and demerits, individualized goals and contracts—as well as an atmosphere of support, concern, friendliness, and warmth help about 75 percent of patients. The process of recovering cognitive abilities, relearning practical and social skills, and dealing with the psychological impact of traumatic brain injury can take four to six years. The nature and extent of the brain damage the person has suffered determines the ultimate outcome; some return to near-normal functioning, whereas others require lifelong care.

STROKE

When the blood supply to the brain is blocked, a cerebrovascular accident (CVA), or stroke, occurs. About half a million people suffer strokes each year; and strokes rank third, after heart disease and cancer, as a cause of death. After decades of steady decline, the number of strokes per year has begun to rise. The chief reasons for this are that Americans are living longer, more people are surviving with heart disease, and the diagnosis and detection of strokes that might not have been discerned in the past have greatly improved.

Strokes can be caused by the blockage of a brain artery by a thrombus or blood clot (cerebral thrombosis) or by the rupture of a diseased artery in the brain that floods the surrounding area with blood (cerebral hemorrhage). When deprived of oxygen as a result of a stroke, brain tissue begins to die. The effects of a stroke depend on the area of the brain in which it occurs and the extent of the damage. The effects can be temporary or permanent, slight or severe, and range from impairments in motor activity, such as walking, to functional difficulties in speaking, finding the right words, or recalling names, places, or events. (See Chapter 20 for a discussion of mini-strokes and vascular dementia.)

Strokes can be psychologically as well as physically disabling. Those that affect the left side of the brain are likely to produce a catastrophic reaction, characterized by irritability, anxiety, tearfulness, intense emotionality, restlessness, and uncooperativeness. When a stroke involves the right side of the brain, the person is more likely to have an indifferent reaction, with apathy, denial of illness, and undue cheerfulness.

Depression is common after stroke and may be related to physical disability or brain damage caused by the stroke. Many individuals become depressed while hospitalized; others may develop major depression or dysthymia in the two years following the stroke. Treatment with medication, psychotherapy, or a combination is often extremely beneficial.

There has been great progress in the treatment of stroke, including the use of clot-dissolving, or *thrombolytic*, drugs which can restore brain blood flow, or other medications, called *heparinoids*, which reduce the blood's tendency to clot. To be effective, these medications must be administered soon after a stroke: thrombolytics within ninety minutes and heparinoids within twenty-four hours. Prompt treatment can make an enormous difference in the prognosis for stroke victims.

EPILEPSY

Derived from a Greek word meaning "seizure," *epilepsy* is the term used to refer to a variety of seizure disorders caused by abnormal electrical discharges in the brain. Severe forms of epilepsy are characterized by sudden attacks (seizures) of violent muscle contractions and unconsciousness. Between 0.5 and 1 percent of all Americans have recurrent seizures. They are rarely fatal; the primary danger is suffering an attack while driving or swimming.

Seizures are classified as major (*grand mal*), minor (*petit mal*), and psychomotor. In a grand mal seizure the person loses consciousness, falls to the ground, and experiences convulsive body movements. Petit mal seizures are characterized by a brief loss of consciousness for ten to thirty seconds, eye or muscle flutterings, and occasionally a loss of muscle tone. A psychomotor seizure may involve both a loss of muscle tone and confusion.

About half of all cases of epilepsy have no known cause (*idiopathic epilepsy*); others stem from conditions that affect the brain, such as trauma, tumors, congenital malformations, or inflammation of the membranes covering the brain. Anticonvulsant drugs can control seizures in most people, but an estimated 10 to 20 percent of epileptics continue to have seizures despite drug therapy. Because technological advances are now making it possible for physicians to pinpoint exactly where seizures originate in the brain, surgery may offer new hope for epilepsy.

Mental disorders are common in those with persistent seizure disorders. In various studies, more than half also suffered from major depression, bipolar disorder, panic attacks (which may be hard to differentiate from seizures), and other problems requiring psychiatric treatment. The severity of depression is related to the duration and frequency of seizures. In some cases there is a greatly increased risk for suicide.

Some antiseizure medications, particularly when used in combination, can cause psychiatric side effects including irritability, aggression, and cognitive difficulties. Conversely, some psychiatric drugs, particularly certain antidepressants, increase the risk for seizures. Psychiatrists who are experienced in treating medically ill patients and are up to date in psychopharmacology can often substitute medications less likely to cause serious problems.

SURGERY

Surgery, the most direct and invasive of all therapies, can cause many indirect effects. Surgeons have long contended that patients who expect to die during an operation will do so, and studies have confirmed that there is some truth to this statement. Persons who are depressed or extremely anxious before surgery are indeed more likely to develop serious, even fatal complications. Those who go into surgery with a positive attitude fare better. Ample information about a planned operation, explanations of the procedure, and understanding of how they will look, feel, and function afterward can greatly enhance their mental state. Nevertheless, regardless of prior preparation, patients who experience surgical complications may develop delirium, dementia, depression, mania, anxiety, or adjustment disorders.

By their very nature, some types of surgery have a greater psychological impact than others. Women who undergo mastectomy may have difficulty in dealing with the loss of a breast as well as the reality of having cancer. For men, urological surgery that may affect potency, such as certain prostate operations, may be particularly distressing. Kidney donors may feel ambivalent or anxious before surgery and depressed or troubled by feelings of loss afterward. After their initial euphoria at getting a new lease on life, recipients of transplanted organs, whether kidneys, hearts, livers, or lungs, often go through a period of disillusionment when they realize that life will never be exactly the way it was before they became ill. They have to deal with both the emotional and the medical realities of living with a transplanted organ, as well as with concerns about body image and sexuality. Many medical centers or communities offer support groups for individuals undergoing specific operations. For many people, this is one of the most effective ways of dealing with practical concerns and emotional issues.

Medications that cause psychiatric side effects

Many common medications, including drugs for high blood pressure, heart disease, asthma, epilepsy, arthritis, ulcers, anxiety, insomnia, and depression, can cause psychiatric side effects. Even medications such as antibiotics, which do not usually cause problems, can generate psychiatric side effects in sensitive individuals. Many problems that can be attributed to drugs, particularly subtle ones like forgetfulness or irritability, are often ignored or dismissed.

Because neither patients nor their physicians usually connect psychiatric symptoms with medications, no one knows precisely

DRUGS THAT CAN CAUSE PSYCHIATRIC SIDE EFFECTS*

TYPE OF DRUG	COMMON NAMES	EFFECTS ON MIND AND BEHAVIOR
Anti-anxiety drugs	**Valium, Librium** (benzodiazepines)	**During use or withdrawal: depression, disorientation, delirium**
Anticonvulsants	**Dilantin, Tegretol**	**Depression, disorientation, delirium, hallucinations** (usually with high doses)
Antidepressants	**Prozac, Wellbutrin, MAO inhibitors, Cyclic antidepressants**	**Agitation, restlessness, anxiety**
	Lithium	**Disorientation, delirium**
Antihistamines (often in OTC cold remedies and sleeping pills)	**Benadryl** (diphenhydramine)	**Disorientation, delirium, hallucinations** (with higher doses)
Antihypertensives	**Reserpine, Aldomet, Guanethidine, Catapres, Inderal**	**Depression, delirium**
Anti-inflammatories	**Indocin, Naprosyn**	**Depression, confusion, paranoia, delirium** (especially in the elderly)
	Corticosteroids	**Depression** (during or after use), **anxiety, delirium, hallucinations** (with high doses), **paranoia**
Antimicrobials	**Acyclovir (Zovirax) Amphotericin B, Keflin, Flagyl**	**Confusion, delirium, paranoia** (with high doses)
Asthma drugs	**Theophylline, aminophylline**	**Anxiety, insomnia**

how many individuals develop such side effects. In one study of nine thousand hospital patients taking drugs for medical problems, about 3 percent developed agitation, anxiety, bizarre feelings, depression, hallucinations, delusions, and other psychiatric symptoms. In at least some of these cases, these symptoms may have been drug-related, although medical problems themselves can cause such problems.

Certain medications—for example, antihypertensives (drugs that lower blood pressure)—trigger depression in more than 10 percent of those who use them. Others, such as the powerful

DRUGS THAT CAN CAUSE PSYCHIATRIC SIDE EFFECTS* (continued)

TYPE OF DRUG	COMMON NAMES	EFFECTS ON MIND AND BEHAVIOR
Decongestants	**Any preparation containing pseudoephedrine**	**Anxiety, restlessness, insomnia**
Estrogen	**Oral contraceptives, Estrogen replacement**	**Mood changes, depression** **Depression** (during or after use)
Glaucoma	**AK-Zol, Dazamide, Diamox**	**Depression, disorientation**
Heart medications	**Digitalis**	**Depression, anxiety, disorientation, delirium**
	Inderal	**Depression**
	Xylocaine	**Depression, delirium**
Painkillers	**Opiates** (meperidine, Percodan) **Salicylates** (aspirin)	**Agitation, delirium** **Agitation, confusion, hallucinations, delirium** (with chronic use)
Parkinson's disease drugs	**Cogentin, Akineton, amantadine**	**Depression, delirium, hallucinations, nightmares** (in elderly and with high doses)
Sleeping pills	*OTC:* **Compoz, Excedrin-PM, Sleep-Eze, Sominex, etc.** *Prescription:* **Dalmane, Halcion, and others**	**Disorientation, delirium** **Depression, confusion, delirium, memory loss, disorientation**
Stimulants	**Amphetamines** **Ritalin**	**Anxiety, paranoia** **Hallucinations** (in children)
Ulcer medications	**Tagamet**	**Disorientation, delirium, hallucinations** (with high doses and in elderly)

*These drugs can also affect physical function; this chart lists only their effects on the mind.

hormones called corticosteroids used in treating severe asthma, autoimmune diseases, and cancer, can cause different psychiatric symptoms in different persons and in different doses.

Unfortunately, physicians may not forewarn patients about possible psychiatric side effects because they themselves are unaware of the danger or because they don't want to scare them away from what may be a very effective treatment. The unhappy consequence is that many people suffer unnecessarily. In almost every case, psychiatric side effects can be avoided, eliminated, or overcome *if* they are recognized.

WHO'S AT RISK?

Anyone, at any age, can develop psychiatric side effects from drugs. However, the following groups are especially vulnerable:

Older men and women. The elderly, who make up only 11 percent of the population, take about 25 percent of all prescription drugs. In one study, 83 percent of the elderly were taking from two to six drugs per day. The use of multiple medications and changes in the way the aging body metabolizes drugs make older persons more prone to psychiatric side effects. Many medications should be prescribed in significantly smaller doses for older men and women.

Children and adolescents. Because their brains and central nervous systems are still developing, children often respond differently to drugs than do adults. Many antibiotics, including penicillin, can cause delirium in youngsters. Even aspirin can be dangerous. Most parents of young children are aware of the potential risk for Reye's syndrome (a dangerous brain inflammation) if they use aspirin for their child's flu or fever. This is why acetaminophen (Tylenol) is recommended instead. However, teenagers often medicate themselves, and they are just as vulnerable to Reye's syndrome as younger children are.

Individuals who have had a psychiatric illness or developed psychiatric drug reactions in the past. In people with a history of depression, certain medications, including common antihypertensive drugs, may be more likely to bring out depressive symptoms. Those who experienced psychiatric side effects from previous drugs they had taken may also be more vulnerable.

Those with serious physical conditions. Persons with problems that affect the brain itself, such as traumatic brain injury, or that affect the way the body metabolizes drugs, such as liver diseases, are highly susceptible to the psychiatric side effects of medications.

Those taking multiple medications. Individuals taking many different drugs are at greater risk for all types of side effects.

Those under great stress. People who have not slept for days, who are isolated from friends and family, or who are in a frightening, unfamiliar environment, such as a hospital intensive care unit, may be more vulnerable to a drug's psychiatric effects.

PREVENTING PROBLEMS

The best safeguard against the psychiatric side effects of medications is awareness that they can develop. The following recommendations can help protect both your mental and your physical well-being:

- Always ask your doctor about possible psychiatric side effects of a medication. Find out whether any alternative medicines that do not induce such side effects might be equally effective.

- Inform your physician of *all* other medicines you are taking including birth control pills and over-the-counter preparations.

- Ask specifically about alcohol and caffeine. Report exactly how much you usually consume every day. Find out how these substances might interact with the medication.

- Check on timing. For example, drugs with sedating effects should not be taken during the day, and those with stimulating effects should be avoided at bedtime.

- If you are taking other medicines, make up a daily calendar and check off each dose of each drug as you take it.

- If you have had a psychiatric problem such as depression in the past, or if you have ever experienced psychiatric side effects from drugs, let your doctor know. You may also want to consult a psychiatrist to find out which medications are recommended to lower the risk for psychiatric side effects.

- If you have any reason to suspect that a medication is affecting your mind or behavior, tell your doctor exactly how you feel. Find out if such side effects are temporary. Many symptoms develop in the first week or two on a medication, then disappear. Sometimes you have to hang in there for a little while, keeping in mind that you will feel better soon.

- If psychiatric side effects do not go away, ask whether you can switch to a lower dose or an alternative medication.

- Get a second opinion. Doctors are often accustomed to doing things one way and may not be flexible. If your physician says there is no other option, consult a psychiatrist.

- Don't suddenly stop taking any medication on your own. If you abruptly discontinue certain medications, you may endanger your physical well-being and end up feeling even greater anxiety, depression, or confusion.

Elderly individuals with mental and emotional problems may:

☐ **Frequently find it difficult to complete a sentence because they forget what they want to say or the words with which to say it**

☐ **Misplace important items, such as money or bank records**

☐ **Often seem confused**

☐ **Forget how to use common items or perform simple tasks**

☐ **Get lost or disoriented in familiar places, especially at home**

☐ **Not be able to identify the month or season**

☐ **Suffer dizzy spells or severe headaches along with memory loss**

☐ **Have a depressed or sad mood, lose appetite or weight, lack interest or pleasure in usual activities, feel hopeless or worthless, have problems in concentrating or making decisions, be indecisive or irritable, complain of chronic exhaustion, aches, and pains, be preoccupied with death or thoughts of suicide (signs of possible depression)**

☐ **Be very restless, tremble, twitch, feel shaky, or show other signs of increased muscle tension; have difficulty in breathing, heart palpitations or an accelerated heart rate; have sweaty or cold, clammy hands; become dizzy or light-headed; develop nausea, diarrhea, or other digestive problems; have trouble with swallowing; feel keyed up or on edge; have exaggerated reactions to sudden sounds (signs of a possible anxiety disorder)**

Even checking a single box may indicate a possible problem. The more boxes that you check, the more reason you may have to be concerned. This chapter describes the most common problems of the elderly and provides guidance on seeking help and appropriate treatments.

Mental Health and Problems in the Elderly

Tom Nelson was the very model of a modern senior citizen. After retiring from an international shipping business in his mid-sixties, he remained active in community organizations. A lifelong athlete, he swam and played tennis or golf several times a week. He and his wife took long trips to Europe and Asia. Although he had some health problems, they didn't undermine his energy or enthusiasm for living.

When Tom was seventy, his older brother and one of his closest friends died within months of each other. For a long time afterward, he seemed distracted and withdrawn. The following year he underwent heart bypass surgery. Recovering in the cardiac care unit, he became delirious. His wife and adult children were frightened to see Tom, who had always been so calm and rational, completely out of touch with what was going on around him. Although his delirium cleared in a few days, his recovery was slow, and he never went back to the sports he had loved.

Over the next two years, Tom developed other health problems, most requiring medication. Unable to sleep through the night, he would go the kitchen for some brandy and fall asleep on the living room sofa. Instead of making plans for each day, he would sit in front of the television for hours at a time. His memory began to falter. He couldn't remember his grandchildren's names or recall conversations he'd had the week before. Increasingly irritable, he often snapped at his wife and quarreled with store clerks and waiters, accusing them of shortchanging him.

"Is something wrong with Dad?" his concerned daughter asked. "He's just getting old and crotchety," her brother replied.

"How can we know for sure?" she said. "Maybe it's not just old age."

After talking with their mother, all three urged Tom to get a complete check-up from specialists in geriatric medicine. Consulting with a geriatric psychiatrist, his physicians realized that many of Tom's symptoms—insomnia, memory problems, irritability, suspiciousness—were the result of a mix of physical ailments, depression, medications, and alcohol.

Like Tom, many older Americans suffer from a combination of physical and mental symptoms that can be effectively treated. All too often, however, such problems are never recognized. Many older men and women are too embarrassed to admit that they are having difficulty or to seek help. Often they, and their relatives, mistakenly believe that depression, confusion, anxiety, or memory problems are the inevitable consequences of old age. This is not the case, and with treatment the elderly are just as likely to improve or recover from these conditions as younger adults.

Optimal aging

We are getting older, not just as individuals but as a society. Men and women over the age of fifty-five make up more than a fifth of our population. By the year 2010, one in four Americans—some 74.1 million people—will be over fifty-five; one in seven will be sixty-nine or older. Just as the number of senior citizens is growing every day, so is their life expectancy. Today's sixty-five-year-olds, far healthier than were their parents and grandparents who survived that long, can expect to live nearly two more decades. The "old" old —those over eighty-five—are the fastest growing segment of the population; by the year 2000 they will number almost 5 million.

For years, the process of getting older was viewed only in terms of deterioration, frailty, and the erosions of time. Today, instead of focusing on the minority of the elderly who have progressive or irreversible conditions, gerontologists—specialists in late life—are studying the majority of men and women who remain vital and resilient in their later years. Increasingly, they emphasize *optimal aging*, which focuses on ways to enhance the well-being and preserve the abilities of older people. Its goal is to enable people to live through old age with the best possible quality of life and the least possible premature disability.

Successful aging demands a redefinition of who a person is and what makes that person's life worthwhile. Some sources of satisfaction, such as physical challenges or professional achievements, diminish later in life. Yet, as social psychologist Carin Rubinstein, author of *In Search of Intimacy*, a study of loneliness in America, comments: "Old people in general feel psychologically better than young people. They have fewer worries about themselves and how they look to other people; they have higher self-esteem; they aren't as lonely as people think they are."

As they age, many individuals find increasing gratification from intimacy with a spouse or partner, and their relationship, enriched by decades of companionship and honest communication, can serve as a powerful buffer against stress. Of course, not all older couples grow closer as they grow older. Some have different values or lack mutual interests; indeed, retirement may reveal problems that had never seemed troublesome during the busy years of child-rearing and career building. Marital counseling can help couples work through the adjustments they face as individuals and as partners in their later years.

Sexual activity typically decreases in the elderly, but it does not end. According to a survey by the National Opinion Research Center at the University of Chicago, more than one third of American married men and women older than sixty make love at least once a week, as do 10 percent of those older than seventy. Even in those with sexual dysfunctions or without partners, romantic and sexual feelings often continue well into old age. Flirtatiousness, ranging from coquettish smiles to hugging and kissing, is common at senior centers, particularly during games, singing, or dancing. There is a longing for physical contact by the elderly that one therapist describes as "touch hunger." For as long as they live, men and women yearn for physical closeness with partners, friends, children, grandchildren, or pets.

Social intimacy, like physical intimacy, can be a source of solace and strength in late life. However, loneliness is an undeniable problem for those who do not have a spouse or partner or who retire to distant regions or move to be closer to their grown children, leaving behind old friends and social networks. Even those who establish new friendships or maintain old ones must face the sadness and loneliness that come as death claims an ever-increasing number of their contemporaries.

Yet whatever their social and emotional ties or the circumstances of their daily lives, some older men and women enjoy much greater emotional well-being than others. What is their secret? According to a long-term study of 173 Harvard College graduates begun in the 1940s, the key factor is an ability to cope with life's setbacks without blame or bitterness. In these men, problems in childhood (such as being poor or orphaned) had almost no effect on psychological health at age sixty-five. Many things that had seemed so important at college age, such as making friends easily, also became unimportant later in life. However, students who had been good at practical organization were among the mentally healthiest at sixty-five, as were those initially rated by psychiatrists as "steady, stable, dependable, thorough, sincere, and trustworthy." Although these individuals changed through the years, their psychological core remained the same.

Even though they are biologically nearer to death, most older men and women do not fear dying more than young people do. In fact, over time many seem to develop an acceptance of death, which they think and talk about more than when they were young. Death may be less frightening to contemplate in old age than in youth or midlife, possibly because of religious beliefs, a sense of having accomplished life goals, or the gratification of having lived a life with purpose and meaning.

The aging brain

Although the brain literally becomes smaller as we age, basic mental abilities do not necessarily diminish. Reaction time, intellectual speed and efficiency, nonverbal intelligence, and the maximal speed at which we can work for short periods may decline somewhat by the age of seventy-five. However, understanding, vocabulary, the ability to remember key information, and verbal intelligence remain about the same. A grandfather playing a computer game with his fourteen-year-old grandson will lose every time, because instead of responding in a fifth of a second like the boy, he needs two-fifths of a second. But when it comes to tests that involve experience and acquired knowledge, the grandfather has the edge.

Although certain aspects of memory falter with time, most people can compensate by relying on simple coping strategies, such as taking notes, making lists, or—if they arrive in a room only to forget what they wanted there—retracing their thoughts and actions before heading there. Some people have better memories in their sixties than others do in their thirties. And at any age, people can improve their recall.

Middle-aged and older individuals may find it more difficult to recall newly learned information than younger ones because they have not learned it well in the first place. Older people often fail to spend as much time organizing the material they want to master as young people do. In preparing for a written driving test, for example, they may not use learning skills, such as highlighting key words or making a list of key points, that could enhance their mastery.

The most common problem for people over sixty is remembering what to call an object or a person. They recognize the person or know how to use the object, but they can't produce the word for it, especially if it's someone or something they don't refer to often. For example, trying to think of the word for a game played with a small white ball and paddles, they think of tennis rather than ping-pong. Running into an old acquaintance, they frantically flip through their mental Rolodex, trying to match the face with a name. The more anxious they get, the more difficult remembering becomes.

Although occasional forgetfulness, memory lapses, and misplacement of everyday objects are common at any age, about 5 to 15 percent of people over the age of seventy develop more serious symptoms of diminished mental capacity, such as errors in judgment and impaired thinking. A number of illnesses, including depression, kidney disease, alcoholism, and Alzheimer's disease, can cause these symptoms. Thorough medical and neurological examinations may be able to pinpoint the specific problem.

Mental and emotional problems in the elderly

Older persons can face a variety of medical, economic, social, and psychological challenges. They may not get adequate nutrition. They may become increasingly isolated. Impaired mobility or vision may interfere with their ability to function from day to day. Hearing loss can be particularly devastating. They may think that others are talking about them in deliberately low tones so as not to be overheard. Unable to discern what others are saying, they may withdraw and become isolated and depressed. With the passage of time, many older people develop serious diseases such as arthritis, arteriosclerosis, cancer, and osteoporosis. A hospitalization, the loss of a home in a fire or flood, or other unexpected catastrophes can have a much greater impact than they would at earlier stages of life. The cumulative impact of stressful events, one often following another before the individual has had time to adjust, can take a toll on physical and emotional well-being.

The American Psychiatric Association estimates that 15 to 25 percent of the elderly have significant symptoms of mental illness. As many as half of all older people hospitalized for medical or surgical reasons develop psychiatric difficulties, such as delirium. Some of these symptoms are caused by abnormal thyroid activity, brain tumors, drug side effects, or depression, and can be reversed. Severe mental illnesses, including delusions and paranoia, affect 1 million elderly Americans. Many more suffer milder forms of mental disorders.

LOSS AND GRIEF

Life's final years, once described as "the season of loss," may mean the gradual loss or end of many things: gratifying work, cherished friendships, financial and physical independence. Retiring after a successful career can seem like the end of purposeful existence. As friends and family die or move away, social networks can disintegrate. Diminished physical abilities can change the way in which individuals view themselves and their future. Those who can no longer see, hear, or get around as well as they once did may mourn the loss of the sense of safety and freedom they once had. Even senior citizens without physical limitations may be fearful—often justifiably so—of venturing out after dark or walking through certain parks or neighborhoods. Regardless of their current health, many worry about what the future might bring, such as the loss of financial, social, domestic, or physical independence. Developing effective coping strategies and reaching out for support from family and friends can be crucial in dealing with these difficult issues.

Regardless of age, the loss of a loved one is always the most stressful of life's traumas. This remains true later in life, when grieving survivors drink more alcohol, take more anti-anxiety drugs, and require more frequent hospitalization than others their age. The phases of grief are common to all ages. Initially, individuals feel shock, disbelief, emptiness, confusion, numbness, and free-floating anxiety. They have problems sleeping, lose their appetites, and experience muscle aches and pains. It takes about four to six weeks for the finality of the loss to hit. They cry, cannot sleep, lose interest in daily activities, and find it hard to concentrate. They yearn to be reunited with the person they have lost, yet feel anger at being abandoned and left behind. Hallucinations, such as seeing the dead person seated in a favorite chair, are common.

During the initial months after a death, survivors may question or blame others as they think of ways it might have been prevented. Often grieving individuals focus almost obsessively on the details of the loved one's final moments; this is part of the process of coming to terms with their loss.

After six months to a year, intense feelings of grief usually subside, although they may return on the anniversary of the death. Although individuals may remain emotionally involved with memories of the deceased for months or even years, ultimately most redefine their image of themselves in the world and decide that it is time to get on with their lives. For some, however, grief, always painful, can become pathological. About 15 to 25 percent of bereaved individuals show signs of significant distress, particularly major depression, a year or two after a loss.

Pathological grief can take both a physical and a psychological toll, damping the immune system and increasing susceptibility to disease in bereaved spouses or partners. In general, bereaved women are more susceptible to mental health problems, such as depression and anxiety disorders, whereas bereaved men tend to develop more physical illnesses, particularly heart disease and, at least initially, to lack the network of friends and acquaintances that provide social support to their married counterparts. Widowers have a higher than expected mortality rate from both natural causes and suicide during the first year after a wife's death. Two years after a loss, older men and women seem to fare about the same in terms of depression, life satisfaction, and resolution of their grief.

Older men and women benefit just as much as younger ones from grief counseling and therapy, including psychodynamic or cognitive-behavioral therapy. One helpful approach is regular telephone or in-home therapy for grieving seniors, which can reduce their incidence of minor illnesses and the number of medications they take.

DEPRESSION

Most elderly people do *not* become clinically depressed, although symptoms of depression frequently occur. According to a 1992 report by the National Institutes of Health consensus development panel on depression in late life, about 15 percent of men and women over sixty-five living in the community experience actual depression. In nursing homes the rate ranges from 15 to 25 percent. Recurrences are common, with 40 percent suffering repeated bouts. Older men and women who become depressed are more likely to develop psychotic symptoms, such as hallucinations and delusions, than younger ones.

In late life, as at other times, the causes of depression are complex. Some older individuals have a biological predisposition or a history of depression that makes them vulnerable. Others often have lost a spouse or have few social supports. Health problems and restrictions, or a sense of not having fulfilled life expectations, may contribute to depression. Some medications, including common drugs taken for high blood pressure, can also play a role.

Late-life depression can be particularly hard to identify. Some of its classic signs—appetite changes, weight loss, insomnia, and fatigue—may be mistakenly attributed to medical problems, medications, or old age itself. Psychiatrists experienced in geriatric care can sort out the underlying causes of telltale symptoms; other physicians may not be able to do so. In one study of 150 older individuals admitted to a hospital for medical reasons, the examining physician did not detect a single case of depression, yet a psychiatrist who interviewed the same individuals found that 15 percent were severely depressed. In older men and women, psychological symptoms such as tearfulness or sadness may be absent or denied, whereas symptoms such as lack of pleasure and physical complaints are more frequent or intense.

The consequences of not recognizing and treating depression that occurs late in life can be tragic. Depression that develops after an illness or injury, if not identified, can hinder recovery; depression following a heart attack or stroke can increase mortality. Older Americans have the highest suicide rate in our society, with some 8,500 elderly persons killing themselves every year. The suicide rate at age sixty-five is five times higher than that of younger individuals. It continues to increase with age, especially among white men. Mental health professionals who are working with a depressed elderly person often meet with family members and enlist their aid in getting their older relatives involved in activities and monitoring them for any signs of suicidal thoughts or behavior.

More than 70 percent of the depressed elderly improve dramatically with treatment, which usually consists of a combination of psychotherapy and medication, often along with family counseling. (Similar improvement occurs when cognitive impairment is treated.) Various methods of psychotherapy, including cognitive and behavioral therapies, have proved effective with older men and women. Common issues that treatment addresses include rapid and cumulative losses and a sense of defenselessness and hopelessness.

Antidepressant drugs can help, but psychiatrists pay special attention to the increased risk of side effects, such as dizziness on sitting or standing abruptly, in selecting a medication for older patients. Often lower doses are adequate. Another strategy for decreasing side effects is dividing the dose by taking half the usual amount twice a day rather than the full dose at one time.

Because of physiological differences caused by age, older individuals usually respond more slowly to antidepressants than younger persons, and it can take from six to twelve weeks for benefits to be apparent. Maintenance therapy can prevent recurrences. For persons with severe depression who do not improve after a trial of at least two medications, electroconvulsive therapy (ECT) is considered safe and beneficial. It can also improve mental abilities in those with cognitive impairment (see Chapter 28).

ANXIETY DISORDERS

Anxiety disorders can occur at any age, but in general their incidence decreases with age. According to the National Institute of Mental Health's (NIMH) epidemiological data, the older individuals are, the less the likelihood of their developing a serious anxiety disorder. However, anxiety itself is a common symptom among older persons, with about 20 percent reporting some physical or psychological signs of anxiety. (Chapter 7 discusses the anxiety disorders.) In late life, anxiety symptoms often occur along with depression.

Sometimes particular circumstances, such as a neighborhood crime or increased difficulty in driving, cause episodic anxiety that abates under different circumstances. Caffeine is a common culprit, particularly when individuals combine their usual coffee intake with over-the-counter medications, such as analgesics that contain caffeine or cold remedies with ephedrine. In cases of more intense and persistent anxiety, health problems such as hyperthyroidism or cardiac arrhythmias may be responsible. Withdrawal from certain substances after long use, among them alcohol and the benzodiazepines, can also cause significant anxiety in the elderly.

Counseling that emphasizes behavioral and relaxation techniques can be very helpful. Medication also has proved effective. Because many drugs remain active in the elderly for much longer periods than in younger people, psychiatrists usually prescribe short-acting benzodiazepines for treatment of anxiety. These drugs must be reduced or discontinued after a few weeks because long-term use can produce cumulative harmful effects, including confusion and psychosis. To avoid withdrawal symptoms, psychiatrists taper the dose gradually over a week or so. Another anti-anxiety agent, buspirone (BuSpar), is not sedating, does not interact with alcohol, has no potential for abuse, and does not interfere with a person's ability to perform motor tasks or drive a car. Its chief disadvantage is that it may take somewhat longer than the benzodiazepines—about two to four weeks—for individuals to experience its full benefits.

SLEEP DISORDERS

Sleep changes drastically in both quality and quantity over the course of a lifetime. A twenty-year-old falls asleep in about eight minutes and spends half an hour or longer in the deepest, most restful sleep stages. An eighty-year-old takes eighteen minutes to fall asleep and spends only a few minutes, if any, in deep sleep. The young person spends 95 percent of the night asleep, racking up an average of seven and a half to eight hours. The older person spends only 80 percent of the night asleep, with a total sleep time of about six hours.

In epidemiological surveys, about one-third of older men and women report sleep problems. The most common are insomnia (difficulty falling or staying asleep), breathing related disorders (such as sleep apnea), periodic leg movements that disturb sleep (nocturnal myoclonus), and a mismatch between sleep-wake patterns and the environment, which in the elderly most often involves falling asleep in the early evening and waking before dawn. Medical and mental disorders, including depression and anxiety, and medications can also contribute to sleep disturbances. (Chapter 15 discusses sleep disorders.)

Treatment often depends on identifying and correcting an underlying problem, such as depression or alcohol dependence, that may be causing the insomnia. Improved sleep habits, sometimes combined with relaxation techniques, are the best long-term option for insomnia. For older men and women, the most helpful guidelines are:

- Establishing regular hours for waking, meals, and bedtime
- Not spending too much time in bed during the day
- Not going to bed too early
- Not drinking alcohol to get to sleep
- Getting some exercise every day
- Cutting down or eliminating stimulants, including caffeine.

Although sleeping pills are effective as a short-term therapy, they have many drawbacks, especially for the elderly. They interfere with the brain's signals to the body to resume breathing, which can be critical in sleep apnea, a breathing disorder that is more common in older persons. They can also cause complications in those who have high blood pressure, heart disease, and other chronic medical conditions. Troubling side effects include impaired memory and daytime drowsiness. Older men and women who take sleeping pills are in danger of hurting themselves if they wake up in the night confused and disoriented. When medications are necessary, psychiatrists may prescribe low-dose tricyclic antidepressants rather than conventional sleep medications or may choose sleeping pills that do not have long half-lives.

PROBLEMS WITH ALCOHOL AND MEDICATIONS

Alcohol dependence and abuse are less common among older men and women than among younger individuals. Less than 5 percent of men and less than 1 percent of women over the age of sixty-five abuse alcohol. Nevertheless, sleeping difficulties and increased stress caused by retirement, illness, isolation, or bereavement may lead to drinking problems.

Alcohol abuse can be particularly harmful for older people because it increases the likelihood of malnutrition, liver disease, heart damage, digestive problems, cognitive impairment, and dementia. Almost any amount of alcohol can make mental confusion and memory problems worse. When severe alcohol dependence or abuse develops, older individuals may require close supervision in a hospital during withdrawal. Possible complications include agitation, delirium, and hallucinations.

Treatment for alcohol abuse depends on the individual's motivation and family support (see Chapter 10). Some psychiatrists prescribe disulfiram (Antabuse) but usually require that a family member take responsibility for administering the daily dose. Self-help groups, such as Alcoholics Anonymous, can be essential for long-term abstinence, although older people may initially refuse to go to such meetings, often because they deny that they have a problem or believe that they can deal with it on their own. Family counseling sessions can help in encouraging them to participate.

Older people, who are more likely to have physical ailments requiring treatment, use one-quarter of all drugs prescribed in the United States and often inadvertently misuse them. Some take ten or more prescription and over-the-counter agents each day. The more medications any person takes, the greater the chance of error. It is wise for the elderly to keep a medication chart, organized by days of the week, on which they check off each dose and drug when taken, and to keep their primary physician or their pharmacist aware of all the drugs they consume, both prescription and over-the-counter, so that these professionals can watch out for possible harmful interactions.

Cognitive problems are the number one psychiatric side effect of drugs in the elderly. When older people become confused, forgetful, or paranoid, family members should find out what medications they are taking and check their alcohol intake. Another not uncommon problem that can cause these symptoms is dependence on sleeping pills or pain medications. Withdrawal from some of these drugs, primarily those in the benzodiazepine family, can be potentially life-threatening and may require careful monitoring in a hospital.

CONFUSION AND DELIRIUM

An estimated 30 to 50 percent of older individuals hospitalized for surgery or a medical problem develop delirium, a state of acute confusion and disorientation characterized by fluctuations in mental state from day to day, hour to hour, or even minute to minute.

Medical conditions, high fever, substance abuse, medications, mental disorders, surgery, or the stress of being hospitalized or in an unfamiliar environment may lead to delirium. Because the elderly are often acutely sensitive to any changes in or around themselves, even simple health problems, such as urinary tract infections or slight metabolic imbalances, can cause symptoms of delirium, such as not thinking coherently, having difficulty taking in new information, and not being able to carry on a conversation without losing the train of thought or shifting from subject to subject.

Usually delirium develops quickly, and typically lasts for hours or days rather than for a prolonged period. Its possible causes include:

- Medical problems such as infection, fever, congestive heart failure, burns, systemic lupus erythematosus, and liver, kidney, or lung disorders

- Metabolic imbalances such as hypothyroidism (low levels of thyroid hormone) or hypoglycemia (extremely low blood sugar)

- Neurological disorders such as traumatic brain injury, stroke, or meningitis

- Reactions to certain medications such as L-dopa, digitalis, sedatives, tricyclic antidepressants, antipsychotic drugs, and corticosteroids

- Surgery (particularly heart operations)

- Withdrawal from alcohol or other addicting substances.

Reassurance and a safe, structured environment are essential for a person with delirium. As described in Chapter 20, a team of physicians in different specialties—such as a psychiatrist, internist, and neurologist—usually work together to identify and treat the underlying medical cause of the delirium.

DEMENTIA AND ALZHEIMER'S DISEASE

About 15 percent of older Americans lose previous mental capabilities and develop an organic brain disorder called dementia. Fifty to 60 percent of these individuals—a total of 4 million men and women over the age of sixty-five—suffer from the type of dementia called Alzheimer's disease, a progressive deterioration of brain cells and mental capacity. About 20 percent have vascular dementia, in which the person suffers a series of small strokes that damage or destroy tissue in the affected areas of the brain. Parkinson's disease can also cause dementia in the elderly.

There have been major advances in unraveling the keys to

Alzheimer's disease, a disorder that robs individuals of their memories, their intellects, their personalities, and eventually their lives. Often the illness progresses slowly, stealing bits of a person's mind and memory a little at a time. Individuals who realize that something is going wrong may make initial efforts to cope by establishing a rigid schedule for daily life and avoiding any changes in that schedule. As the disease progresses, those who have periods of awareness of their condition can become upset and depressed. In time, these lucid periods become less frequent, memory is severely impaired, and eventually the ability to recall words or form sentences is lost.

The personalities of individuals with dementia often change. Its victims may withdraw into a world of their own, become quarrelsome or irritable, and say or do inappropriate things. Some become more stubborn or impulsive, others apathetic. Those who develop increasing suspiciousness may accuse others of thefts, betrayal, or plotting against them. As cognitive impairment worsens, inhibitions often loosen; demented persons may masturbate or take off their clothes in public. Some become aggressive or violent. Eventually individuals may forget the names of their close relatives, their former occupations, occasionally even their own names. Because they may wander away from home and get lost, close supervision may become necessary, either at home or in a nursing facility.

The early signs of dementia—insomnia, irritability, increased sensitivity to alcohol and other drugs, and decreased energy and tolerance of frustration—are usually subtle and insidious. Diagnosis requires a comprehensive assessment of an individual's medical history, physical health, and mental status, often involving brain scans and a variety of other tests.

Even though no one can restore a brain in the process of being destroyed by an organic brain disease such as Alzheimer's, medications can control difficult behavioral symptoms and enhance or partially restore cognitive ability. Low doses of antipsychotic medications ease symptoms such as agitation, wandering, hallucinations, paranoid delusions, and hostility. A drug called tacrine (Cognex), the first specific treatment for Alzheimer's, produces some cognitive and behavioral improvement in about a third of patients. Often therapists find other medical or psychiatric problems, such as depression; recognizing and treating these conditions can have a dramatic impact. Antidepressant drugs, for example, may improve sleep, appetite, energy, and involvement with others.

For those with vascular dementia, low-dose aspirin can help to prevent blood clots and recurrent brain damage. Other medications may also be helpful; as in Alzheimer's, antipsychotic drugs may lessen agitation, wandering, and paranoid delusions. As many as 30 percent of those with dementia that is not related to Alzheimer's also suffer from depression, but there are few data on whether antidepressants are beneficial in these individuals.

Adequate rest, exercise, intellectual stimulation, social contacts, balanced and regular meals, and elimination of nonessential drugs can help even those with severe dementia. Most people with dementia do best in consistent, familiar surroundings, with daily routines, prominently displayed clocks and calendars, night-lights, checklists, and diaries to help them with orientation.

SUSPICIOUSNESS AND PARANOIA

Suspiciousness in the elderly is a common symptom not limited to dementia. It can range from increased wariness to intense distrust of family members to, more rarely, paranoid delusions, psychotic beliefs that usually focus on being threatened or developing a serious illness and that have no basis in reality. Elderly people who live alone, especially those with vision or hearing problems, are particularly prone to suspiciousness. If they have difficulty comprehending what they see and hear, they may assume that something harmless—a neighborhood boy running through the yard, for example—is a potential threat. Often they need only reassurance, correction of vision or hearing problems, and treatment of any underlying medical problems to ease their fears. Usually their suspiciousness does not reach the point of being delusional.

One relatively uncommon disorder, unique to the elderly, is called *paraphrenia*. Its primary symptoms are paranoid delusions, which usually develop slowly, always after the age of sixty. At first, affected individuals seem preoccupied with harassment or assault. They complain to the police, retaliate against neighbors for supposed grievances, try to escape by fleeing or attempting suicide, or withdraw from others, eating little, pacing about their homes, scurrying out secretively, paying no attention to their appearance. Family members who suspect this problem should make sure that their relative sees a geriatric psychiatrist as soon as possible.

The prognosis is best for those who are married, have had symptoms for only a brief time, have experienced a stressful incident, and also have depressive symptoms. However, many individuals who develop paraphrenia initially refuse to comply with treatment, which usually consists of antipsychotic drugs. With treatment, more than half recover completely, although there is a high relapse rate.

Delusional disorders (described in Chapter 17) can develop in late life. Often individuals focus on a single theme, such as the delusion that their adult children are trying to steal their money. Even detailed explanations and objective evidence may not persuade them that this is not the case. Some delusions are caused by medications and by conditions such as chronic alcohol abuse. On occasion, suspiciousness and paranoid delusions can lead to extreme agitation, a state of almost frenzied restlessness that may require emergency treatment.

In moderate to severe cases of delusional disorders, medication, usually with antipsychotic drugs, is the primary treatment. The prognosis is good for individuals who receive adequate treatment and maintenance therapy for a period that may range from a few months to several years.

Treating psychiatric problems in late life

Older men and women who develop mental and emotional problems are just as likely to improve with treatment as younger individuals. Only recently have mental health profession- als realized this fact, however, and are now devoting time, energy, and resources to the psychiatric needs of the elderly. Geriatric psychiatry, although growing, remains a comparatively new field, and physicians may not be aware of how much it has to offer their older patients.

Another barrier to treatment is the reluctance of the elderly to seek help when they need it. Only 4 percent of individuals seen at community mental health centers and 2 percent of those seen by private practitioners are over sixty-five, and these figures by no means represent the numbers of those who would benefit from help. Some older men and women may feel ashamed to admit they have a psychiatric disorder; others may not realize that the under- lying problem is mental or emotional; some may doubt that any- one can help them or fear that they will not be able to afford treatment. Their children may attribute their parents' symptoms to old age and dismiss them as inevitable and incurable. Their pri- mary care physicians may fail to recognize a problem or to provide adequate treatment. Yet once individuals overcome these obstacles and receive professional help, they can benefit enormously.

PSYCHOTHERAPY

A combination of supportive and insight-oriented psychotherapy often works best for older men and women. For those with cogni- tive impairments or debilitating diseases, mental health profes- sionals may take a more active role, offering concrete suggestions and taking into account any limitations in the person's thinking or memory. They may encourage individuals to express pent-up feel- ings and reminisce about life experiences, as well as educating them about their condition and affirming their continuing value and worth.

Research studies indicate that about 70 percent of older individuals are helped by cognitive, behavioral, and psychodynamic psychotherapy. The very old improve just as much as those who are somewhat younger. Cognitive therapy may be especially helpful for depressive disorders. Behavioral therapy works well with specific problems such as anxiety.

One approach tailored specifically for older men and women is life review therapy, which makes the most of the universal tendency of aging individuals to look back on their lives. By reminiscing, they remind themselves of a time when they felt valued and vital and reflect on their experiences, instilling them with new significance. Working with a mental health professional, they can resolve or come to terms with old problems, work through guilt and fears, and come to accept the present. Therapy can include trips to places where a person once lived, autobiographical tapes, reunions with families and friends, looking through albums and scrapbooks, and summing up an individual's life work, either verbally or in writing. The benefits of such reminiscences extend beyond the older person to others in the family by establishing connections between the generations that might otherwise not be recognized and by enriching the relationship between parents, their children, and their children's children.

MEDICATION

Because the capacity to metabolize or break down drugs within the body declines with age, medications may remain active in the elderly for a longer period than in younger adults. As a result, older men and women are more sensitive to certain side effects, such as drowsiness or a drop in blood pressure that can cause dizziness and light-headedness on sitting or standing (orthostatic hypertension). Usually psychiatrists prescribe lower doses for older individuals, often about half the amount they would give a younger person, or choose particular agents considered safer for the elderly. They also monitor blood levels of psychiatric medications more frequently in older men and women.

Physical problems can complicate drug treatment of psychiatric symptoms. A heart condition may make the use of certain antidepressants risky. Older men with enlarged prostates may develop serious complications from tricyclic antidepressants and many antipsychotic drugs. A careful assessment of the person's medical condition is necessary before medications are prescribed.

HOSPITALIZATION

Hospitalization on a psychiatric or geropsychiatric unit may be necessary when older men and women develop symptoms that severely impair their daily functioning, that threaten their safety or the safety of others, and that require a complete evaluation by a team that includes both an internist and a psychiatrist. The team approach ensures that health care providers do not miss anything that might be interfering with a person's ability to function well psychologically. If, for example, there is a possibility that a medication to lower blood pressure may be contributing to depression, the psychiatrist and the internist can work together to adjust the dose or can try a different drug, so that they are treating both the medical and the emotional problem.

The treatment team also may include psychiatric nurses, a social worker, an occupational therapist, and consultants from the hospital's pastoral service and family therapy clinic. "We start out looking for a person's strengths," says one social worker who works with the elderly. "These individuals are survivors. They've been through wars, depressions, all sorts of traumas. We try to find what's kept them going: their sense of humor, their pride in something they can do, maybe a cherished friend or pet. We pay very close attention to their life stories, not just because they're often fascinating, but because they reveal the wellspring of their lives. And that helps give them what they need to flourish again."

Often elderly persons admitted to a psychiatric unit turn out to have a number of relatively minor problems. They may be a little dehydrated, a little malnourished, a little anemic. They may not have been eating adequately or taking their medications properly. Once those problems are taken care of, they can work with a therapist to deal with the psychological issues in their lives, such as loneliness or anxiety. Adjunctive forms of therapy include occupational therapy and crafts activities, such as working with wood or stained glass. These treatments underscore individuals' sense of accomplishment, help them to structure their time, and allow them to interact with other people.

NURSING HOMES

Ninety percent of those over the age of sixty-five live in the community, either in their own homes or with relatives. However, some older individuals are no longer capable of living independently. Falls, wanderings, accidental burns while cooking, incontinence, episodes of extreme agitation or aggressive behavior, serious medical illness, or physical disability can all lead family members to consider the various options available. Home-care services, adult day care centers, and foster and group homes help growing numbers of the elderly by filling the gap between living at home and entering a nursing home. Social workers or counselors from a local hospital or community mental health center may be able to help families sort through these alternatives, as well as facilities with more extensive services and medical resources if they are needed.

The decision to place an elderly relative with a severe, debilitating illness such as Alzheimer's in a nursing home can be a complex one influenced by financial limitations, insurance coverage, and other practicalities. There also are many difficult emotional issues, both for elderly persons, who, if mentally aware, may resist institutionalization for what is clearly the last stage of their lives, and for family members, who may feel guilt, anguish, or helplessness. Again, counselors experienced in working with the elderly can provide perspective and support.

▼

Self-help   The same strategies that enhance psychological well-being at younger ages remain beneficial in old age. Exercise, appropriately adapted to physical limitations, has such powerful effects on mind and body that some researchers have called it "the closest thing we have to an anti-aging pill." Good nutrition, particularly a balanced, low-fat, high-fiber diet, helps to maintain physical and psychological well-being.

Equally important is feeding the mind and spirit. Just as older men and women have to use their bodies to keep them in good shape, they must exercise their brains regularly. Most people have a certain level of intellectual stimulation at which their minds function best. This may change with age, but it remains essential for mental fitness.

Social ties also are crucial. As noted earlier in the chapter, losses are frequent in old age, as family members or friends move away or die and old networks falter or disappear. Older men and women may have to take active steps to create new circles and relationships if they are to avoid or overcome loneliness. Church activities, neighborhood groups, and volunteer programs offer opportunities to reach out to others and to enjoy regular interactions. In some communities, support groups for the elderly—some focusing on specific issues, such as recent retirement, and some dedicated to sharing perspectives on a wide range of mutual problems—help older people to deal with psychological problems.

▼

Impact on the family   About 80 percent of all older people have adult children, but few live with them. When two or three generations do live under the same roof, everyone has to make substantial adjustments, from the older parent or parents accustomed to independence and doing things their way to their adult children who may find themselves "sandwiched" between the needs of their aging parents and those of their own growing children. But there can be benefits for all, such as the immense gratification senior relatives may feel by contributing to the household—for example, by baby-sitting—and the close ties that develop between grandparents and grandchildren. There can also be difficulties. The elderly parents may be physically frail and require considerable care. If they have suffered some mental decline, they may be increasingly dependent on their adult children, who can feel overwhelmed in trying to take care of several generations at one time. Financial problems may need to be addressed. Family counseling can be of great help in resolving conflicts and enabling all the members of the family to communicate more effectively and cope better.

Even when aging parents live on their own, in group homes, or in other facilities, adult children may face difficult emotional issues. Progressive illnesses such as Alzheimer's disease may present the most difficult challenge. Often relatives must watch helplessly as a loved one slowly becomes a stranger to them and as they become strangers to a parent. Many hospitals and community mental health centers provide counseling and support groups for spouses and children whose parents have Alzheimer's. (See Chapter 30, When Someone You Love Has a Mental Disorder. The Resource Directory at the back of this book lists national support organizations.)

▼
Outlook Like every other age, late life has its unique challenges and rewards. Although some losses and declines are inevitable, many are not. Being aware of this fact can be critically important. In older individuals, even minor physical problems can interfere with mood, memory, and thinking; conversely, depression or anxiety can undermine physical well-being. But if problems are recognized, a great deal can be done to maximize physical *and* psychological potential so that older men and women can function at the highest possible level for the longest possible time. Life may not end with the vigor, joy, and excitement with which it begins, but it can end with dignity, peace, and acceptance.

Youngsters with mental or emotional problems may:

☐ **Fidget or squirm constantly and find it hard to sit still**

☐ **Be impulsive or aggressive**

☐ **Have difficulty concentrating and be easily distracted**

☐ **Frequently lose their temper and get into fights or arguments**

☐ **Defy rules or refuse to do chores**

☐ **Show a marked change in activity level or school performance**

☐ **Eat or sleep much more or less than usual**

☐ **Seem listless, lack energy, or complain of always being tired**

☐ **Feel sad or discouraged; need a great deal of reassurance**

☐ **Be extremely irritable or negative**

☐ **Criticize everything they do; often put themselves down**

☐ **Fail to gain weight as expected**

☐ **Be extremely shy and apprehensive about any new situation**

☐ **Have difficulty forming relationships with peers, relatives, or adults**

☐ **Not get along with other children**

☐ **Refuse to go to school or leave a parent**

☐ **Always seem tense**

☐ **Withdraw from friends or usual activities**

☐ **Lack bladder or bowel control after the age of five or six**

☐ **Fail to develop physical, intellectual, or academic skills at the same time as most children of the same age**

Even checking a single box may indicate a possible problem. The more boxes that you check, the more reason you may have to be concerned about your youngster. This chapter describes the most common problems of childhood and provides guidance on seeking help.

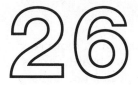

Is Something Wrong with My Child?

At two, Alyssa hasn't said a word. Six-year-old Jeremy is still wetting the bed. Zander's first-grade teacher reports that he has problems concentrating in class. Jasmine's behavior is perfect, but the ten-year-old worries so much about her parents' divorce that she can't get to sleep at night. Surly and defiant at twelve, Max sasses back, swears, refuses to obey house rules, and explodes in fury when his parents try to discipline him. Fourteen-year-old Krista, miserable ever since her family moved away from the only home she'd ever known, locks herself in her room for hours and avoids any conversation with her parents.

Adults like to think of childhood as a kingdom in which the sun always smiles. Children know better. (Adults, remembering their own childhood, know better, too.) The challenges they face—controlling their impulses and behavior, separating from their parents, acquiring the fundamental skills of living, forming relationships with peers—are far from simple or easy, and any child can run into difficulties along the way to adulthood. According to recent surveys, mental or emotional problems affect as many as one in every five children.

For years no one acknowledged, let alone explored, the darker regions of a child's world. Today, thanks to advances in the fields of child psychology and child psychiatry, two of the youngest behavioral sciences, both youngsters and parents can get help in coping with the critically important early years of life. Diagnostic criteria have become more precise, and there has been more research into various therapies. Increasingly, mental health professionals have been able to tailor treatments to specific problems and to the needs of specific children.

Although there has been little long-term research on youngsters who develop emotional difficulties in childhood, most of those who receive help improve greatly. Early identification of problems and appropriate treatment can be critical in preventing a wide range of complications and in getting youngsters back on the track of normal development.

What's normal and what's not

It can be very difficult for a parent to judge whether something is amiss and whether a child needs professional help. A "normal" childhood is punctuated with ups and downs, occasional peaks and a lot of valleys, and parents may not know whether a youngster is acting out a painful emotion he or she cannot express in other ways, "going through a phase," or reacting to some upsetting experience, such as bullying at school, that the parents may not even be aware of.

What makes the parents' job harder is the fact that children can rarely put their emotional distress directly into words. Young children may cry, whine, or hit, or they may communicate in more subtle ways, such as becoming unusually lethargic or not wanting to play with others. Teens may complain of being bored or say they don't care. When pressed, they may not be able to find words to describe what's really troubling them.

Just as with adults, the key factors to keep in mind are the severity and duration of a problem. Is the troublesome behavior or problem having a significant impact on family life, schoolwork, or a child's normal activities and relationships? Has it persisted for more than a few weeks? Does it recur fairly regularly? Does it have an effect on all aspects of a child's life—at home, at school, and with peers? If the problem is pervasive, persistent, and affecting a child's happiness, parents should take it seriously.

Talking with a youngster's teachers, whether in preschool, grade school, or high school, can help. Because teachers see children every day in varied learning and social situations, they can offer valuable perspective. Many books provide insight into the emotional life of children of various ages, and they, too, may be useful. A family doctor or pediatrician who knows a youngster well and sees children of all ages can help in sorting out what is normal and what is not.

If there is a possible problem, parents should consider a professional assessment. Keep in mind that an evaluation by a child psychiatrist or psychologist cannot hurt and may prove to be more helpful than anything else a parent might do to aid the youngster. To find a qualified specialist, parents can ask their pediatrician, a child's teacher or guidance counselor, the local mental health association, or a local community mental health center. It is advisable to get several names and to check credentials. We recommend seeking out psychiatrists, psychologists, or clinical social workers with training and experience in working with children and adolescents, rather than those who work primarily with adults.

To gather information, the therapist may ask questions— always using age-appropriate words and concepts—and also have youngsters draw pictures, tell stories, or choose dolls or toys to play with. Careful observation can provide clues to emotional issues that the child may not be able to put into words. Sometimes a single consultation is sufficient to identify what is wrong and obtain recommendations for a plan of action. If the child is jealous of a new sibling, for example, the therapist may provide parents with specific guidelines for handling the problem on their own. In other cases, the consulting professional may recommend therapy, either with the consultant or with another therapist. If medication may be needed, a child psychiatrist, who can prescribe drugs, would be the best choice.

If the assessment doesn't strike the parents as being on target, they may want to get a second opinion or to interview other mental health professionals to make sure there is a good fit between child and therapist. Like adults, children need therapists they feel comfortable with and can trust. Since parents will also be working closely with the therapist, they need to establish a good rapport and have confidence in the therapist's ability.

NORMAL DIFFERENCES IN TEMPERAMENT

A few decades ago many experts in child psychology believed that children's personalities were shaped almost entirely by their family and environment. Since then researchers have proved what any parent with more than one child knows: that babies are born different. One is lively, another listless; one easygoing, another fussy; one fearful, another feisty.

"Children aren't blank slates written upon by their parents," observes Sandra Scarr, Ph.D., a professor of psychology at the University of Virginia, whose research has documented nature's influence and nurture's limits. "Children enter the world with a certain temperament, a built-in way of interacting with their environment. We have a responsibility to help our children become the most they can with what they've got, but we can't ignore what they've got."

The scientific study of temperament dates back to the 1950s, when a husband-and-wife team of psychiatrists in New York City, Stella Chess, M.D., and Alexander Thomas, M.D., began to suspect that there was something wrong with the premise that parents should and could be blamed for everything a child did wrong. Launching a thirty-year study that has followed more than 130 youngsters into adulthood, Chess and Thomas asked parents whether their babies were constantly squirming or relatively calm, if they had regular or erratic biological rhythms (such as sleep and hunger), if they responded intensely or quietly to new sounds and sights.

About 40 percent of the group had "easy" babies who ate and slept regularly, had mild mood swings, and were generally tranquil. About 10 percent of the infants were "difficult": intensely negative, extremely active, and highly irregular in sleeping and eating patterns. Thirty-five percent had mixed traits, some easy and some difficult. The remaining 15 percent were termed "slow to warm up" children, whose style of getting to know new people or situations was to proceed slowly but without anxiety or fear.

Although some temperaments may be easier to live with than others, none is completely negative. Just as important as temperament is what Chess called the "goodness of fit," the compatibility of parent and child. In a good fit, the parents' expectations dovetail with their child's abilities. In a bad fit, parents and children misunderstand each other, and may make each other miserable.

Here are some of the most common temperament types and some practical recommendations for bringing out the best in each:

Active. These youngsters need outlets, activity, and space to release their extra energy. Parents should watch out for situations in which young children get overly revved up because they don't know when to stop the activity they are engaged in and should intervene before a child loses control.

Intense. Whether happy, sad, or angry, an intense child vents feelings at full volume. From early childhood, parents can help by labeling emotions: "You are very upset." "You are angry." "You are frightened." This gives children the vocabulary they need to understand and express what they are feeling. When these youngsters are upset, parents should take them to a quiet place to help them calm down.

Distractible. From infancy, these children have a hard time concentrating on one thing for more than a few seconds. Parents can work with a baby by focusing on a single toy, talking about it, and extending the time spent playing with it. As the child grows, parents should be alert for early signs of restlessness during play or homework and suggest a short break.

Irregular. Children who do not become hungry or sleepy at predictable intervals can be very hard to live with. The rest of the family may gather for lunch or dinner, but one child may not be hungry. At bedtime, he or she may not be tired. It can help if parents separate eating from mealtimes and sleeping from bedtimes. This means that a youngster may sit down for meals with the rest of the family but eat only as much as he or she wants. Similarly, the child gets into bed at a regular time but can read or play until drowsy.

Negative. These youngsters are usually irritable or unhappy and whine or complain a lot. Although it is easy for parents to become exasperated, they need to point out to such children the pleasurable aspects of an outing or activity and to highlight the positive things they love and appreciate in the child.

Sensitive. These children have a low level of tolerance for new tastes, smells, textures, colors, or lights—whatever impinges on their senses. They may seem picky, but in fact they cannot control their reaction to such experiences as tasting unusual foods or wearing new clothes that irritate their skin. Parents will find it helpful to introduce novel items slowly and gently.

Shy. Fearful or shy children pull away from new places or cry or cling if forced into new situations. Advance preparation, such as reading books or telling stories to prepare a young child for an airplane trip or a family reunion, can help. Pretend games, in which they act out new situations, such as going to a summer day camp, are valuable for older youngsters.

Persistent. These children do not adapt easily; they find transitions and change difficult. Extremely single-minded, they hew to one activity and cannot switch gears smoothly. Young children need warnings of up to ten minutes before a change in activities. For older children, a clock can help alert them to switches or changes.

NORMAL STAGES OF DEVELOPMENT

At a child's birthday, parents often mark the preceding year's growth on a height chart, tracing the rate at which their boy or girl is sprouting toward physical maturity. Just as the body grows and changes, a child's personality also develops. Many key figures in psychiatry and psychology have charted normal psychological and mental development. Each of these authorities provides a different kind of insight into a child's evolution.

Freud's view: psychosexual development   Sigmund Freud argued that the events of the first five years of life, especially sexual desires and conflicts, form the basis for the ego's behavior throughout life. He established six stages of psychosexual development:

1. *Oral phase* (infancy to eighteen months): Primary satisfaction comes from sucking, crying, chewing, etc.

2. *Anal phase* (eighteen months to three years): Anal functioning is the source of sexual pleasure. During this time, the main issues revolve around control—not only controlling one's bowels but control in general: who's the boss, who's in control, temper tantrums over control.

3. *Phallic phase* (three to four years): The genitals are the focus of sexual interest.

4. *Oedipal phase* (four to six years): The child becomes possessive of the opposite-sex parent.

5. *Latency phase* (school age): The sexual conflicts of early childhood lessen.

6. *Genital phase* (puberty and adolescence): Children again focus on the genitals as they mature into sexual adults.

Erikson's perspective: ego development   Erik Erikson provided a picture of how the ego can develop successfully in a good environment. He identified several stages of ego development from birth to death, with positive and negative aspects, each affected by society and each marked by a key developmental crisis. The stages of childhood are:

1. *Trust versus mistrust* (birth to eighteen months): If their needs for care and stimulation are met, babies develop a basic trust in self and the world. If care is inconsistent, impaired, or lacking, babies develop a fundamental mistrust of the world.

2. *Autonomy versus shame and doubt* (eighteen months to three years): As children develop control over more aspects of their lives, including their bladders and bowels, they gain confidence in their abilities, especially in their capacity for controlling themselves. But if they are made to feel ashamed or foolish, they distrust their own judgment and develop self-doubts.

3. *Initiative versus guilt* (three to six years): Capable of initiating physical and intellectual activity, children grow in curiosity about the outside world. If they can explore their environment and satisfy their curiosity, their initiatives toward independence flourish. If they are made to feel bad about new behaviors and interests, their initiative is stifled.

4. *Industry versus inferiority* (six years to puberty): Children develop confidence in their abilities to function in the outside world. Peers and school become important. If they can master the challenges of

the outside world, children become confident in their industriousness; if thwarted in their quest for mastery, they feel inferior.

5. *Ego identity versus role confusion* (teen years): Struggling to develop a personal identity, adolescents must separate psychologically from their parents and develop a stable social and sexual identity. Suspended between childhood morals and the ethical values they will eventually develop in adulthood, they cling to each other. Their peers are all-important.

Piaget's research: cognitive development In extensive studies of children at various ages, the Swiss psychologist Jean Piaget concerned himself more with how than with what they think. He identified a sequence of stages in cognitive ability:

1. *Sensorimotor stage* (birth to two years): Piaget was the first to show that babies are active, competent learners who seek out stimulation and explore the world with all their senses. Infants have no sense of object permanence—that is, an object exists only when they see or touch it. At about eighteen months, they begin to develop mental images of objects that are not within sight. By the age of two they can use words and visual images to recall the past and to think about objects they cannot see.

2. *Preoperational thought* (two to six years): Preschoolers judge everything from their own perspective and cannot understand another's point of view. Capable of dealing with only a limited amount of data, they tend to focus on one aspect of an object and ignore others.

3. *Concrete operations* (seven to twelve years): Children at this stage can cope with several dimensions of a problem at once, and can deal with them mentally. They begin to focus on changes rather than states of being and have more flexible thinking patterns.

4. *Formal operations* (adolescence onward): Teenagers can think abstractly and deal with complex problems of reasoning. They can formulate hypotheses and conceive of many interpretations of a single event.

Many others have contributed important insights into childhood development. Margaret Mahler, for example, developed the theory of separation-individuation, in which a child moves from a state of complete psychological enmeshing with the mother in infancy to increasing curiosity about the world, and ultimately, at about twenty-five months to three years, a sense of the mother as separate. John Bowlby, who worked with children separated from their parents during World War II, underscored the importance of an infant's attachment to its mother and the impact of separation. He suggested that early attachment served as a crucial basis for emotional security and social autonomy later in life.

THE MODERN AMERICAN FAMILY

America's families aren't what they used to be. Less than 10 percent of the population now live in traditional families with a working husband, homemaker wife, and 2.2 children. More than half of the children born in the 1990s will spend at least one year living in a single-parent household before they turn eighteen. Three in every ten households consist of "blended" families formed by two divorced partners who remarry.

But even as "norms" or expectations about families have changed, values and ideals have not. Whatever form a family takes, the basic job of parents remains the same: meeting the needs of their children. Children have tangible needs for food, shelter, and protection that must be met, or their physical welfare will be at risk. Children also have psychological and emotional needs that must be met, or their ability to have fruitful lives and satisfying relationships may be in jeopardy.

A child's greatest need is for love—the feeling of being wanted and cared for, of being special, and of realizing that the parents genuinely like and accept the child for him- or herself. According to a study that followed 379 kindergarten-aged children for thirty-six years, warm, loving parenting—the kind that comes with plenty of hugging, kissing, holding, and cuddling—had more influence on adult social adjustment than any other parental or childhood factor. The individuals whose mothers and fathers were openly affectionate were able to sustain long and relatively happy marriages, develop close friendships, and enjoy varied activities outside of their marriage. By comparison, cold parenting led to feelings of depression and a lack of psychological well-being.

Of course, children need many other things too: the security that comes from knowing their parents will be there when needed most; protection; a feeling of belonging; a set of standards and human values; and a sense of clearly defined limits and controls. Children also need role models, for the family serves as a training ground for living. Youngsters use their experience in the family to learn how to behave in other groups and with other individuals. If parents behave lovingly and with respect toward each other and their children, their youngsters are likely to learn how to have loving and healthy relationships with others. If children are victims of abusive parents at home, they may become someone else's victim—or abuser—elsewhere. A family is a society in miniature, and children's experience in this one unit gives them a way of perceiving how they fit into the larger system.

Children of divorce   Each year the parents of more than a million children divorce. The grown-ups aren't the only ones to feel the pain of a dream that died. After divorce, very young children may become more babyish, irritable, and dependent. Preschool or young school-age children often blame themselves, feeling that "Daddy left because I was bad." School-age children may feel lonely, helpless, and depressed; some develop illnesses or have problems in their friendships. Preteens may experiment with alcohol, drugs, and sex. For teenagers, divorce can make separating from the family and establishing an adult identity even harder than it usually is.

Classes, seminars, and other programs that deal with the psychological effects of divorce on children are springing up around the country. Many use role playing, films, and lectures to give parents a child's-eye view of the trauma of their breakup. The goal is to help parents communicate better and stop the bickering and bitterness that can be especially harmful for youngsters.

According to various reports, 15 to 20 percent of all children whose parents divorce may require professional therapy. Several studies suggest that the impact of divorce is more intense for boys than for girls. One long-term effect of divorce that affects girls more than boys, however, is a greater likelihood of divorce themselves when they marry.

After a divorce, parents may have difficulty accepting and respecting the relationship between the child they love and the spouse they no longer love. Family therapists advise divorced parents not to fight in front of youngsters or use them as ammunition in ongoing battles. Although honesty is best in explaining why a couple separated, children should be spared the nasty details. Above all, youngsters should be reassured that both parents love them and that it's okay for them to love both their parents. They also need to spend time with each parent, and to have a chance to talk about how they feel without worrying that what they say will hurt or anger their parents. The more constructively a mother and a father can work together as parents after the divorce, the better off their children will be.

Children in single-parent and blended families   As divorce rates have climbed, the percentage of children in single-parent homes has grown. A recent poll suggests that as many as 18 percent of parents may be raising their children alone for some period of time. Like two-parent families, one-parent families are all different. An educated divorced woman in her thirties with one school-age child has many more options and opportunities than a young, unskilled, never-married woman with three preschoolers.

At every economic level, the amount of time single parents spend with their children is not significantly different from that spent by parents in two-parent families, and psychologists have found no negative impact of a single-parent family on a child's intellectual or academic achievement. The National Longitudinal Survey of Youth, one of the largest and most comprehensive studies of children of divorce, followed some 1,700 children, aged five to eight, for nine years. According to its findings, most of the youngsters who grew up in single-parent homes fared just as well academically as those from intact families.

"The conventional wisdom is that when a father leaves, the people in a family have problems, at least for a while," says sociologist Frank Mott, Ph.D., director of the Center for Human Resources Research at Ohio State University. "That probably is still valid. The bigger question, though, is what happens down the road."

Initially, youngsters without a live-in dad seemed to not do as well on standard math and reading tests as those from two-parent homes. These differences disappeared almost entirely once the researchers factored in the mothers' backgrounds. The children of more highly educated mothers consistently did better in school than those whose mothers had less formal education. "How children do academically seems fairly independent of a father's presence or absence," says Mott, who notes that divorced parents should find the study findings reassuring. "This is one thing they don't have to feel guilty about. The bottom line is that academically the kids will be okay."

There also have been optimistic findings about children who become part of new, blended families when their parents remarry. Over the years, many studies have found significant differences in these families, but psychologist James Bray, Ph.D., of Baylor College of Medicine has found that some of these differences diminish over time. After following 198 children and their middle-class families for seven years, he concluded that, initially, step-families have "more negative family relationships and more problematic family processes" and stepchildren have more behavioral problems and more life stress. However, 80 percent of these children function within a normal range, and if they master skills for better communication and more effective problem solving, blended families are usually able to work through their problems in time.

Mental and emotional problems

Many of the problems that occur in adults also develop in children: depressive disorders, anxiety, attention disorders, eating disorders, adjustment disorders, sleep problems, substance abuse disorders, psychosomatic illnesses, personality disorders, and psychotic disorders. (The individual chapters on each of these conditions, found in Part II of this book, provide detailed discussions of their causes, symptoms, and treatments.)

Other disorders are unique to childhood and adolescence or require special consideration in young people. These include disruptive behaviors—problems of attention, conduct, or opposition—that can be difficult for parents to assess. Some youngsters may simply be testing the limits to find out what is acceptable and accepted behavior and what isn't. In other cases, there may be an underlying problem that is responsible for a child's extreme physical activity, defiance, or aggression.

ATTENTION-DEFICIT/HYPERACTIVITY DISORDER

The term *hyperactive* has been used so loosely over the years that parents may hear it applied to any child who seems particularly energetic or rambunctious. Although all children become restless and fidgety at times, relatively few—an estimated 3 to 5 percent of school-age children—suffer from an actual disorder. These youngsters are not merely squirmy or distractible. Some consistently cannot focus their attention, and others are unable to resist an impulse to blurt out what's on their mind or to grab what they want. At home and at school, the behavior of these youngsters isn't simply more active than that of others their age; it is more chaotic, reckless, and disorganized.

Psychiatrists themselves have used different terms to refer to attention and activity problems in children: minimal brain damage, minimal brain dysfunction, hyperactivity, hyperkinetic syndrome. Attention-deficit/hyperactivity disorder (AD/HD), the current diagnostic term, refers to a spectrum of problems, from impulsivity to distractibility, that may or may not include hyperactivity per se. (Hyperactivity is characterized by excessive running, jumping, climbing, etc.)

Boys, who usually have more visible—and more vexing—symptoms, such as extremely active behavior, are diagnosed as having AD/HD far more often than girls, who tend to develop more subtle signs, such as an inability to concentrate. Many youngsters have symptoms, such as being impulsive or inattentive, but do not meet the diagnostic criteria for AD/HD.

For years scientists have debated possible causes for childhood attention problems, including food additives, excessive sugar intake, lead poisoning, head trauma, and dysfunctional families. Carefully controlled studies have failed to show any significant link between sugar consumption, once theorized to be a culprit, and AD/HD, nor have any of the other supposed factors proved to be responsible.

AD/HD probably has multiple causes. Genetics plays a role in

Is it attention deficit/ hyperactivity disorder?

According to the DSM-IV, a diagnosis of AD/HD should be based on these criteria:

■ **EITHER:**

1. *Inattention.* At least six of the following that occur often and persist for at least six months to a degree that is maladaptive and inconsistent with developmental level:

- Failing to pay close attention to details or making careless mistakes in schoolwork, work, or other activities
- Difficulty sustaining attention in tasks or play activities
- Not seeming to listen when spoken to directly
- Not following through on instructions and failing to finish schoolwork, chores, or duties in the workplace (not because of oppositional behavior or failure to understand instructions)
- Difficulty organizing tasks and activities
- Avoidance, dislike, or reluctance to engage in tasks that require sustained mental effort, such as schoolwork or homework
- Losing things necessary for tasks or activities (e.g., toys, school assignments, pencils, books, tools)
- Easily distracted
- Forgetful in daily activities

OR

2. *Hyperactivity-impulsivity.* At least six of the following that occur often and persist for at least six months to a degree that is maladaptive and inconsistent with developmental level:

Hyperactivity

- Fidgeting with hands or feet or squirming in seat
- Leaving seat in classroom or in other situations in which remaining seated is expected
- Running about or climbing excessively in situations where it is inappropriate
- Difficulty playing or engaging in leisure activities quietly
- Acting as if "driven by a motor"; "on the go"
- Excessive talking

Impulsivity

- Blurting out answers to questions before the questions have been completed
- Difficulty awaiting turn
- Interrupting or intruding on others (e.g., butting into games)

■ Development of symptoms before age seven

■ Impairment in two or more settings (e.g., school and home) as a result of symptoms

■ Clinically significant distress or impaired ability to function in social settings, school, or work

■ Does not occur exclusively during a pervasive developmental disorder, schizophrenia, or another psychotic disorder and cannot be better accounted for by another mental disorder

Adapted from the Diagnostic and Statistical Manual of Mental Disorders, 4th Edition. *Used with permission.*

about 40 percent of cases, and youngsters with AD/HD often have several close biological relatives with the same problem. In some cases a viral infection may play a part. The incidence of AD/HD increases after an outbreak of encephalitis. Other cases may stem from an occurrence in pregnancy—possibly exposure to infection, alcohol, nicotine, cocaine, toxins, or environmental factors—that affected the prenatal development of key areas in the brain that regulate movement and attentiveness. Researchers at the National Institute of Mental Health (NIMH), using positron emission tomography (PET) scans, have found that children and adults with attention disorders are slower to metabolize glucose, the brain's main energy source.

▼

Seeking help Often parents aren't sure whether their pint-sized perpetual motion machine is hyperactive or simply energetic. It is very difficult to diagnose AD/HD prior to age four or five because preschoolers typically are active and impulsive and may not be able to focus their attention for a sustained period of time. If you are trying to get a handle on your child's behavior, ask yourself whether your child:

- Fidgets or squirms constantly
- Has a hard time sitting still
- Is easily distracted
- Can't wait for a turn in games or groups
- Blurts out answers to questions before they've been completed
- Is unable to follow through on instructions from others
- Finds it hard to concentrate on tasks or play
- Shifts from one uncompleted activity to another
- Has difficulty in playing quietly
- Talks excessively
- Interrupts or intrudes on others
- Often doesn't seem to be listening or paying attention
- Constantly loses toys, pencils, books
- Does dangerous things, like running into the street, without considering the consequences.

If you answer "yes" to several of these questions, the problem could be AD/HD. However, the range of symptoms of this disorder is broad, and even mental health professionals may find it hard to distinguish between normal and abnormal behaviors. In making an evaluation they rely on a comprehensive interview with the child, as well as evaluations from teachers and parents and standardized assessment scales. For a diagnosis of AD/HD, the behaviors must persist for at least six months and be so severe that they cause severe distress or impair a child's functioning at home or school or in social situations. (See the table, Is It Attention-Deficit/Hyperactivity Disorder? on page 658.) In making the diagnosis, therapists distinguish types of AD/HD, depending on whether symptoms of inattention, hyperactivity-impulsivity, or a combination predominate.

▼

Treating AD/HD

A combination of medication, remedial education, behavior modification, individual counseling, and family therapy is most effective in treating this disorder. Parents can help by learning as much as possible about AD/HD, avoiding stressful situations that may cause fatigue, frustration, or overstimulation for the child, and establishing regular routines and consistent limits. Many find classes in parenting skills or programs for parents of hyperactive children useful.

The primary drugs used in treating AD/HD are stimulants—methylphenidate (Ritalin), dextroamphetamine (Dexedrine), and pemoline (Cylert)—which have a paradoxical effect on individuals with AD/HD and reduce rather than heighten their activity level. Rather than stimulating them, as they do in those without the disorder, these medications improve performance of various tasks, possibly by enhancing concentration.

Youngsters who do not respond to a particular stimulant may improve with another one or with the antidepressants desipramine (Norpramin), imipramine (Tofranil), or nortriptyline (Pamelor). Short-term side effects, which occur in less than 5 percent of youngsters, include insomnia, loss of appetite and weight, headaches, and stomachaches. Clonidine (Catapres), a drug used to treat hypertension, is sometimes used, usually along with a stimulant, for youngsters with AD/HD who are extremely agitated, hyperactive, impulsive, or defiant. It often helps them to fall asleep, overcomes their refusal to go to bed, and counteracts the effects of stimulants. However, it can make children drowsy, at least during the initial weeks of treatment.

In follow-up studies, parents, teachers, physicians, or therapists have rated 75 percent of hyperactive children given stimulants as improved, compared to 40 percent given a placebo. Nevertheless, although medication helps, particularly in decreasing physical activity, these children typically continue to have some problems. A therapist can teach parents behavioral techniques, such as sending children to a quiet spot for a time-out if they become disruptive, that improve academic performance. Supportive

A PARENT'S GUIDE TO STIMULANT MEDICATIONS

Methylphenidate (Ritalin)

daily dose range: 10 to 60 mg, two to four times a day

Dextroamphetamine (Dexedrine)

daily dose range: 5 to 40 mg, two to four times a day

Pemoline (Cylert)

daily dose range: 37.5 to 112.5 mg, one or two times a day

POTENTIAL BENEFITS

Reduced physical overactivity; less talking and disruptive behavior at school; more focused classroom behavior; greater ability to sustain attention; less distractibility; improved capacity for independent play and work; reduced anger and impulsivity; improved quality and quantity of completed schoolwork; better fine motor control and handwriting; reduced aggressive behavior—verbal and physical—and bossiness with peers; less impulsive stealing or destruction of property; reduced defiance and refusal to obey parents and teachers; better use of thinking skills and strategies

POTENTIAL SIDE EFFECTS

Common (usually developing early in treatment and improving with lower doses)
Loss of appetite and weight; irritability; abdominal pain; headaches; heightened emotional sensitivity and crying

Less common

Insomnia; less interest in socializing; less-than-expected weight gain for normal development; anxiety; nervous habits, such as pulling hair or biting nails; increased activity and irritability as the medication wears off; a generally bad mood or impaired performance on standardized cognitive tests (with high doses)

Rare

Tics; depression; interference with normal growth; rapid heart beat; high blood pressure; compulsions or repetitive activities; Tourette's syndrome; psychotic hallucinations

MONITORING

The child's physician or psychiatrist should regularly assess height, weight, blood pressure, pulse, mood, tics, and, with pemoline, test for liver enzymes and check involuntary movements, night terrors, and licking or biting of the lips.

---

psychotherapy helps to deal with low self-esteem and other problems related to AD/HD. Family therapy can also be beneficial.

About 25 percent of children with AD/HD have specific learning disabilities; 40 percent have a pattern of starting fights, stealing, and lying (conduct disorder) or of defiance, disobedience, and rule-breaking (oppositional disorder); these problems are discussed later in this chapter. Those with both AD/HD and a conduct disorder are more likely to drop out of school, abuse drugs or alcohol, or break the law. Those who do not have a conduct disorder have a better prognosis than those who do, although they also are more likely than unaffected children to develop problems such as anxiety and mild depression. About one-third of children with AD/HD continue to show some signs of this disorder in adolescence and adulthood. (Chapter 14 discusses adult attention disorders.) Teens and young adults with AD/HD are much more likely to cause or be involved in auto accidents than other young drivers. A national support and educational organization, Children with Attention Deficit Disorders (CHADD), can provide helpful information and referrals. (See the Resource Directory at the back of the book.)

OPPOSITIONAL DEFIANT DISORDER

From the time they can say "no," youngsters may refuse to do what their parents want. Tantrums and other forms of defiance are considered normal in children before age three. Throughout their school years, it is common for boys and girls occasionally to be uncooperative, disobedient, or hostile.

Oppositional defiant disorder (ODD), a relatively new psychiatric diagnosis, refers to a persistent pattern of frequent negativity, defiance, hostility, disobedience, and provocative behavior. Irritable and resentful, children with this disorder quickly take offense at anything parents and others may say or do. They may blame others for their mistakes and deliberately annoy people. They swear, make threats, and refuse to comply with the simplest rules. However, their bad behavior, although extremely frustrating and infuriating, stops short of harming others (although they may be verbally aggressive).

Boys with this problem outnumber girls until puberty, when both genders may be equally likely to develop ODD. Youngsters who had difficult temperaments as babies and small children may be more likely to develop ODD. This disorder, which usually develops by the age of eight, may stem from an inherited predisposition. It seems more common in families with a parent who has a history of ODD, AD/HD, conduct disorder, antisocial personality disorder, substance abuse, or a mood disorder. Parents who do not reward good behavior or set firm, fair, and consistent limits to control unacceptable behavior may contribute to the problem.

Seeking help It can be difficult for parents, who may be extremely provoked by their child's defiance, to be objective in assessing how serious a problem it is. If you are concerned about a possible oppositional defiant disorder, ask yourself whether your child frequently or persistently:

- Loses his or her temper
- Argues with adults
- Defies rules or refuses to do chores
- Deliberately annoys others
- Blames others for his or her mistakes

- Is easily irritated
- Seems spiteful or vindictive
- Swears or uses obscenities.

If you answer "yes" to several of these questions, the problem could be oppositional defiant disorder. In making an evaluation, mental health professionals conduct a comprehensive interview with the child (who may be on his best behavior—as the therapist realizes) and also rely on reports from parents and teachers and psychological tests.

▼

Treating ODD   Behavioral therapy is the usual treatment. Parents (and some-times teachers, too) use some form of reward tokens, such as points or stars, which are given for desired behaviors and taken away for undesirable ones. The rewards may consist of money, food, toys, television, privileges, or being allowed to participate in a pleasant activity with an adult. Time-outs also may be used as punishments or negative reinforcers. Treatment does result in improved behavior, although its effectiveness over the long haul has not been studied.

CONDUCT DISORDERS

Some youngsters go beyond defiance and consistently behave in deliberately disruptive ways that violate the rights of others and the rules of society. They feel no guilt, remorse, or empathy with others, nor do they take responsibility for their own behavior. They do not get along well with other children or adults and can be cruel to animals or people. Unable to tolerate any frustration or to delay gratification, they are often irritable and try to provoke others. Children with a conduct disorder may bully or threaten others or get into fights, acting alone or with a gang. They may steal, set fires, destroy property, assault, rape, or, rarely, murder. Those who engage in a variety of serious misbehaviors are most likely to develop antisocial personality disorder or alcoholism as adults. Conduct disorder is associated with early onset of sexual behavior, drinking, smoking, use of illegal drugs, and reckless or risky acts. It may lead to suspension or expulsion from school, problems with the law, sexually transmitted diseases, unplanned pregnancy, physical injuries, and an increased risk of suicide.

Sometimes youngsters with conduct disorders first develop AD/HD or ODD. Other problems, including depression, bipolar illness, or psychosis, may also play a part in the development of a conduct disorder. Additional factors that may contribute to a con-

*According to the
DSM-IV, a diagnosis
of ODD should be
based on these
criteria:*

■ **A pattern of negativistic, hostile, and defiant behavior that lasts at
least six months, during which at least four of the following occur
often:**
   1. **Loss of temper**
   2. **Arguments with adults**
   3. **Active defiance or refusal to comply with adults' requests or
   rules**
   4. **Deliberate annoying of other people**
   5. **Blaming others for his or her mistakes or misbehavior**
   6. **Touchiness; easily annoyed by others**
   7. **Anger and resentment**
   8. **Spitefulness or vindictiveness**

■ **Significant impairment in social, academic, or occupational
functioning**

■ **Does not occur exclusively during the course of a psychotic or
mood disorder**

■ **Symptoms do not meet the criteria for conduct disorder (see
page 666) or, if eighteen years or older, antisocial personality
disorder (see page 528).**

Adapted from the Diagnostic and Statistical Manual of Mental Disorders,
4th Edition. *Used with permission.*

duct disorder include difficult temperament, lower-than-average
intelligence, poor academic achievement, parents who ignore good
behavior and focus only on bad behavior, lack of consistent limits
or adequate supervision, marital conflict, physical or sexual
abuse, removal from a home for any reason, poverty, and brain
damage. Mentally retarded youngsters may steal or become aggressive because they do not have other coping skills or because
they are led into such activities by other children.

▼
Seeking help   If you suspect a possible conduct disorder, ask yourself whether
your child:

- Bullies or threatens others

- Gets into frequent fights

- Has ever used a dangerous weapon

- Steals

- Stays out past curfew

- Has run away from home overnight at least twice

- Lies frequently

- Sets fires

- Skips school repeatedly

- Has vandalized property or broken into a car, home, or building

- Is cruel to animals or people

- Is physically aggressive or violent

- Has deliberately destroyed property.

If you answer "yes" to several of these questions, the problem may indeed be a conduct disorder. Usually mental health professionals evaluating youngsters receive reports of bad behavior from several sources—parents, teachers, police, or other community members. In making their assessment, they screen for other problems, including AD/HD, anxiety, depression, substance abuse, brain damage (especially in violent children), and developmental disorders (see the table, Is It a Conduct Disorder? on page 666). Therapists make note of whether a conduct disorder begins in childhood (prior to age ten) or later. Those with early onset tend to be male, physically aggressive, and have disturbed relationships with peers. Those who develop symptoms after age ten are less likely to be aggressive and have more normal peer relationships.

▼

Treating conduct disorders

Youngsters with a conduct disorder usually do not benefit from individual psychotherapy. However, group or family therapy, with a focus on improved communication and healthier patterns for interacting, can be effective. Parents learn to use clear and consistent rules, reinforce good behavior, and set limits to restrict negative behavior. Behavioral approaches are also helpful. Youngsters may be taught cognitive techniques, such as problem-solving skills, as an alternative way of resolving conflicts.

Community services, such as Big Brothers and Big Sisters, or special outdoor or sports programs can help. Youngsters with learning disabilities as well as conduct problems may benefit from remedial education. For others, vocational training can be a good option. For some young people, particularly those who are violent or have gotten involved in criminal activities, therapists may recommend a residential treatment program that provides close supervision, behavior modification, and instruction in social and educational skills. Some problems are so overwhelming that it takes a twenty-four-hour-a-day team approach over several months to turn a child around.

The long-term success of all these interventions is not known.

Is it a conduct disorder?

According to the DSM-IV, a diagnosis of conduct disorder should be based on these criteria:

- A repetitive and persistent pattern of violating the basic rights of others or age-appropriate societal norms or rules, with at least three of the following occurring in the past twelve months and at least one present in the last six months:

Aggression to people and animals:
1. Often bullying, threatening, or intimidating others
2. Often initiating physical fights
3. Use of a weapon that can cause serious physical harm to others (e.g., a bat, brick, broken bottle, knife, gun)
4. Physical cruelty to people
5. Physical cruelty to animals
6. Stealing in a confrontation with a victim (e.g., mugging, purse snatching, extortion, armed robbery)
7. Forcing someone into sexual activity

Destruction of property:
8. Deliberate fire setting with the intention of causing serious damage
9. Deliberate destruction of others' property in other ways

Deceitfulness or theft:
10. Breaking into someone else's house, building, or car
11. Frequent lying to obtain goods or favors or to avoid obligations (e.g., "conning" others)
12. Stealing items of nontrivial value without confronting the victim (e.g., shoplifting, forgery)

Serious violation of rules:
13. Often staying out at night despite parental prohibitions, beginning before age thirteen
14. Running away from home overnight at least twice (or once without returning for a lengthy period)
15. Frequent truancy from school, beginning before age thirteen

- Significant impairment in functioning socially or at school or work

- In individuals age eighteen or older, symptoms do not meet criteria for antisocial personality disorder (page 528).

Adapted from the Diagnostic and Statistical Manual of Mental Disorders, 4th Edition. *Used with permission.*

Some youngsters seem to outgrow their "bad" behavior. In others, nothing seems to have a lasting impact. Those who get involved in serious violations of social and legal norms are likely to get into further trouble as they grow older. As teenagers, they may join gangs and commit crimes. In adulthood, they have a higher incidence of alcoholism and antisocial personality disorder.

DEPRESSIVE DISORDERS

Like adults, children can have mood swings and feel down in the dumps or blue. Although symptoms of being depressed, such as feeling sad, are common among youngsters of all ages, major depression is more intense, more enduring, more disabling, and more serious. Depression takes different forms in children of different ages. A preschooler may become listless, lose interest in playing, and cry easily and often. A grade-schooler may pull away from family and friends, have problems with schoolwork, and seem sad and discouraged. A teenager may argue with parents and teachers, refuse to do chores or homework, and drop out of sports or other favorite activities. At any age, depressed youngsters may be irritable and extremely self-critical. Parents may not be able to tell whether their child is "going through a phase" or struggling with depression; mental health professionals experienced in evaluating and treating children and teenagers can.

By conservative estimates, about 2 percent of children and 4.7 percent of adolescents develop major depression. An additional 3.3 percent of teenagers suffer from chronic mild depression, or dysthymia. Some investigators believe that the incidence of depressive disorders in the young is much higher than these figures suggest. In a study of 508 boys and girls in elementary school who were followed for five years beginning in the third or fourth grade, researchers from Stanford University and the University of Pennsylvania found that 10 to 15 percent were moderately to severely depressed. In a 1988 study of almost 1,500 boys and girls, the percentage of depressed girls zoomed up from about 8 percent in the preteen years—about the same as for boys in childhood and adolescence—to 16 percent among those between the ages of fourteen and sixteen.

As in adults, the causes of depression in children are complex. Some may inherit a biological predisposition, and depressed children often live with a depressed parent, usually their mother. Depression also may develop after extreme stress or a traumatic loss, experiences that can lead to deep feelings of helplessness and hopelessness.

Different factors may have more of an impact at different ages. Among younger children, "the major predictors of depression are negative life events, such as parental divorce, a close relative's death, or a major financial setback for the family," says Susan Nolen-Hoeksema, Ph.D., assistant professor of psychology at Stanford University. "But as youngsters get older, another variable becomes equally important: their explanatory style or way of interpreting what happened."

Children who blame themselves (for example, concluding that

they got a poor report card because they're "stupid" rather than because they didn't study hard), or who take the pessimistic view that more bad things will happen to them in the future, are most likely to develop depression. In a study of third, fourth, and fifth graders rejected by their classmates, those who blamed the rejection on something wrong with them were likely to become depressed, whereas those who felt they might be able to turn things around were not.

Depression in children can interfere with their personal development and their acquisition of basic social skills. Moreover, once youngsters become moderately depressed, they often stay that way for a very long time. "Our study showed that kids don't just 'get over it,'" says Nolen-Hoeksema. "Negative life events or distress early in life can affect self-concept in such a way as to make a child more vulnerable to depression throughout life."

▼

Seeking help   If you suspect that depression may be a problem, ask yourself whether your child:

- Seems sad, discouraged, bored, or irritable
- Has lost interest in favorite activities
- Has stopped taking part in after-school sports or hobbies
- Is not gaining weight at the expected rate
- Is sluggish and lethargic or becomes agitated and restless
- Feels tired all the time
- Has withdrawn from family and friends
- Pretends to be sick to stay away from school, sports, or play
- Seems to cover up sadness with lots of activity or aggression
- Argues over everything
- Cries easily and often
- Has poor self-esteem and negative feelings about him- or herself and others
- Has no interest in food
- Sleeps much more or less than usual
- Has nightmares or is extremely restless while sleeping
- Gets poor grades
- Argues with teachers
- Cannot get schoolwork done
- Refuses to do chores
- Expresses feelings of hopelessness.

If the answer is "yes" to several of these questions and the symptoms have persisted for two weeks or more, the problem could be a depressive disorder. Mental health professionals base their diagnosis on a careful interview with the child, asking questions about his or her mood in age-appropriate terms, such as using the word *cranky* rather than *irritable* with a younger child. In making the diagnosis, they consider all aspects of a child's functioning and physical and mental state (see the table, Is It Major Depression? in Chapter 5). The key differences in diagnosis in children are that their mood may be irritable rather than sad and that they may fail to gain weight as expected rather than actually lose weight.

Depression can be a fatal disease. More than half of all teens who attempt suicide are depressed. Because of the risk of suicide (discussed in Chapter 22 and later in this chapter), therapists ask depressed children or adolescents whether they have thought about dying or killing themselves, whether they wish to die, and whether a friend or relative has recently committed suicide.

Dysthymia (chronic mild depression) in children and teens can impair schoolwork and relationships with peers and adults. The symptoms of this disorder in youngsters are similar to those in adults, except that their mood may be irritable rather than depressed and they feel this way for one year, rather than two. In addition to being depressed or irritable, children with dysthymia tend to react to almost everything, including praise or an invitation to participate in a fun activity, in a negative way. They may also eat and sleep much more or less than usual, have little energy, have poor self-esteem, have problems concentrating, and feel hopeless. (See the table, Is It Dysthymia? in Chapter 5.)

▼

Treating depressive disorders

The primary treatment for depression in children and teens is psychotherapy: individual, family, or both. Family therapy is especially helpful if other family members also suffer from depression. Interpersonal therapy, which has proved effective in adults and is described in Chapters 5 and 27, also holds promise for children by helping them to express feelings and communicate better with others, particularly their parents.

Mental health professionals who work with children usually modify the same approaches used for adults—for example, using children's drawings, story telling, and play to help youngsters express difficulties. A child's comments about a figure in a drawing or a doll may indicate low self-esteem or feelings of loneliness. Through their interactions, the therapist can point out the many good things about the child or teach him or her ways of reaching out to others. With older children, therapists might use cognitive-behavioral techniques in the same way they would with adults. If a teenager believes that no one likes her because one group of girls has snubbed her, the therapist might point out that she is generalizing and encourage her to focus on the much larger number of her peers who are friendly.

For youngsters who do not improve within four to six weeks, child psychiatrists may prescribe antidepressant medications. Psychotherapy continues to remain an important part of therapy, not only to help youngsters deal with psychological issues that may have contributed to the depression but also to deal with what it means to a child to have a "condition," take a pill, and work through problems in therapy.

"Based on clinical experience, there seems to be a subset of kids who respond beautifully to medications," says Susan Friedland, M.D., a child psychiatrist at California Pacific Medical Center in San Francisco. "However, we don't yet know how to identify these kids beforehand. With adolescents, it has been difficult to document the effectiveness of drugs because teenagers have a very high placebo response, and in clinical trials tend to improve whether they are given an antidepressant or a placebo."

Before prescribing medication, a child psychiatrist may check pulse and blood pressure and order various tests, including a baseline electrocardiogram (ECG), complete blood count, and blood chemistry. Usually an antidepressant is prescribed for eight to twelve weeks to see if it helps. "If it proves useful, drug treatment continues for nine to twelve months; then the medication is gradually reduced to see if the child can do without it," says Friedland. "If not, the youngster goes back on medication for another six to twelve months." Maintenance therapy, which has proved very helpful in preventing recurrences in adults, has not been studied in children.

Children are at risk for the same medication side effects as adults (described in Chapter 28). Parents should closely supervise administration of medication and keep the pills in a secure place. Youngsters taking certain drugs, such as tricyclic antidepressants, will need monitoring of their blood and heart rates. "The selective serotonin reuptake inhibitors seem to be very well tolerated and do not require extra monitoring," Friedland notes. "There is some evidence that they may be especially useful in treatment-resistant depression."

▼

Outlook Without treatment, an episode of major depression in children can last eleven months or longer. As in adults, depression in children usually improves with treatment. The risk for relapse is high. In the first major study to follow 134 children into adulthood, researchers at Western Psychiatric Institute in Pittsburgh found that about three of four children who had a first episode of major depression between the ages of eight and thirteen had a recurrence later in life. Those with dysthymia, or mild depression, had a high risk for developing an episode of major depression—so-called *double depression*—within two years. The increased risk for depressive disorders continued into young adulthood.

"Generally, the earlier in life that depression develops, the more severe its course over a lifetime," says Friedland. "The prognosis is better if childhood depression is recognized and treated quickly because then development proceeds more normally."

A particularly hopeful development has been a new focus on preventing depression in children, usually between the ages of ten and thirteen, who are considered at risk. One approach involves special "antidepression" classes in which small groups of youngsters learn to think before acting, to challenge self-critical thoughts, and to handle disputes with others. Practical coping skills like these may be especially helpful for youngsters entering the rocky emotional territory of adolescence. Rates of depression among "graduates" have proved to be lower than among teens in comparison groups.

ANXIETY DISORDERS

Although adults may like to think of children as carefree, worry is common at every age. However, the nature of youngsters' worries and fears varies as they grow. A two-year-old may be terrified of the vacuum cleaner, and a four-year-old may be afraid of the dark. In elementary school, children may come to worry most about tests and school performance. In high school, teenagers may worry about being liked by their peers.

Whatever the source of their apprehensiveness or fear, there is a difference between feeling anxious and an anxiety disorder, which is a more serious, longer-lasting problem. The anxiety disorders—the most common mental disorders among children as well as adults—include phobias, such as intense fear of insects or dogs, extreme anxiety when separated from loved ones (usually parents), excessive shrinking from contact with unfamiliar people, or persistent and unrealistic overanxiousness. (Chapter 7 provides a more comprehensive discussion.)

Two to 8 percent of children and adolescents develop anxiety disorders, which often overlap with depression. After puberty these are more common in girls than boys. Many more children suffer from undue anxiety, even though they may not have a true anxiety disorder, and they, too, can benefit from treatment.

Separation anxiety Separation anxiety and fear of strangers are normal phases of infant development, usually beginning between the ages of seven and nine months. There can be recurrent bouts of such anxiety as young children venture into each new world of play, preschool, kindergarten, and grade school. Most quickly get over their initial apprehensiveness, but some become so fearful of leaving their parents (or others to whom they are deeply attached) that they cannot participate in normal play and other activities.

About 4 percent of children and young adolescents develop a separation anxiety disorder. Worried that something terrible will happen to them or their parents, they may refuse or be reluctant to go to school or to sleep alone or away from home. They often avoid being alone, have nightmares about separation, and experience extreme distress or physical symptoms before or during a separation from parents. (See the table on the opposite page.) There may be a relationship between separation anxiety in childhood and the development of agoraphobia in adulthood.

School phobia Because youngsters with separation anxiety disorder often do not want to go to school, this specific problem is sometimes called school phobia. However, some degree of anxiety about school is normal. Grade-schoolers may not cling like toddlers when it's time to leave their parents behind, but the start of the school year often triggers an unsettling mix of anticipation and apprehension. Kindergartners and first graders, who are making the enormous leap into "big-kids' school," may face the most stressful transition, but each year brings new anxiety. Some children seem especially vulnerable and continue to have problems at the beginning of every school year until they reach their teens.

Parents can help to prevent a serious problem at the beginning of the school year by making the transition as smooth as possible and by spending extra time with their children in the initial weeks. They should not criticize or make fun of an anxious child for "acting like a baby," but neither should they overreact. It is much more reassuring for children if parents don't buy into their anxiety and become anxious themselves. Although parents should offer sympathy and reassurance, as a rule they should never allow a child to stay home rather than go to school.

Sometimes youngsters show their anxiety by a reluctance to get dressed and leave the house. Getting up five or ten minutes earlier to allow a more relaxed morning routine can make a difference. Children also feel more secure if they know exactly when they will see their parents again. If a child is anxious about separation from one parent in particular, that parent might pick the child up after school occasionally or spend some special time together. Some-

■ Developmentally inappropriate and excessive anxiety concerning separation from home or from those to whom the child is attached, as demonstrated by at least three of the following:

1. Recurrent and excessive distress when separation from home or major attachment figure occurs or is anticipated
2. Persistent and excessive worry about losing, or about possible harm befalling, these individuals
3. Persistent and excessive worry that an untoward event, such as getting lost or being kidnapped, may lead to separation from a major attachment figure
4. Persistent reluctance or refusal to go to school or elsewhere because of fear of separation
5. Persistent and excessive fearfulness or reluctance to be alone or without major attachment figures at home or without significant adults in other settings
6. Persistent reluctance or refusal to go to sleep without being near a major attachment figure or to sleep away from home
7. Repeated nightmares involving separation
8. Repeated complaints of physical symptoms (headaches, stomachaches, nausea, vomiting) when separation occurs or is anticipated

■ Recurrent distress in anticipation of or when separation occurs

■ Disturbance continuing for at least four weeks

■ Development of symptoms before age eighteen

■ Significant distress or impaired functioning as a result

■ Does not occur exclusively during the course of a pervasive developmental disorder, schizophrenia, or other psychotic disorder, and, in adolescents and adults, not better accounted for by panic disorder with agoraphobia

Adapted from the Diagnostic and Statistical Manual of Mental Disorders, 4th Edition. *Used with permission.*

times there is a problem at school that parents and teachers can identify and deal with: a playground bully, for instance, or a learning difficulty that could be helped with extra tutoring.

Most children get over school-related anxiety fairly quickly; when they don't, there may be a disorder in need of further probing. In such cases there are almost always other things going on in the greater fabric of a child's life than a fear of school or of leaving his or her parents. If, for example, a grandmother has recently moved from the youngster's house into a nursing home, or a parent has left on an extended business trip, the child may hide his real feelings because he thinks it is more acceptable to say that the problem is school. In sessions with a therapist, children often reveal their real concerns, which can then be dealt with directly. Some therapists prescribe medication, such as imipramine (Tofranil), for children who are resistant to other treatments for extreme separation anxiety.

Phobias Some children develop specific phobias—intense fears far out of proportion to any actual danger. The most common phobias involve animals (most often dogs or snakes), insects, spiders, the dark, water, or thunderstorms. Youngsters with such phobias are typically so scared that they avoid going near the feared object, such as a dog, and may become upset even at the sight or sound of a dog. According to the National Institute of Mental Health's (NIMH) epidemiological data, specific phobias are the most common anxiety disorders, and many, especially those involving animals, begin in childhood, most before age seven.

Youngsters also may develop social phobia, a general fear of potentially humiliating situations in which others may observe them. The most common fears in social phobia in children are of answering questions or speaking in front of the class. (Chapter 7 has a comprehensive discussion of phobias.)

Overanxious disorder (generalized anxiety disorder in children)
Some children develop extreme and unrealistic worries about almost everything. They may fear for the future, worry about something that happened in the past, and doubt their own ability to deal with the present. Often self-conscious about their appearance, they seek constant reassurance and may develop physical symptoms. Often they bite their nails, suck their thumbs, pull or twist their hair, or have problems falling asleep. Overanxious children are often described as overly mature. Determined to be perfect, they are extremely sensitive to criticism and often have their feelings hurt. Although they have warm, close relationships, they worry about doing well and being accepted and liked. Sometimes the parents of overanxious youngsters are also anxious and may, without realizing it, put excessive pressure on them to succeed.

This problem can vary greatly in severity. Some children manage to function, but often only with difficulty. Treatment is essential when the problem persists for six months or more, significantly affects a child's functioning at school or home, interferes with friendships, interrupts academic or social development, or causes family disruption. Overanxious disorder can persist into adulthood as generalized anxiety disorder.

▼

Seeking help for anxiety-related problems

Parents can easily empathize with the fears and worries that their youngsters develop, but they may not be able to sense how serious these are. If you are concerned about separation anxiety or school phobia, ask yourself if your youngster:

- Cannot function normally because of incapacitating fear
- Has unrealistic fears that parents will be harmed or not return
- Refuses to go to school because it means leaving a parent
- Will not sleep away from home without a parent
- Clings to or "shadows" parents
- Suffers nightmares about separation
- Complains of physical symptoms, such as headaches or stomachaches, when anticipating a separation
- Wants social involvement only with familiar people.

If you think that the problem might be a specific phobia, ask yourself whether your child:

- Is terrified of a particular object or situation
- Becomes extremely scared almost every time he or she confronts it
- Becomes intensely anxious and fearful even before actually confronting it
- Tries to avoid whatever frightens him or her so intensely
- Does not want to engage in usual activities because of this fear.

If you are concerned about overanxiousness, ask yourself whether your child:

- Worries excessively about future events or past behavior
- Is extremely self-conscious
- Constantly needs reassurance
- Seems tense and unable to relax.

If you answer "yes" to several of the questions under any of these headings, your child may well benefit from professional assessment and treatment. A complete evaluation should consist of a comprehensive interview with a child psychiatrist or psychologist, as well as a medical examination and history to check for physical causes for problems such as headaches, stomachaches, nausea, or vomiting. Therapists will also look for patterns in the child's behavior, such as a flare-up of anxiety symptoms on mornings before school.

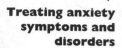

Treating anxiety symptoms and disorders

Children with anxiety symptoms or an anxiety disorder can benefit greatly from treatments that help them to relax, bring their fears out into the open, and teach them practical coping skills. They often respond well to behavioral techniques such as relaxation training, systematic desensitization, and assertiveness training. In individual psychotherapy, therapists may use verbal and play techniques to deal with underlying conflicts and teach more adaptive ways of coping. With dolls or puppets, for example, youngsters can act out a scene that makes them fearful; the therapist can suggest ways of dealing with the situations that frighten them. Cognitive therapy, for children old enough to grasp the basic concepts, may reduce anxiety by changing negative, self-defeating thoughts. A youngster who constantly criticizes himself—for example, saying, "I'm such a klutz" or "I'm so stupid"—can be taught thought-stopping techniques that help him to break out of the cycle of constantly putting himself down. Family therapy that brings parents, the anxious child, and, if appropriate, siblings or other close relatives together can also be useful in dealing with issues that affect them all and in reducing parental anxiety.

POSTTRAUMATIC STRESS DISORDER

Children who survive an extremely frightening, stressful, or shocking experience—one so out of the ordinary, such as a school-yard shooting or an earthquake, that anyone would be deeply upset by it—may develop long-lasting emotional and behavioral symptoms (see Chapter 12 on stress-related disorders). They may re-experience the trauma in daydreams or nightmares and try to avoid any reminder of what happened. Youngsters may also develop such symptoms after experiencing a trauma such as being raped or kidnapped, watching another person being injured, as in a serious car accident, or learning that something terrible has happened to a relative or friend.

Children respond differently to trauma than adults do. Initially, they mainly feel fear—fear of leaving or losing their parents, of dying, of still more fear—and may withdraw from new experiences. They usually remember many details of the experience accurately, but their sense of the sequence or duration of events may be distorted. Often they re-enact what happened in symbolic play or in actual behavior. Physical symptoms, such as headaches and stomachaches, are common. They may have sleep problems and generally regress—that is, act as if they were younger and less mature. Because of difficulties in concentrating and a drop in motivation, they may perform poorly at school.

Youngsters often blame themselves for what happened and assume that they are responsible even when there is nothing they could have done to prevent or avoid the trauma. If anyone else was hurt, they may feel guilty about not having been able to protect or save the other person. Many traumatized children develop a sense of hopelessness and pessimism about the future. Even four or five years afterward, they may feel deep shame about their own helplessness.

Although any child or teenager can develop psychiatric symptoms or posttraumatic stress disorder (PTSD) after a trauma, those who have pre-existing anxiety or depression or who have experienced previous stresses or losses are at highest risk. Symptoms may intensify if a child's living circumstances change as the result of the trauma, as when, for example, the family must move because their home was destroyed in a fire or earthquake.

Individual psychotherapy, including play therapy, is the usual approach to treatment. Group therapy, organized in schools or the community, can help children who were exposed to the same trauma, such as a flood or hurricane. A stable, supportive family can ease symptoms. However, if the family is in turmoil or when the trauma involves child abuse (discussed in Chapter 24), family therapy is likely to be essential. Even in stable families, supportive treatment for parents and siblings who went through the same traumatic experience, but bounced back from it more quickly, can help them to understand the child's symptoms and behavior.

OBSESSIVE-COMPULSIVE DISORDER

Various studies have shown that 0.4 to 1 percent of youngsters develop obsessive-compulsive disorder (OCD), a malfunction of information-relaying mechanisms within the brain that causes repetitive thoughts or ritualistic behaviors to spin out of control. However, many therapists believe that this problem is far more common than these percentages support. (Recent research has shown that one in every forty adults may have OCD.) Chapter 8 discusses OCD in depth; this disorder is similar in children and adults.

OCD can run in families. About 20 percent of affected children have a family member with the disorder. In a study of seventy children with OCD, conducted by the Child Psychiatry Branch of NIMH, the mean age at onset was 10.2 years, and boys outnumbered girls by more than two to one. Most children develop a single obsession or compulsion and then shift to another after a period of months or years. At least three-quarters wash their hands excessively. Teenagers may develop obsessive sexual thoughts, such as fear of AIDS, that trigger the washing. As in adults, obsessions and compulsions can become so severe that they interfere with normal living and make children miserable.

Treatment with clomipramine (Anafranil) or fluoxetine (Prozac), combined with behavioral therapy and psychotherapy, leads to improvement in 75 percent of youngsters with OCD. In severe cases, medications are used for children under ten as well as for older ones. Although symptoms are rarely eliminated entirely, the medication can reduce the force of obsessions and compulsions and greatly improve the quality of a child's life. OCD tends to be chronic, although symptoms may come and go over the years, often flaring up during times of change or crisis.

ELIMINATION DISORDERS

A problem with bladder or bowel control is often extremely embarrassing for youngsters and exasperating for parents. However, such difficulties are common and, with time and patience, are highly treatable.

Bed-wetting Most children learn to control their bladders somewhere between the ages of eighteen months and four years. Usually, daytime control comes before nighttime dryness. At age five, 7 percent of boys and 3 percent of girls wet the bed occasionally. The percentage of children with a bed-wetting (or enuresis) problem declines with age. By age ten, 3 percent of boys and 2 percent of girls are unable to control their bladders.

Children who have never been able to control urination during the day or at night have *primary enuresis*; those who begin to wet their beds after at least one year of bladder control have *secondary enuresis*. Children occasionally regress as a result of illness or psychological stress; this is considered normal rather than a sign of a disorder.

Most cases of enuresis stem from delayed maturation of bladder control mechanisms, a condition that runs in families; 75 percent of children with this problem have a close biological relative with a history of enuresis. A small bladder capacity or lack of systematic training may contribute to the problem. Sometimes children with other psychiatric problems may wet themselves. A child with AD/HD, for example, may wait too long to head for the bathroom and lose control on the way, and one with ODD may refuse to use the toilet as part of a battle for control.

Pediatricians handle most enuresis problems. Their usual advice for parents with youngsters under age seven is to be patient, not to punish the child, to teach him or her how to change pajamas and bed linens, and to restrict fluids before bedtime. Exercises, such as waiting as long as possible before urinating after drinking water during the day, or stopping and starting the flow of urine to strengthen the bladder sphincter muscles, may help.

Older children often improve with behavior modification techniques, such as a chart with stars or stickers for each dry night and rewards for achieving a certain goal. Parents also have tried specialized urine alarms, with a bell that rings when a pad gets wet; little is known about their effectiveness.

Some children who wet their beds regularly may not produce adequate amounts of antidiuretic hormone (ADH), a natural substance that limits urine production during sleep. Their bladders fill completely every few hours during the night because they keep producing urine at the same rate as during the day. If they are very deep sleepers, as many bed-wetters are, they do not respond to the sensation of having a full bladder and end up wetting the bed. For them, a new treatment option is a nasal spray that contains a synthetic form of ADH called desmopressin acetate (DDAVP), which lowers urine production. The most common side effect is a runny nose in the morning; occasionally youngsters complain of a headache or stomachache. Many doctors prescribe the spray for three months and then see how youngsters do without it. Eventually children produce adequate ADH on their own.

Some physicians prescribe low doses of tricyclic antidepressants for special occasions, such as an overnight visit at a friend's house or vacation at summer camp. These are partially effective at controlling nighttime wetting, but when discontinued, the children usually wet their beds again until maturation occurs.

Encopresis Most children achieve bowel control between the ages of two and a half and five. About 1 percent of five-year-olds cannot control their bowels, with boys outnumbering girls.

Encopresis is the medical term for involuntary passage of feces into clothing or other inappropriate places occurring at least once a month for at least three months in children older than four. Youngsters who have never had bowel control have *primary encopresis*; those who had been able to control their bowels for at least one year may develop *secondary encopresis*.

Medical problems, including abnormalities in the digestive tract, hypothyroidism, and lactase deficiency, can lead to encopresis. One very common cause is chronic severe constipation, which impairs the usual movements and contractions of the colon and leads to a fecal obstruction. As feces become impacted, loose stool leaks around the obstruction into the child's underpants or clothing. A lack of systematic toilet training, delays in physical maturation, other psychiatric disorders such as AD/HD or ODD, and mental retardation also can contribute to a bowel control problem.

Children with encopresis should undergo a complete medical history and physical examination. Medical treatment is essential for those suffering from chronic constipation. It usually consists of bowel "retraining" with mineral oil, a high-roughage diet, and a regular toileting routine. Enemas are discouraged because they do not improve bowel function and can create difficulties and conflict between parents and children.

Children who continue to have soiling problems after age six often have psychiatric symptoms as a consequence of harsh discipline imposed on them for soiling themselves or of rejection or humiliation by their peers. Psychotherapy can help them to deal with anger, embarrassment, and low self-esteem.

Substance abuse

Drugs have become a fact of life for children growing up in the United States. "It's not a question of whether kids will be exposed to drugs but how they'll deal with it when they are," says Lee Dogoloff, former executive director of the American Council on Drug Education, "Every child in our society has to make a decision about using alcohol, marijuana, and tobacco, usually before the age of twelve. Some youngsters are more vulnerable than others, but there's a lot we don't know about risk factors. The most salient one is a family history of alcohol or drug abuse, extending even beyond parents to grandparents, uncles and aunts." (Chapters 9 and 10 discuss drug and alcohol abuse in detail.)

Other predictors of drug use in young people include learning disabilities, low grades or poor school performance, aggressive or rebellious behavior, excessive peer influence, lack of parental warmth, support, or guidance, and behavior problems at an early age. "But it's not just problem kids who get in trouble with drugs," says Dogoloff. "Most kids try drugs for two reasons: First, they're available, and adolescence is a time of experimentation with all sorts of things. Second, no one has told them not to."

Almost always drug use starts with legal substances, such as alcohol, the number one drug of abuse. Young substance abusers, particularly during the early stages of drug experimentation, typically feel invulnerable, as if nothing could ever harm them and they could never lose control. Yet before they even realize what's happening, they may become psychologically or physiologically hooked. As drug prevention experts emphasize, there are no safe drugs. All psychoactive substances, including alcohol, target the brain, affect judgment, and can lead youngsters to do things they otherwise wouldn't do. With continued use, schoolwork suffers. Psychological problems worsen. The risk for accidents, pregnancy, sexually transmitted diseases (including HIV infection and AIDS), and suicide increases.

▼

Seeking help

Often parents find it hard to admit to anyone, including themselves, that their children may be using drugs. If you have any reason to be suspicious, ask yourself whether your child:

- Often seems vague or withdrawn or has sudden outbursts of anger
- Loses interest in activities he or she once enjoyed
- Has been skipping classes or has had a sudden decline in school performance
- Suddenly resists discipline or reacts strongly to criticism
- Makes secretive phone calls or arranges mysterious meetings
- Demands greater privacy concerning his or her room or personal possessions
- Changes sleeping and eating habits or loses weight suddenly
- Often borrows or steals money
- Disregards personal appearance
- Ignores deadlines, curfews, or other regulations
- Has more difficulty getting along with family and old friends
- Has made new friends and feels staunchly loyal to them.

If the answer is "yes" to several of these questions, your child may be experimenting with drugs. However, it is not uncommon for parents to notice many of these telltale indicators yet try to ignore them. "Denial is a key feature of chemical dependence, by family members as well as users," notes Dogoloff. "If you have a gnawing sense that something is wrong, it's probably true, and you've got to do something about it."

The actual problem underlying the troubling behavior may not be drugs, but a physical or emotional disorder, such as depression. "You still have to check it out," says Dogoloff. "Sometimes parents hesitate to take a child to a doctor for urine testing or to a drug counselor for an evaluation because they worry about how the child will feel if it turns out negative. My response is, 'Wouldn't that be wonderful?' There is no downside to checking out a possible drug problem. What you tell a child is, 'This is my job. If I saw you sleeping all the time and drinking a lot of water, I'd get your blood sugar tested for diabetes. I wouldn't assume it would go away on its own. I've got to do the same when I see signs that could indicate drug abuse.'"

Coming to grips with the fact that your child uses drugs can be heart-wrenching. "It was one of the most painful things I ever experienced as a parent," says Dorothy Hudson, a member of the board of the National Federation of Parents for Drug-Free Youth.

"But you've got to push past your shame and denial so you can help your child."

The first step is confronting youngsters, calmly and frankly, at a time when they are not high or drunk. "What I did was gather my evidence very carefully," says Hudson. "Then I said to my son, 'I know what you're doing. I love you, but I will not tolerate drug use in this family. I'm here to help you, but you have to make the decision to stop.' The most important thing is to make sure your youngsters understand that you still love them, that you're rejecting the drug use, not the child."

▼

Treating substance abuse

The earlier parents recognize a problem and get treatment, the brighter the prognosis for their youngster. As soon as they realize that there is a problem, parents need to find out how serious the problem is and what the options for treatment are. (Chapter 9 describes therapies for overcoming drug use.) Treatment must always be based on the particular youngster and his or her circumstances. In some cases, individual, group, or family therapy can be effective. In others, children or teens may have to be placed in a residential or day treatment center. The outlook for young people who receive treatment for substance abuse is very good. As one mental health professional puts it, "With youngsters, treatment is more a matter of habilitating rather than rehabilitating. Since they're more or less blank stones, you can do a lot more molding than with adults."

Dorothy Hudson, whose son completely turned his life around after drug treatment, can testify to its success: "Drug use is treatable and curable. It's not impossible for anyone to become drug-free. When a child uses drugs, it can tear a family apart. But if the right steps are taken, they can put the family together again in a better way."

DEVELOPMENTAL DISORDERS

One in every ten youngsters may not develop physical, intellectual, or academic skills at the same time as most children of the same age. These children may have difficulty with coordination, language and speech (including stuttering), or school subjects (arithmetic, expressive writing, and reading). As a result, they may feel demoralized, develop low self-esteem and behavioral problems, and refuse to apply themselves at school.

Different types of developmental problems often run in families, suggesting a genetic cause. Early diagnosis, usually by testing and assessments by teachers, parents, and others, is crucial in preventing harmful emotional and behavioral complications. Remedial training, such as tutoring, weekly speech therapy, or special classes or schools, is the primary treatment. Supportive psychotherapy can help with problems of low self-esteem, lack of motivation, anxiety, or depression. Family therapy can deal with issues such as parental styles of criticism.

Boys and girls often acquire certain skills at different ages. "We know that physiologically girls develop a little faster than boys, and the same may be true of brain structures," says psychologist Jack Naglieri, Ph.D., a professor at Ohio State University, who has found that girls in the early elementary years have a greater natural ability to plan ahead. (Boys do catch up.) "Planning really is the key to school performance," says Naglieri. "It serves as the control center that allows us to make good decisions, to recognize bad ones, and to modify what we're doing."

Yet some stereotyped gender differences in academic abilities, such as reading problems, may be overstated. In general, boys are three to four times more likely to be identified as having reading problems as girls, but that may be simply because educators expect more boys to be "reading disabled."

"There seems to be a definite bias," says Sally Shaywitz, M.D., an associate professor of pediatrics at Yale University School of Medicine, who directed a study of 215 girls and 199 boys. Using subjective assessments of behavioral, academic, and cognitive skills, teachers found that boys performed more poorly in each area and that far more boys than girls had reading difficulties. Yet objective, highly reliable tests of actual reading ability and achievement found no difference in reading skills between boys and girls.

"We found significant gender differences in behavior between *normal* boys and girls," says Shaywitz, noting that boys are more active, less attentive, and less dexterous. "Normal boys may be held to a standard that's more appropriate for girls so teachers label their behavior as abnormal." As she notes, gender-based assumptions also put girls at a disadvantage because teachers are less likely to pick up on actual reading problems they may have and to provide whatever extra help such girls may need. Among the factors that increase the likelihood of reading disability in both sexes are prior difficulties with language, fine-motor coordination, or attention.

Mental retardation   About 1 percent of children have lower than normal intellectual functioning. Most of them (85 percent), who have IQs in the range of 50–55 to 70, are considered mildly retarded. Another 10 percent, with IQs from 35–40 to 50–55, are moderately retarded. Those with IQs from 20–25 to 35–40 are severely retarded, and those with IQs below 20–25 are considered profoundly retarded. Mental retardation has multiple causes, including genetic abnormalities, metabolic disorders, injuries, and exposure to toxins. Psychosocial factors, such as neglect, lack of stimulation, and poverty, also may contribute to it.

Although their mental retardation cannot be reversed, a great deal can be done to help youngsters maximize their potential. Many are helped by specialized training programs, such as the use of exercises and various forms of play to stimulate infants' minds. Adolescents and young adults may benefit from vocational training and, depending on the degree of retardation, opportunities to live in group homes in the community.

For the most part, psychiatry has not played a major role in the treatment of mental retardation. Specialists in a variety of other disciplines, often working with families and advocates, have developed many of the innovations, such as community care, that have brought new hope to the mentally retarded. However, advances in neuropsychiatry are now fueling fresh optimism and scientific interest among psychiatrists, and the future may well bring even more effective ways of helping individuals with mental retardation live to the fullest of their potential.

Certainly, there are many remaining challenges. The incidence of mental disorders, behavior problems, and psychiatric symptoms is much higher in the retarded, regardless of age, than in the general population. An estimated 1 million Americans suffer from both mental retardation and a mental disorder, yet there has been little research in this area. Mental disorders appear to be more severe and more common in those with the greatest intellectual impairment. The prognosis is less favorable for those with the most severe mental handicaps than for those with milder retardation.

Mental retardation may increase vulnerability to mental illness because of underlying abnormalities in brain anatomy and function. In addition, it increases daily challenges and stresses. Individuals must struggle constantly to understand a world that seems confusing and frightening. They may be isolated, lonely, and frustrated by their inability to express their feelings or meet unrealistic expectations. In addition, many never receive psychiatric care or see mental health professionals with special training in understanding their needs. All too often their problems, including such common conditions as depression, are never diagnosed. Medications may be prescribed by physicians in other fields who are not familiar with the most recent data on drugs of choice, doses, or duration of treatment, particularly for children.

Except in cases of profound retardation, many families rear children at home. This experience is often both rewarding and enormously stressful, causing great strain on a marriage and on family dynamics. Parents may constantly be torn between their "special needs" youngster and his or her siblings, who may feel embarrassed, resentful, or guilty about their brother or sister. Inevitably, parents also worry about the future, especially about providing for the costs of caring for their child in adulthood if they become too old or ill, and what will happen after their deaths.

In some circumstances, parents wrestle with the decision of whether or not institutionalization would be best. This choice always depends on what seems best for the individual and the family. A realistic assessment—often with the help of a professional experienced in working with the retarded—is essential in determining which environment would be most beneficial.

Family therapy can help parents to deal with their feelings and with any developmental crises that arise throughout their youngster's childhood and adolescence; it can be helpful for siblings as well. Many parents have found that political and social activism is an effective way of helping their children—and themselves. One of the most powerful forces in improving services for the retarded and their families has been the National Association for Retarded Citizens, which has state and local chapters throughout the country. By uniting families and lobbying intensively, this group has promoted dramatic changes in educational policy, disability legislation, housing options, community services, and public attitudes and acceptance (see the Resource Directory at the back of the book).

Autism and other pervasive developmental disorders   Some children seem to live in a world of their own, unable to connect with other people. Even as infants they do not make eye contact or respond to cuddling. As they grow they do not interact or play with others. Compared with others of their age or developmental stage, their speech and language may be delayed or abnormal. They appear to be incapable of recognizing others' thoughts or feelings and cannot see things from another's view. They are prone to repetitive motions, which may change over the years. Head banging is particularly common among infants and very young children; older youngsters may rock back and forth.

Youngsters with these behaviors may suffer from a profound developmental disorder called *autism*. (See the table on page 686.) This problem is often evident before the age of one and can cause moderate to severe impairment.

In the *DSM-IV*, the category of pervasive developmental disorders (PDDs) also includes other conditions characterized by severe, persistent impairment in various areas of development, social interaction, communication skills, or stereotyped behavior, interests, or activities. In *Rett's syndrome*, which has been reported only in girls, the head growth of youngsters under age four slows and they develop specific deficits, such as a loss of pur-

Is it autistic disorder?

According to the DSM-IV, a diagnosis of autistic disorder is based on these criteria:

■ **At least six of the following from (A), (B), and (C), with at least two from (A) and one each from (B) and (C):**

(A) Qualitative impairment in social interaction, as manifested by at least two of the following:

1. **Marked impairment in the use of multiple nonverbal behaviors such as eye-to-eye gaze, facial expression, body postures, and gestures to regulate social interaction**
2. **Failure to develop peer relationships appropriate to developmental level**
3. **Lack of spontaneous seeking to share enjoyment, interests, or achievements with other people (e.g., not showing, bringing, or pointing out objects of interest)**
4. **Lack of social or emotional reciprocity**

(B) Qualitative impairment in communication as manifested by at least one of the following:

1. **Delay in or total lack of the development of spoken language (not accompanied by an attempt to compensate through alternative modes of communication, such as gesture or mime)**
2. **In individuals with adequate speech, marked impairment in the ability to initiate or sustain a conversation with others**
3. **Stereotyped and repetitive use of language or idiosyncratic language**
4. **Lack of varied, spontaneous make-believe play or social imitative play appropriate to developmental level**

(C) Restricted repetitive and stereotyped patterns of behavior, interests, and activities, as manifested by at least one of the following:

1. **Encompassing preoccupation with one or more stereotyped and restricted patterns of interest that is abnormal either in intensity or focus**
2. **Apparently inflexible adherence to specific, nonfunctional routines or rituals**
3. **Stereotyped and repetitive motor mannerisms (e.g., hand or finger flapping or twisting, or complex whole body movements)**
4. **Persistent preoccupation with parts of objects**

■ **Delays or abnormal functioning in at least one of the following areas, with onset prior to age three: social interaction, language as used in social communication, or symbolic or imaginative play**

■ **The disturbance is not better accounted for by other disorders.**

Adapted from the Diagnostic and Statistical Manual of Mental Disorders, 4th Edition. *Used with permission.*

poseful hand skills and poor coordination of movements, after a period of at least five months of normal development after birth. In *childhood disintegrative disorder*, youngsters between ages two and ten regress after a period of normal development, losing previously acquired skills in communicating, relating, controlling their bladders or bowels, playing, and moving. In *Asperger's disorder*, children suffer severe, persistent impairment in social interaction and develop repetitive patterns for behaviors, interests, and activities, but do not experience significant delays in language development.

Developmental disorders appear to be the result of genetic or chromosomal defects. Magnetic resonance imaging (MRI) scans of autistic individuals have found abnormalities in specific areas of the cerebellum. There is no evidence that parenting styles contribute to autism or other PDDs, and such theories, once prevalent (and anguishing for the parents of these children), have been discredited. Rather than blaming parents, specialists in caring for youngsters with these disorders enlist their aid as important resources in helping their children reach their fullest potential. Families are viewed as a critical support system and parents as highly effective and valuable co-therapists and teachers.

Education, mandated by federal law as a right for youngsters with autism and pervasive developmental disorders as well as other conditions, is the most common "treatment." Specialized educational programs emphasize social, language, and behavioral skills, beginning as early as possible (before age four or five) and continuing through adolescence. Some parents have reported success from intensive behavioral therapy beginning early in a child's life. Early intervention can prevent the need for institutionalization for most youngsters with autism or PDD. The goal of educational programs for these children, as for others, is to prepare them to function as independently and as productively as possible in adulthood.

Group therapy, either with other autistic youngsters or with normal children, can help to improve social skills. Parents or teachers taught behavioral techniques can use them to increase learning and limit harmful behaviors. No medications directly treat autistic disorders, although child psychiatrists may prescribe antipsychotic medications such as haloperidol (Haldol) to decrease symptoms such as aggressiveness, temper tantrums, or withdrawal, or stimulants to reduce overactivity and improve attention. Clomipramine (Anafranil), a medication used for obsessive-compulsive disorder, reduced or stopped symptoms in at least one small study of autistic youngsters.

Dealing with children with these disorders can be extremely trying, regardless of how loving parents may be. From the time they first wonder if something is wrong with their infant, they go through an often grueling process of seeking assessments and getting opinions that may be contradictory or confusing. Those whose babies have an irregular sleep schedule or are extremely active and demanding when awake may struggle against constant exhaustion. Once infancy is over, parents may find it hard to cope with their child's inability to communicate, his or her impulsivity or lack of appropriate caution and fear, and emotional unresponsiveness. Difficulty in finding capable baby-sitters to provide occasional respites can compound the feeling of being overburdened.

As youngsters grow, parental worries shift to concerns such as hyperactive or destructive behavior, rejection by peers, lack of needed services, and continuing problems with eating or toileting. Parents often worry about their other children, who may resent the attention given to an autistic sibling, and about the ever-mounting toll on their own emotional and financial resources.

Problems are common in every family with an autistic child, yet some couples manage to cope so well that researchers describe them as *invulnerable* parents. Faced with extreme stress, they steadfastly refuse to be overwhelmed. Instead, many focus on learning as much as possible about the causes, assessment, and treatment of their child's disorder. Bolstered by this information, they manage to be realistic in terms of the prognosis, yet also consistently compassionate in dealing with their youngster. Often these invulnerable parents have dealt with other stresses in the past and can draw on the benefits of this experience.

The vast majority of parents, although not invulnerable, manage to cope fairly well, but some do "burn out." This is most likely to happen when they do not have access to adequate child services. Often a brief period of respite from daily care of the child can help. Counseling, including supportive psychotherapy and participation in support groups, are also essential in helping families who care for an autistic child at home. Families benefit not only from the opportunity to acquire useful information but also from being able to express the strong emotions that dealing with their child can generate.

Siblings, too, can benefit from counseling programs, which increase their understanding of autism, help them to explore both positive and negative aspects of their relationships with an autistic brother or sister, and teach them specific skills to improve their interactions.

YOUTH SUICIDE

To a parent, nothing may be more unthinkable or devastating than a child taking his or her own life. In the hollowness that grief leaves in their hearts, one question echoes again and again: Why? There are theories, speculations, research data. Ultimately, none provides an adequate answer. Some youngsters subjected to troubled or disruptive childhoods commit suicide; most do not. Most children who grow up in loving, stable homes do not take their own lives; some do. Suicide by the young is unpredictable. Often there is nothing parents should have noticed but didn't, nothing they could have done but didn't.

Although growing up never has been easy, these days it may be especially hard. Adolescence is a time of rapid change—physically, emotionally, intellectually, socially. The mobility of modern life, economic demands, sexual dangers, and substance abuse all add to the stress teens feel. According to some experts, many young people have a sense of immortality and do not believe, in their heart of hearts, that death is final; others may not be able to see any other way out of whatever difficulties they find themselves in.

Substance abuse may play a major role. Naturally impulsive, young people who drink or take drugs may be especially likely to act without thinking and take their lives in a burst of rage or frustration. Those who first turned to drugs or alcohol as a way of easing their anxiety or escaping pressures may feel increasingly desperate as they realize that their problems haven't gone away or that they are losing control over their drinking or drug use.

More than half of all teens who attempt suicide may be clinically depressed. Often they feel that no one needs them or cares. Many have suffered a loss: the end of a romance or friendship, the death of a loved one, their parents' separation or divorce. According to recent studies comparing adolescents who attempted suicide, those considered at risk, and other teens, two key factors are feelings about hopelessness and about suicide. Young people who had tried to kill themselves reported feeling more hopeless than any of the other groups and also answered "yes" more often to the question, "Have you ever felt life wasn't worth living?"

In one review of suicides over the last twenty years, 36 percent of the young people who tried to kill themselves were breaking up with a boyfriend or a girlfriend; 22 percent of the girls were pregnant or thought they were; 40 percent had a relative or close friend who had attempted suicide; and 72 percent were living in households in which at least one biological parent was absent because of separation, divorce, or death.

Studies have found a higher rate of parental alcoholism, family arguments, and disruption in the homes of young people who attempt or commit suicide. Sometimes teens who attempt suicide are locked in conflict with their parents over poor grades, skipping school, delinquent behavior, or drug use, and then encounter a final straw: being grounded, breaking up with a boyfriend or girlfriend, or any incident that intensifies their feelings of despair, humiliation, rejection, fear, and inadequacy. They may see suicide as an act of revenge, a way of getting back at parents or friends who have hurt them.

In some circumstances, the thought of suicide seems to capture the imagination of young people. When one suicide occurs in a community, it can spark a cluster of similar teen deaths. Studies of the impact of television movies on teen suicides have produced conflicting results, but some therapists feel that teens, more prone to peer influence, may kill themselves more often after watching televised movies that portray suicide victims sympathetically.

▼

Seeking help   The most obvious risk factor is a failed attempt at suicide. If nothing changes afterward, if young people do not get the help they need, if parents or friends believe there is no ongoing problem, teenagers often try again—and succeed in ending their lives. There are other indicators of danger as well. To determine if a youngster may be at risk, ask yourself whether your child:

- Has made dramatic changes, for no apparent reason, in familiar routines for eating, drinking, and sleep
- Seems increasingly moody, down, discouraged, sad, ashamed, or guilty
- Has threatened suicide
- Has produced writings or drawings revealing a preoccupation with death
- Has been having problems at school, including a decline in quality of work
- May be drinking or using drugs
- Has broken off old friendships
- Has broken up with a boyfriend or girlfriend
- Has dropped out of normal activities
- Seems bored or has become violent, hostile, or rebellious
- Has run away from home
- Is neglecting his or her personal appearance
- Seems to have difficulty concentrating
- Complains about physical symptoms, such as headache or fatigue
- Seems to be experiencing delusions or hallucinations
- Makes statements such as "It's no use" or "Nothing matters anymore"
- Gives away favorite possessions or cleans up a usually messy room
- Suddenly becomes cheerful after a depression.

If you answer "yes" to several of these questions, your number one priority should be contacting a mental health professional. You may want to call a local suicide hotline, a mental health crisis center, or your physician or therapist. In emergencies, call 911 and explain the circumstances to the dispatcher. If you have any reason to worry about suicide or self-destructive behavior, remove all weapons from your home. Teenagers in areas where handguns are readily available commit suicide with these weapons more often than those who cannot obtain guns easily.

Parents must be especially careful about not judging teenagers or dismissing their feelings as "stupid" or "silly." Troubled teens need to know that friends and family care about them and are not going to lecture or criticize them. Keep in mind that appropriate treatment can help as many as 70 to 80 percent of those at risk for suicide. Among young people, early recognition and treatment of depressive disorders and of alcohol and drug use could help to save thousands of lives each year. For more information on suicide and on what to do if a loved one may be considering suicide, see Chapter 22.

Psychiatric treatment

Mental health professionals who work primarily with children and teenagers use the same basic approaches as they might with adults, adapted to the age of the child and the nature of the problem. (The various types of therapy are described in depth in Chapter 27.) However, treating problems in young people always involves some unique concerns. Different mental health professionals deal with children and adolescents. They include school counselors, pediatric social workers, child psychologists, and child psychiatrists.

In preparing younger children for a first visit to a mental health professional, parents can explain that they are going to see a special type of doctor who will want to talk or play with them. One of several excellent books that can prepare a child for seeing a psychotherapist, *A Child's First Book about Play Therapy*, published by the American Psychological Association, explains that child therapists are special helpers or "worry doctors" who help children to deal with problems that make them feel bad. The authors stress to children that they can talk with a therapist about anything, that therapists keep a child's ideas or feelings private, and that as they play, draw, or talk with therapists, their problems will diminish. With older children or teens, parents can provide more explicit information, as well as reassurances that there is nothing shameful about "having problems that make you feel bad" or about seeing a therapist in order to feel better.

Both parents and children should realize that treatment is always tailored to the child's age, physical health, mental and emotional development, and language skills. Since children are less able to use abstract language than adults, play often serves as a means of expressing feelings, describing past events, and working through traumatic experiences. Young children and grade-schoolers may choose dolls, puppets, drawings, paintings, or clay. Teens may prefer creative writing, painting, or sculpting.

Often neither parents nor the child know precisely what is causing a youngster to feel or act in a troubling way. Discovering the nature and sources of the problem is an integral part of therapy. In assessing a child or adolescent, mental health professionals rely on many sources: the youngsters themselves, parents, and, with the parents' consent, teachers or caregivers. A physical examination may reveal medical conditions that may be related to a behavioral problem. Psychological evaluation, including intelligence and achievement tests, are helpful if there is any question about the child's IQ or learning ability. Once therapists diagnose what's wrong, they consider which treatment or combination of treatments might be most useful in helping the child to achieve greater control and mastery.

There have been very few systematic, prospective studies comparing various treatments in children and adults. In most cases, therapists weigh the relative risks and benefits, advantages and disadvantages, of various approaches and discuss them with the parents. The American Academy of Child and Adolescent Psychiatry has completed practice guidelines for the treatment of disorders such as AD/HD and conduct disorder, and parents might want to ask whether the recommendations are in line with these conditions. As in adults, children often benefit most from a combination of treatments. For example, those with oppositional or conduct disorders may do best with a combination of individual therapy, group play, and parental training in behavioral techniques. Youngsters with AD/HD respond best to medication plus behavioral modification.

Confidentiality is a subject that parents and children should discuss openly with a therapist. Adolescents usually are more sensitive about this issue than younger children. However, therapists should make clear that whenever youngsters are involved in potentially dangerous activities or have serious thoughts of harming themselves or others, their parents will be informed. Usually both parties—parents and youngsters—are told if or when information they have given the therapist will be passed on to the other. Often, rather than relaying information, therapists will bring parents and children together and encourage them to speak for themselves.

Siblings, teachers, and pediatricians may also play some role in the treatment process.

PSYCHOTHERAPY

Individual therapy uses attention, encouragement, and suggestion to instill hope and pride, to help children achieve greater control and mastery, to bolster their ability to cope, to enable them to return to normal developmental processes, and to encourage them to abandon or modify unrealistic expectations of themselves or their environment. Treatment, which may combine supportive and psychodynamic approaches, may be brief or long-term. Time-limited treatment, usually for six months or less, appears as effective as longer therapy for children with relatively recent and limited problems. Those who have suffered serious losses or neglect or who have more severe disorders may require more intensive and extensive treatment.

Individual psychodynamic therapy is more helpful for youngsters in emotional distress or struggling to deal with a stressful event, such as their parents' divorce or remarriage. Those with AD/HD or oppositional or conduct disorders usually do better in group or family therapy. Supportive psychotherapy seems especially helpful for children who do not have satisfying relationships with adults, sometimes because parents are unavailable physically or emotionally and sometimes because their symptoms make it hard to establish a good relationship.

BEHAVIORAL THERAPY

Behavioral approaches are the most widely studied forms of therapy for youngsters. Ideally, parents learn basic principles, such as giving tokens (stars, stickers, points) to reward good behavior and taking them away to discourage undesired behavior. The keys to success are cooperation by parents (and teachers, in some instances), focusing on specific behaviors, and making sure that consequences occur quickly and consistently after a specific behavior. Working with a therapist, parents also learn to give clear instructions and to use punishments, such as time-outs, effectively. In addition, therapists may teach problem-solving and self-control skills to youngsters who are aggressive, hyperactive, or impulsive.

Behavioral therapy is the most effective treatment for simple phobias, enuresis, and encopresis, and for the refusal to comply that occurs with oppositional defiant and conduct disorders. In AD/HD, behavioral therapy can help in both academic achievement and behavior. The drawbacks of behavioral therapy are that children may fail to generalize or to use what they have learned in one setting in other situations. In addition, they may not maintain their improvement over time unless there is continued parental involvement.

GROUP THERAPY

Since children are often more willing to share their thoughts with their peers than with adults, group therapy can be very helpful. In addition, many youngsters with mental disorders find it difficult to establish and maintain friendships. In a group, they can observe and practice social skills while also benefiting from companionship and mutual support.

Often combined with individual therapy or drug treatment, group therapy is usually tailored to the ages and needs of youngsters; group members are generally of similar ages and may have similar problems. Among the situations that respond best to group therapy are difficulty in getting along with peers, aggression, social timidity or withdrawal, and poor social or problem-solving skills. Groups have proven useful for treatment of eating disorders and substance abuse in teens. They are not suited to very hyperactive or aggressive youngsters, those with antisocial behaviors who may victimize other members, and those with psychotic symptoms.

Even very young children in the preschool years may benefit from groups. Since small children cannot verbalize extensively, these groups—which usually involve structured play—can serve as a means for teaching social skills and language. This may be particularly important for autistic or developmentally delayed youngsters.

For school-age children, groups may involve games and crafts. The therapist makes sure that playing does not become the sole focus of the group and uses cognitive problem-solving techniques, such as soliciting youngsters' ideas about how to deal with a conflict, or behavioral modification. If successful, children are able to use the skills learned in a group to form friendships elsewhere.

Because adolescents place such importance on their peers, groups are especially effective for teens. Indeed, many youngsters who do not have mental disorders or psychiatric problems can benefit from "human development" groups that focus on issues such as sexuality or stress.

PARENTAL COUNSELING

Often therapists recommend that parents attend educational programs, either alone or in groups, to learn about normal child development. Parents of youngsters with psychiatric or learning problems need to learn about the nature of their child's disorder, how to evaluate treatments, and how to manage difficult behavior. This approach helps parents to understand their child and his or her problems and to learn how to modify behavior that may be contributing to the current difficulties. Sometimes this serves as a first step into family therapy. Such training also helps parents to become advocates for their children, which may be necessary to ensure that they receive the schooling and treatment they need.

FAMILY THERAPY

The family is crucial in the treatment of any child or adolescent because what affects any one family member—whether it is the result of normal development, medical illness, a psychiatric disorder, or treatment—affects the entire family unit. Therapists may suggest counseling sessions that include parents along with the child who is undergoing treatment or the entire family. Meeting together with a therapist is particularly useful in helping families to improve the quality of their communication and interactions and to deal with life changes such as a divorce or remarriage.

Family therapy also helps when there is impaired communication among family members or when the problem is related to difficulty or a change in the family, such as adoption of another child or a parent's severe illness. If more than one member of the family is having problems, family therapy may be more efficient and effective than individual approaches.

Sessions may also teach parents some basic behavioral therapy principles that can help families negotiate and solve problems together. For example, a parent and teen may learn how to work out a written contract that spells out behaviors both agree to change, with specified consequences for failure to do so.

PSYCHIATRIC DRUGS

Medications can play a useful role in relieving symptoms of certain problems, such as AD/HD, depression, and certain anxiety disorders, enabling children to benefit from psychotherapy and other approaches. Because many medications have not been tested in children, often little is known about possible side effects or optimal doses.

The use of medication in children can be complicated. Every drug has more than one effect, and children metabolize and respond to drugs differently from adults. They may have rapid and unpredictable swings in blood levels of a medication, from too much to too little. In addition, youngsters are growing physically, mentally, and emotionally, and medication must not interfere with their development.

We feel that child psychiatrists are best qualified to prescribe and supervise the use of medications in children. They are most experienced in weighing the risks of a disorder with what is known about the relative efficacy and the side effects of medication. Frequent follow-ups are an important part of treatment.

Parents and, to whatever extent is possible, children should learn about how a specific medication works and what its effects and side effects are. Parents need to be informed about the complete range of possible effects, including those involving thinking and behavior as well as physical reactions, and must know when they should call the psychiatrist. It is critical that they be aware of any dangers of abuse or overdose. Except for certain anti-anxiety agents, psychiatric medications are not addictive. There is no evidence that children who take medications for a mental or emotional disorder are more likely to develop drug abuse problems later in life.

Medication schedules should be followed conscientiously, with parents supervising their children's taking of the drugs. Taking medications as directed often requires the cooperation not only of the youngster but also of the parents and possibly of teachers, too. If a child refuses medication, if parents don't believe that their child really needs a drug, or if school personnel cannot follow a schedule for giving medication, many of the potential benefits of drug therapy may be lost.

DAY TREATMENT

In general, youngsters do best with treatments that do not disrupt their daily lives, but some children and adolescents require more intensive care than outpatient visits to a therapist can provide. In a day treatment program they continue to live at home but spend all or part of the day in a specialized center that usually provides schooling as well as counseling. When children and teens have been hospitalized, day programs can help them to make the transition to their own or a foster or group home.

There are specialized intensive summer day treatment programs for children with AD/HD and other behavioral and learning problems. They provide positive social and recreational experiences for youngsters who might not otherwise be able to attend a summer camp. In addition, they provide some classroom instruction and an opportunity for staff members to assess the efficacy and side effects of medications.

HOSPITALIZATION OR RESIDENTIAL TREATMENT

Treatment at a residential facility may be best for youngsters with severe disorders or problems, such as substance abuse, aggression, running away, or self-destructive acts, that the family cannot manage. In general, youngsters need hospitalization only if there is active psychosis (for instance, if they hallucinate and lose touch with reality), a risk of their harming themselves or others, a need for systematic and detailed observation and evaluation, or when parents find it impossible to cope with the child, possibly because of extremely aggressive or disruptive behavior or drug dependence. The duration of hospitalization depends on the nature and severity of the problem as well as on practical concerns, such as health insurance coverage. Most stays tend to be fairly short, usually less than a month. Within the structured environment of a hospital or residential center, young people may learn about their problem, and participate in individual and group psychotherapy and family counseling, in addition to taking medication, if needed. After discharge, they may continue treatment at a day center or see a therapist on an outpatient basis.

▼

Impact on relationships

Many parents worry about their children's feelings, fears, and emotional well-being. Such concern comes with the territory of parenting. Parents of youngsters with psychiatric problems share these emotions but also may blame themselves needlessly for conditions that almost invariably have multiple, complex causes. The severity of an acute problem or the sheer unremittingness of a persistent disorder—along with the guilt and self-blame that so often accompany such problems—can create enormous tensions for parents and between parents, as well as uncertainties about what to do. Yet parents need to present a consistent, unified front so that they can nurture their youngsters and effectively handle daily challenges as well as cope with crises.

For parents with more than one child, there is worry about meeting the needs of the other youngsters, who may react to their brother's or sister's problem in various ways, from acting out, to becoming disruptive, to doing poorly at school, to becoming "too good" or withdrawing. Family therapy can be the ideal way of dealing with such issues. (Chapter 30 focuses on what happens within families when a loved one has a mental disorder, including the impact on siblings and parents.)

The issues for families vary according to the age of the child and the nature and severity of the problem. A lag in academic skills may cause great concern but have little impact on day-to-day family life. On the other hand, a severe behavioral or developmental disorder can shatter home routines, create an atmosphere of heightened tension, and lead to resentment and conflict.

Sometimes the process of obtaining a diagnosis—or a string of inconsistent diagnoses—is itself frustrating and upsetting. In certain disorders, seemingly mundane matters such as toileting, eating, or sleep patterns turn into intense and exhausting struggles. Although parents may feel great compassion for their child, the behaviors they have to deal with may be so emotionally trying that they have to struggle to control their own powerful feelings. Moreover, the more difficult or demanding a child's needs are, the harder it can be to find adequate child care so that parents can get much-needed time alone to renew their own relationship and bolster their coping ability.

Most families, including those facing extreme stress, do manage to cope. Various factors seem to help: ample information about their child's disorder so they can have realistic expectations, a feeling of partnership with the professionals involved in their child's care, occasional periods of respite, and empathy and support from families dealing with similar problems.

Nevertheless, when a child faces a serious difficulty, marriages typically show some strain. Partners may criticize each other's handling of the situation or have very different ideas about treatment. Some forms of therapy, such as behavioral techniques, require patience and consistency, often over a long period, and this, too, can be demanding. If spouses stop talking, distance themselves, or blame each other, the relationship can be jeopardized.

Counseling sessions—whether in the form of educational groups, one-on-one meetings with the child's therapist, or family therapy—can help parents to develop ways of meeting each other's needs for intimacy, sexuality, and emotional support. Parents often benefit from participating in the education and support groups that have been set up by groups such as Children with Attention Deficit Disorders (CHADD), the Learning Disabilities Association of America, and the Autism Society of America.

PART IV

Healing the Mind

27

The Talking Therapies

In the beginning there was only the word. Long before they had the knowledge, skill, or medicines to treat physical or mental illness or to relieve pain, healers listened to those who were suffering and offered reassurance and hope. A century ago Sigmund Freud, whose theories shaped modern psychiatry and psychology, discovered that words could do more than comfort: They could serve as a tool for exploring the unconscious mind. Since Freud's development of the first "talking cure," generations of therapists have created and refined an enormous variety of approaches and techniques that all have one thing in common: the power of the word.

The term *psychotherapy* refers to any type of counseling based on the exchange of words in the context of the unique relationship that develops between a mental health professional and a person seeking help. The process of talking and listening can lead to new insight, relief from distressing psychological symptoms, changes in unhealthful or maladaptive behaviors, and more effective ways of dealing with the world.

There are many different and distinctive forms of psychotherapy, and some are clearly more effective for certain problems, or for certain people, than others. Most mental health professionals today are trained in a variety of psychotherapeutic techniques and tailor their approach to the problem, personality, and needs of each person seeking their help. Because skilled therapists may combine different techniques in the course of therapy, the lines between the various approaches are often blurred.

This chapter outlines the most common and widely accepted forms of psychotherapy. The chapters on specific disorders in Part II explain how these therapies are used in treating different problems.

Basics of psychotherapy

Psychotherapy strives to influence thoughts, behavior, emotions, and attitudes through talking and other psychological techniques. Some people think that this makes psychotherapy different from "biological" treatment with psychiatric medications. Yet in psychotherapy, just as with drug therapy, the brain is the target. Only the approach is different. The ultimate goal is to change the way a person feels, thinks, acts, and relates to others so that he or she can discover and pursue new options, gain new insight into behavior, and acquire new skills for coping.

Mental health professionals today are endeavoring to apply therapeutic approaches with greater precision and consistency than in the past. However, psychotherapy never can nor will be as uniform as the standard treatments for many medical problems. No two patients or therapists are alike, and the art of therapy is as important as the science. In ways that research may never be able to quantify or qualify, the success of psychotherapy depends on the intangible factors involved in forging a connection, building trust, and establishing a cooperative partnership.

TRANSFERENCE

Individuals undergoing therapy unconsciously project or "transfer" their wishes, needs, hopes, and desires, which often are related to significant people in their past, onto their therapists. This transference of long-submerged feelings and thoughts reveals patterns of behavior that continue to cause emotional distress. In turn, therapists, who are just as human as those they help, project emotions, thoughts, and wishes from their own past onto their clients. This reaction is called *countertransference.* During therapy, mental health professionals constantly monitor their internal responses to make certain that they do not impose their values or interject their own concerns or issues into their interactions with those they are treating.

THERAPEUTIC ALLIANCE

The relationship that develops between the individual and the therapist—the so-called *therapeutic alliance*—allows them to work together in a cooperative manner. The individual must feel sufficiently comfortable with and trusting of the therapist to reveal what is troubling him or her and to be able to understand and accept the therapist's interpretations or analyses of the significance of particular events or behaviors. Without this trust, a person cannot confide his or her innermost feelings. It is the therapist's responsibility to nurture this alliance by being caring and respectful and by never emotionally, sexually, or financially exploiting those who seek help.

CONFIDENTIALITY

The relationship between mental health professionals and the individuals who seek their help is confidential. Therapists are bound by ethical principles not to divulge any information without the person's consent, and must seek permission if they want to share information with family members, another professional, or an insurance company. The wishes of those who refuse permission must be respected. The only exceptions are cases in which individuals are in danger of hurting themselves or others, whether in the form of suicide, violence, or the abuse of a child, a partner, or an elder.

EFFICACY

Careful scientific studies have shown that psychotherapy can indeed help overcome many mental disorders. However, it is not always clear which form of psychotherapy may be most helpful to which individuals for which problems. Thus, behavioral therapy has proved extremely beneficial in treating specific phobias, but supportive therapy also can be helpful. In many cases, a combination of several approaches, such as medication and psychotherapy, is most effective. The decision of which treatments to use often depends on the therapist's preferences and experience, as well as the individual's personality, preferences, and needs.

DURATION OF TREATMENT

Because of increasing pressures to contain costs, insurance companies and health care plans often limit the duration of psychotherapy as well as the amount of reimbursement for each session. At least in part because of these economic pressures, mental health professionals are adopting a "time-limited" attitude that aims at getting the most out of every session, regardless of the duration of treatment.

In some cases, even a single session of psychotherapy can make a difference. In the past, therapists viewed individuals who never returned after an initial session as treatment failures. In follow-up studies, however, these "dropouts" often said that the reason they didn't return was not because they weren't helped but because they were. The single meeting with a therapist had given them the reassurance, confidence, information, or insight that they needed to cope with the problem that had brought them to the therapist.

Brief psychotherapy is an excellent approach for individuals who are functioning well at work, have good relationships with others, can think in psychological terms, and are motivated to change. Time-limited treatment can foster changes in behavior and thinking, enhance coping skills, and instill a better sense of self. It provides an opportunity for the individual to begin a process of change that continues long after therapy is over, a process that can turn a half-lived life into a rich and fulfilling one. Those most likely to benefit are interested in solving immediate problems rather than in changing their basic character. Nevertheless, mental health professionals caution that it is very difficult to identify which individuals will benefit most from brief therapy. Sometimes dealing with a particular problem brings up underlying issues and problems that may require additional exploration.

The distinctive features of brief therapy include a focus limited to a central theme, problem, or topic, and time limits. Most clinicians set twenty-five sessions as a maximum, although some may go as high as forty. The therapist takes a more active role than in open-ended, long-term therapy.

The question of how much therapy is enough always depends on the individual and on the nature and severity of the problem. In one analysis that plotted improvement rates in a large number of previous studies as a function of time, 50 percent of patients showed significant improvement by the eighth session and 75 percent by the twenty-sixth. It may be that obvious symptoms tend to diminish fairly quickly, whereas substantive personality change may take longer.

Those whose disorders are more intractable or who need to deal with issues that go beyond their immediate problem may well benefit from long-term therapy. Given insurance coverage restrictions and depending on the type of health insurance they have or the health care plan they belong to, individuals or their families may have to assume the full cost of treatment if therapy sessions extend beyond a set number. Some, sadly, may not be able to afford the more extensive care they need.

Psychodynamic treatments

For the most part, today's mental health professionals base their assessment of individuals on a "psychodynamic" understanding that takes into account the role of early experiences and unconscious influences in *actively* shaping a person's behavior. This is the "dynamic" in psychodynamic. Psychodynamic treatments are among the most widely used psychotherapies, and many of the principles of psychodynamic therapy have been incorporated into other approaches.

PSYCHODYNAMIC PSYCHOTHERAPY

Goal	To provide greater insight into problems and bring about behavioral change
Techniques	Face-to-face interactions with therapist
	Development of a therapeutic alliance
	Free association
	Interpretation and clarification of what the individual says
	Focus more on the "here and now" than the distant past, as in psychoanalysis, although less so than in other brief therapies
Most likely to benefit	Individuals with sufficient understanding to experience and explore intense emotions
	Individuals with certain personality disorders
	Individuals with chronic mental disorders who want to deal with the psychological and social dimensions of their illness
Duration	Brief, consisting of fewer than twenty-five sessions, or longer term, lasting for several years

This approach, also called *insight-oriented, psychoanalytic,* or *exploratory* psychotherapy, uses free association, in which individuals report all thoughts that enter their mind (without censoring or dismissing them) as a way of discovering and understanding unconscious conflicts that arose in childhood and have continued into adulthood. These conflicts, which affect a person's patterns of behavior, feelings, thoughts, fantasies, and actions, may pit aggressive wishes against anxiety about retaliation, or a desire for sexual and emotional gratification against a fear of loss. In psychodynamic terms, libidinal wishes include all longings for happiness, excitement, pleasure, anticipation, or love. Aggressive wishes include the desire to destroy or the experiencing of pleasure from anger, hate, or pain.

As individuals talk, remember, and express intense feelings, the therapist listens without judging and interprets what they are saying. Often these interpretations reveal that the individual is using a defense mechanism, a maladaptive way of dealing with a difficult situation that interferes with psychological well-being. The most common defense mechanisms are:

- *Repression*, the underlying basis of all defense mechanisms, in which individuals keep threatening impulses, fantasies, memories, feelings, or wishes from becoming conscious.

- *Denial*, the inability to accept a painful reality, such as the death of a loved one or the diagnosis of a debilitating disease. This is not an unusual temporary reaction, but it can indicate a serious emotional problem if it persists for a prolonged period after the initial shock.

- *Rationalization*, which substitutes "good," acceptable reasons for the real motivations for our behavior.

- *Projection*, which attributes unacceptable feelings or impulses to someone else.

- *Reaction formation*, which occurs when an individual adopts attitudes and behaviors that are the opposite of what is really felt.

- *Displacement*, which redirects feelings from their true object to a more acceptable substitute.

- *Regression*, which is a return to a less mature and adaptive way of responding to overwhelming stress.

- *Splitting*, in which an individual who cannot cope with ambivalent feelings about others deals with these conflicting emotions by compartmentalizing such people as all good or all bad.

- *Undoing*, the substitution of one behavior for another for the sake of changing or modifying the original action.

- *Intellectualization* or *isolation*, an attempt to avoid painful feelings by taking an objective or abstract view of them.

In psychotherapy, individuals work toward developing more mature and adaptive ways of dealing with stressful situations. Since such mechanisms also ward off unpleasant emotions, they usually are helpful rather than harmful. They include:

- *Sublimation*, the redirection of any drives considered unacceptable into socially acceptable channels.

- *Humor*, which counters painful feelings by focusing on the comic aspects of a situation.

- *Altruism*, which takes a negative experience and turns it into a positive one.

- *Mastery and control*, in which individuals confront a painful situation directly and develop ways of facing it without feeling overwhelmed.

Psychodynamic psychotherapy may be brief, consisting of less than twenty-five weekly sessions, or long-term, with two or three sessions a week over a period of several years. Medications may be used as part of a combined treatment plan. Compared with psychoanalysis (described below), psychodynamic psychotherapy focuses more on the present than on the developmental origins of conflicts, and it does not center on transference issues.

Both brief and long-term psychodynamic therapy rely on the same principles as psychoanalysis, such as the importance of childhood experiences, unconscious influences on behavior, and transference. However, in short-term therapy the goals are more limited, and the therapist is more involved and active, pointing out denial or avoidance, expressing direct support, yet taking care not to be overly controlling. Long-term therapy aims at broader goals, and the therapist's approach may be more indirect. There has not been extensive or conclusive research on the relative benefits of short versus longer-term psychodynamic psychotherapy. Many questions remain unanswered, including whether longer-term therapy may result in greater or more enduring therapeutic gains.

Specific schools of psychodynamic psychotherapy have different roots and approaches to treatment. *Jungian* analysis, based on the theories of Carl Jung (once a student of Freud), pays greater attention to the mythical dimensions of dreams and fantasies. *Gestalt therapy*, developed by Fritz Perls, focuses on integrating emotions and hidden feelings into harmony in the here and now. *Human-potential* or *client-centered* therapy, largely developed by Carl Rogers, encourages individuals to explore their emotional needs, and, with the warm support of the therapist, to work toward self-actualization or realization of their greatest potential.

PSYCHOANALYSIS

Goal	To rework aspects of an individual's personality related to childhood conflicts
Techniques	Free association while lying on a couch
	Development of a therapeutic alliance
	Frequent sessions
	Focus on fantasies, transference, slips of the tongue
	Dream interpretation
Most likely to benefit	Individuals with the ability to understand, experience, and explore strong emotions
	Those whose problems stem from childhood conflict
Duration	Three to six years

Classical psychoanalysis, developed by Freud, is a complex, lengthy process that deals with long-repressed feelings and issues. Less widely used than briefer forms of psychotherapy, it remains an option best suited for high-functioning individuals who want to explore distressing patterns in their lives, such as chronic difficulties in establishing successful relationships.

Psychoanalysis is based on Freud's realization that the "psychic reality" of childhood events—the subjective experience of the individual, regardless of whether an event actually happened—is critical to development. Psychoanalysis uses techniques such as free association and dream interpretation to bring unconscious and unremembered experiences of childhood into consciousness. Awareness and understanding of the conflicts experienced in childhood (what is called the *childhood neurosis*) become the foundation for understanding and changing present behavior.

"Analysands" lie on a couch, looking away from the analyst, and free-associate, that is, they say whatever comes to mind. The analyst remains neutral and relatively passive in order to encourage transference, which is the key component of psychoanalysis. Through transference, individuals become aware of unconscious drives and emotions that have been troubling them. As the analyst makes interpretations that aid in this awareness, analysands are able to gain insight and modify their way of dealing with the world.

Modern psychoanalysis requires frequent meetings, usually four or five per week (Freud met with his patients six times a week), for an average of three to six years. This intensity is necessary for individuals to develop sufficient trust to explore their inner fantasy life. Traditionally, medications have not been combined with this approach, although some analysts are now experimenting with the use of antidepressants for individuals with depressive disorders who may be interested in psychoanalysis as a way of exploring troubling issues in their lives.

INTERPERSONAL THERAPY

Goal	To enhance relationships and social interactions and improve interpersonal skills
Techniques	Reassurance and support Clarification of feelings Emphasis on improving interpersonal communication and skills
Most likely to benefit	Individuals with major depression, including adolescents and the elderly Those with chronic difficulties developing relationships and interacting with others Individuals with dysthymia or bulimia Couples dealing with marital problems and depression
Duration	Twelve to sixteen sessions, longer for continuation or maintenance treatment for major depression

This approach, originally developed for research into the treatment of depression, focuses on relationships in order to help individuals deal with unrecognized feelings and needs and improve their interpersonal and communication skills. Unlike other psychodynamic treatments, it does not deal with the psychological origins of symptoms but focuses on current interpersonal problems. The supportive, empathic relationship that the person develops with the therapist, who takes a more active role than in other forms of psychodynamic psychotherapy, is the most crucial component of this therapy. The emphasis is on the here and now and on interpersonal rather than intrapsychic issues.

Interpersonal therapy (IPT) can be either brief or longer term and may be combined with medications, particularly in treating major depression. There are three phases of treatment. In the first, which may consist of one to three sessions, therapists gather diagnostic information, evaluate symptoms, assess the need for medication (as based on severity of symptoms, psychiatric and medical history, treatment response, and individual preference), and outline a framework for therapy. They look at an individual's beliefs, thoughts, dreams, or defense mechanisms mainly in terms of interpersonal relations and try to identify characteristic difficulties related to one of four problem areas: grief, interpersonal role disputes, role transitions, or deficiencies in interpersonal skills.

In the second or middle phase of treatment, therapists direct their attention to the specific problem area. For those suffering from unresolved grief, therapists may help them deal with their loss and develop new activities and relationships. If the problem involves disputes with a spouse, other family members, a friend, or co-workers, therapists help individuals explore the nature of the conflict and consider options for resolving it. Men and women going through transitions—starting or ending a relationship, moving, retiring, graduating, learning that they have a serious illness—may get help in recognizing positive and negative aspects of what they're leaving behind and what they're going toward. For those lacking in social skills, IPT focuses on providing help in starting or maintaining relationships. In the final phase of treatment, therapists help individuals recognize and reinforce what they have learned and develop ways of identifying and countering any symptoms of depression that may arise in the future.

Interpersonal therapy has proved especially effective in reducing the symptoms of major depression and improving an individual's relationships and social functioning. In comparisons of various treatments, the combination of IPT and medication has led to the best outcomes. In a three-year study of maintenance treatment for major depression, monthly IPT sessions without medication had a modest but significant beneficial effect, preventing the recurrence of depressive symptoms for a mean time of eighty-two weeks. The effects of more frequent (biweekly) IPT sessions are currently being studied.

In a review of the literature, IPT was described as "a promising but still not fully tested treatment" for depressed adolescents or elderly men and women, HIV-positive, depressed individuals, those with dysthymia or bulimia, those with mild depression diagnosed by a primary care physician, and couples dealing with depression and marital problems.

SUPPORTIVE PSYCHOTHERAPY

Goal	To maintain or restore an individual's highest possible level of functioning
Techniques	Concern, advice, reassurance, suggestion, reinforcement
	Little, if any, focus on transference
	Discussion of alternative behaviors
	Teaching of social/interpersonal skills
	Assistance in problem solving
Most likely to benefit	Healthy individuals in highly stressful situations
	Those with serious medical conditions
	Those with serious psychiatric disorders who are unable to benefit from other approaches
Duration	Brief (a single session or several sessions over a period of days or weeks) to very long term (over many years), depending on the nature of the problem

In a sense, any form of psychotherapy or counseling that offers reassurance, empathy, and education is supportive. However, mental health professionals distinguish between treatments that work toward change and those that help individuals through difficult situations, although in practice these approaches often overlap. Some compare change-oriented treatments to antibiotics used to eliminate a bacterial infection, whereas supportive psychotherapy is analogous to the indirect measures, such as bed rest, that help a person recover from a viral infection.

The goal of supportive psychotherapy is to help individuals to adapt and to return to their usual or previous best level of functioning to the extent possible given personality, life circumstances, ability, or illness. Although many people think of supportive psychotherapy as simply providing comfort and advice, the process is far more complex than that and can include many therapeutic techniques, among them education, suggestion, reassurance, reinforcement, setting limits, social skills training, and medication.

Although it may sound contradictory, supportive psychotherapy, which may be brief or long term, is used most often for those considered quite healthy and those considered quite ill in terms of mental well-being. Men and women with no psychiatric problems may temporarily feel unable to cope during a time of great stress, for example, after surviving an accident or learning that they have a serious physical illness. Supportive psychotherapy may speed their recovery, relieve stress-related symptoms such as disturbed sleep, strengthen self-awareness, and help them integrate and learn from their experience.

Supportive psychotherapy can also help those with severe or chronic psychiatric illnesses, such as schizophrenia, who lack the ability to communicate thoughts and feelings or who cannot handle the stress of change-oriented treatments. Therapists serve as surrogate emotional parents, and it often takes them months to establish a good working relationship with individuals who have these conditions. Once the therapists prove themselves safe, predictable, and reliable, they provide encouragement and direction and model skills for their patients, such as self-observation.

Supportive therapy draws on a psychodynamic understanding of the individual's development, conflicts, and current circumstances. Although therapists may make interpretations of what the person says or does and may offer insights that help to make the individual aware of unconscious factors associated with these behaviors, this is done only to a limited extent, if at all. The therapist's primary role is to serve as a trustworthy guide toward improved mental health and as a mentor who can help individuals face challenges or difficult decisions. In working with persons with schizophrenia, for example, a psychiatrist may provide reassurance that, with medication, frightening symptoms of psychosis can be controlled, and also help in sorting out issues such as whether to return to college or to move back into the family home.

There have been few scientific studies of supportive therapy per se, although the available data show that what therapists describe as "sophisticated support" can improve an individual's ability to function and can bolster mental well-being, sometimes almost as much as change-oriented therapies. In studies of individuals with anxiety disorders (see Chapter 7), for example, supportive therapy, based on psychodynamic principles and used along with medication, was as helpful as a combination of behavioral therapy and medication. It may be that both of these forms of therapy help by encouraging individuals to confront situations that they fear. Although medication is the most effective treatment for schizophrenia, the addition of supportive therapy has been shown to lead to somewhat better outcomes than certain medications alone.

Supportive therapy has proved very useful for many patients with medical illnesses such as ulcerative colitis and cancer. There also have been reports of beneficial effects, such as less pain, fewer complications, and briefer hospital stays, in those recovering from heart attacks and surgery. In such cases, supportive therapy typically includes education about the illness and its treatments, along with reassuring and encouraging the person to express feelings. Appropriate cognitive and behavioral techniques, described below, also may be used.

Cognitive-behavioral therapy

Although cognitive and behavioral techniques were developed as separate, distinctive approaches to psychotherapy, therapists increasingly use both methods in a *cognitive-behavioral* approach that recognizes the complex interrelation of thoughts and behavior.

COGNITIVE THERAPY

Goal	To identify and change distortions in thinking
Techniques	Identification of the individual's beliefs and attitudes
	Recognition of negative thought patterns
	Education in alternative ways of thinking
	Cognitive rehearsal
	Homework assignments
Most likely to benefit	Individuals with major depression, anxiety disorders, or other mental disorders, including eating disorders and substance abuse
Duration	Brief, usually involving fifteen to twenty-five sessions

The aim of this approach, which focuses on inappropriate or inaccurate thoughts or beliefs, is to help individuals break out of a distorted way of thinking. The techniques of cognitive therapy are based on the assumption that certain thought patterns, called *cognitive structures* or *schemas*, shape the way people react to the situations in their lives. Each individual's cognitive structures are unique, formed by factors such as physical health and early losses, achievements, and failures. These structures can interact with biological, social, and interpersonal factors and can lead to maladaptive behaviors, especially in times of stress.

Developed by psychiatrist Aaron Beck, M.D., and his colleagues, cognitive therapy has proved particularly effective for persons with depression. As Beck found, very often individuals who are depressed have three major thought patterns, which he called the *cognitive triad*: a negative view of themselves, a negative interpretation of experience, and a negative view of the future.

During therapy, individuals learn to recognize distorted ways of thinking that produce negative attitudes. Some of the most common are:

- *All-or-nothing (dichotomous) thinking,* in which an individual sees things only in terms of extremes. For example, if a person gains two pounds, he concludes that he is fat and utterly lacking in willpower.

- *Magnifying* or *minimizing,* in which an individual either over-states or underestimates the significance of an event. For example, a sales representative concludes that not meeting a single monthly sales quota means that she is incompetent and deserves to be fired or, when she does exceed a sales goal, downplays it as no more than a lucky break or a fluke.

- *Overgeneralization,* in which an individual makes far-reaching, global conclusions based on a single interaction. A college student who does badly on a test may say, "I'm stupid; even if I studied harder, I could never figure this stuff out." In addition to this nega-tive self-view, he might take a negative view of his entire academic experience and see all his classes as too difficult, or, looking ahead, may think, "I'll probably flunk out of college—and even if I squeak by, I'll probably never get a decent job."

- *Arbitrary inference,* in which an individual draws a mistaken con-clusion from an experience. When a coworker suggests a revision in a memo or report, for example, the person concludes that the co-worker considers her incompetent.

- *Selective abstraction,* in which individuals base their view of themselves or a situation on a single negative detail taken out of context. Thus, someone who knocks over a drink at a party con-cludes that he is hopelessly clumsy and that the entire evening was a humiliating experience.

- *Personalization,* in which individuals see events that have nothing to do with them as somehow reflecting on them. A waiter's surli-ness, for example, may be interpreted as testimony to their own unattractiveness or lack of appeal.

- *Automatic thoughts,* spontaneous negative statements directed at the person that break into his or her stream of consciousness. Typical ones include "You're stupid," "You can't do anything right," or "You've screwed up again."

Cognitive therapy helps people to identify and restructure these negative ways of thinking. One specific strategy is cognitive re-hearsal, in which individuals envision a troubling situation, imag-ine how they would master it, break this process down into small, manageable steps, and rehearse each step mentally. Therapists may also use behavioral techniques for these problems, such as exposure therapy and social skills training.

Cognitive therapy is relatively brief, usually requiring ten to twenty highly structured sessions. The focus is on problem-solving in the here and now. Psychoeducation is a major component of therapy, with therapists teaching individuals new ways of thinking about current dilemmas and managing problems in the future. Homework assignments may include monitoring thoughts, keeping a diary, and performing specific activities. For example, a depressed woman who has pulled away from her friends might keep a diary of all her activities during one complete week. After reviewing the diary, her therapist may "prescribe" certain tasks for her, such as telephoning a friend or going out in a group. As she does so, she makes notes of her expectations (negative or positive) and the outcomes of these social encounters. At the next session she reviews her notes with the therapist, who may point out that most of the experiences turned out pleasantly even when her expectations were bleak. In the course of therapy, her confidence grows, and the therapist assigns her more challenging tasks. The diary serves as a reminder of successes, and when something negative does occur, helps to put that experience into perspective.

In addition to treating depression, cognitive therapy combined with behavioral approaches has proved beneficial in treating anxiety disorders, including panic attacks, social phobia, and generalized anxiety. Although its use has been less extensively studied in other conditions, it has shown promise in the treatment of eating disorders, substance abuse, chronic pain, and possibly personality disorders.

BEHAVIORAL THERAPY

Goal	To substitute healthier ways of behaving for maladaptive patterns used in the past
Techniques	Behavior modification
	Systematic desensitization
	Relaxation or social skills training
	Graded exposure or flooding
	Modeling
	Paradoxical intention
Most likely to benefit	Individuals who want to change habits
	Those with anxiety disorders, such as phobias or panic attacks
	Those with substance abuse or eating disorders
Duration	Brief, usually involving less than twenty-five sessions

Behavioral therapy focuses not on what individuals say but on what they do. The premise is that, like all behavior, distressing psychological symptoms are learned responses that can be modified or unlearned. Some therapists believe that changing behavior also changes the way people think and feel. As they put it, "Change the behavior, and the feelings will follow."

Behavioral therapies work best for disorders characterized by specific abnormal patterns of acting, such as alcohol and drug abuse, eating disorders, anxiety disorders, and obsessive-compulsive disorder. Often they are used in combination with other approaches, especially cognitive therapy.

A basic concept in behavioral therapy is conditioning. As Pavlov demonstrated, individuals learn to respond in a consistent way to a specific stimulus, just as his dogs learned to salivate at the sound of a bell even when no food was forthcoming. In his landmark research, the psychologist B.F. Skinner, who demonstrated that the environment alters voluntary behavior, introduced concepts such as reinforcement, punishment, and stimulus control. He theorized that the environmental consequences of a particular behavior determine which of these behaviors are strengthened over time and which are extinguished.

Social-cognitive learning theory, at present the most widely accepted theoretical foundation for behavioral therapy, incorporates both Pavlovian and Skinnerian theories but moves beyond them to explore the interaction among environment, behavior, and cognitive processes. The basic techniques of behavioral therapy include:

- *Behavior modification,* which focuses on a negative habit or behavior, such as a child's disobedience, and aims to reduce or eliminate it by the use of reinforcement; that is, rewarding a desired behavior or punishing unwanted ones. For example, parents can learn to use "time-outs" when a child disobeys and to provide reinforcements, such as stickers or tokens that can be traded in for a special reward like an outing, for good behavior.

- *Systematic desensitization,* which teaches individuals how to reduce or control fear triggered by specific stimuli. People afraid of flying might first look at pictures of planes in flight and use relaxation techniques to diminish the feelings of anxiety or panic that these evoke. They then might imagine themselves flying and learn to control any anxiety associated with this imagined flight, usually by means of relaxation techniques. Gradually they build up to more challenging situations, such as going to an airport, then actually getting on a plane, then taking a short flight. This approach, although still used with extremely fearful individuals, is now employed less frequently than exposure therapy for the treatment of phobias.

- *Relaxation training,* which helps individuals to control their physical and mental state. Although there are many different techniques, most involve the alternate tensing and relaxing of different muscle groups, along with visualization of a pleasant scene or the use of a simple mantra to control distracting thoughts. With practice, often with an instructional audio- or videotape, most people master the basics quite quickly. (Chapter 29 provides more information on relaxation techniques.)

- *Exposure therapy,* which involves gradual stages of direct exposure to a feared object or situation to control anxiety without the use of relaxation techniques. Most often used in treating phobias, including agoraphobia, this approach, which has several variants, always begins with the construction of a hierarchy of feared situations. Thus, in agoraphobia, a house-bound individual may prepare a list of increasingly fearful situations—for example, first walking a few yards from the front door, then walking half a block, then walking a full block. Each day the person walks as far as possible until he feels mildly anxious. He repeats this same walk daily until the anxiety eases, then begins to walk further. A diary records daily progress, which tends to be slow at first. Although most individuals experience setbacks, eventually they make faster and faster progress. In some cases a therapist may accompany a person to a feared situation—for example, into an elevator—and provide direct support by challenging the person's distorted thoughts of danger. Exposure therapy may also be conducted in groups made up of individuals with similar fears.

- *Flooding,* which exposes individuals to whatever they fear most and keeps them in this situation until their fear dissipates. In this way, they learn that the consequences they dread are not going to occur. Thus, persons with a phobia about heights might go to the top of a high building (usually accompanied by the therapist), face the fear of something awful happening, and feel their anxiety ease when it doesn't. This approach is quicker than graduated exposure, but it causes such extreme anxiety that it is no longer widely used.

- *Modeling,* a procedure in which a therapist performs a desired behavior that individuals then copy. As they master the desired behavior in therapy sessions—for example, directly expressing a negative emotion—they are encouraged to do the same at home and in other situations.

- *Social skills training,* a process that begins by identifying undesirable behaviors, such as avoiding eye contact or speaking too softly or too loudly, and then teaches individuals new ways of acting. Basic techniques of this training are modeling and rehearsal, often in a group setting so that individuals can try out the new behaviors and act out real-life problems before others under a therapist's supervision.

- *Paradoxical intention,* in which a person is encouraged to engage in whatever behavior he is trying to stop. For example, a compulsive hand-washer might be instructed to wash even more frequently. This helps because it often illustrates the irrationality of the behavior and reduces resistance to change.

Behavioral medicine utilizes the techniques of behavioral therapy for the relief of medical problems, such as hypertension, insomnia, or chronic pain. In particular, biofeedback, which uses devices that detect subtle changes in brain waves or muscle tension, has proved beneficial for such conditions. Other strategies, including yoga, meditation, and deep muscle relaxation, also can be helpful.

Couples, marital, and family therapy

Goal	To change relationships, improve communications and interactions, and learn better ways to resolve conflicts
Techniques	Basic approaches of supportive, cognitive-behavioral, psychodynamic, or interpersonal therapy
Most likely to benefit	Couples or families who want to change their basic ways of interacting Children or teenagers with mental disorders or troubling psychological or behavioral symptoms
Duration	Weeks to months

In individual psychotherapy, the focus is on the person. In couples, marital, and family therapy, the unit or system is the focus. However, these forms of treatment are not mutually exclusive. Depending on the nature of the problem, therapists may suggest a combination of individual and couples or family therapy.

Although some mental health professionals work with individuals as well as with couples and families, many specialize in this type of therapy. Marriage and family therapists, who may be psychiatrists, psychologists, social workers, or nurses, have a graduate degree plus at least two years of supervised training in dealing with relationship problems. The American Association for Marriage and Family Therapy provides referrals to local therapists with this expertise. (See the Resource Directory at the back of the book.)

Just as it can be difficult to determine when an individual's symptoms are serious enough to warrant professional treatment, it can be hard for couples or families to determine whether they should seek help for their problems. The complaints may seem trivial: a wife feeling that her husband doesn't pitch in or pick up after himself; a husband thinking that his wife nags him constantly; parents uncertain how to deal with a child's unruliness or defiance. However, trivial complaints can sometimes be indications of a more serious underlying problem. As with individual symptoms, the key issue is how severe or how enduring the difficulty is. If it is serious enough to interfere with the couple's or family's normal functioning, or if it persists day after week after month, it may signify or lead to deeper problems.

Couples who are having difficulties in their relationship may seek out a marital therapist on their own. Sometimes therapists treating an individual recommend couples or family therapy as an additional form of treatment. Very often families do not seek family counseling themselves but are steered to therapy after a child is diagnosed as having a problem, such as a conduct disorder, by the child's therapist, school counselor, or pediatrician. As always, it is important that couples or families choose mental health professionals with whom they feel comfortable and whom they can trust and work with cooperatively. (Chapter 4 provides guidelines on finding a therapist.)

Therapists who work with a couple or a family look beyond an individual's feelings or behavior to the impact of these feelings or behavior on others. This *systems orientation* is not simply a therapeutic method but is an important conceptual way of evaluating human problems in the context of a couple, a family, or a larger group. Systems theory operates on the assumption that all couples and families have both strengths and vulnerabilities and are affected by their interactions with larger social systems, such as school or the workplace. It recognizes that any couple or family can run into difficulties in certain situations or at certain stages of family or individual development, difficulties that range from external stresses, such as financial setbacks or the loss of a job, to an internal crisis, such as the illness or injury of a family member. A comprehensive discussion of systems theory is beyond the scope of this book, but knowing some of its key principles can be helpful to those considering or engaged in couples and family therapy. These include:

Context. According to systems theory, a change or a mental or emotional problem in any one individual always affects the other family members *and* the family as a whole. For example, if a husband becomes depressed, his wife may try to cheer him up. He may find this irritating and angrily tell her to leave him alone. When she does, he feels more isolated and despondent than ever, and she feels frustrated and helpless. In turn, their child may begin to misbehave as a way of getting more attention or as a reaction to the heightened tension at home.

Interaction. Systems theory emphasizes the importance of the interplay between biological, psychological, and social factors and family transaction patterns—the processes by which family members communicate and relate to each other. These processes are given as much attention as the content of a specific problem.

Fit. From a systems perspective, behavior is not normal or abnormal in itself but must be considered in relation to the fit between an individual and family and the context or psychosocial demands of a situation. Thus, a passionate display of emotion that would be considered normal and welcome in one family may be entirely inappropriate in another one.

Causality. Systems theory does not take a linear perspective and look at a particular cause as having a particular and direct effect. Rather, it considers that psychological problems develop as the result of a circular process involving mutual reinforcement. For example, when parents start having more than their usual number of disagreements, one of their children may "act out" by skipping school or getting into playground brawls. Forced to focus on the youngster, the parents stop fighting and tension in the home eases.

Triangulation. According to systems theory, there is a tendency for any two-person system, such as a couple or a parent and a child, to draw in a third person whenever tension develops. Every time a couple has an argument, for example, one spouse may turn to his or her parent for support or comfort, interfering with the couple's ability to learn how to resolve problems on their own.

Adaptability. In evaluating couples and families, therapists consider various components of functioning. One of the most important is adaptability, which refers to the ability of a couple or family to respond flexibly to changing demands or circumstances while also maintaining stability, predictability, and consistency. Some families are extremely rigid and find any change difficult; others are so chaotic in their organization that change seems the norm rather than the exception.

Cohesion. This system refers to the balance between connectedness and separateness in a couple or family. There is no single ideal for either of these components of functioning, which often reflect the stages of the relationship, the ages of the children, and cultural as well as personal values. However, a family's normal adaptability or cohesiveness may not work in certain situations. Thus, a family in which each person usually fends for himself in a highly independent manner may find it hard to cope when a crisis, such as the loss of their home in a fire or flood, forces them to pull together. Family therapy may help them acknowledge their interdependence and can offer guidance on how to provide mutual support and work cooperatively.

COUPLES OR MARITAL THERAPY

According to the American Association for Marriage and Family Therapy, at least one out of every five couples in this country would benefit from professional counseling. After moving in together, two partners, married or not, may find themselves fighting constantly about money and possessions. A husband's intense jealousy may be making both him and his wife miserable. Over the years, one or both partners may lose interest in sex. In each of these situations, couples or marital therapy can be helpful.

Couples who seek help may be heterosexual or homosexual, married, living together, contemplating marriage, or committed to each other in some other fashion. Depending on the circumstances and nature of the problem, one or both partners also might undertake individual psychotherapy.

Couples counseling tends to be relatively brief, lasting for a period of weeks to months. Common issues include communication difficulties, sexual problems, and differing expectations of the relationship. The goal is to identify and resolve specific problems as quickly as possible. If the issues are primarily sexual, sex therapy may be advised. If children are involved, marital therapy may lead to family therapy. However, since couples often enter therapy because of a crisis or estrangement, the two partners may not be equally committed to overcoming their difficulties and saving their relationship. If the partners decide to end the relationship, the focus may shift to divorce mediation.

Therapy typically begins with the partners identifying specific problems or areas in which they would like to see some change. A husband may complain that his wife is always berating him for not doing his share of child care, while the wife may feel overwhelmed by the demands of their young children. The therapist may help them to identify specific target behaviors that need to be changed and contract with each other to modify these behaviors in small, specific ways. For instance, the husband may agree to take over responsibility for giving the youngsters their evening baths. In return, the wife agrees to allow him fifteen minutes of peace and quiet to regroup when he gets home. As therapy continues, the couple makes more such changes, while also discussing their hopes and expectations, their prior family experiences, their role expectations about men and women, changing social norms for gender roles, and their needs for both intimacy and independence (see the box, "Lessons from Couples Therapy," on page 722).

Recent research indicates that the relationships of about two-thirds of those who receive counseling do improve—both in the couples' own judgment and according to objective measures of marital satisfaction. Whenever partners find themselves struggling to stay close, a well-trained counselor can help by spotting destructive behavior patterns and viewing troubling situations in a new light. Therapy often helps stop spouses from completely destroying the relationship. At the least, it can help both partners decide whether to stay together.

Mental health professionals working with couples always tailor their advice to the individuals and their unique situation. However, they often stress the importance of some fundamental principles for strengthening or saving a relationship, such as:

- Make sure your expectations are realistic. Persons who assume that their partners will always agree with them, automatically see their point of view, or be able to meet all of their needs are doomed to disappointment because no one could ever live up to such expectations.

- Train yourself to notice what's right with your partner rather than what's wrong.

- Learn to negotiate for what you want. One effective approach is offering your mate what he or she wants in return.

- Look for the problem behind the problem. Often an affair or a lack of sexual interest is merely a symptom; the real question is why this problem has developed.

- Keep your perspective. Uncapped toothpaste tubes or socks on the floor may be annoying, but are they worth a fight?

- Rather than thinking of all the things your partner is or is not doing, focus on what *you* can do to make your marriage better.

FAMILY THERAPY

Family therapy, by simplest definition, is psychological treatment involving a person identified as the patient or client and at least one member of his or her family. Often the entire family is involved. The therapist may meet with various family members separately, as well as with the entire family. The focus is on the *interaction* between individuals rather than on processes within a single person's psyche or even on the content or nature of a specific problem.

There is limited research concerning situations in which family therapy is the best option, and most clinicians recommend this approach on the basis of their experience and judgment. It seems particularly helpful when there are communication or interaction problems within a family, especially when these develop at a significant stage, such as a remarriage or after the birth of a new sibling. Family therapy is an efficient approach when more than one individual in a family has a problem or when a family is "scapegoating," that is, blaming complex problems on one of its members rather than acknowledging the ways in which others in the family contribute to these problems. For individuals who are not motivated to participate in individual therapy or are wary of it, family therapy may seem less threatening, and it can prove to be just as effective, if not more so, than individual therapy. Family therapy is also extremely beneficial when one family member has a serious mental illness, such as recurrent depression or bipolar disorder.

Lessons from couples therapy

Arguing is not in itself a sign of trouble in a relationship. According to a report from the National Institute of Mental Health, couples who fight fairly and effectively have a 50 percent lower divorce rate than those who haven't mastered the art of disagreeing. In an ongoing study of 150 couples from premarriage through the first ten years of marriage (the highest risk period for divorce), researchers found that "nondestructive" arguing lowers the likelihood for physical violence, helps couples stay together longer, and benefits the children by modelling negotiating skills and preparing them to build good intimate relationships as adults.

The art of arguing is a skill, like bicycle riding, that anyone can master with time, patience, and plenty of practice. Here are some guidelines:

☐ Start your sentences with "I," not "you." Instead of attacking with a statement like "You're jealous and immature," say "I feel hurt when you quiz me about my old relationships."

☐ Focus on the issue at hand.

☐ Don't embarrass each other by fighting in front of others.

☐ Avoid generalizations, such as "You always interrupt me."

☐ Be fair. Whenever there's a cheap shot, one of you should stop the fight by crying "Foul!"

☐ Think before you open your mouth.

☐ Learn to listen. Rather than thinking about what you're going to say next, tune in to your partner's words, gestures, or expression.

☐ If you can't come to terms on a particular issue, agree to disagree or to keep talking about your differences in the future.

Many marital disputes center on money. While it may make the business world go round, money has the opposite effect on marriages, knocking them off their tracks, bringing them to a halt, turning them inside out. More money doesn't necessarily make things better. The amount of money couples have has almost nothing to do with why they fight about it. Couples are just as likely to have money conflicts whether they're earning $20,000 or $200,000. Attitudes are as important as assets. Money is a metaphor for power, self-esteem, and love. What matters most is what money means to both partners: Does each person use money to meet emotional needs? Who decides how the money is spent? Who keeps track? Until they resolve these issues, couples may quarrel over money as long as they are together.

Here are some guidelines for tackling money issues:

☐ Try to understand that having different values or expectations about money doesn't make one of you right and the other wrong.

☐ Recognize the value of unpaid work. A spouse who's finishing school or taking care of the children is making an important contribution to the family and its future.

☐ Go over your finances together so you have a firm reality base for what you can and can't afford.

☐ Talk about the financial goals you hope to attain five years from now. Set priorities to meet them.

☐ Set aside money for each of you to spend without asking or answering to the other.

Like every other aspect of a relationship, sex evolves and changes over the course of marriage. The red-hot sexual chemistry of the early stages of intimacy invariably cools down. Even among happy couples, at least 40 percent report a reduction of sexual interest and desire over the course of time. Yet, according to the National Opinion Research Center at the University of Chicago, the happiest couples have sex more often (74.8 times a year) than unhappily married pairs (who have sex 42.9 times a year).

What matters most isn't quantity alone, but the quality of sexual activity and intimacy. Are both partners satisfied with their sexual relationship? Does one partner always initiate sex? Do the partners talk about their preferences and pleasures? Sexuality, like personality, is dynamic and changes throughout life. Do the partners acknowledge and adapt to these changes? Do they feel sufficiently at ease with each other to discuss anxieties about sex? The answers to these questions can determine how sexually gratifying a marriage is for both spouses. Many couples do not realize that sexual problems, like others, are both common and treatable. Chapter 13 discusses the most common sexual disorders and offers guidance on seeking help.

It helps to educate the entire family about the illness, minimizes feelings of guilt and scapegoating, and helps the individual with the disorder and the family to find constructive methods of coping.

There are many different approaches to family therapy. Some emphasize problem-solving and tend to be brief, focused, and highly pragmatic. Others are more exploratory or insight-oriented. In clinical practice, therapists often combine techniques from the various approaches. Family therapy, like individual therapy, may be brief or longer-term. Brief treatment is most useful for a specific, focused problem, such as a school phobia (see Chapter 26). Very often a child-centered problem is what brings a family into therapy, and once this difficulty is addressed, the focus switches to a marital problem. The major approaches include:

- *Structural family therapy,* which emphasizes the importance of family organization for the functioning of the family unit and the well-being of its members. This approach, the most widely used and studied, views symptoms as the result of an imbalance in family structure. A family therapist counseling a family with a parent who has a substance abuse disorder, for example, may find that a child has crossed over the appropriate boundaries and taken on parental responsibilities. In therapy, the family comes to recognize what has been going on in the *structure* of the family. The goals are to reorganize this structure by shifting the relative positions of the members, enhancing parental leadership, creating clear boundaries, and promoting more adaptive coping. The emphasis is on the present and on action and change, not on exploring the origins of a problem.

- *Strategic* or *systemic family therapy,* which views a problem as both a symptom and a response to family interactions. This approach pays special attention to the family's unsuccessful attempts to solve its problems, which may inadvertently make them worse or create new difficulties. Thus, the parents of a teenage girl with anorexia nervosa may spend a great deal of time buying and preparing special foods to entice her to eat more, a response that only intensifies the household's focus on eating. The therapist may explain that such attention only reinforces the child's anorexia, and may recommend that they not allow her anorexia to dominate daily life or to dictate eating patterns for the entire family.

  Strategic family therapy tends to be practical, focused, and action-oriented. The therapist helps the family develop a clear plan and initiate change to get "unstuck" from the patterns of interacting that have been perpetuating the problem. One specific technique used in this approach is paradoxical instruction, in which the therapist makes a recommendation that seems to oppose or contradict the stated goals but actually serves to move the family toward them. For example, if the family complains about a lack of communication, the therapist may urge them to do even less talking, knowing that ultimately this will overcome their resistance to communication and help them to become more open. Paradoxical instruction requires skillful therapists but can be useful when families are resistant to more straightforward techniques.

- *Behavioral family therapy*, which views problem behavior as the result of reinforcement through family attention and rewards. Its goal is specific behavioral change. The therapist serves as an educator, model, and reinforcer, teaching negotiating and problem-solving skills and guiding the family in learning more effective ways of dealing with one another, often by reinforcing desired behavior in a positive way through acknowledgment and approval. For example, if the problem is bad conduct, parents would use negative reinforcers, such as time-outs, when a child disobeys and positive reinforcers, such as an incentive chart in which they might agree to spend extra time with the youngster after he earns a certain number of stars or stickers.

- *Psychoeducational family therapy*, which looks at problems in terms of stress and adaptive challenges. This approach has proved very helpful for families with a child with schizophrenia or another serious or chronic problem, such as eating disorders, attention-deficit/hyperactivity disorder (AD/HD), or depression. It is also used for families who are dealing with unexpected challenges, such as divorce or remarriage. Its goal is to reduce stress and help families adapt. Therapists serve as "respectful collaborators" who provide useful information about the psychological issues the family is facing and offer support and practical guidelines for handling a crisis, solving problems, and reducing stress. This approach has been used in one-time consultations with an individual family and in multifamily groups that meet at critical transitions or stages, such as shortly after the diagnosis of a mental illness or a child's discharge from a psychiatric facility.

- *Psychodynamic family therapy*, which applies psychodynamic as well as family system theories to therapy. This approach traces problems in a family to unresolved conflicts or losses in the parents' families of origin—for example, child abuse or divorce. Its goals are to confront and resolve these issues and to promote individual and family growth. Therapists work toward greater insight by family members, particularly the development of conscious awareness of the links between the dynamics that operated in their families of origin and those of the present.

- *Multigenerational family therapy*, which focuses on how current patterns in families repeat the past, rather than emphasizing unresolved conflicts as in psychodynamic family therapy. As the parents develop insight into their families of origin, they recognize the impact on their own nuclear families. Grandparents may be included in the sessions, which look at intergenerational difficulties and patterns of interpersonal behavior.

- *Experiential family therapy,* which sees symptoms as nonverbal messages that develop as a reaction to current problems in communication. Therapists work to change interactions in sessions in which family members share their feelings, engage in role-playing, and learn ways of communicating more spontaneously and nondefensively.

Group therapy

Goal	To change ways of interacting with others and relieve distressing psychological symptoms
Techniques	Basic approaches of supportive, cognitive-behavioral, psychodynamic, interpersonal or psychoanalytic therapy
	Self-disclosure and catharsis
	Sharing of insight and information
	Feedback from peers and the therapist
Most likely to benefit	Individuals who have a similar mental or physical disorder
	Adolescents
	Hospitalized psychiatric patients
	Families of individuals with mental disorders
Duration	Brief to long-term

There are many types of group therapy, using a variety of methods that range from role-playing to free conversation to sensitivity exercises. This section deals only with groups led or facilitated by mental health professionals. Lay groups—which are discussed in Chapter 29—operate on many of the same principles as psychotherapy groups and use similar techniques, but they are not led by a therapist or a team of co-therapists.

Individuals with problems such as substance abuse, compulsive gambling, social anxiety, or chronic illness may participate in both psychotherapy and support groups. In both settings, the members of these homogeneous groups play a crucial role themselves. Because they are too knowledgeable to "con" one other, they quickly spot a statement that doesn't ring true with their own experience. Thus, binge eaters might confront and challenge a group member who denies gorging and vomiting by asking about the amount of money he or she spends on food or how much time is spent thinking about food. The therapist also plays a critical role by helping the group to move beyond confrontation and confession toward insight and change.

Group therapy, the most widely used form of psychotherapy today, works toward the same goals as individual therapy: self-understanding, self-acceptance, and the modification of distressing behavior. Rigorous studies have shown that it is often as effective as individual therapy. Indeed, for some people, it can be even more effective because it allows them to see themselves as others do, to explore the motivations and personalities of others as well as themselves, and to learn new ways of interacting within a supportive environment.

The therapist organizes each session, prescribes exercises within the session, establishes ground rules, resolves conflicts between members, and provides summaries of the sessions. By their very nature, groups create a wide range of emotionally charged situations in the here and now. The members may find themselves struggling for dominance, vying for the therapist's attention or approval, and revealing attitudes and behaviors, such as arrogance or obsequiousness, that might well stay hidden under other circumstances. Individuals in a group almost invariably act out the problems they have with other people and receive immediate feedback from the therapist and others in the group.

As they observe themselves and others, group members become conscious of blind spots—aspects of their behavior that are visible to other people but that they were not aware of—and develop a better sense of how their behavior affects others' feelings and opinions. As they come to understand the way in which they are regarded, their sense of self-worth alters, and they begin to take greater responsibility for what they say and do, gradually coming to believe in their ability to change. This entire process is likely to be intensely emotional. In fact, the more emotional and "real" it is, the greater the potential for change.

Mental health professionals have identified several other key therapeutic factors in group therapy that contribute to improvement in psychological well-being. They include:

Self-disclosure. Revealing personal information to a group fosters feelings of acceptance and belonging.

Insight and information. As they talk and listen, group members gain a better understanding of themselves. If the groups include lectures or discussions of particular aspects of a disorder by the therapist, more formal education may also occur. Members also freely offer advice to one another.

Cohesiveness. As they share their problems, group members develop a sense of belonging and being valued. This camaraderie grows out of acceptance of one another, support, and the meaningful relationships that form as the group works together. For individuals who may not have had much experience in "belonging," the experience of being a valued, participating member of a group can be very beneficial.

Lessons in relating to others. As they interact, group members learn how to adapt and communicate effectively. They also give of themselves, offering support, providing reassurance, and making suggestions. People who feel demoralized or worthless discover that they have something valuable to offer others: the benefit of their experiences. This can be especially helpful for individuals who have been totally absorbed in their own misery.

Social learning. Many groups use role-playing, and individuals may be able to act out situations that terrify them in real life. They also learn about appropriate behavior by getting feedback from other group members, who are often able to make comments, such as mentioning a disconcerting habit of avoiding eye contact or speaking very loudly, that might sound like a criticism in another context.

Catharsis. Ventilating feelings and admitting or acknowledging behaviors that one is ashamed of or knows to be destructive can be an intensely emotional experience that leads to a sense of enormous relief. In itself, this rarely leads to lasting change, but the realization that it is possible to show strong emotions without losing the acceptance of others is immensely valuable, especially to people who had been feeling unlovable or repulsive.

As they discover that others have similar problems, individuals feel less alone. Often for the first time, they can talk openly about behaviors, such as bulimia, that they may have kept secret for years. This in itself provides great relief. In addition, by reaching out and trying to help others, group members feel that they, too, have value. As they listen and watch the therapist and fellow group members, they acquire insights into the behaviors of others—and their own. Groups also instill a sense of hope about the future, because individuals often are encouraged not just by their own progress but by the improvement they observe in those about them.

Groups take place in many settings: psychiatric hospitals, community mental health centers, health maintenance organizations, teaching hospital clinics, private offices. Hospital inpatient groups, composed of patients with acute problems, often meet daily and are a required form of therapy in the treatment program. In mental health clinics or outpatient treatment centers, many groups, especially those for individuals with chronic psychiatric disorders, focus on a particular problem, such as medication, and set a specific limit on the number of sessions. These sessions tend to be highly structured; their objective is to educate patients about their medications and to solve practical problems.

Mental health professionals in private practice may organize groups based on similar issues or needs. Psychotherapy groups that usually meet once a week can be an important part of the treatment of a wide range of common psychiatric problems, including eating disorders, depression, and anxiety disorders. Because adolescents place such great importance on peers, groups are especially effective for teens, who face tumultuous physical, social, intellectual, and emotional changes whether or not they suffer from mental disorders.

Group therapy may be an individual's only form of treatment or may be combined with individual therapy, either with the group leader (in what is called *combined* therapy) or another mental health professional (*concurrent* or *conjoint* therapy). What happens within a group can vary greatly, depending on the goals and the techniques the therapist chooses. Some use mainly cognitive-behavioral strategies; others focus on interpersonal therapy. Although groups organized around a particular problem may require members to meet certain criteria, such as having an eating disorder of a certain duration or severity, the most important qualification for joining is usually the ability to work within the group toward the shared goals of the members.

Videotaping of group sessions has become increasingly common, and some mental health professionals make video recording of the group a major feature of therapy. Watching the tape together provides feedback that individuals can perceive for themselves. Initially, they may focus superficially on how they look or gesture, but with subsequent sessions, they begin to notice more substantive factors, such as how aloof or argumentative they seem. Whereas a group member may have felt at the time that others' comments about his or her behavior were off base, seeing a videotape afterwards can show that these observations were indeed correct.

Given the new climate of cost control, groups, which were originally developed to serve large numbers of patients as cost-effectively as possible, may become even more popular. They enable large numbers of people to receive professional therapy with positive results in a very efficient manner. But the benefits of groups go well beyond their economic advantages, because they can be used in an enormous variety of settings for an equally varied array of psychiatric problems.

Hypnosis

Hypnosis is a state of intense concentration that alters the way the brain processes perceptions. In a hypnotic "trance," individuals focus so intently that they are unaware of sounds, sights, sensations (including pain), and other occurrences around them. In experimental studies, EEGs have shown clear changes in the electrical activity of the brain in hypnotized subjects. Individuals vary in their capacity for focused concentration, or hypnotizability. About one of every four adults is not hypnotizable; one of every ten is highly hypnotizable.

"Hypnosis may control the number of neurons that are recruited and deployed to focus on a stimulus," observes David Spiegel, M.D., professor of psychiatry at Stanford University. "Hypnotizable people can narrow the focus of their attention by turning down the noise in their minds." In essence, they "dissociate," so that they are no longer aware of routine experiences that would normally enter their consciousness.

In itself hypnosis is not a form of therapy, but it can be used in therapeutic ways. Because of their intense absorption, hypnotized individuals are more suggestible and accepting of instructions. Hypnosis does not take away their will; instead, it suspends the tendency to challenge or criticize. Therefore, it is particularly effective for breaking bad habits, such as smoking and overeating. In restructuring, an approach developed by psychiatrists David Spiegel and Herbert Spiegel, individuals focus on a positive affirmation of what they are for, such as a healthy body, rather than what they are against—for instance, cigarettes or overeating.

Mental health professionals use hypnosis in the treatment of various problems, including anxiety, phobias, and insomnia. It can be remarkably effective in pain control in situations such as labor and delivery, cancer or burn therapy, or relief from chronic arthritis or other painful conditions. Hypnosis is also proving useful in helping trauma victims to work through upsetting memories of what happened to them. During a trance, they may visualize an imaginary screen, a technique that provides a comforting sense of distance. On one half of the screen they may picture some aspect of the event, such as a rapist's face; on the other they project an image of something they did to protect themselves, whether it was struggling, running away, or talking. This can enable trauma victims to reframe their view of what happened so they feel less helpless and vulnerable. (Chapter 12 provides more information on the treatment of stress disorders, including posttraumatic stress.)

Expressive or creative treatments

Therapists may use any spontaneous form of creativity, such as art, music, drama, poetry, or dance, as an element in treating mental disorders. Sometimes drawings express feelings and fears that cannot be put into words, particularly by children. Dance therapy, which encourages free, expressive movements, can also release pent-up emotions. Almost always these approaches are used together with other forms of individual or group therapy.

The creative therapies can be very effective in many different settings. For a woman with dissociative identity disorder hospitalized because of a suicide attempt, painting or drawing may be a way in which her various "alters" communicate with each other and the therapist. For a man with an avoidant personality disorder whose inability to relate to others has brought him to outpatient therapy, sculpting small clay figures may be a means of connecting with the therapist. For an elderly woman with dementia who lives in a retirement home, dance therapy may be a way of tuning in to the past and becoming more aware of the present. All of these therapies can be valuable adjuncts in a comprehensive treatment program.

Is therapy working?

If you or someone close to you has been troubled by a problem and finds an empathic therapist, there can be a feeling of great relief as psychotherapy begins. If problems don't disappear, however, or if painful symptoms persist, it is common to wonder whether therapy is helping. Even those who do feel that they are getting better may find it a good idea to stop every now and then and take stock. In fact, some therapists schedule regular reviews or evaluations. Such sessions can help prevent a person from getting "stuck" or unconsciously falling into an unwanted pattern of behaving, for example, automatically responding to a conflict by pulling away from others or becoming abusive. Individuals in therapy should always feel free to ask to review their progress when they feel that there is a good reason to do so.

Although there are no consistent markers to indicate that therapy is on course, there are red flags that suggest that it is not proceeding as it should. Because of the nature of psychotherapy itself, these may be so subjective that only the person in therapy can sense their presence. They include:

- An intuitive sense that the therapist doesn't understand the problem
- Difficulty communicating with or confiding in the therapist
- Sexual advances or any seductive statements or behaviors
- Feeling uneasy about the therapist's ethics, competence, integrity, or behavior
- Dreading each session, or feeling "stuck," upset, adrift, or bored and unchallenged

- A sense of getting worse rather than better, or of not making any progress at all
- The perception of increasing time and attention being spent on the therapist's concerns, needs, or personal life
- Insulting remarks by the therapist
- The development or persistence of thoughts, impulses, or behaviors that might be dangerous, such as suicidal or violent thoughts or actions, drug or alcohol abuse, abuse of others (especially children), severe depression or anxiety, confusion, disorientation, a sense of losing control, or the inability to work or function normally. In these circumstances, immediate help is critical. Those whose condition is worsening may require the more intense and continuous care available only in a hospital.

A person who feels stuck or does not think he or she is making progress should tell the therapist. Once informed of this concern, the therapist may suggest an additional form of treatment, such as psychiatric medication, or a change in the frequency of sessions. Occasionally the therapist may not have the skills or expertise to deal with the person's symptoms and may refer the individual to a mental health professional who specializes in a particular problem.

If a therapist has made sexual advances at any time or acted in ways that seem improper, individuals should seek out another mental health professional to continue treatment. They also should contact the local chapter or the national office of the appropriate association—for example, the American Psychological Association, the American Psychiatric Association, or the American Association for Marriage and Family Therapy—for information and guidance on filing a complaint. These groups have adopted policies and spelled out protocols for the investigation and censure of members who violate professional ethics. State licensing agencies should also be notified. If such action is indicated, individuals may file criminal charges or civil suits against therapists.

Even if no problems or improprieties occur, it is still possible to feel dissatisfied or unsure about the course of therapy. Negative feelings about therapy do not necessarily mean that it isn't working. In fact, they may be a sign that it is. Confronting long-buried emotions and dealing with difficult issues is not easy. When one begins to explore problems, they may seem so large and forbidding that overcoming them seems impossible. Later, as therapy continues and change does seem conceivable, this prospect, too, may be frightening. Adding to the problems that bring a person into therapy is the anxiety of facing the unknown. Sometimes people become most angry with their therapists when they are at the brink of a breakthrough. Such resistance is a normal part of the psychotherapeutic process and indicates that the person is indeed dealing with matters that are important.

If you or someone close to you feels that something more than resistance is interfering with therapy, these are the questions that should be asked in evaluating the experience:

- Do you have a clear goal for therapy?
- Does the therapist know what you want and expect?
- Have you been completely open about your feelings, thoughts, and behavior?
- Have you listened to the therapist's comments and considered them carefully?
- Have you offered feedback about your perspective on the therapy?
- Does your therapist seem warm and caring or aloof and critical?
- Does your therapist seem to believe in your ability to change?
- Do you feel treated with respect and acceptance?
- Are your ideas challenged in a way that is constructive?
- Is your therapist available and dependable?
- Have you had appointments canceled abruptly?
- Are your phone calls returned within a reasonable time?

Your answers to these questions should be discussed with the therapist. It can be useful to find out his or her opinion about the way you are working together, your shared understanding of your goals, and your ability to deal with misunderstandings or disagreements.

If there seem to be real difficulties, you may want to consider consulting another therapist to get a different perspective. It is usually best to talk with your therapist first about why you think there is a problem and why you would like another opinion. Many therapists welcome such additional insight, particularly if they, too, feel that the therapy is not going well or that another therapist may have something to offer that they can't. However, not all therapists respond positively. Some may see it as a challenge to their competence or an accusation that they have failed in some way. They may argue that it is part of your resistance and something to discuss rather than act on. Although you and your therapist should indeed talk, you should persist and follow through on a consultation if your gut feeling is that you could and should be getting better and you aren't.

When you do see another therapist, describe yourself, your history, and your goals for treatment, as well as your concerns about your current therapy and your reason for wanting a second opinion. Ask for the consultant's candid evaluation of whether the therapy seems to be working and what might be done to improve it. Afterwards, consider his or her recommendations carefully. You may want to pass them along to your therapist, readjust your goals for therapy, continue therapy with him or her despite some reservations, or change therapists or the type of psychotherapy. All of these options are within your rights, and you should feel free to make the choice that seems best for you.

Ending therapy

Termination—the process of bringing psychotherapy to a close—is an important and unique stage in treatment. Individuals who have contracted formally or informally for a set number of sessions may know precisely when treatment will end. In such circumstances therapists often allot a certain amount of time for dealing with termination. In open-ended therapy, mental health professionals usually wait for the person to bring up the issue of ending therapy. There are good and bad, appropriate and inappropriate reasons for doing so. Sometimes individuals want to stop prematurely because they are reluctant to tackle difficult issues, are frustrated with the progress they have made, are fearful of becoming too dependent, or are angry or hurt because of something the therapist has said. Some are repeating a pattern of quitting difficult endeavors or sabotaging relationships. An impulsive urge to quit is more likely to stem from issues like these than is an evolving sense that it may be time to stop.

Individuals who are ready to end therapy usually feel that they have made progress. They may feel more confident, hopeful, accepting, and aware of their emotions and needs. It may be easier for them to get along with others, to recognize and avoid potential emotional pitfalls or self-defeating behavior, to accept responsibility rather than blame others. They realize that challenges, disappointments, and setbacks are inevitable but feel they will be able to deal with them. Often they have also changed their views of the therapist and of therapy itself. Rather than imbuing the therapist with awesome powers, they are realistic about what he or she can do, and they put increasing trust in their own judgment. Some find that they feel restless during therapy sessions.

Although many people feel awkward or anxious about bringing up the subject of termination, it is a normal part of the process. Raising the issue allows the therapist to voice any reservations or concerns he or she may have and enables both parties to reflect on the progress that has been made and the work that may still remain. It is extremely helpful for an individual and the mental health professional with whom he or she has been working to devote some time to summing up their experiences together, dealing with inevitable feelings of loss, and providing "closure" for the psychotherapy.

In therapy, as in other relationships, endings don't necessarily last forever. People who engage in fairly brief psychotherapy that focuses on a specific problem or crisis often return to therapy to deal with new issues as their life circumstances change. Individuals who have a mental disorder, such as depression, that can recur—as many illnesses often do—may find that periodic sessions with a therapist can help to maintain mental health or can serve as an early intervention if and when symptoms begin to develop. Just as they may have a primary physician to whom they turn for periodic medical evaluations, advice, and treatment if trouble arises, individuals may develop a long-term relationship with a mental health professional who is there to provide support when needed and treatment when appropriate.

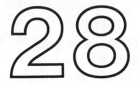

Psychiatric Drugs and Electroconvulsive Therapy

A college student with schizophrenia, once so agitated that his nonstop shuffling would wear out the soles of his shoes in a matter of days, can sit quietly and study. A woman who had lived in constant dread of terrifying panic attacks feels in control. A mathematician whose obsessive rituals consumed hours of his day can devote his energies to his work and family. A physician whose depression had sapped her stamina and energy feels like her "old" competent and confident self again.

Medications that alter brain chemistry and relieve psychiatric symptoms have brought great hope and help to millions of people like these. Thanks to the development of a new generation of more precise and effective psychiatric drugs, the success rates for treating many common and disabling disorders—depression, panic disorder, obsessive-compulsive disorder, schizophrenia, and others—have soared. Often used in conjunction with psychotherapy, sometimes used as the primary treatment, these medications have revolutionized mental health care.

Yet many who could benefit from drug therapy are not receiving it. "In part, this is because many psychiatric conditions are underdiagnosed, and people are unaware of what is wrong with them and what can be done about it," says Stephen Dubovsky, M.D., professor and vice-chairman of the Department of Psychiatry at the University of Colorado in Denver. "Many also are reluctant to take psychiatric medications, because of the stigma attached and because of the negative things they've read about drugs like Halcion and Valium."

Most certainly, mental disorders are complex problems, and drugs may not be the best or the only solution for some of them. Moreover, like all medications, psychiatric drugs have side effects and must be used with care. When they are taken appropriately, however, these agents can alleviate tremendous suffering and re-duce the financial and personal costs of mental illness by lessen-ing the need for hospitalization and by restoring an individual's ability to live up to his or her potential, to work, to relate to others, and to contribute to society.

Understanding psychiatric drugs

Psychiatric medications can affect every aspect of a person's physical, mental, and emotional functioning, including alert-ness, attention, coordination, energy, mood, judgment, sleep pat-terns, and interpersonal relationships. Some of these medications take effect at once; others do not have an immediate effect; some continue to exert their effects long after an individual discontinues their use.

In prescribing these medications, physicians must consider many factors, including the person's general health, history, aller-gies, and lifestyle. Age can be an important consideration because older individuals may metabolize certain drugs more slowly or may be more susceptible to medication side effects. A thorough history, including the presence of any emotional disorders in family mem-bers, and an assessment of the person's general medical condition to rule out any illnesses that might be causing psychiatric symp-toms are essential. Individuals who have not recently had a full medical evaluation may have to undergo a complete physical ex-amination and a variety of blood and laboratory tests, possibly including brain-imaging scans (described in Chapter 2).

The prescribing physician must also weigh the benefits and risks of specific medications. Although many psychiatric drugs are not habit-forming, others can be addictive and must be prescribed and taken with appropriate caution. Many can cause side effects that range from mildly irritating (such as dry mouth) to more bothersome (dizziness or constipation) to life-threatening (seizures or arrhythmias). In general, side effects tend to be most common and troubling when the drugs are first taken and most usually diminish or disappear after a few weeks. However, long-term use of certain types of drugs, such as conventional antipsychotic medications, can lead to serious adverse reactions, such as a chronic neuromuscular condition called *tardive dyskinesia* (discussed later in this chapter).

Most prescriptions for psychiatric drugs are written not by psychiatrists but by primary care physicians. Some who are not experienced or up to date in psychopharmacology may not prescribe the most effective or appropriate medication, may select an agent solely because it is simple to take and requires little monitoring, may recommend lower dosages than needed, or may not continue therapy for an adequate period. Determining the right drug in the right dose for any individual requires expertise in treating mental disorders, in-depth understanding of the latest advances in psychopharmacology, and close cooperation between the individual, the physician, and often the family as well.

Because adequate information about psychiatric drugs can help individuals and family members to make wise decisions, comply with medical instructions, and handle possible side effects, these are some of the questions consumers should ask before beginning drug therapy:

- Why is medication necessary?
- What specific symptoms will it relieve?
- What are the other possible benefits?
- What are the possible side effects and risks?
- How long will it be before the medication begins to help?
- How often must the drug be taken?
- Is there a preferred time of day or night for taking it?
- Do I have to avoid eating before or after taking it?
- Should it be taken with food?
- Will it affect my ability to drive or operate machinery?
- Will it affect my ability to work?
- What is the initial dosage?
- How can I tell if the drug is working?
- Should I call you if any particular side effects develop?
- Is there any danger from skipping a dose? From taking a double dose?
- What are the risks of overdosing?

Questions about medicine

Here are some of the questions that patients often ask when they are taking medicines. There is space after each question to write down the answers you receive, and a place to add any additional questions of your own.

Name of medicine (both chemical and brand names):

_____

_____

Dose/Instructions:

_____

_____

Questions about taking the medicine:

1. When and how often do I take the medicine? On an empty stomach or with food?

_____

_____

2. What are the side effects? Will I be tired, hungry, thirsty?

_____

_____

3. Are there any foods or drinks I should not use while taking the medicine?

_____

_____

4. Can I have beer, wine, or other alcoholic beverages?

_____

_____

5. Can I take the medicine together with the other medicines (including over-the-counter drugs) I am taking?

_____

_____

- Does this medicine interact with any other medications?
- Can I drink alcohol while taking this medication?
- Are there any foods or substances I should avoid?
- How long will I have to take this medication?
- Is there a danger that I'll become addicted?
- What are the alternatives to using this drug?
- What are the odds that this medicine will help me?
- What if this drug doesn't work?

6. What should I do if I forget to take my medicine?

_____

_____

7. How long will I have to take the medicine?

_____

_____

8. What are the chances of my getting better with this treatment?

_____

_____

9. How will I know if the medicine is or is not working?

_____

_____

10. What does the medicine cost?

_____

_____

Write your own questions here:

_____

_____

_____

_____

_____

_____

Adapted from Depression Is a Treatable Illness: A Patient's Guide. _U.S. Department of Health and Human Services, 1993: AHC PR 93-0553._

As a rule, only physicians are permitted to write prescriptions. Nonmedical therapists (such as psychologists, social workers, and psychiatric nurses) who are treating persons who may require medication often work closely with psychiatrists. The individual continues psychotherapy with the therapist but also consults a psychiatrist, who determines the need for medication, ensures that it is working, and monitors for side effects or medical complications.

If a particular psychiatric drug does not help, there are alternatives, and also alternatives to the alternatives. One should not become discouraged if the initial medication, or even the second or third, does not produce the desired results. Almost always, psychiatrists with expertise in pharmacotherapy can ultimately recommend a medication that will work. Indeed, the failure of a particular drug may provide some insight into the way an individual's illness will respond to treatment, increasing the likelihood that the next one will be more effective.

In some cases, psychiatrists prescribe a combination of medications. For example, depressed individuals who recover only partially after treatment with a single antidepressant may take an additional agent, such as lithium or a thyroid supplement, to boost their chances for complete recovery. The use of combined-medications requires clinical expertise and close supervision to ensure maximal benefits and minimal complications.

If the cost of a medication is a concern, talk to your physician about the possibility of using less expensive equivalents, such as generic drugs. In some cases there is no reason not to use these agents; in others the brand-name medication may be far more reliable and effective. In addition, it is essential to get precise instructions about doses, timing, and other details related to correct use of the medication (see the box, "Questions About Medicine," on the two previous pages).

If your primary care physician has prescribed a psychiatric medication for depression or an anxiety disorder and you have not noticed significant improvement within two months, ask about a consultation with a psychiatrist. Increasingly, many insurance and health care plans are discouraging primary care physicians from referring patients to specialists, including psychiatrists, but if you are not feeling better or if improvement is only slight, be insistent about seeing someone who is skilled in determining whether the problem might be the illness, the drug, the dose, or a need for a different or additional form of medication or therapy.

Drugs used to treat depression

S erendipity led to the discovery of the first antidepressant medications in the 1950s. In one instance, researchers working to develop a new antipsychotic drug that might also help depression discovered a compound called imipramine—which was to become the first tricyclic antidepressant—that had a beneficial effect on mood. In another instance, physicians who gave a new antituberculosis medication, isoniazid, to TB patients in sanatoriums in Europe found not only that it was effective in treating this major illness but also that it made the patients so ebullient that some reportedly danced in the hallways. Isoniazid is chemically similar to the drugs now known as monoamine oxidase (MAO) inhibitors.

The tricyclic antidepressants and MAO inhibitors can be considered the first generation of antidepressant medications. Trazodone (Desyrel), with a different chemical composition, could be considered a second-generation antidepressant. The selective serotonin reuptake inhibitors (SSRIs)—fluoxetine (Prozac), paroxetine (Paxil), and sertraline (Zoloft)—and the atypical antidepressant bupropion (Wellbutrin) represent a third generation. The most recently released fourth-generation drugs include nefazodone (Serzone) and venlafaxine (Effexor).

It was long believed that all antidepressants work by increasing or decreasing levels of various neurotransmitters involved in depression, such as serotonin and norepinephrine. "Now we know that the therapeutic effects of these drugs have more to do with cellular function and the transmission of impulses via receptors than with neurotransmitter levels per se," says Dubovsky.

Most of today's antidepressants are about equal in effectiveness. About 60 to 70 percent of individuals respond to the first medication prescribed for them; a greater percentage eventually improve with an alternative drug. Combined treatment, which involves both drug therapy and psychotherapy, has proved most effective in overcoming depression and in lowering relapse rates.

Many medications classified as antidepressants are also effective for treatment of other mental disorders. The tricyclics are used to treat panic disorder, posttraumatic stress disorder, generalized anxiety disorder, and various physical problems, such as chronic pain and migraine headaches. MAO inhibitors may be prescribed for panic disorder and social phobia. The SSRIs have proved beneficial in treating obsessive-compulsive disorder and bulimia nervosa; they also appear helpful for panic disorder, certain impulse control disorders, and posttraumatic stress disorder.

A PRACTICAL GUIDE TO ANTIDEPRESSANTS

In choosing an antidepressant, physicians weigh many factors, including the individual's medical status, history of manic or hypomanic episodes, previous depressions, prior responses to an antidepressant, and the presence of "atypical" symptoms such as increased sleep, weight gain, or anxiety, or psychotic symptoms such as delusions or hallucinations. It is important for consumers to understand why their doctor recommends a particular medication and to be informed about its possible side effects as well as its potential benefits.

Because individuals vary widely in their responses to different medications, they must work closely with their psychiatrists in choosing and using an antidepressant. In general, starting doses are low and are gradually increased so that it can take several weeks before a full dose is reached. Both the initial dose and the "therapeutic" or effective dose vary from person to person. Younger adults typically need higher doses than older ones. For several of the tricyclic antidepressants (imipramine, desipramine, and nortriptyline), monitoring drug levels in the blood helps to ensure the greatest benefits with the fewest side effects.

A critical fact about antidepressant treatment is that it takes time. Although a few individuals may experience some improvement, such as increased energy, by the end of the first week, most do not see significant benefits for three or four weeks. Because doses are increased gradually, five or six weeks may pass from the time a person takes the first pill until the symptoms are substantially relieved, and eight weeks or longer for the medication to have its full impact. The reason for this delay may be that several weeks of drug therapy are required to either increase or decrease the receptors' ability to bind to selected neurotransmitters.

Doctors should keep in touch with individuals taking antidepressants to make sure that the drugs are having an effect. Within two weeks, many people find they are sleeping better. After about four to eight weeks of treatment, psychiatrists can determine if individuals have experienced a full or partial response or have failed to improve at all. For those with an initial episode of a mild to moderate depression, medication is usually continued for six to twelve months and is then tapered off. For those with more severe depression or who have had prior depressive episodes, treatment may continue for a longer time. As explained in Chapter 5, recent studies have revealed a high rate of recurrence in major depression, and maintenance drug treatment, which can prevent another episode of depression, has become increasingly common.

"We do not know of any long-term risks in keeping people on antidepressants for prolonged periods, but we do know that there are risks in *not* treating them," says Dubovsky, who is an expert in psychopharmacology. "The depression could come back. The medication that worked in the past might not work. The depression could be harder to treat. If it becomes severe, it could be life-threatening."

Individuals who do not improve on one type of antidepressant are usually switched to another type, for example, from a tricyclic to an SSRI or from an SSRI to bupropion (Wellbutrin). An estimated 60 to 65 percent of individuals who do not respond to one of these classes of medication will improve with another.

Those with a partial response may benefit from a switch in medication or from *augmentation therapy*, the addition of other agents to enhance or magnify the beneficial effects of an antidepressant. As discussed in Chapter 5, the agents used for augmentation therapy include the mood stabilizer lithium, T_3 thyroid hormone supplements, anticonvulsants (carbamazepine and valproic acid), and stimulants (although there are no scientific guidelines for how long these should be used). If other approaches fail, psychiatrists may try a combination of antidepressants, such as an SSRI along with a tricyclic antidepressant, or electroconvulsive therapy (ECT), discussed at the end of this chapter.

▼

General precautions Individuals should let their doctors know if they have ever had an allergic reaction to an antidepressant or any other medication, if they are taking any other prescription or nonprescription drugs or vitamins, if they are planning to undergo surgery or medical tests or procedures in the coming months, and if they have *any* concurrent or chronic medical conditions, such as a seizure disorder. All antidepressants may slightly increase the risk for developing seizures; this danger is greatest with bupropion and, to a lesser extent, with maprotiline. It is always wise to check with a physician before using any other medication. Another standard—and sound—recommendation is to stop smoking; nicotine lowers the levels of antidepressants in the blood and may reduce their beneficial effects.

The various types of antidepressants produce different side effects (these groups are listed later in the chapter). Many common side effects, such as dry mouth or nausea, subside after several weeks. Moreover, although bothersome, these effects do have a positive aspect: They indicate that a drug is working and that blood levels of the drug are rising. Even when side effects are annoying, it is critical to continue to take the medication long enough for it to be beneficial and to keep increasing the dose as directed until symptoms improve.

In the elderly, not only must dosages be lower than those for younger persons but the side effects of certain antidepressants can also be more difficult for them to tolerate. In women who are pregnant or trying to conceive, the question of initiating or continuing antidepressant treatment is a difficult one. Clinical reports are very limited. In a Canadian study of fluoxetine (Prozac) use in the first trimester of pregnancy, no higher rate of birth defects was associated with the drug. The women taking fluoxetine had a higher incidence of miscarriages, but it is not clear whether this was related to the medication, to the depression, or to other factors. Reports on tricyclics suggest that they do not cause birth defects. However, most physicians prefer not to prescribe or continue any medications, including antidepressants, during pregnancy unless they are absolutely essential.

"Some depressions get better in pregnancy and do not require treatment; some get worse," says Dubovsky. "Even if there is no effect on organ formation, antidepressants may have what is called behavioral teratogenicity—an effect on behavior that we may not find out for decades—and it may be positive or negative. We also don't know what impact depression itself, which alters hormone levels, may have on a fetus. The best a psychiatrist and a woman can do is look at the potential risks and benefits and make what seems to be the best determination for her."

Individuals taking antidepressants should avoid alcohol, which depresses the central nervous system and stimulates enzymes that break down the medication, lowering the amount in the blood and making it more difficult to maintain therapeutic levels. Alcohol can enhance the sedating effects of the antidepressants that cause drowsiness as an initial side effect, and may interfere with recovery. "I have had patients who drank a glass or two of wine a week and remained depressed," says Dubovsky. "When they stopped drinking, they got better." Individuals who are continuing drug treatment but no longer have depressive symptoms should also be cautious about alcohol use. "If a patient wants to have an occasional glass of wine, I say, 'Try it and see,'" says Dubovsky. "If you start feeling depressed again, you know it's not a good idea." Individuals taking MAO inhibitors should avoid drinking beer, including nonalcoholic varieties, which could cause a dangerous rise in blood pressure.

Overdoses of the tricyclic antidepressants can be fatal, and psychiatrists often initially prescribe only small quantities of a tricyclic to avoid this possibility or else choose newer antidepressants, such as the SSRIs, trazodone, or nefazodone, which are considered less likely than the tricyclics to be lethal in overdoses.

Another risk is suicide. Although most studies indicate that all antidepressants decrease suicidal thoughts, some individuals paradoxically consider suicide or attempt to kill themselves (sometimes successfully) *after* they begin taking medication. It is possible that, in this early stage of treatment, depressed persons with suicidal thoughts have the energy, because of the medication, to act on self-destructive impulses. In some cases hospitalization may be necessary to prevent a suicide attempt.

Antidepressants should not be stopped suddenly but must be gradually tapered off. As many as half of all people taking antidepressants experience withdrawal symptoms when they reduce the dosage. The most common of these are insomnia, increased anxiety, a flu-like malaise, diarrhea, and the recurrence of depressed mood. Often, a very gradual lowering of the dose can avoid these problems.

SELECTIVE SEROTONIN REUPTAKE INHIBITORS

The best known of the selective serotonin reuptake inhibitors (SSRIs) is fluoxetine (Prozac), a drug that has attained celebrity status (see box on page 748); others include sertraline (Zoloft), paroxetine (Paxil), and fluvoxamine (Luvox). The SSRIs primarily affect the neurotransmitter serotonin; they are, as their name states, selective.

The SSRIs have become very popular, largely because they cause fewer side effects than other antidepressants and are easy to prescribe and to take. (Often they can be taken in a single dose in the morning.) "It's important to keep in mind that their popularity far outstrips the scientific basis for their use," notes Dubovsky. "They have been conclusively demonstrated to be effective in mild to moderate depression, but there have not yet been large-scale studies of their efficacy for severe depression." The SSRIs are often the best choice for individuals with medical problems such as heart disease, dementia, or Alzheimer's disease, and certain other mental disorders such as bulimia nervosa or PTSD. They also are a good option for depressed individuals who have difficulty tolerating any medicine, who are extremely irritable, or who tend to ruminate or obsess constantly.

The SSRIs are also used to treat obsessive-compulsive disorder, phobias, panic disorder, and trichotillomania. Some psychiatrists have used fluoxetine to treat depression in individuals with borderline and schizotypal personality disorders and, in small clinical studies with no control groups, have reported significant decreases in symptoms of depression and improvement in difficult characterologic traits that may have been aggravated by the depressive episode.

The SSRIs may not be the best choice for people who suffer from migraines (which may get worse), who become nauseated easily, or who have a sexual dysfunction such as impotence or difficulty achieving orgasm. (Depression itself can cause sexual dysfunction, which for many people improves as their depression lifts.)

▼

Side effects   The SSRIs are usually less sedating than tricyclic antidepressants, although fluvoxamine may produce significant somnolence in selected patients. The SSRIs do not lower blood pressure or trigger heart arrhythmias. The most common side effects are nervousness, restlessness, problems in sleeping, headaches, nausea, diarrhea, and other gastrointestinal symptoms. Some individuals complain of "jitters" or restlessness; caffeine can contribute to such "hyper" feelings. Starting with low doses of the drug and increasing it gradually can also help.

The SSRIs can cause sexual dysfunction, in particular retarded ejaculation in men and delayed orgasm in women, or, as noted above, intensify a preexisting dysfunction. Such side effects occur in at least 10 to 20 percent of individuals and may abate over time (usually a year or more). Most people report a very slight weight loss of a pound or so, although some have reported gaining substantial amounts of weight. Although the SSRIs usually do not provoke cardiac arrhythmias, they can increase heart rate and blood pressure. They are less likely to cause postural hypotension (dizziness on sitting up or standing up suddenly) than the tricyclics, but this problem has occasionally been reported.

The SSRIs can increase the blood levels of other medications metabolized in the liver by inhibiting their metabolism. For example, fluoxetine has been shown to increase the levels of warfarin (Coumadin), an agent that blocks the clotting capacity of blood. Sertraline, which may be less likely to do so, may be chosen as an alternative medication.

Individuals who are taking two or more drugs that boost serotonin levels, such as an SSRI together with the antidepressant trazodone, may develop an uncommon condition dubbed *serotonin syndrome*, caused by excessive stimulation of the serotoninergic system. This syndrome can also occur in those taking a single SSRI, especially at higher doses (such as 60 mg or more of fluoxetine). Initial symptoms include lethargy, restlessness, confusion, flushing, sweating, tremor, and involuntary muscle jerks. Over time, a small percentage of patients may develop muscle disorders, hyperthermia, and rigor, which may lead to respiratory problems, increased platelet clotting, destruction of red blood cells and their excretion by the kidneys in urine, and kidney failure. This potentially deadly syndrome requires emergency medical treatment and discontinuation of the serotonin-boosting medications.

None of the SSRIs should ever be used with an MAO inhibitor. Overdoses with the SSRIs have rarely proved fatal, but further research is needed for adequate assessment of the danger. The symptoms of a possible overdose include agitation, nausea, and convulsions. Immediate emergency treatment is essential.

SELECTIVE SEROTONIN REUPTAKE INHIBITORS

CHEMICAL NAME
Fluoxetine

BRAND NAME
Prozac

DOSAGE The initial dose is usually between 10 and 20 mg once a day. If there is no improvement in depression within two or three weeks, the dose can be increased by 10- to 20-mg increments every one to two weeks, to a maximum of 60 mg per day. Individuals taking this medication for obsessive-compulsive disorder (OCD) may require higher doses (80 to 100 mg) than those being treated for depression.

SPECIAL CONSIDERATIONS Fluoxetine is the most stimulating of the SSRIs; individuals taking it may experience nervousness, restlessness, and sleep disturbances. Other side effects include nausea and tremor. Its metabolites remain in the body for a week or more; because of this long half-life, missing a single dose is not likely to cause problems. Fluoxetine is more likely to interfere with the liver's ability to metabolize certain other drugs, which can keep the blood levels of the other medications high and increase their effects. In cases in which a change in medication is indicated because fluoxetine does not prove helpful, individuals should wait a full four weeks after discontinuing fluoxetine before switching to an MAO inhibitor, and one to four weeks before switching to any other antidepressants.

CHEMICAL NAME
Fluvoxamine

BRAND NAME
Luvox

DOSAGE The recommended starting dose for fluvoxamine is 50 mg a day, administered at bedtime. The dose is usually increased in 50 mg increments every week, as tolerated, until maximum therapeutic benefit is achieved. Once the total daily dose exceeds 100 mg, the medication should be given in two divided doses, with the larger dose (if applicable) given at bedtime. The maximum recommended daily dose is 300 mg.

SPECIAL CONSIDERATIONS Fluvoxamine is an SSRI similar to fluoxetine (Prozac), sertraline (Zoloft), and paroxetine (Paxil). It is probably as effective as other SSRIs in treating major depression, phobias, panic disorder, bulimia nervosa, PTSD, and trichotillomania. However, the FDA has approved its use only for the treatment of obsessive-compulsive disorder.
Fluvoxamine's major side effects are nausea, somnolence, insomnia, dry mouth, nervousness, and dizziness. It produces much more sedation than fluoxetine and sertraline and is usually more sedating than paroxetine. Its half-life is approximately fifteen hours in younger adults and about a day in elderly patients.

CHEMICAL NAME
Paroxetine

BRAND NAME
Paxil

DOSAGE The initial dose is usually 10 to 20 mg once a day. If there is no improvement within two or three weeks, the dose can be increased by 10-mg increments weekly to a maximum of 50 mg per day.

SPECIAL CONSIDERATIONS Paroxetine is slightly less activating than fluoxetine. It may be associated with a higher incidence of headaches, nausea, dry mouth, and sedation. Its metabolites do not remain in the body as long as fluoxetine's; its half-life is approximately one day.

CHEMICAL NAME
Sertraline

BRAND NAME
Zoloft

DOSAGE The initial dose is usually 25 to 50 mg. If there is no improvement within two or three weeks, the dose can be increased by 25- to 50-mg increments weekly to 100 mg or, occasionally, to a maximum of 200 mg per day.

SPECIAL CONSIDERATIONS Sertraline produces less nervousness or agitation than fluoxetine and may be less likely to interfere with the metabolism of other drugs by the liver. Side effects include nausea, diarrhea, sleep disturbances, restlessness, and nervousness. It has a half-life of about one day.

The Prozac phenomenon:
A new era of cosmetic pharmacology?

It is the Madonna of psychiatric drugs, a green-and-beige capsule that has become famous for being famous. Introduced in 1988, Prozac was first hailed as a breakthrough antidepressant, then damned as a trigger for violence and suicide, and ultimately vindicated and elevated to cult status. Users say it makes them less of the things they hate being and more the way they'd like to be: upbeat rather than morose, easygoing rather than irritable, eventempered rather than moody.

"If my doctor told me that if I continued Prozac, I would feel as well as I do now but be dead in two years, whereas without it I'd feel the way I used to but not die, I'd take death," says one man who suffered from depression for decades before starting on the medication. "I wouldn't live in that kind of torture again."

Prozac has indeed proved effective against depression, obsessive-compulsive disorder, panic disorder, and bulimia nervosa. What sets it and the other new antidepressants apart is that they are more precisely targeted so that they cause fewer troublesome side effects and are easier for people to tolerate. Moreover, because they are safer and require fewer dose adjustments than older medications, they are also easier for physicians to prescribe and monitor. Most prescriptions for Prozac are written by nonpsychiatrists, many for individuals with no diagnosable mental disorder.

Do "healthy" individuals who respond to Prozac actually have mild forms of mental illness? Should they keep taking it for indefinite periods of time, despite unknown long-term risks? Is this drug therapy or a new type of drug dependence? In *Listening to Prozac*, a book as popular and provocative as the drug that inspired it, psychiatrist Peter Kramer, M.D., mused about the coming of an era of "cosmetic pharmacology," in which individuals might transform their personalities as readily as they now change their hair color. Given the choice, he asks, who could resist the opportunity to live, not just as a blond, but as a perky, carefree, confident blond?

This possibility—tantalizing to some, threatening to others—has been greatly overblown in the media. "Almost always, people take psychiatric drugs because they need them," observes Steven Dubovsky, M.D., professor and vice-chairman of psychiatry at the University of Colorado, who notes that these medications, like others, have side effects and other disadvantages that must be outweighed by their benefits. For some, the benefits have been enormous indeed.

"Until I started on medication, I thought everyone was basically miserable," says a woman with chronic depression. "A month later I was telling people, 'So this is how the rest of you feel!' I'd had no idea."

Individuals taking other psychiatric drugs for problems such as attention deficit disorders, panic disorder, and social phobias report a similar sense of finally achieving a psychological state that others take for granted. "We are not sedating or tranquilizing these people; we are making them normal," says neuropsychiatrist Stuart Yudofsky, M.D., of Baylor College of Medicine, co-author of *What You Need to Know about Psychiatric Drugs*. "Appropriate psychopharmacotherapy is like giving insulin to diabetics."

In the future, new psychiatric drugs will be able to fine-tune the neurobiology of mood to a degree not even imaginable today, bringing long-awaited relief to the millions of mentally ill who have been helped only a little, if at all, by current therapies. Some new agents may also offer others the chance to be, as one of Kramer's patients described himself, "better than well"—calmer, braver, brighter, even nicer than might otherwise be possible.

Will legions of eccentric, ill-at-ease, unhappy men and women turn to these agents to smooth away the rough edges of their personalities or buffer every setback life hands them? We doubt it. The world isn't filled with self-created blonds, perky or otherwise, but with individuals struggling to come to terms with who they are and what they might become. Perhaps the psychiatric drugs of the future will serve as tools not to avoid or mask this struggle but to work through it.

ATYPICAL ANTIDEPRESSANTS

Some medications used to treat depression are "atypical," or chemically different from the SSRIs, tricyclic antidepressants, and MAO inhibitors. Bupropion (Wellbutrin) may affect the neurotransmitter dopamine. Trazodone (Desyrel) targets serotonin.

CHEMICAL NAME
Bupropion

BRAND NAME
Wellbutrin

DOSAGE Unlike the tricyclics or SSRIs, which can be taken in a single daily dose, bupropion must be taken two or three times a day. The initial dose is usually 100 mg twice a day. It can be increased gradually to 300 mg or, in some cases, to a maximum of 450 mg a day. To minimize the risk for seizures, no single dose should exceed 150 mg, and there should be intervals of four hours or longer between doses.

SPECIAL CONSIDERATIONS This drug, originally developed for individuals who did not benefit from other antidepressants, may affect the neurotransmitter dopamine. Bupropion is nonsedating, and causes fewer side effects than the tricyclics and MAO inhibitors. It does not make users drowsy, does not cause weight gain, does not affect the heart, and does not cause postural hypotension. The risk for sexual dysfunction is lower than with other antidepressant medications. It may be especially beneficial for depressed individuals with HIV infection. In research studies, bupropion has proven as effective as other antidepressants.

Like other antidepressants, bupropion does pose a risk for seizures, which develop in about four of every one thousand individuals (0.1 percent) taking these medications. (To put this risk in perspective, one of every one thousand people not taking any medicine develops seizures.) With daily doses of bupropion higher than 450 mg, or with single doses of more than 150 mg, the risk for seizures rises to 5 percent. Consequently, the standard of practice is not to prescribe daily doses greater than 450 mg. Individuals with bulimia nervosa should not take high doses of this medication because they are especially likely to develop seizures.

Like the SSRIs, bupropion cannot be used in combination with an MAO inhibitor. Individuals taking bupropion should always check with their physicians before taking other medications, which may affect blood levels of this agent.

CHEMICAL NAME
Trazodone

BRAND NAME
Desyrel

DOSAGE When used as the sole agent for depression, trazodone is usually prescribed in an initial dose of 50 mg, twice a day. It can be gradually increased in 100-mg daily increments to 300 or 400 mg per day; some individuals may require a higher dose, up to 600 mg. When it is used together with an SSRI (primarily to aid sleep), the dose is usually 50 to 100 mg.

SPECIAL CONSIDERATIONS Trazodone, which affects serotonin receptors, is one of the most sedating antidepressants and can help those who have difficulty in falling asleep. Often a bedtime dose is prescribed as a sleep aid for individuals taking SSRIs or MAO inhibitors.

Side effects include dizziness, dry mouth, blurred vision, constipation, and urinary retention. In those over the age of sixty, postural hypotension is possible. When used in combination with an SSRI, trazodone can enhance sexual interest and orgasmic functioning, especially in women with sexual dysfunction caused by the SSRI. A very small number of men taking this drug (about one in six thousand) may develop prolonged and painful erections (*priapism*), which may require emergency surgery that can lead to permanent sexual impairment. The risk for lethal overdoses is much lower than with the tricyclic antidepressants.

FOURTH-GENERATION ANTIDEPRESSANTS

Nefazodone (Serzone) and venlafaxine (Effexor), which were approved for release by the FDA in 1994, have different mechanisms of action. Nefazodone blocks a specific serotonin receptor subtype in addition to blocking serotonin reuptake. Venlafaxine acts on both serotonin and norepinephrine.

CHEMICAL NAME
Nefazodone

BRAND NAME
Serzone

DOSAGE The initial dose is 100 mg twice a day, usually taken in the morning and at night. After one week, the dose is increased to 150 mg twice a day. The usual adult dose is between 300 and 600 mg a day, equally divided between morning and night.

SPECIAL CONSIDERATIONS Nefazodone blocks a specific serotonin receptor subtype (abbreviated 5HT-2) and inhibits serotonin uptake. Because of this dual effect on serotonin, it may be described as a serotonin receptor modulator. It produces less sedation than trazodone and has not been associated with priapism. In contrast to the SSRIs, nefazodone has not been reported to produce sexual problems and does not cause anxiety or insomnia. In clinical trials, its major side effects were dry mouth, nausea, drowsiness, dizziness, and light-headedness.

CHEMICAL NAME
Venlafaxine

BRAND NAME
Effexor

DOSAGE The usual starting dose is 37.5 mg twice a day. Doses are increased by 37.5 to 75 mg once a week. The usual therapeutic dosage is 75 to 225 mg a day; the maximal daily dosage is 375 mg in three divided doses.

SPECIAL CONSIDERATIONS This antidepressant has shown promise in helping individuals who do not improve with other antidepressants. At high doses it is very activating. Its most common side effects are sweating, nausea, nervousness, sleep disturbances, weakness, and constipation. At higher doses it may increase blood pressure.

TRICYCLIC ANTIDEPRESSANTS

These medications, also called *cyclic* or *heterocyclic* antidepressants, block the recapture or reuptake of the neurotransmitters serotonin and norepinephrine so that they remain in the synapse longer. Once the agents of first choice in treating depression, they have been largely replaced as first-line drugs by the SSRIs, atypical antidepressants, and nefazodone.

General precautions Because of the risk for postural hypotension, individuals, especially those over the age of sixty, should never rise to their feet suddenly, as when the telephone or the doorbell rings. They should change from a lying position to a standing one in two stages, first moving slowly to a sitting position and then waiting sixty seconds— or longer if feeling light-headed—before slowly standing up.

The tricyclic antidepressants can interact with any medications that affect the central nervous system, including allergy drugs, muscle relaxants, and sleeping pills. Check with a physician before taking any such substances, whether prescription or over-the-counter. Alcohol intensifies sedation and impairs driving ability. The tricyclics should not be discontinued abruptly; sudden stopping can cause a worsening of the original disorder, headache, restlessness, and flu-like physical symptoms. Their effects may last for up to seven days after use is stopped.

As noted earlier, the major drawback of the tricyclic antidepressants is the risk for unintentional overdose or suicide. Taking a large quantity of any of these medications can be fatal. Because a person with depression is at high risk for suicide, psychiatrists may try to minimize the danger of overdose by prescribing no more than a few days' supply of the drugs at a time. With frequent visits, psychiatrists also can provide support and counseling.

The first symptoms of overdose, which typically develop one to four hours after the drug is taken, are difficulty in breathing, dangerous changes in heart rhythm, agitation, lowered blood pressure, garbled speech, high fever, confusion, disorientation, and coma. Immediate emergency treatment at a hospital can prevent permanent damage or death.

▼

Side effects In addition to increasing the levels of norepinephrine and serotonin, the tricyclic antidepressants lower levels of the neurotransmitter acetylcholine, producing various *anticholinergic* side effects. Many of these effects—dry mouth, blurry vision or difficulty focusing at close range, constipation, and problems in urinating—are caused by decreased stimulation of the nerves that affect the muscles controlling these functions. Other common side effects include postural hypotension, drowsiness, and confusion. Many of these initial side effects usually abate by the third week of use. In the meantime, practical coping strategies can help (see Chapter 5). Because these drugs are sedating, taking them before bedtime helps; indeed, the drowsiness often is considered a plus for those who have trouble sleeping. If coping strategies are not effective and reducing the dosage or trying alternative antidepressants does not help, some physicians prescribe medications such as bethanechol chloride to relieve troubling dry mouth, constipation, and urinary hesitancy and retention.

Weight gain is a common problem; most individuals put on several pounds while using tricyclics. Particularly among women, this is the most common reason for discontinuance. At the beginning of treatment, many people complain of feeling dizzy or "foggy"; this usually lessens over time. If individuals become confused or forgetful, their psychiatrists may recommend an antidepressant less likely to produce these effects.

Less common side effects associated with the tricyclic antidepressants include flushing, sweating, allergic skin reactions, photosensitivity (rashes or painful sunburns after exposure to the sun), blood abnormalities (such as reduced production of white blood cells and platelets), tremor, speech impairment, increased insomnia or anxiety, increased appetite, and cardiac arrhythmias.

CHEMICAL NAME
Amitriptyline

BRAND NAMES
Elavil, Endep

DOSAGE Amitriptyline is usually prescribed in an initial dose of 50 to 75 mg and is gradually increased to 150 mg or, in some cases, 200 to 300 mg daily.

SPECIAL CONSIDERATIONS Amitriptyline, the most sedating antidepressant, is primarily used to treat pain in depressed individuals and as a sleep aid. Taken in the daytime, it causes severe drowsiness, especially during the first weeks of use. Amitriptyline is usually not prescribed as an antidepressant for the elderly because of the risk for memory problems, confusion, and falling.

CHEMICAL NAME
Amoxapine

BRAND NAME
Asendin

DOSAGE Amoxapine is usually prescribed in an initial dose of 50 to 75 mg and gradually increased to 150 mg or, in some cases, to as much as 600 mg daily.

SPECIAL CONSIDERATIONS Unlike other tricyclic antidepressants, amoxapine is a metabolite of the antipsychotic agent loxapine, which is used to treat schizophrenia, and some physicians believe that it may be particularly effective for treatment of psychotic depression. It is the only antidepressant that works by itself for psychotic depression; others must be combined with an antipsychotic drug. Because amoxapine, like many antipsychotic drugs, blocks the reuptake of dopamine, users may develop tardive dyskinesia (see page 775). The risk increases with the length of treatment and the cumulative dosage; it is greater in the elderly, although it can occur at any age. Amoxapine is generally used only for psychotic or treatment-resistant depression.

CHEMICAL NAME
Desipramine

BRAND NAMES
Norpramin, Pertofrane

DOSAGE The initial dose is usually 50 to 75 mg, gradually increased to 150 mg or, in some cases, to 200 to 300 mg daily.

SPECIAL CONSIDERATIONS Desipramine is less sedating and more stimulating than most tricyclics, and some depressed individuals cannot tolerate the nervousness and muscle twitches that may occur with this drug. In addition to its use in treating depression, this medication may reduce the craving for cocaine in addicts undergoing withdrawal. There is less likelihood of significant weight gain than with other tricyclics.

CHEMICAL NAME
Doxepin

BRAND NAMES
Adapin, Sinequan

DOSAGE The initial dose is usually 50 to 75 mg, which can be gradually increased to 150 mg or, in some cases, to 200 to 300 mg daily.

SPECIAL CONSIDERATIONS This sedating tricyclic, similar to amitriptyline, should be taken at bedtime. Sometimes doxepin is used as a sleep aid along with an SSRI for individuals who develop sleep disturbances as a side effect or whose sleep problems worsen. Like trimipramine (Surmontil), doxepin has antihistamine effects and is as effective as standard anti-ulcer medications, such as cimetidine (Tagamet), for ulcers.

These medications may aggravate an eye condition called narrow-angle glaucoma and may trigger seizures in susceptible individuals. In general, sexual dysfunctions are less common than with the SSRIs, although problems, including retrograde ejaculation (in which sperm is forced back into the bladder rather than out of the penis), can occur.

CHEMICAL NAME
Imipramine

BRAND NAMES
Tofranil, Janimine

DOSAGE The initial dose is usually 50 to 75 mg, which is gradually increased to 150 mg or, in some cases, 200 to 300 mg daily. The dosages used for panic disorder are usually smaller than those initially used for depression, although they may be increased gradually to the same level as in depression or even higher.

SPECIAL CONSIDERATIONS Imipramine, the "gold standard" for evaluation of antidepressants in clinical trials, is more likely to be used in research than in clinical practice because of its troubling side effects. However, it is effective as a treatment for depression, panic disorder, and uncomplicated PTSD. In addition, imipramine can be used in the treatment of individuals undergoing cocaine withdrawal. Its use as a treatment for chronic bed-wetting in youngsters over the age of six years is controversial. If prescribed for depressed children or teenagers, a child psychiatrist should always monitor its use to ensure that the child is taking the drug properly.

CHEMICAL NAME
Maprotiline

BRAND NAME
Ludiomil

DOSAGE Individuals usually take an initial dose of 50 to 75 mg, which is gradually increased to 150 mg or, in some cases, up to a maximum of 225 mg daily.

SPECIAL CONSIDERATIONS A risk for seizures is associated with high doses of this tricyclic. The likelihood is low, but the risk increases if the dose is increased rapidly, if dosages exceed the recommended ranges, or if individuals take other medications that interact with maprotiline.

CHEMICAL NAME
Nortriptyline

BRAND NAMES
Aventyl, Pamelor

DOSAGE The usual starting dose is 25 to 50 mg, which is gradually increased to a maximum of 150 mg daily.

SPECIAL CONSIDERATIONS Like imipramine and desipramine, this tricyclic is an effective treatment for people with panic disorder. Some psychiatrists also feel that it is a good choice for individuals with depression and anxiety and for the elderly, since it is less likely to cause postural hypotension.

CHEMICAL NAME
Trimipramine

BRAND NAME
Surmontil

DOSAGE The initial dose is usually 50 to 75 mg, which is gradually increased to 150 mg or, in some cases, 200 to 300 mg daily.

SPECIAL CONSIDERATIONS Trimipramine, more sedating than many other tricyclic antidepressants, should be taken at bedtime to help with sleep difficulties and to avoid daytime drowsiness. Like doxepin, trimipramine has antihistamine effects and is as effective as standard anti-ulcer medications such as cimetidine (Tagamet) for ulcers. This makes it a good choice for depressed individuals with ulcers.

MONOAMINE OXIDASE INHIBITORS

MAO inhibitors, the oldest antidepressants, are as effective against depression as tricyclic antidepressants and the SSRIs. However, they work in a different way, by inactivating monoamine oxidase, an enzyme that breaks down neurotransmitters in the synapse, so these chemical messengers remain intact longer.

The MAO inhibitors are usually not the first drugs of choice for treatment of depression, primarily because of their potential for serious adverse effects and the requirement that individuals taking them avoid some common foods and beverages. They are prescribed most often for individuals who develop atypical depression (see Chapter 5), which is characterized by oversleeping, overeating, extreme lethargy, great sensitivity to rejection, and highly emotional reactions to life experiences. The MAO inhibitors may also be effective in treating symptoms of panic disorder or specific phobias.

Isocarboxazid (Marplan), a well-known MAO inhibitor, is no longer on the market. A new "reversible" MAO inhibitor, moclobemide, is in use in Canada. It does not require dietary restrictions, but there are questions about its efficacy. It has not been approved for use in the United States.

▼

General precautions

For individuals taking these drugs, it is essential (though not always easy) to avoid foods containing tyramine, an amino acid found in many common foods, which can interact with the MAO inhibitors and produce potentially toxic effects, including sudden, extremely dangerous surges in blood pressure (hypertension). This is sometimes called the *cheese reaction* because aged cheese contains relatively high concentrations of tyramine. The reaction can range from mild to severe, producing symptoms such as sweating, palpitations, headache, and, in severe cases, a rise in blood pressure and possible bleeding within the brain caused by rupture of cerebral arteries.

Recent studies that measured tyramine in foods found little need to avoid some previously banned substances. The primary foods to avoid are avocado, fava beans, cheeses (except cream, cottage, and ricotta), chocolate (in large amounts), overripe bananas, sauerkraut, shrimp paste, sour cream, and soy products, including tofu. MAO inhibitors can also interact harmfully with certain over-the-counter and prescription medications and with illegal drugs, especially cocaine.

Individuals should alert their doctors if they have high blood pressure or heart problems, if they often have severe headaches, and if they may be undergoing anesthesia, surgery, or medical testing in the coming months. Anyone using an MAO inhibitor

Dietary and drug restrictions when taking MAO inhibitors

Foods that MUST be avoided:

☐ Cheese (except ricotta, cottage cheese, and cream cheese)

☐ Cheese-containing foods (e.g., pizza, fondue, many Italian dishes, and some salad dressings)

☐ Fermented or aged foods (especially fermented or aged meats or fish, e.g., corned beef, salami, pepperoni, and sausage)

☐ Liverwurst

☐ Broad bean (fava) pods

☐ Meat extracts or yeast extracts, such as Bovril and Marmite (yeast and baked goods containing yeast are safe)

☐ Overripe or spoiled fruits (e.g., bananas, pineapples, avocados, figs, and raisins)

☐ Soy sauce, tofu, fermented bean curd (an ingredient in soybean paste and miso soup)

☐ Sauerkraut

☐ Shrimp paste (shrimp are safe)

☐ Beer and ale (including nonalcoholic varieties)

☐ Vermouth, sherry, cognac

☐ Sour cream

Foods that may lead to medical complications if consumed in large amounts:

☐ Coffee, caffeine

☐ Chocolate

☐ Red wine (especially Chianti)

Foods that are now considered safe:

☐ Pickled herring (brine is unsafe)

☐ Smoked salmon, smoked whitefish

☐ Yogurt (unless unfresh; check expiration date)

Drugs that MUST be avoided:

☐ Cold medications (e.g., Dristan, Contac)

☐ Nasal decongestants and sinus medications

☐ Asthma inhalants

☐ Allergy and hay fever medications

☐ Demerol

☐ Cocaine

☐ Amphetamines

☐ Anti-appetite (diet) preparations

☐ Local anesthetics with epinephrine

☐ Levodopa for parkinsonism

☐ Dopamine

These restrictions should be followed from one day before to two weeks after taking an MAO inhibitor.

Adapted from Hales, R. E., Yudofsky, S. C., and Talbott, J. A. (editors). The American Psychiatric Press Textbook of Psychiatry, 2nd Edition. *Washington, D.C.: American Psychiatric Press, Inc., 1994.*

should check with a physician before using *any* drug, including prescription and over-the-counter cold medications, cough syrups, decongestants, nose drops or sprays, treatments for sinus conditions or hay fever, or preparations that suppress appetite or claim to reduce weight. Antihistamines are not a danger unless combined with decongestants.

If surgery is necessary, the anesthesiologist should be informed before the operation that the patient is taking an MAO inhibitor; the medication may have to be discontinued at least ten days before surgery. The use of procaine (Novocain) for dental procedures may be dangerous, and individuals anticipating dental work should consult with their dentist and psychiatrist about potential risks. Persons who have not been helped by a MAO inhibitor must wait fourteen days after discontinuation of these drugs before starting another antidepressant, including another MAO inhibitor, or using any foods, beverages, or drugs containing tyramine.

▼

Side effects   Drowsiness is common, especially early in treatment. Individuals should avoid driving or operating machinery until they are confident that they can do so safely. Other side effects include blurred vision, weakness, weight gain, sexual dysfunction, a rapid or slow heartbeat, and dry mouth. In those over the age of sixty, postural hypotension is a major concern. Less common side effects include constipation, diarrhea, rashes, chest pain, severe headache, chills or shivering, and jaundice.

Individuals taking an MAO inhibitor who develop an extremely painful or unremitting headache should immediately seek medical help, including blood pressure monitoring. A very high blood pressure reading may require emergency medical treatment. Persons taking MAO inhibitors should carry an identification card or wear a Medic Alert bracelet that notifies health personnel that if they develop a hypertensive reaction, therapy consists of 2 to 5 mg of phentolamine (Regitine), and that they should *not* be given meperidine (Demerol). All illegal or "recreational" drugs should be avoided. The use of cocaine can lead to an extremely dangerous increase in blood pressure.

The symptoms of an overdose include drowsiness, low blood pressure, difficulty breathing, convulsions, and coma. Immediate emergency treatment is essential.

MAO inhibitors should not be discontinued without consulting a physician, and use should be gradually reduced to avoid withdrawal symptoms. After discontinuation, individuals must continue to follow the dietary restrictions for at least two weeks to avoid possible toxic reactions.

COMMON MAO INHIBITORS

CHEMICAL NAME
Phenelzine

BRAND NAME
Nardil

DOSAGE Phenelzine is usually prescribed in an initial dose of 15 to 30 mg, which can be gradually increased to 45 to 75 mg. This medication has a cumulative effect, and doses may be cut after an individual has experienced a positive response. As a treatment for social phobia or panic attacks, the initial dose is usually 15 mg a day, with gradual increases to 45 mg. If symptoms persist, the dosage can be increased to 90 mg.

SPECIAL CONSIDERATIONS All illegal or "recreational" drugs should be avoided. This medication is extremely dangerous when combined with cocaine. Individuals taking phenelzine should not undergo any dental treatment requiring the use of procaine (Novocain) or any surgery requiring certain types of general anesthesia.

CHEMICAL NAME
Tranylcypromine

BRAND NAME
Parnate

DOSAGE The initial dose is usually 10 mg, taken twice a day. It can be gradually increased, usually no higher than to 50 mg.

SPECIAL CONSIDERATIONS In rare cases this drug may cause agitation or restlessness or reduced urinary output, in addition to the other side effects commonly associated with MAO inhibitors.

Drugs used to treat bipolar illness

The primary medications used for bipolar disorders are lithium, anticonvulsants, and antidepressants. Lithium carbonate, a naturally occurring salt, helps to treat both manic and depressive episodes and to prevent recurrences of both.

As noted in the American Psychiatric Association's practice guidelines for the treatment of bipolar illness, the anticonvulsants carbamazepine (Tegretol) and valproic acid (Depakene) have proved useful in manic depression. Because antidepressants can push bipolar individuals into a manic phase or speed up the cycling, psychiatrists usually first prescribe lithium, carbamazepine or valproic acid. Sometimes one of these mood stabilizers alone proves adequate; often, an antidepressant is added later.

Lithium usually diminishes manic symptoms after seven to ten days of use. Individuals with milder forms of bipolar disorder, such as cyclothymia, also may benefit from this medication. When individuals do not improve on lithium, they may be given an anticonvulsant as well. Other drugs being used experimentally to treat mania in bipolar illness include clonazepam (Klonopin), a benzodiazepine, and verapamil (Isoptin or Calan), a treatment for arrhythmias (irregular heartbeats) and high blood pressure.

LITHIUM CARBONATE

Some researchers theorize that lithium regulates the movement of calcium in and out of nerve cells; others contend that it controls the sensitivity of various receptors on the nerve cells. Whatever the mechanism of action, a number of studies have shown that lithium successfully reduces both the number and the intensity of manic episodes for as many as 70 percent of those with bipolar illness. About 20 percent become completely free of symptoms.

Individuals with less severe bipolar disorders, such as cyclothymia or bipolar type II disorder—in which major depressions alternate with hypomanic (less than full-blown manic) episodes—also can benefit from lithium. Those with rapid cycling disorder who experience four or more mood disorder episodes a year may not respond as well. Lithium can be used as an adjunct to antidepressant treatment for individuals who improve only partially. It may also be helpful as a maintenance treatment after ECT.

If administered early in a hypomanic episode, lithium can produce results in a few days. If not given until full-blown mania develops, lithium alone may not be a sufficient therapy. As the 1994 APA treatment guidelines note, "both benzodiazepines and neuroleptics have been shown to be helpful and often necessary for extremely agitated and psychotic patients." Although neuroleptic drugs, such as haloperidol (Haidol), have been used and studied more widely, the guidelines recommend consideration of benzodiazepines—most often clonazepam (Klonopin) and lorazepam (Ativan)—as an alternative. These agents are frequently as effective as neuroleptics in treating acute mania and do not pose the risk of tardive dyskinesia (discussed on page 775).

General precautions

The gap between the therapeutic and the toxic level of lithium is very narrow. Adequate fluid intake is essential to prevent toxicity, and individuals should take care to drink ample amounts of fluid and make sure their salt and water intake is sufficient during hot weather and exercise. Using careful trial-and-error testing, doctors usually prescribe the lowest possible dose that will prevent episodes of mania and depression. Lithium requires extremely conscientious monitoring by a psychiatrist or another physician experienced in the use of psychiatric drugs. Regular tests of the level of lithium in the blood and assessments of kidney and thyroid gland function are essential. Monitoring for potential toxic effects, particularly those involving the central nervous system, such as slurred speech, dizziness, vertigo, incontinence, somnolence, restlessness, confusion, stupor, and seizures, is also important.

Taking lithium at the time of conception or during the first trimester of pregnancy has been linked to heart defects in the fetus, although data now suggest that this risk may be less than had been estimated in the past. ECT is a safer treatment alternative for women who want to have a child. Those who receive lithium are advised to wait until they have taken it for at least two years without any episodes of mania or depression before discontinuing the drug. In the event of a serious relapse, lithium or certain antidepressants can be used later in pregnancy but must be stopped two weeks before delivery. Women taking lithium should not breast-feed their babies.

▼

Side effects   According to the APA practice guidelines, as many as 75 percent of individuals treated with lithium experience some side effects. Most are minor and can be reduced or eliminated by lowering the dose or changing the timing of the medication. The most common side effects of lithium include hand tremor, fatigue, weight gain, nausea, diarrhea, and skin rashes.

About 60 percent of those taking lithium experience increased thirst and frequent urination and should drink ten to twelve glasses of water a day to reverse dehydration. A single daily dose (rather than a divided one) or a lower dose may help to relieve these problems. Some lithium users, most often women or those with thyroid abnormalities, may experience depressed thyroid function (hypothyroidism). Hypothyroidism tends to appear after six to eighteen months of lithium treatment. Some may require thyroid hormone replacement treatment. Others may experience changes in their parathyroid glands, which can affect their blood levels of calcium and parathyroid hormone, and may be given medication to lower their calcium blood levels. About 5 percent develop psychological symptoms (mood changes, anxiety, delirium, aggressiveness, sleep disturbances, apathy, or confusion).

Half of those taking lithium develop a hand tremor. This often becomes less noticeable after several weeks on the drug; if it does not, the beta-blocker propranolol (Inderal) can be used to treat the tremor. Other possible side effects include an increase in white blood cells, impaired memory and concentration (particularly in those with neurological disorders), changes in heart rhythm (usually harmless), hair thinning or straightening, and, less commonly, changes in kidney form and structure, which may affect kidney function.

▼

Overdose risk   Because of the narrow gap between therapeutic and toxic levels of lithium, there is a high risk for accidental overdose. Symptoms include confusion, delirium, seizures, and coma. If not treated, overdoses can be fatal.

ANTICONVULSANT MEDICATIONS

Carbamazepine (Tegretol) and valproic acid (Depakene) are anticonvulsants used both to treat and to prevent manic behavior. They have proved as effective as lithium and often help individuals who do not respond to this agent. Although these anticonvulsants have various effects on the central nervous system and neurotransmitters, they may help in treating bipolar illness by controlling *kindling*. In this process, repeated electrical stimulation of the brain, possibly triggered by psychological stresses, produces activity in pathways of the nervous system that transmit impulses that may lead to seizures and manic behavior.

The anticonvulsants are effective for mania, and other treatments may be needed if the person becomes depressed. In some cases, an anticonvulsant may be added to an antidepressant for treatment of refractory depression. An anticonvulsant can be used in combination with lithium for individuals who do not improve on lithium alone, or as a single medication for those who develop serious side effects while taking lithium. Anticonvulsants may also be the first choice for those who experience rapid cycling or frequent episodes of mania.

▼
General precautions

Persons taking carbamazepine must undergo regular blood tests because of its most serious adverse effect, aplastic anemia. This condition, in which the bone marrow stops making blood cells, is rare; it occurs in only one of 125,000 individuals taking this drug, but it can be fatal. A somewhat more common risk is leukopenia, a drop in total white blood cells, which occurs in about 10 percent of patients. All individuals taking anticonvulsants should undergo liver function tests before treatment because these drugs can damage the liver, and preexisting liver disease may preclude their use.

Carbamazepine and valproic acid have been linked to spina bifida and other neural tube defects in the babies of women who take these drugs during the first trimester, and should therefore be avoided during pregnancy. Women who use them after delivery should not breast-feed their babies.

▼
Side effects

Carbamazepine may cause blurred vision, constipation, dry mouth, dizziness, drowsiness, rash, and difficulty in awakening. As with many other drugs, these side effects tend to be more common and more serious during the early phases of treatment and diminish as therapy progresses. The drug can also cause severe allergic reactions. The most common of these is *dermatitis* (skin rash), which often goes away when the drug is discontinued and then restarted. If periodic tests indicate the development of liver abnormalities, the drug cannot be used again.

The side effects of valproic acid include indigestion, heartburn, and nausea, which may be alleviated by taking the medication with food. About 18 percent of individuals, particularly women, experience some weight gain. Other possible side effects include tremor, drowsiness, and hair loss.

▼

Overdose risk   The first symptoms of an overdose may appear one to three hours after taking too much of an anticonvulsant. These include difficulty in breathing, muscle twitching, drowsiness, dizziness, tachycardia (rapid heartbeat), and coma, and require immediate emergency treatment.

Drugs used to treat panic disorder

The primary drug treatments for panic disorder are antidepressants and anti-anxiety drugs. As discussed in Chapter 7, all antidepressants except bupropion work well for panic disorder. Imipramine (Tofranil), the tricyclic antidepressant that has been most commonly used to treat panic disorder, has proved effective in 50 to 90 percent of those treated. Desipramine (Norpramin, Pertofrane) and nortriptyline (Aventyl, Pamelor) are also effective. In the future, SSRIs may become the preferred treatment for panic disorder. Although conclusive research has not been completed, they appear as effective as the tricyclic antidepressants and have fewer side effects. MAO inhibitors are equally effective. Although they are used less often because of the need for dietary restrictions, they are an excellent alternative for those who cannot tolerate the side effects of other agents or who do not respond to them.

Most individuals with panic disorder take antidepressant medications for at least six months. About two-thirds experience panic attacks when they reduce or stop the drugs, and usually must go back on medication for at least one more year.

The benzodiazepine drug clonazepam (Klonopin) is increasingly being used for panic disorder. Its chief initial side effect is sedation, but most individuals can adjust to this over time. Like alprazolam (Xanax), which was more widely used in the past, clonazepam is effective in blocking panic; it works faster and has fewer side effects than the tricyclic antidepressants. Compared with alprazolam, clonazepam is longer acting, produces more sedation, and causes fewer withdrawal problems.

Clonazepam can be used for individuals who have severe anticipatory anxiety (fear of having a panic attack) and those whose panic or phobic symptoms intensify during the early stages of antidepressant treatment for panic disorder. As the antidepressant takes effect, the dose of clonazepam is gradually tapered.

Drugs used to treat social phobia

Some people with social phobia may require medication as well as psychotherapy. The standard choices are tricyclic antidepressants, SSRIs, or MAO inhibitors. However, since individuals with social phobia tend to be sensitive to the side effects of the tricyclics and may develop irritability, insomnia, and jitteriness even at low doses, an SSRI or phenelzine (Nardil), an MAO inhibitor, is often the first choice. The main drawback of phenelzine is the need for dietary restrictions (see page 755).

BETA-BLOCKERS

Beta-adrenergic receptor blocking agents (beta-blockers) have proven especially helpful in treating individuals with a particular form of social phobia, performance anxiety. These medications work by blocking the beta-receptors in the nervous system, which are responsible for producing physical symptoms of anxiety such as racing heart, butterflies in the stomach, rapid breathing, dry mouth, and tingling in the hands, and can lessen these physical manifestations of anxiety. Although the beta-blockers have not been approved as a treatment for social phobia, a number of studies have assessed their effectiveness in individuals in various stressful or competitive situations such as performing music, taking examinations, or giving speeches. In more than half, the beta-blockers relieved anxiety and improved performance.

By far the most widely used beta-blocker for performance anxiety is propranolol (Inderal), which lowers blood pressure and heart rate and prevents constriction of blood vessels in the lungs. Psychiatrists may prescribe a low dose of the drug to be taken an hour or two before an activity that normally causes mild anxiety.

For particularly severe performance anxiety, some psychiatrists suggest long-term preventive treatment with higher doses of propranolol; the dosages vary depending on the individual but usually range from 40 to 120 mg. Frequent monitoring of blood pressure and heart rate is necessary to make certain that they do not drop too low. Individuals should report any dizziness, loss of coordination, or wheezing. It may take six to eight weeks to determine whether beta-blockers are having an effect. These medications should never be discontinued suddenly; the dosage should be reduced gradually to avoid possible complications, such as rebound hypertension.

The beta-blockers have some potentially serious side effects. They constrict breathing passages, which can be dangerous for those with asthma. They decrease heart rate, a problem for individuals with congestive heart failure. Insulin-dependent diabetics must be careful because the beta-blockers increase levels of blood sugar. They can mask the symptoms of hyperthyroidism. They also can increase the risk for a depressive episode in persons with a prior history of depression.

Beta-blockers should never be taken without a complete medical evaluation and should be used only under the direct care of a psychiatrist or another physician with experience and expertise in this area. Women who are pregnant or planning a pregnancy should avoid these medications. Individuals over the age of sixty may be more prone to side effects, particularly dizziness when sitting or standing up.

It is difficult, although not impossible, to overdose on beta-blockers. The symptoms include slow heartbeat, dizziness, difficulty breathing, and convulsions, and require immediate emergency treatment.

Drugs used to treat generalized anxiety disorder

The primary medications used to relieve the symptoms of generalized anxiety disorder are the benzodiazepines, which are among the most widely prescribed psychiatric medications, and buspirone (BuSpar). Because of their safety, benzodiazepines have largely replaced older anti-anxiety (anxiolytic) medications, such as the barbiturates and meprobamate (Miltown). Because it does not produce dependence and hence does not lead to addiction, buspirone is frequently used for longer-term treatment of anxiety. According to recent reports, most tricyclic antidepressants (discussed on pages 750–753) appear to be just as effective for individuals with generalized anxiety disorder and those with symptoms of both an anxiety disorder and depression.

BENZODIAZEPINES

The benzodiazepines include drugs highly effective in relieving anxiety symptoms, such as alprazolam (Xanax), clonazepam (Klonopin), and lorazepam (Ativan), as well as others with different effects. Neuroscientists have located receptors for benzodiazepines in the brains of both animals and humans. The more likely a benzodiazepine is to bind with these receptors, the greater its therapeutic effects on anxiety.

The use of some benzodiazepines that had revolutionized the treatment of anxiety disorders in the 1960s—including diazepam (Valium) and chlordiazepoxide (Librium)—has declined with the development of newer drugs that are equally if not more effective and that cause fewer side effects or withdrawal symptoms.

▼

General precautions   For most people, moderate doses of benzodiazepines for no more than two weeks carry little risk of dependence. However, use beyond this, even for as brief a period as two to four weeks, can induce both physical and psychological dependence. Because the risk for dependence is so high, benzodiazepine use should be supervised and limited. Psychiatrists prescribe these medications with caution, especially in individuals with a family or personal history of alcoholism or substance abuse. Individuals taking benzodiazepines should not drink alcohol, which interacts with benzodiazepines and can lower blood pressure to a dangerous level, decrease the breathing rate, and cause loss of consciousness and possibly death. Men and women already dependent on alcohol or drugs may become addicted to benzodiazepines after no more than one or two doses.

Interactions with other drugs, such as marijuana, sedatives, narcotics, and other benzodiazepines, are also dangerous and in some cases potentially fatal. In addition, many other medications, especially those that affect liver function, can increase the actions and side effects of the benzodiazepines. Among these are birth control pills; ulcer drugs such as cimetidine (Tagamet); propranolol (Inderal), a beta-blocker; and disulfiram (Antabuse), which is used to treat alcoholism. Individuals should always consult their physicians before taking any of these medications. The only benzodiazepines that do not interact with these drugs are lorazepam (Ativan), oxazepam (Serax), and temazepam (Restoril), a sleeping pill used for treating insomnia.

Persons who take benzodiazepines for three or four weeks or longer and then stop abruptly may experience withdrawal symptoms, including anxiety, irritability, restlessness, insomnia, impaired memory and concentration, and panic attacks. Among these symptoms are some that led them to take the drugs in the first place. Withdrawal can begin from one to ten days after discontinuation, depending on the particular benzodiazepine. All of these drugs require slow, carefully supervised tapering over a period of weeks or even months.

The benzodiazepines vary widely in their half-lives and potency (that is, in how long their metabolites remain active in the body and how powerful their impact is). Half-life is an especially impor-

DRUGS COMMONLY USED FOR GENERALIZED ANXIETY DISORDER

CLASS AND MEDICATION	TRADE NAME
Short half-life benzodiazepines[a]	
Alprazolam	Xanax
Lorazepam	Ativan
Oxazepam	Serax
Temazepam	Restoril
Triazolam	Halcion
Long half-life benzodiazepines[b]	
Chlordiazepoxide	Librium
Clonazepam	Klonopin
Clorazepate	Tranxene
Azaspirone	
Buspirone	BuSpar
Beta-adrenergic blockers	
Propranolol	Inderal

[a]*Half-life, 5–20 hours.*
[b]*Half-life, 20–200 hours.*

tant consideration for the elderly, who may become drowsy or confused by medications that remain in the body for a long period. Also, longer-acting agents have more of a tendency to build up in the body and produce sedation and confusion. The benzodiazepines that are eliminated very quickly from the body are less likely to cause side effects. However, withdrawal symptoms can be more acute than those of benzodiazepines with longer half-lives.

If your psychiatrist has prescribed a benzodiazepine, take the first dose at home at a time when you do not have to drive or operate machinery; these medications can impair coordination and mental alertness. Report your reaction to your psychiatrist, who can advise you on when and how often to take subsequent doses. Women who arc hoping to conceive or who are pregnant or nursing should not use benzodiazepines.

It is not easy to overdose on benzodiazepines. Although they are often used in suicide attempts, they rarely cause death unless they are combined with alcohol, sedatives, or narcotics. Signs of overdose include sedation, reduced coordination, slurred speech, poor concentration, decreased breathing rate, confusion, and memory problems. Immediate treatment at the nearest emergency room is critical.

Side effects   Benzodiazepines can cause drowsiness (particularly in the first few days of use): impaired coordination, memory disturbances, and problems in concentration; and muscle weakness. If these effects persist, reducing the dose or switching to another benzodiazepine can minimize some of them. Another option is to use buspirone (BuSpar), a completely different type of anti-anxiety agent (see page 768), instead of a benzodiazepine.

Some individuals taking benzodiazepines have *paradoxical* responses—that is, reactions opposite to those that might be expected—including a loss of inhibition that can lead to bizarre behavior, intense anger, outbursts of rage or violence, intense feelings of depression, and extreme anxiety or irritability. These reactions may be more likely to occur in the elderly, people with brain damage, and those who have a prior history of hostility, poor impulse control, antisocial or borderline personality disorder, or aggression. If a paradoxical reaction develops, the drug should be discontinued, and another agent, such as buspirone, should be used instead.

CHEMICAL NAME
Alprazolam

BRAND NAME
Xanax

DOSAGE Alprazolam is usually prescribed in an initial dose of 0.25 to 1.5 mg a day; doses may be increased gradually to a maximum of 6 to 8 mg a day. Most individuals who will benefit from this drug experience a reduction in anxiety within a week of beginning treatment. Some feel better within a day or two. It usually takes longer, two to three weeks, for the drug to have an effect on depression or panic disorder.

SPECIAL CONSIDERATIONS The primary advantage of this medication is the rapidity with which it begins to relieve anxiety and panic symptoms—much more quickly than the tricyclic antidepressants, which can take two or three weeks to produce benefits. Because alprazolam also can relieve the symptoms of depression, it may be prescribed for individuals suffering from both an anxiety disorder and depression, most often for those who do not improve after treatment with other antidepressants. However, individuals who stop taking it often report that their anxiety symptoms return as intensely or even more so than before. Alprazolam can be highly addictive, and withdrawal is difficult. The drug should never be discontinued abruptly; doses should gradually be reduced to minimize withdrawal symptoms.

CHEMICAL NAME
Chlordiazepoxide

BRAND NAME
Librium

DOSAGE The initial dosage is usually 15 to 75 mg per day, with increases as needed to a daily maximum of 300 mg.

SPECIAL CONSIDERATIONS Introduced in 1960, Librium revolutionized the drug treatment of anxiety. Its use has declined with the development of agents that are equally effective and pose less risk for physical and psychological dependence. It is now mainly used to treat alcohol withdrawal symptoms.

CHEMICAL NAME
Clonazepam

BRAND NAME
Klonopin

DOSAGE Clonazepam is usually prescribed in an initial dose of 1.5 mg a day, which can be increased, as needed to control symptoms, to a usual maximum of 8 to 10 mg. Many people feel the effect of this medication within the first day or within a few days of treatment.

SPECIAL CONSIDERATIONS Clonazepam is used to treat panic disorder and other mild to moderate anxiety disorders and may be useful in treating mania, tics, tremors, and movement disorders. Long-term use can lead to physical and psychological dependence. Some people feel lethargic and less alert or able to concentrate when taking this medication. It also can affect physical coordination. For panic disorder, the general recommendation is that clonazepam be used for six months to a year. However, panic disorder often recurs, and doctors may recommend continuing treatment for a year or more to ensure that symptoms do not recur.

CHEMICAL NAME
Clorazepate

BRAND NAME
Tranxene

DOSAGE Clorazepate is usually prescribed in an initial dose of 15 mg a day, with increases up to a maximum of 60 mg to control symptoms.

SPECIAL CONSIDERATIONS This benzodiazepine is used for short-term treatment of mild to moderate anxiety symptoms, alcohol withdrawal, and seizure disorders.

CHEMICAL NAME
Diazepam

BRAND NAME
Valium

DOSAGE The initial dose is usually 2 to 5 mg a day, with increases to a maximum of 40 mg to control symptoms.

SPECIAL CONSIDERATIONS Once one of the most widely prescribed drugs, Valium as a treatment for anxiety has been supplanted by drugs that are equally effective but carry fewer risks for physical and psychological dependence and problems of withdrawal. It is now used primarily for alcohol withdrawal, muscle spasms, and epilepsy.

CHEMICAL NAME
Lorazepam

BRAND NAME
Ativan

DOSAGE The initial dose is 2 to 3 mg a day, with increases of up to 10 mg to control symptoms.

SPECIAL CONSIDERATIONS This agent is used primarily in medical settings, e.g., given in injection form before surgery to relieve apprehension. Because it is metabolized differently from other benzodiazepines, it has less effect on the liver, and therefore may be a better choice for those taking medications that can affect liver function, such as birth control pills, propranolol, disulfiram, and ulcer drugs.

CHEMICAL NAME
Oxazepam

BRAND NAME
Serax

DOSAGE The initial dose is usually 30 to 60 mg a day, with increases as needed to a maximum of 120 mg.

SPECIAL CONSIDERATIONS Like other benzodiazepines, this drug is used to treat mild to moderate anxiety symptoms; it is also sometimes prescribed for alcohol addiction or withdrawal. It is considered a good choice for older patients because it has a gradual onset of action and a short half-life, so is cleared from the body reasonably quickly. Like lorazepam (Ativan), it is metabolized differently by the liver, and therefore causes fewer interactions with other drugs.

BUSPIRONE (BuSpar)

It is thought that buspirone, which belongs to a family of medications called *azaspirones,* may relieve anxiety symptoms primarily by altering serotinin receptor sensitivity and increasing serotonin activity in the brain. It is used for treatment of generalized anxiety disorder, social phobia, and refractory obsessive-compulsive disorder, usually in combination with an SSRI. It is also a good choice for individuals with a personal or family history of alcohol or substance dependence or abuse. It is especially useful in treating anxiety with associated depressive symptoms.

Although it has a chemical structure completely different from the benzodiazepines, buspirone is equally effective for most kinds of anxiety disorders, except panic disorder. It is less sedating, does not cause memory loss, does not impair coordination or driving skills, does not interact dangerously with alcohol, appears to have little risk for overdose, and has little danger of dependence. However, because it has a slower onset of action than the benzodiazepines, it may take up to a month for its full effects to be felt. Buspirone should never be used in combination with an MAO inhibitor.

CHEMICAL NAME
Buspirone

BRAND NAME
BuSpar

DOSAGE Buspirone is usually prescribed in an initial daily dose of 10 to 15 mg, taken in divided doses of 5 mg each two or three times a day, with increases as needed to a maximum daily dose of 60 mg. There can be a lag time of three to four weeks between the time individuals take their first doses and when they begin to feel better. At higher doses (10 to 60 mg) buspirone may be an effective antidepressant.

SPECIAL CONSIDERATIONS Side effects, which include dizziness, nausea, diarrhea, headache, nervousness, light-headedness, and insomnia, are usually mild and temporary. There is little danger of overdosing, but if this occurs, the signs include increased dizziness and nausea, confusion, and sleepiness.

Drugs used to treat obsessive-compulsive disorder

Although obsessive-compulsive disorder (OCD) is considered an anxiety disorder, the drugs that have proved most effective in treating it are antidepressants. The three agents currently approved in the United States for treatment of OCD are clomipramine (Anafranil) and the SSRIs fluoxetine (Prozac) and fluvoxamine (Luvox). Clomipramine has been used to treat depression and OCD in Europe for more than twenty years, and was the first drug to win FDA approval as a therapy for OCD. Fluoxetine has since been approved for this purpose as well, and fluvoxamine was approved for treating OCD in 1995. The other SSRIs may also prove useful. Scientists do not yet know why medications that block serotonin reuptake are effective, but they relieve symptoms in 60 to 70 percent of those who take them.

When clomipramine, fluoxetine, or fluvoxamine alone fails to help or causes troubling side effects, psychiatrists may prescribe combinations of two of these agents together or augment these drugs with other medications, selecting a specific agent based on an individual's symptoms. Examples might include buspirone (BuSpar) for associated anxiety, fenfluramine (Pondimin) for symptoms of depression, trazodone (Desyrel) for those with insomnia and depression, clonazepam (Klonopin) for panic attacks or anxiety disorder, or lithium for mood swings and other signs of bipolar illness. Antipsychotics may be recommended if individuals become delusional. Although these combinations have proved clinically helpful, they have not been fully tested, and they should be carefully monitored by a psychiatrist experienced in their use.

CHEMICAL NAME
Clomipramine

BRAND NAME
Anafranil

DOSAGE Clomipramine is usually given in a divided dose of 50 to 75 mg a day; this can be gradually increased to 150 mg daily. Some people may require a higher dose of 200 or 300 mg.

SPECIAL CONSIDERATIONS Clomipramine is a tricyclic antidepressant, most closely related to imipramine, and has a powerful effect on serotonin reuptake. It is usually prescribed for a period of six to nine months and does not cause dependence. The side effects of clomipramine are similar to those of other tricyclics: sedation, trembling hands, dry mouth, dizziness, constipation, headache, decreased sex drive, insomnia, sweating, weight gain, blurred vision, and problems with ejaculation. Some individuals become anxious or nervous. Less common side effects include memory impairment, muscle twitching, rash, diarrhea, loss of appetite, flushing, sore throat, runny nose, impaired urination, menstrual changes, impotence, muscle pain, and changes in taste perception.

Clomipramine should be used with caution in the elderly, who may require lower doses. It should not be used concurrently with MAO inhibitors or within fourteen days of taking these drugs. Overdoses can be dangerous and sometimes fatal. Symptoms include difficulty in breathing, shock, agitation, delirium, and coma. Emergency medical treatment is essential.

Selective serotonin reuptake inhibitors, such as fluoxetine (Prozac) and fluvoxamine (Luvox), are also commonly used in treating individuals with OCD (see pages 745–747).

Drugs used to treat insomnia

Sleeping pills may be used for limited periods when individuals are temporarily under great stress, when prescribed by a psychiatrist at the beginning of treatment for depression or an anxiety disorder, or when there is a medical problem that interferes with sleep. They also can help to overcome the effects of jet lag.

There is no perfect sleeping pill, and behavioral approaches usually are the best long-term solution to sleep difficulties (see Chapter 15). The sleeping pills chiefly in use today are benzodiazepines, which are safer than earlier medications used, such as barbiturates. They decrease the amount of time it takes to fall asleep and increase total sleep time. Physicians often choose one over the other on the basis of its half-life and the effects individuals may feel the next day. Those with long half-lives remain in the body for a long period and may cause drowsiness and confusion. Some with short half-lives have been linked to other problems, including amnesia and agitation. For individuals who also suffer from depression, psychiatrists may use a sedating antidepressant, either alone or with another antidepressant, to improve sleep.

▼

General precautions   Dependence develops if benzodiazepine sleeping pills are used for more than two weeks. As these drugs lose their effectiveness as sleep inducers, users may develop tolerance and increase their doses in an attempt to replicate the initial effectiveness. Those who stop taking them after prolonged use typically develop rebound insomnia, in which sleep is even more disturbed than before the drugs were used. Careful tapering of dosages over the course of a few nights can prevent these problems.

The elderly metabolize sleeping medications more slowly so that they remain in the body longer, and are more prone to the side effects noted below and to an increased risk of falling. A National Institutes of Health (NIH) consensus conference on treating sleep problems in the elderly recommended that clinicians consider sleeping pills only after a thorough assessment of the possible causes of the insomnia, improvements in sleep hygiene, and behavioral treatments. If these efforts prove unsuccessful, sleeping pills are recommended, but only in low doses and for short periods of time.

Although it is difficult to overdose on benzodiazepines, combining them with alcohol, barbiturates, or narcotics can be fatal. Immediate emergency treatment is essential.

Side effects The benzodiazepines may interfere with breathing, especially in people with chronic respiratory problems. They may also impair daytime coordination, memory, driving skills, and thinking, and may disrupt normal sleep stages. Confusion, hallucinations, and other psychiatric disturbances may occur, especially in the elderly. These drugs should not be used in pregnancy because of the risk for birth defects in the fetus.

CHEMICAL NAME
Estazolam

BRAND NAME
ProSom

DOSAGE For the elderly, I mg is usually effective. For adults, 2 mg is recommended.

SPECIAL CONSIDERATIONS This medication has an intermediate half-life of ten to twelve hours. Therefore, it causes fewer day-after and rebound side effects than longer-lasting sleeping pills.

CHEMICAL NAME
Flurazepam

BRAND NAME
Dalmane

DOSAGE The usual dose is 15 mg a night; this can be increased to 30 mg if required.

SPECIAL CONSIDERATIONS Flurazepam, with a long half-life of between two and four days, is rarely prescribed. With daily use, the amount of drug in the body builds up rapidly and can cause daytime drowsiness and impair performance.

CHEMICAL NAME
Temazepam

BRAND NAME
Restoril

DOSAGE The usual dose is 15 to 30 mg; 15 mg in the elderly.

SPECIAL CONSIDERATIONS Temazepam, absorbed slowly by the body, can take thirty minutes to induce sleepiness. With a half-life of about twelve hours and no active metabolites, it causes fewer day-after and rebound side effects than sleeping pills with longer or shorter half-lives and is considered a good choice for older individuals.

CHEMICAL NAME
Triazolam

BRAND NAME
Halcion

DOSAGE Recommended doses have been lowered to between 0.125 and 0.25 mg. This lower dose has proved effective in the elderly but not in younger adults.

SPECIAL CONSIDERATIONS Triazolam has a short half-life of three to six hours and does not linger in the body. In the 1980s, users of this once-popular agent began reporting side effects, including amnesia, agitation, paranoia, depression, and hallucinations. In 1991, triazolam was banned in Britain. After an investigation, the FDA recommended that it be used only in lower doses and for limited periods of time.

CHEMICAL NAME
Zolpidem

BRAND NAME
Ambien

DOSAGE The recommended dose is 10 mg for adults and 5 mg for the elderly.

SPECIAL CONSIDERATIONS Although not considered a benzodiazepine, zolpidem, with a half-life of 3.5 to 5.5 hours, is similar in many ways. It has fewer anticonvulsant and muscle-relaxing effects than the benzodiazepine sleeping pills, and may cause somewhat fewer central nervous system and withdrawal side effects, such as daytime drowsiness, dizziness, fatigue, depression, amnesia, and risk of falling. For patients with early morning awakening, a longer-acting agent may be prescribed.

NONPRESCRIPTION SLEEP AIDS

Antihistamines, usually the main ingredient of over-the-counter (OTC) sleep products, produce drowsiness as a side effect. If taken for several weeks, these drugs can be habit-forming and can cause troubling complications such as dizziness, impaired coordination, confusion, memory disturbances, and thickening of lung secretions. Very high doses of over-the-counter sleeping pills can produce nausea, vomiting, hallucinations, delirium, and convulsions.

OTC painkillers containing salicylates, such as aspirin, can help to improve sleep for a night or two. However, they should not be used by people with certain medical problems, such as ulcers. The amino acid L-tryptophan, once a popular OTC sleep aid, was taken off the market after contaminated batches led to dangerous blood abnormalities, and is no longer available.

Drugs used to treat psychotic disorders

Antipsychotic drugs do not cure schizophrenia and other psychotic disorders but make individuals with these serious mental illnesses feel more comfortable and in control of themselves, help to organize chaotic thinking, and reduce or eliminate delusions or hallucinations. Because tranquilization or sedation is a common side effect, these drugs used to be called "major tranquilizers." They are now referred to as *antipsychotics* or *neuroleptics*; the latter term is based on the fact that their side effects can mimic neurological diseases such as parkinsonism.

Although neuroscientists do not completely understand how antipsychotic drugs work, many believe that psychotic symptoms result in part from an excess of the neurotransmitter dopamine, increased sensitivity of the dopamine receptors, or altered activity in specific dopamine pathways within the brain. Antipsychotic drugs may work, at least to some extent, by preventing dopamine from binding to dopamine receptor sites in the brain. The new "atypical" antipsychotic agents also may have an effect on serotonin receptors.

In most cases, hallucinations and delusions decrease in intensity after one or two weeks of treatment with an antipsychotic medication. However, almost one-third of those given conventional antipsychotics continue to have residual or negative symptoms, such as apathy and lack of motivation (see Chapter 19). A relatively new medication, the atypical antipsychotic drug clozapine (Clozaril), can help to relieve both positive and negative symptoms for individuals who do not improve with standard medications or who develop intolerable side effects. Another recently released medication, risperidone (Risperdal), has also shown promise in treating negative symptoms such as apathy and withdrawal.

CONVENTIONAL ANTIPSYCHOTIC DRUGS

Over the last thirty years, many studies have confirmed the efficacy of antipsychotic medications in treating psychotic symptoms, such as delusions, hallucinations, and disorganized speech and thinking, in individuals with schizophrenia, major depression, bipolar illness, and brain disorders such as Huntington's disease or traumatic brain injury. Antipsychotic drugs may also be used in the treatment of borderline or schizotypal personality disorders, somatization disorder, severe obsessive-compulsive disorder, and a neurological disorder known as Tourette's syndrome. These drugs have proven valuable for treating individuals who become aggressive or intensely agitated, but they should not be used as a treatment for chronic aggression or agitation.

Antipsychotic drugs are categorized either by their chemical similarities or by their potency (low, intermediate, or high), which depends on the dosage required to achieve a desired effect. Thus, haloperidol (Haldol) is called a high-potency neuroleptic because less of it is needed to reduce psychotic symptoms. Chlorpromazine (Thorazine) is a low-potency neuroleptic because more of the drug is required to achieve a similar benefit.

Often the reversal of psychotic symptoms is gradual, occurring over a period of several weeks to several months. Without continued treatment after the remission of acute psychotic symptoms, the relapse rate for individuals with schizophrenia can be as high as 15 percent per month. By comparison, those who continue to take antipsychotic medication have a relapse rate of 1.5 to 3 percent per month. Individuals with chronic, relapsing schizophrenia may take the lowest possible dose of medication for years.

Although some antipsychotic medications act more rapidly than others, overall, most are equally effective, differing only in dosages, side effects, and costs. Nevertheless, for unknown reasons, different individuals often tend to respond better to one drug than another. The only way to determine which drug and which dose will help a person most and be best tolerated is by trial and error, a process that, although necessary, can be time-consuming and sometimes distressing.

▼

General precautions   Individuals taking antipsychotic medications should be careful about using other medications and should avoid alcohol, which not only makes psychotic symptoms worse but can also be dangerously sedating. The question of continued use during pregnancy must always be decided on a case-by-case basis.

▼
Side effects   Antipsychotic drugs differ in the side effects they produce. Low-potency antipsychotics tend to be very sedating and often lower blood pressure. High-potency medications can cause abnormal movements such as parkinson-like trembling and involuntary movements, but are less sedating and less likely to lower blood pressure. Dry mouth, blurred vision, constipation, dizziness on sitting or standing (orthostatic or postural hypotension), and drowsiness are most likely to occur during the first few weeks of therapy. These usually disappear, or the individual adjusts to them, after a few weeks. Other side effects include difficulty in urinating, increased heart rate, rash, sensitivity to sunlight or heat, weight gain, muscle spasms in the head or neck, slowing and stiffening of muscle activity in the face, body, arms and legs, drooling, hand tremor, and seizures in seizure-prone individuals. Although some of these effects are obviously uncomfortable, they do not cause lasting impairment. In some cases additional medications are used to prevent or relieve troubling side effects. For example, beta-blockers can relieve *akathisia*, a condition in which individuals become so restless that they constantly need to move and are unable to sit still.

Some persons develop what is called an *acute dystonic reaction* during the first hours or days of treatment. They may experience tightening of the face and neck and spasms of the muscles of the head and/or back. Sometimes the eye muscles are affected, causing the eyes to roll upward and "lock" in this position. This problem can be rapidly alleviated by the intramuscular injection of an anticholinergic drug such as diphenhydramine (Benadryl).

Antipsychotic drugs affect many hormones in the body, especially the sex-related hormones. Both men and women may develop enlargement of the breasts and occasional fluid discharge from the nipples. The medication amantadine (Symmetrel) can alleviate these side effects. Antipsychotics can also affect sexual desire and performance. Some men may have difficulty achieving or maintaining an erection, may experience retrograde ejaculation, or may develop priapism. Both men and women may have trouble achieving orgasm.

After several weeks of drug therapy, some individuals may talk and gesture less, seem apathetic, and have difficulty initiating usual activities. This condition, called *akinesia*, is sometimes mistaken for depression. On occasion, long-term drug treatment can lead to *rabbit syndrome*, which consists of lip movements that mimic the chewing of a rabbit. It can be treated effectively with anticholinergic drugs such as diphenhydramine.

The most disabling and difficult-to-treat side effect of the traditional antipsychotic medications is *tardive dyskinesia*, a neurological disorder marked by involuntary movements that can affect any muscle group in the body, most often the face. According to the American Psychiatric Association Task Force on Tardive Dyskinesia, 15 to 20 percent of individuals undergoing long-term treatment with traditional antipsychotics show some signs of this problem. The incidence among young adults is about 5 percent per year of treatment and rises with age. The most significant risk factors are increasing age and duration of treatment.

Individuals with tardive dyskinesia may, without meaning or wanting to, frown, blink, grimace, smile, pout, pucker, smack their lips, bite, clench, chew, or stick out their tongues. Others may rock, twist, squirm, tap their fingers, or shrug their shoulders. This condition does not affect mental function but it can be so severe that walking, eating, and even breathing become difficult. There is no known cure, although scientists are studying various medications that may prove useful. Some cases are irreversible.

Because of the risk of tardive dyskinesia, some states, among them California and New Jersey, require that individuals give informed consent specifically for this condition, before antipsychotic drugs can be prescribed. If it is not possible to obtain consent because an individual is acutely psychotic, psychiatrists educate family members about the risk and obtain their consent. The patient is then informed when symptoms ease.

Regular examinations every six months can check for early signs of the disorder, such as small, wormlike movements under the surface of the tongue. In some cases individuals with tardive dyskinesia who are switched from a traditional antipsychotic to clozapine or risperidone show improvement. In other cases it becomes necessary to weigh the therapeutic benefits of the antipsychotic medication against the risk for tardive dyskinesia and to decide which course to pursue on the basis of this risk/benefit assessment.

A rare but life-threatening side effect of conventional antipsychotic medications is *neuroleptic malignant syndrome*, in which the person becomes rigid and develops a fever, rapid heartbeat, abnormal blood pressure, rapid breathing, heavy sweating, and changes in mental state ranging from confusion to coma. This condition, a medical emergency requiring immediate hospitalization, can occur with any traditional antipsychotic drug but is more common with high-potency agents such as haloperidol.

LOW-POTENCY ANTIPSYCHOTIC DRUGS

These medications include chlorpromazine (Thorazine), chlorpro-
thixene (Taractan), mesoridazine besylate (Serentil), and thioridazine (Mellaril). All of the low-potency medications require more
milligrams of medication to achieve a similar therapeutic response
compared with other antipsychotics. They are often used in the
early treatment of an otherwise healthy young person who becomes psychotic and agitated, and can help to control physical
activity that might harm the individual or others. In addition to
sedation, side effects include low blood pressure, photosensitivity,
sexual dysfunction, constipation, and blurred vision.

INTERMEDIATE-POTENCY ANTIPSYCHOTIC DRUGS

These medications include loxapine (Loxitane), molindone (Moban),
and perphenazine (Trilafon). They are less sedating than the low-
potency drugs and cause fewer movement abnormalities than
high-potency antipsychotics. Some must be used with caution
in seizure-prone individuals. Molindone is the only antipsychotic
agent that does not cause weight gain, and it is associated with
less risk of seizures.

HIGH-POTENCY ANTIPSYCHOTIC DRUGS

These medications include fluphenazine (Permitil, Prolixin), haloperidol (Haldol), pimozide (Orap), thiothixene (Navane), and tri-
fluoperazine (Stelazine). High-potency antipsychotics are less
sedating and less likely to lower blood pressure. However, they
can cause abnormal movements, such as parkinson-like trembling
and involuntary movements (these are called *extrapyramidal
symptoms*), and agitated restlessness. Psychiatrists often prescribe
an additional medication—usually drugs called anticholinergic
medications, such as benztropine (Cogentin) or trihexyphenidyl
(Artane)—to reduce these side effects.

Pimozide (Orap) has proved helpful for delusional disorders, such
as erotomania and involuntary tics, and has shown promise for
treatment of both negative and positive symptoms in schizophrenia.

CLOZAPINE

Almost one-third of individuals given conventional antipsychotics
continue to experience residual symptoms, such as apathy and
social withdrawal. In the past, little if anything could be done to
relieve these negative symptoms. A major breakthrough in treatment came with the development of a different type of antipsychotic. The atypical antipsychotic agent clozapine (Clozaril) can
help with both positive and negative symptoms, such as lack of

motivation and withdrawal, for individuals who do not improve with standard medications or who develop intolerable side effects. In one study, 30 percent of those with so-called refractory schizophrenia who were not helped by other antipsychotics improved with clozapine. It may also be useful in refractory cases of schizoaffective disorder and psychotic depression.

Clozapine, which is believed to act on receptors for subtypes of dopamine and serotonin, is less likely to cause neurological side effects such as tardive dyskinesia. Its side effects include heavy salivation, sedation, increased heart rate, low blood pressure, and seizures.

Although clozapine is highly effective and helps to reduce the length of hospital stays, it has one serious drawback. About 1 percent of those who use it may develop agranulocytosis, a potentially fatal reduction in infection-fighting white blood cells. For this reason, individuals taking this drug must have their blood checked regularly and must discontinue it if their white blood counts drop dangerously low. The need for frequent monitoring makes use of this drug very costly, an estimated $5,300 to $9,000 annually. Mental health advocates argue that only a fraction of those who might benefit from clozapine have been able to afford it.

RISPERIDONE

A newer medication, risperidone (Risperdal), which also blocks receptors for subtypes of serotonin as well as dopamine, became available in the United States in 1994. In clinical trials, this antipsychotic, unrelated chemically to other antipsychotic drugs, has shown fewer neurological side effects such as acute dystonic reactions (muscle spasms), tremors, and akathisia (subjective sense of motor restlessness). Side effects include agitation, anxiety, and insomnia.

Although less is known about risperidone than about older antipsychotics, it has shown promise in significantly reducing both positive and negative symptoms of schizophrenia. It produces fewer side effects than clozapine (and the conventional antipsychotics) and it does not require intensive—and expensive—weekly blood monitoring. According to manufacturer estimates, the cost of a year's dose is about $2,500.

ON THE HORIZON: THE MEDICATIONS OF TOMORROW

Advances in molecular biology and neuroscience are bringing the development of drugs for disorders of the brain and mind into a new phase through what is called "rational drug design." According to the theory behind this approach, if the structure of a specific drug receptor is known, it should be possible to design tailor-made drugs to selectively interact with and modulate its functions. If this proves true, the psychiatric medications of the future may well be safer, easier to take, more precise, specific, and effective, and more likely to point the way to even better therapies.

Electroconvulsive therapy

Electroconvulsive therapy (ECT)—the passage of a controlled electrical current through the brain to induce a brief seizure—is not only one of the most controversial psychiatric treatments, but also one of the most effective for serious mental disorders, especially severe major depression. The mild electrical stimulation affects many of the neurotransmitters and receptors involved in depression, including serotonin, dopamine, norepinephrine, and epinephrine, as well as other brain chemicals. Because anesthesia and muscle-relaxing drugs are used before the electrical current is administered through electrodes attached to the scalp, patients do not experience any pain during the procedure, and their muscles do not shake or jerk. As many as 80 to 85 percent of depressed persons who undergo ECT improve.

Despite its documented benefits as a safe, reliable, and effective treatment, ECT is still regarded with suspicion by much of the general public. This attitude stems largely from outdated misperceptions of ECT as a painful, often dangerous treatment that leaves patients in a zombielike state. It is true that in the 1940s and 1950s ECT was sometimes used inappropriately, sometimes for illnesses it could not help and sometimes for patients whom psychiatric hospitals found difficult to control. In addition, a much stronger electrical charge was employed, and fewer precautions were taken to prevent injury.

All this has changed. Today, ECT involves a briefer, less intense electrical charge, varied electrode placement, and the use of muscle relaxants, oxygenation, and a short-acting general anesthetic before the brief pulse passes through the brain. The level of the current is tailored to the individual, unlike the practice in the past of administering maximal doses. Women typically need less current than men; older individuals need more than younger ones. ECT can be safely used for pregnant women, enabling them to avoid psychiatric drugs that might affect the fetus.

ECT is usually administered no more than three times a week, for a lower total of treatments (typically twelve or fewer) than in the past. (Some centers continue to administer ECT more than once a day, but this has been shown to cause greater post-ECT confusion without increasing the benefits of treatment.) *Unilateral* ECT, application of electrodes to the non-dominant hemisphere, usually the right side of the head, can significantly reduce the temporary memory loss because the brain's verbal center, in the left hemisphere, is bypassed. There have been questions as to whether this approach is as effective as *bilateral* ECT.

Typically there is a period of confusion after each treatment, which lasts for about half an hour. Some individuals also complain of headaches and muscle aches. Although individuals may not be able to remember the hours immediately before therapy, they usually show no signs of cognitive problems two or three weeks after treatment. A small number of people, estimated at about one in every two hundred, report persisting memory problems that may take six months to clear. A very few have lasting impairment of memories of certain important personal events.

ECT is the treatment of choice for individuals with severe depression who are suicidal, delusional, or whose disorder is life-threatening, possibly because they refuse to eat and drink. Other individuals likely to benefit are depressed men and women who:

- Do not improve with other approaches, including psychotherapy and a trial of at least two antidepressant drugs
- Have psychotic symptoms, such as delusions
- May not be able to tolerate the side effects of psychiatric medications, often because of their advanced age
- Need a treatment that produces rapid results because of the danger of suicide or harm to themselves
- Have had previous depressions that did not improve when treated with antidepressant drugs
- Have improved with ECT in the past.

Individuals at high risk for recurrence, often because of a history of previous depressive episodes, may receive maintenance ECT treatments every two weeks to every few months or may take antidepressant medications after ECT to prevent another episode of depression.

In individuals with mania that does not subside with drug treatment or who cannot tolerate the side effects of medications, one to three ECT treatments can be highly effective.

ECT helps about 15 percent of those with schizophrenia. It is most likely to be beneficial in cases in which:

- There was acute onset of schizophrenia, with confusion and affective symptoms

- Psychotic symptoms are out of control or are causing extreme suffering that does not improve with drug treatment
- Catatonic symptoms are jeopardizing health and life
- There also are symptoms of depression or mania.

Before undergoing ECT, individuals should have a complete medical and neurological examination, including an electrocardiogram, a chest x-ray, and blood tests. Informed consent is essential, and they and/or their families should be fully briefed on the procedure. (Sometimes they are also shown a videotape of an ECT treatment.) They should make certain that all their questions and concerns have been fully answered.

29

Self-Help Strategies for Better Mental Health

No one lives in a state of constant or complete mental health. By its very nature, life challenges us. We worry. We weep. We encounter frustrations and setbacks. Just as we can do a great deal to preserve our physical health, we can take steps to meet and solve day-to-day psychological problems more effectively.

One way to begin is by gaining an understanding of what mental health truly is. Freud defined the essence of psychological well-being as the ability to love and to work. Tolstoy put it more poetically when he wrote, "One can live magnificently in this world if one knows how to work and how to love, to work for the person one loves and to love one's work." In *The Sane Society*, Erich Fromm observed, "The criterion of mental health is not one of individual adjustment to a given social order, but a universal one, valid for all men, of giving a satisfactory answer to the problem of human existence."

The answer that each person comes up with is unique. Yet in every time and every culture, regardless of the variations of that time or culture, mentally healthy individuals share certain common characteristics. They are in touch with their feelings and can acknowledge and express them. They can perceive reality as it is, respond to its challenges, and develop rational strategies for living. Although not immune to problems or conflicts, these individuals can cope with them in ways that allow psychological growth. They can deal reasonably with others. And because they value themselves and their role in the world around them, they feel a sense of fulfillment that makes the routines of daily living and the effort these require worthwhile.

One of the core elements of mental health is self-esteem, the sense of belief or pride in oneself that gives each person confidence to strive toward a goal or to reach out to others to form friendships and close relationships. Self-esteem makes each of us feel significant as a human being who has unique talents, abilities, and a role in life. It is the small voice that whispers, "You're worth it. You can do it. You're okay."

Self-esteem is not based on external factors, such as wealth or beauty, nor is it something we are born with or can obtain from others. Self-esteem develops over time. We begin to build it as babies if we are nurtured and loved as we develop basic skills, such as our ability to walk and talk. It is fostered when, as young children, we learn to take care of our bodies and control our impulses—provided that we receive positive feedback about these accomplishments. Low self-esteem is more common in people who have been psychologically or physically abused as children, and it may increase susceptibility to mental illnesses, such as depression, anxiety disorders, and substance abuse. By comparison, those with good self-esteem, although they occasionally suffer the feelings of self-doubt that go with being human, focus on what's good about themselves and accept their limitations. Although this does not mean that they are immune to distressing problems, evidence suggests that a positive perspective may be beneficial for mental health.

There is a fine and not always clear line between mental health and mental illness, between reactions to a temporary crisis and a chronic pattern of negative feelings and destructive behavior. Some problems can be solved on one's own or by talking through the issues with trusted friends. Others require professional treatment because only a trained therapist can provide the type of help needed to restore mental well-being. The techniques described in this chapter are valuable aids to psychological health whether or not one is troubled, and they can also be helpful additions to professional therapy.

Self-help strategies

Self-care can contribute enormously to both physical and psychological health. Some of the most useful approaches for enhancing mental health are discussed below.

EXERCISING

Exercise has proven to be good not only for the body but also for the mind. It is particularly beneficial for mild depression. A number of studies of its psychological impact indicate that aerobic workouts such as walking or jogging can significantly improve the mood of mildly depressed individuals. Even nonaerobic exercise, such as weight-lifting, has been shown to boost spirits, improve sleep and appetite, reduce irritability and anger, and produce feelings of mastery and accomplishment. Exercise can also lower the risk for recurrence in depression. In a major eighteen-year longitudinal study of almost seven thousand adults, researchers at the Human Population Laboratory in Alameda, California, found that inactive men and women were at two to three times the risk for becoming depressed again as those who exercised regularly.

Exercise is also an effective means of anxiety reduction. Walking, swimming, other aerobic activities, and working with exercise equipment are all beneficial.

It may be that working out increases blood flow and oxygenation in the brain and alters the levels of various brain chemicals, thereby causing changes in mood. Beyond its effects on the brain, physical activity may have indirect benefits. In addition to distracting individuals from their troubles and relieving tension, regular workouts enhance the sense of well-being and improve overall health. As people lose weight or firm up flabby muscles, they feel better about their bodies and their lives. Their sense of competence and confidence grows as they see for themselves that they are capable of change.

EATING RIGHT

Both the body and mind require good nutrition to run efficiently. Poor eating habits—skipping meals, wolfing them down, munching on junk foods—can make people physically uncomfortable and psychologically uneasy, unable to concentrate on tasks at hand, relax, or enjoy being with others. A healthful, balanced diet is essential to a feeling of well-being as well as to good health. People who are depressed need to be especially watchful because they may lose their appetite, eat less, and lose weight, and can be at risk for nutritional deficiencies. Although various nutritional "cures" for depression have been touted over the years, none has been scientifically validated. A well-balanced diet should be part of every treatment plan.

Excessive amounts of caffeine can cause many symptoms associated with anxiety or panic, and caffeinated beverages should be drunk in moderation. Individuals troubled by anxiety disorders should not use them at all, restricting themselves to decaffeinated coffee and cola drinks.

Many people increase the amount of alcohol they drink when under stress. Depressed individuals sometimes try to drown their sorrows; those who are anxious may drink to calm their "nerves." Drinking only makes these problems worse. Alcohol, which is a central nervous system depressant, can intensify a depressed mood or exacerbate anxiety, and people with these problems should avoid it completely.

TALKING TO YOURSELF

All of us silently "talk" to ourselves every day, commenting on how we look and act or ruminating over problems. Some people constantly replay scenes from their lives, fretting about what they should or could have done differently. Others criticize or belittle themselves, magnifying the most minor of faults or failures into epic proportion. Negative forms of self-talk like these provide no resolution and only heighten anxiety and tension. It is far better to focus on the things you like about yourself or those that you do well. People who fight off negative thoughts fare better than those who give into them in the face of unhappiness or who rely on others to make them feel better.

As a test of your own self-talk, try tuning in to the "tape" within your brain. If you hear negative messages, talk back to yourself. Here are some suggestions:

- If you usually say, "I always feel awkward at parties," change the message to, "Tonight I'll try smiling at a stranger and maybe even start a conversation."

- Instead of saying, "I'm never going to do well in this job," tell yourself, "No one expects me to be perfect. My best efforts should be enough."

- Instead of, "Things never work out for me; no wonder I'm a nervous wreck," say, "If I'm realistic in my planning I'll feel less anxious."

- Instead of fruitlessly replaying the past by continually thinking, "If only I had said..." or "I shouldn't have done...," plan and develop a better way of handling a similar situation in the future.

As simple as such mental self-corrections may sound, they can be surprisingly effective in reversing negative patterns of thinking.

KEEPING A PSYCHOLOGICAL JOURNAL

A psychological journal is different from a conventional diary. Rather than focusing on the who, where, when, and hows of life, it emphasizes the *why*s. Writing about problems and concerns can ease anxiety and help individuals work through painful feelings. The more honest and probing the journal entries, the better. In a study at Southern Methodist University, for four consecutive days college students wrote for twenty minutes either about traumatic events they had never confided to anyone or about superficial topics. Those who wrote accounts of highly personal and upsetting experiences found that they felt much better psychologically.

To get started, reflect about each day or week, and identify the most meaningful parts of it. If you experience an intense emotion, positive or negative, write down the circumstances and the effects the experience had on you. Analyze recent events to identify possible sources of stress. "Autopsy" any encounter that makes you feel bad. If you find yourself worrying about a particular person or situation, record your concerns in detail. As you read your own notes, try to discern the underlying reasons for your worry.

Keeping a diary may also be a "homework" assignment in certain forms of therapy. Therapists who treat eating disorders may ask individuals to record their food intake and eating behavior, write down their thoughts about food and weight, and try to put what they're feeling and thinking into words. Such entries, which can serve as a starting point for a therapy session, provide additional material and offer insight that the therapist can use in exploring important psychological issues.

TAKING AN OPTIMISTIC VIEW

The dictionary defines optimism as "an inclination to anticipate the best possible outcome." In their book *Healthy Pleasures*, Robert Ornstein and David Sobel redefine it psychologically as "the tendency to seek out, remember, and expect pleasurable experiences. It is an active priority of the person, not merely a reflex that prompts us to look on the sunny side."

When bad things happen to optimists, they tend to see such setbacks or losses as specific and temporary incidents. In their eyes, a disappointment is "one of those things" that happens every once in a while, rather than the latest in a long string of disasters. And rather than blaming themselves (a pessimist might say, "I always screw things up"), optimists look at all the different factors that may have caused the problem.

No one is born optimistic or pessimistic. "We have a choice about how we think," says psychologist Martin Seligman, author of *Learned Optimism: The Skill to Conquer Life's Obstacles, Large and Small.* "We can choose to change the habits of pessimism into optimism." The key to changing is disputing the automatic negative thoughts that flood our brains—self-criticisms, fears, doubts—and asserting our own statements of self-worth. "Optimism is a set of learned skills," says Seligman. "Once learned, these skills persist because they feel so good to use."

CULTIVATING HUMOR

Humor, which often enables us to express fears and negative feelings without causing distress to ourselves or others, is another hallmark of mental health and may, in fact, enhance physical well-being. Thousands of years ago, King Solomon declared that "a merry heart doeth good like a medicine, but a broken spirit drieth the bones." Even in the face of critical or fatal illnesses, humor can help people live with greater joy until they die. Joking and laughing are ways of expressing honest emotions and of overcoming dread and doubt. Since we laugh as often, if not more, with others than by ourselves, humor also helps us in forging supportive relationships.

REACHING OUT

All of life's challenges need not be solved on one's own. As individuals build friendships and intimate relationships, they may find that some problems are easier to put into perspective. There are other dividends as well; people who feel connected to others tend to be healthier physically and psychologically. Social ties can also foster a sense of purpose or meaning, or motivate people to take better care of themselves. Large, carefully controlled studies have identified social isolation as a major risk factor for illness and early death. Individuals with few social contacts have two to four times the mortality rate of others. It is possible that a lack of "connectedness" weakens the body's ability to ward off disease.

Reaching out to help others also is important. Altruism enhances self-esteem and may relieve physical and mental stress. Studies suggest that giving helps those who give as well as those who receive. People involved in community organizations often are healthier and live longer, and they also report a surge of well-being called "helper's high," a sense of calmness and freedom from stress, increased energy, warmth, enhanced self-esteem, and fewer aches and pains.

Self-help groups

An estimated 12 to 14 million Americans belong to support groups, such as those organized by and for individuals who have cancer, arthritis, or other illnesses, who are wrestling with a substance abuse disorder, who have experienced common traumatic experiences such as miscarriage or child abuse, or who are dealing with similar challenges, such as widowhood or racial or sexual discrimination. Often these groups do not have a professional leader or formal structure. Their primary goal is to provide support and encouragement, overcome a sense of isolation, and share information.

Even though they do not aim or claim to cure, peer support groups can be therapeutic. They help by offering empathy, building morale, providing reinforcement, allowing emotional catharsis, and creating a new social world of persons dealing with similar life issues. The most widely studied of these organizations, Alcoholics

Anonymous (AA), has been demonstrated to help alcoholics control or stop their drinking. (Chapter 10 discusses AA and twelve-step programs.)

The members themselves play a crucial role in such groups. Because individuals with similar problems, such as substance abuse, compulsive gambling, or a chronic illness, cannot "con" one another, they can recognize any attempts to gloss over a problem or deny its emotional impact. The process of sharing problems helps group members to develop a sense of belonging and being valued. This camaraderie grows out of acceptance of one another, support, and the meaningful relationships that form as the group works together.

The experience of talking with people who have similar problems is extremely useful for those with mental disorders. Hospitals and community mental health centers often sponsor informal support groups. Such groups, especially those associated with a specific problem such as depression or an eating disorder, can also help in preventing recurrences. By participating, individuals are able to develop a sense of connectedness with others with similar problems and to receive and provide round-the-clock support.

Stress management

Although stress is a very real threat to emotional and physical well-being, what matters most is not the nature of a specific problem or incident but how an individual handles it. One of the best ways to think of stress is captured by the Chinese word for crisis, which consists of two characters: one means danger, the other opportunity.

Psychologist Suzanne Kobasa, co-author of *The Hardy Executive: Health Under Stress*, has found that some people seem to be stress-resistant. Although they confront the same stresses as others, they don't crack under the strain. Kobasa suggests that the reasons for this may lie in three major personality traits, which she calls the three Cs: *commitment* to self, work, family, and other values; *control* over their lives, based on the belief that they can influence their fate; and *change*, seen as a normal but challenging part of life that can bring new opportunities.

Other researchers have identified additional characteristics of stress-resistant individuals. They respond actively to challenges. If a problem comes up, they seek out resources, do reading or research, and try a solution, rather than giving up and feeling helpless. Because they have successfully faced many challenges in the past, they have confidence in their ability to cope. They have formulated defined personal goals, such as reaching a certain level of success or becoming a better parent. They use a minimum of "substances," such as nicotine, caffeine, alcohol, and drugs, and they make time every day for some form of relaxation, such as meditation or exercise. Rather than keeping to themselves, they seek out others and become involved with them.

Sometimes simply becoming aware of potential stressors can help build stress resistance. Psychologist David Elkind describes three daily stress situations:

1. *Stresses that are foreseeable and avoidable.* An example is getting so far behind on a project that it becomes impossible to meet a deadline. If this happens repeatedly, time management skills may be helpful.

2. *Stresses that are neither foreseeable nor avoidable.* These can range from the serious, such as a bad accident, to the minor, such as a delayed plane flight. There is nothing anyone can do to change the situation; the only option is to accept it. Simply realizing this fact can ease anxiety.

3. *Stresses that are foreseeable but not avoidable.* A tax audit is a good example of this kind of stress. Individuals can make even this universally dreaded experience somewhat less stressful by careful preparation beforehand.

Specific strategies can help to manage stress and to minimize its negative effects. Here are some of the most effective:

-   Review commitments and plans, and if necessary, scale them down. Assess what you're doing and ask why. Is it what you want to do or what you feel you *should* do? All of us have to do things we'd rather not do; the strategy is to make sure the *should*s do not overwhelm the *want-to*s in our life.

-   Watch alcohol intake. Many people believe that drinking will make them feel better; in fact, it impairs the ability to cope.

-   Recognize stress signals. Is your back bothering you more? Do you find yourself speeding in your car or misplacing things? Whenever you see these early warnings, force yourself to stop and say, "I'm under stress, and I need to do something about it."

-   Try "stress-inoculation." Rehearse everyday situations that you find stressful, such as speaking before a group. Consider how to handle the situation, perhaps by breathing deeply before you talk, or visualizing yourself speaking with confidence. With practice, you should find situations like these less stressful.

-   Develop alternative plans. You'll feel in greater control once you realize that you do have options.

-   Think of one simple thing that could make your life easier. What if you put up a hook to hold your keys so that you didn't spend five minutes searching for them every morning? *Doing* something, however small, will boost your sense of control.

Relaxation techniques

Special stress-management techniques help to produce a state of relaxation, a physical and mental state of calm that is the opposite of the fight or flight reflex, which is characterized by rapid heartbeat, sweating, and an increase in blood pressure.

PROGRESSIVE RELAXATION

Progressive muscle relaxation involves intentionally increasing and then decreasing tension in the muscles. The individual sits in a quiet, comfortable setting and clenches and releases various muscles, for example, beginning with those of the hand and then proceeding to the arms, shoulders, neck, face, scalp, chest, stomach, buttocks, genitals, and on down each leg to the toes. Relaxing the muscles can quiet the mind and restore internal balance. Here are some basic guidelines:

1. Sit quietly in a comfortable position.

2. Close your eyes.

3. Deeply relax all your muscles, beginning at your feet and progressing up to your face. Keep them relaxed.

4. Breathe through your nose. Become aware of your breathing. At the end of each exhalation, say the word *one* silently to yourself, establishing the following pattern: Breathe in . . . out, "one"; in . . . out, "one." Breathe easily and naturally.

5. Continue to do this for ten to twenty minutes. You may open your eyes to check the time, but do not use an alarm clock. When you finish, sit quietly for several minutes, at first with your eyes closed and later with your eyes open. Wait a few minutes before standing up.

6. Do not worry about whether you are successful in achieving a deep level of relaxation. Maintain a passive attitude and permit relaxation to occur at its own pace. When distracting thoughts occur, try to ignore them by not dwelling on them, and return to repeating the word *one*. With practice, you should be able to reach a state of calm relaxation with little effort. Practice the technique once or twice a day, but not within two hours after a meal because the digestive processes seem to interfere with the ability to achieve deep relaxation.

VISUALIZATION

Visualization, sometimes called *guided imagery*, is another useful stress-management skill. Using your imagination, you can create mental pictures that calm you and focus your mind. Visualization skills take practice and sometimes require instruction by a qualified health professional. However, the following tips can help:

1. Sit or lie down in a comfortable position, with shoes off, clothing loose, lights dimmed, and eyes closed.

2. Take a deep breath, filling your abdominal region as well as your upper chest with air. Slowly let the air out. Repeat, breathing still deeper and feeling yourself relax.

3. Repeat a simple word or phrase (some people use a prayer) to yourself. Concentrate on this phrase, banishing all distracting thoughts.

4. Beginning with the top of your head, tense and relax the muscles in your body.

5. Conjure up a vivid image of a tranquil, quiet, safe place, and visualize yourself in that setting.

6. Practice this procedure from ten to twenty minutes a day.

In addition to its usefulness in promoting relaxation and managing stress, visualization can serve other purposes. Athletes may visualize themselves giving a peak performance. Individuals with illnesses or injuries may promote healing by visualizing themselves returning to full health.

MEDITATION

Literally for ages, people have practiced meditation in a myriad of forms, from the yogi trances of the East to the Quaker silence of more modern times. There is no single correct way to meditate, and many people have discovered how to meditate on their own, often without even recognizing that this is what they are doing.

Most forms of meditation have common elements: sitting quietly for fifteen to twenty minutes once or twice a day, concentrating on a word or image, breathing slowly and rhythmically. In *transcendental meditation* (TM), the main difference is that the meditator silently repeats a mantra or special phrase.

If you wish to try meditation, it often helps to have someone guide you through your first sessions. You can also tape record the mantra in your own voice (with or without favorite music in the background) and play it back to yourself, freeing yourself to concentrate fully on the goal of relaxation.

This step-by-step guide will introduce you to one form of meditation. You may expand on it by repeating some of the steps for each part of your body:

1. Breathe deeply three times, allowing your breath to rise from your abdomen into your upper chest.

2. Exhale slowly through your mouth.

3. Imagine a white beam of light over the top of your head.

4. Allow the light to begin slowly pouring into the top of your head, warming, energizing, and filling your insides.

5. Allow your muscles to be supported by the warm light.

6. Allow the stream of light to move slowly down from your head through your neck, shoulders, and arms—filling your whole chest cavity, abdomen, hips, genitals, buttocks, legs, and feet. As it moves, feel the tension drain away from each part of your body.

7. Continue breathing deeply and slowly.

8. As the light flows through your body, allow "dis-ease" and blocked energy to be pushed slowly out through your hands and dissipate into the atmosphere.

During this process, your body will feel light, tingly, relaxed, and warm. There may be ripples of energy through the muscles. Relax, continue breathing deeply, and enjoy the release of blocked energy. Open your eyes; then sit quietly for a few minutes.

MINDFULNESS

This modern-day form of an ancient Asian technique involves maintaining awareness in the present moment. You tune in to each part of your body, scanning from head to toe, noting the slightest sensation. You allow whatever you experience—an itch, an ache, a feeling of warmth—to enter your awareness. Then you open yourself to focus on all the thoughts, sensations, sounds, and feelings that enter your awareness.

Mindfulness keeps you in the here and now, thinking about what *is* rather than about "what if" or "if only." Medical researchers are experimenting with this approach in overcoming stress, pain, and other chronic problems, including high blood pressure and migraines.

One way to focus your thoughts and create a feeling of being centered is by controlled breathing. Here are some guidelines:

1. With your eyes open, focus on your breathing.

2. Take five slow, deep breaths, pulling air down into your lower abdomen. Concentrate on your breathing. If your mind wanders, empty it of all other thoughts.

3. As you breathe in, picture yourself inhaling warm, soothing air.

4. As you breathe out, visualize yourself exhaling.

BIOFEEDBACK

Biofeedback is a stress-management technique that utilizes an electronic monitoring device, attached to the skin, to provide information about internal bodily functions previously thought to be beyond conscious control, such as temperature, blood pressure, heart rate, muscle tension, and brain waves, that are affected by stress. The sensors communicate the information back to the person through a tone, light, or meter, and by paying attention to this feedback, most people can be trained to gain some control over these involuntory functions.

Biofeedback consists of three stages:

- Developing increased awareness of a body state or function
- Learning to control it
- Eventually becoming able to exert this control without the use of the electronic device.

The goal of biofeedback for stress reduction is a state of tranquility. After several training sessions under the direction of a qualified health professional, most people can induce a sense of serenity more or less at will.

Preventing problems

The self-care strategies described in this chapter work best when they are used as a means of maintaining mental health and preventing problems, rather than in times of crisis or intense distress. All of them stem from one basic principle: the importance of taking good care of yourself. Look for opportunities to do so every day. Take occasional breaks, whether you use the time to eat lunch in the sun or meet a friend for coffee. Allow yourself small indulgences, such as five extra minutes in the shower. If you can't take a week off for vacation, a single day here and there can interrupt the constant rush of modern life and ease the pressure. Seek out pleasant activities, such as hanging out with friends, spending a sunny afternoon in a park, watching a splendid sunset. Learn to appreciate your own company. Try playing a musical instrument or doing some creative writing (including keeping a journal) as a form of psychological release.

Nurturing mental well-being may have an added payoff: You may end up happier. Rarely studied as a scientific phenomenon, happiness is defined by psychologist David Myers, author of *The Pursuit of Happiness: Who Is Happy—and Why,* as "a sense of well-being, a feeling that life as a whole is going well." As he notes, the best predictors of happiness aren't wealth, beauty, or fame. The individuals most likely to describe themselves as happy share certain traits in common: high self-esteem, an optimistic outlook, a network of supportive relationships, and a sense of being in control of their fate. Not coincidentally, these are also the key characteristics of good mental health.

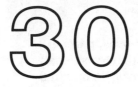

30

When Someone You Love Has a Mental Disorder

A once-dynamic mother spends most of the day in bed with the shades drawn. A teenage son begins to talk of voices that mock everything he does. A husband reaches for his first drink of the day earlier and earlier. A sister tearfully describes the waves of anxiety that make it impossible for her to drive, work, or now even leave her apartment. A close friend who had never ventured onto the water suddenly quits his job, spends his life savings on a boat, and declares he's going to sail the Atlantic.

Watching people you care about change before your eyes is heartbreaking. You keep hoping that they'll go back to normal, but you don't know when. You suspect that something is very wrong, but you don't know what. You want to offer your help, but you don't know how. You may feel desperately alone, but you are not: One in every four families in the United States is affected by mental illness.

The impact of realizing that someone you love has a mental disorder can be as profound as the diagnosis of a grave medical illness. "It's as much of a shock as getting a call saying your child has been shot on the playground," says one mother whose teenage daughter had a psychotic break one day at high school. "From the moment you find out, you start blaming yourself, wondering what it is you could or should have done differently."

Whatever the specific circumstances, the family changes. As one therapist puts it, "the deck gets reshuffled." Everyone close to an individual with a serious mental disorder—spouses, parents, children, brothers, sisters, grandparents, grandchildren—can be affected as intense emotions and fears sweep over them, family dynamics change, and priorities are reassessed. Family members feel vulnerable and confused. Each wants desperately to know when life will return to normal, whether the person will ever be the same, what this will mean for the future.

Many people think that if they can just love enough, care enough, do enough, everything will work out. One woman whose daughter has schizophrenia describes going to see her soon after she was admitted to a psychiatric hospital: "She didn't say a word but smiled beatifically. Her body is here, I thought, but where oh where is my daughter? . . . Like an intravenous line, I tried to pump my love through the limp hand I held in mine."

Family members need to realize, first and foremost, that love alone isn't enough to cure a psychiatric disorder. But this does not mean that love doesn't matter, or that they can't or shouldn't try to help. Loving sympathy and support can indeed light the way from the blackness of despair into a brighter new day for troubled individuals and those who love them.

Is something wrong?

Usually, mental disorders do not appear suddenly. There may be changes in behavior or attitude, subtle at first, that partners, parents, siblings, or close friends notice but attribute to stress or a recent setback. If the changes become more intense or persist over weeks or months, they may worry but still not be able to tell whether there truly is a problem. It helps to pull back and look as objectively as possible at your friend or relative. What precisely seems to have changed? In what ways is this person acting differently? How long have you noticed these changes? Does he or she seem to be getting worse? In particular, ask whether your loved one:

- Has seemed sad, depressed, or moody for several weeks
- Seems to lack energy and feels tired all the time
- Doesn't seem to get any pleasure from enjoyable activities
- Complains of problems in sleeping
- Seems preoccupied with death or talks about suicide
- Displays extreme mood swings
- Seems tense, nervous, or restless
- Appears confused or has problems in concentrating or thinking

- Experiences sudden feelings of panic or terror
- Has become extremely suspicious or fearful of others
- Is unusually irritable
- Has difficulty getting along with people at home or work
- Drinks more than usual
- Uses illegal drugs
- Has not bounced back from a crisis or loss that happened several months ago
- Seems unable to control or stop self-destructive behavior, such as gambling
- Has lost interest in sex or cannot perform as usual
- Complains of troubling physical symptoms that have no known medical cause
- Mentions bizarre or grandiose ideas
- Has become threatening, aggressive, or violent.

If the answers to any of these questions indicate specific signs of trouble, you may want to talk to other family members and friends to see if they, too, have spotted these behaviors. It may be useful to read through the checklists that begin each chapter in Part II of this book to get a better idea of the type of problem your loved one may have. Depending on your relationship with the individual, you may choose different ways of expressing your concerns. A spouse may try to have a quiet, intimate conversation. Parents may want to sit down together with their youngster. Close friends may choose to put their worries into a letter to the person or get together with others to voice their shared concerns.

What is important is to emphasize how much you care and to keep the focus on what you find troubling. Talk about how you feel—worried, frightened, sad, angry, whatever is applicable. Your tone should be compassionate rather than critical. Nevertheless, no matter how difficult it is, be as direct as possible. You might say that you've noticed changes in the person's behavior, or that you're distressed because he or she seems to be pulling away from everyone or is continually making self-critical statements about being stupid or incompetent.

How the affected person will react depends both on the problem and on the individual. Some may be defensive, angry, hurt, or rejecting. A person mired in depression may not show any response at all. Those who are dependent on drugs or alcohol may deny a problem. If your family member dismisses your concerns or keeps coming up with explanations or excuses, ask that he or she simply consider what you've said. Emphasize your worry rather than the fact that you think there is a serious problem. If the person has someone outside the family to turn to in times of crisis, such as a personal physician or a trusted minister, it may be helpful to suggest that he or she talk to this person to get another perspective. If it seems appropriate, you may want to suggest that the individual read the relevant self-assessment checklists in this book. Some people will recognize themselves and finally realize that their troubling symptoms are caused by a real and treatable disorder. Unfortunately, others will not, and may deny even more fiercely that there is anything wrong.

Regardless of the person's response, make it clear that you are not abandoning him or her and that acknowledging that there is a problem is the first step in the process of getting help. You also might want to point out some basic facts about mental disorders: that they are extremely common, that there are many effective treatments, that most people can be helped. Underscore your conviction that whatever is wrong is a challenge that you and your loved one will face and overcome together. If the person agrees that there may be a problem, talk about ways of dealing with it. Try to provide information and point out possible options. If he or she seems too depressed, anxious, or upset to seek help, take the initiative. Suggest seeing a mental health professional for a one-time evaluation or to find out whether therapy has anything to offer. You might also suggest a medical examination to rule out physical problems. For those who balk at any form of individual counseling, it may be useful to suggest couples or family therapy (whichever best fits the situation), which may seem less threatening and can often reveal and deal with many of the issues that may have caused or exacerbated a problem.

If no approach works and your loved one absolutely refuses to hear what you are saying, it is necessary to assess the gravity of the situation. If you perceive danger, whether to the individual because of self-destructive or suicidal behavior or to others, do not hesitate to contact a mental health professional immediately. If the situation is less extreme but the person's behavior is clearly off-base and becoming more so, the best option may be to consult a mental health professional yourself. Often a skilled and experienced therapist can offer insight and advice about dealing with your specific circumstances.

Coping with mental illness in a family

Severe mental disorders such as schizophrenia affect every aspect of a family's life: emotional, social, and financial. The entire family may need help—and time—to come to terms with the fact that the person they love so much may never be the same again, that the family's routines and rituals may be changed forever, and that all of them may have to sacrifice time and energy for the sake of their partner, parent, child, or sibling.

Because even less serious mental disorders almost always interfere with an individual's ability to express love and show affection, spouses, children, and close relatives or friends often feel emotionally abandoned. They also experience periods of intense self-blame for the illness that has afflicted their loved one. Therapy can enable them to deal with their sense of guilt and loss and to give one another psychological support as they face the challenge of caring for the affected person.

The more that family members learn and understand about a loved one's condition, the better prepared they will be to cope. Knowledge about the nature and course of the disorder and the behavior it induces provides both support and reassurance. In some cases, becoming involved in the treatment program enables them to communicate their concerns and work together in overcoming the problem. Even when the person's illness is not curable, as with Alzheimer's disease, family members can benefit not only from practical advice on day-to-day care but from education and counseling about the nature of the illness, the stresses it induces, and the problems that may arise. Whatever the disorder, relatives come to understand that their mate, parent, sibling, or child isn't deliberately acting or talking in hurtful ways.

Families struggling to come to terms with a loved one's mental illness may have to deal with an array of internal problems, from financial worries to emotional and physical exhaustion. Anorexia nervosa, for example, often creates a terrible power struggle between concerned parents and a child who seems to be willfully starving herself. Parents, who often feel demoralized and guilt-ridden, may need permission to get away and restore their own internal reserves.

Difficulties occur whether the person with a mental disorder is a child, partner, or aging parent. "No one else is there twenty-four hours a day to manage or monitor the illness," notes Laurie Flynn, executive director of the National Alliance for the Mentally Ill (NAMI), "so family members become the health professionals and the rest of the relationship suffers. Communication can be reduced to 'Have you taken your pill?' All of the richness of a relationship with a partner or a well child can be gradually squeezed out." Flynn's recommendation is to set aside specific times to talk to the person about something other than the illness. If it is difficult to find any other subject, arrange to go to a movie, shopping mall, or museum together. Work as best you can at keeping alive the bonds that once held you close.

As you focus on your loved one, do not ignore your own needs.

To provide ongoing help, caregivers need support and periodic respites. Seek out support groups, such as those sponsored by NAMI, the National Depressive and Manic-Depressive Association, and the other groups listed in the Resource Directory at the end of this book. Gather information, read books, and talk to people you know who may have faced similar problems. If at any point you feel that your own mental well-being is in jeopardy or that the person you love may be dangerous to himself or others, promptly consult a mental health professional, whether the one providing care for your family member or someone else, to help you decide what the next course should be.

Seeking help when needed is a positive step to take, a way of making the most of both personal and family strengths and coping with the inevitable strain on a marriage or family. Often, dealing with the serious problems associated with a mental disorder forces partners to look at behaviors they never faced before and to learn how to talk and act in ways that are constructive rather than destructive. The very fact that a couple or a family sees each other through a critical time and overcomes a difficulty together can ultimately bring them closer.

When a partner has a problem

A husband may seem distracted or withdrawn. A wife may seem moody or tearful. The spouse can think of plenty of reasons for this—overwork, money woes, constant demands from the children. But when a partner continues to behave in unusual ways, the person who loves him or her most may run out of excuses.

Maintaining an intimate relationship with someone who has a mental disorder is always difficult. Individuals suffering from depression, anxiety disorders, or other psychiatric conditions are often too wrapped up in their own pain to relate to anyone else. Over time, mental illness can erode the intimacy, trust, interdependence, and affection that make marriage rewarding.

Feeling that they cannot simply sit by as their loved one becomes more depressed, anxious, or out of control, many partners fall into the same trap: They start "overfunctioning" and take on more and more of the things their partner once did. But assuming a spouse's usual responsibilities may make a mate feel even more helpless, inadequate, and resentful. In turn, the well-intentioned partner begins to feel frustrated, because no matter how enormous the outlay of emotional energy, nothing seems to help. This pattern often occurs in codependence, a way of interacting that frequently develops in cases of alcohol or drug abuse but is found in other disorders as well.

It is a cycle that can be dangerous for the troubled individual, for the partner, and for their marriage. Yet, although helping a troubled spouse isn't easy, a partner's support can make a crucial difference in recovery if it is offered in the right way. Here are some basic recommendations:

Don't try to treat a problem yourself. If her husband is depressed, a wife may be tempted to try to cheer him up by pointing out what a beautiful day it is or noting that other people have much more reason to feel down in the dumps than he does. The husband of a woman with phobias may dismiss her fears as "silly," tell her why, and advise her to tough it out. Such comments are no more effective than they would be against the flu. Indeed, they can make matters worse. They sound like a dismissal by a spouse who doesn't want to hear bad or unpleasant things. Sometimes individuals with psychiatric problems feel that the only thing they *can* be sure of is how miserable they feel. To insist that they see the bright side makes it sound as if the spouse is trying to take even this feeling away from them.

Don't try to heap compliments and positive remarks on a partner. Reassuring troubled spouses that they're competent, successful, or sexy doesn't help when the distorted internal mirror in which they see themselves magnifies flaws and failures. Contradicting their self-perception may make individuals feel that you are patronizing or lying to them.

Tune in to changes in your partner's life and how he or she feels about them. Many people fail to see the connection between what is happening from day to day in a person's life and the way this is affecting a chronic or recurring problem, such as a depressive or anxiety disorder. If, for example, you know that your partner has suffered an emotional loss, such as the betrayal of a close friend or the collapse of a project that had taken months of work, you might encourage him or her to discuss its impact. This can help the person realize that the issues he or she is facing are very real and may require some assistance to work through.

Encourage your partner to be active. Many mental disorders breed inertia. In the case of depression, there may be near-paralysis. In anxiety, restlessness and agitation may give the impression of activity but in fact there is no actual physical expenditure of energy. Instead of asking whether a person wants to "do something," be specific; say, "We're going for a walk" or "It's time for the movie." Since even mild exercise can help to boost spirits and relieve tension, suggest that both of you head for a bicycle path or a hiking trail.

Give your partner as much control and responsibility as possible. Let the person know that you still expect him or her to function as a partner and parent. Structure time spent at home so that your spouse doesn't ruminate fruitlessly. Insist that partners continue to perform some chores. Don't go to Little League games or teacher conferences in their place. Encourage them to socialize, whether it's playing cards with friends or watching Sunday football at a neighbor's.

Distinguish between the individual you love and his or her illness. Preoccupied with their internal misery, spouses may say hurtful things, such as that they're not sure they ever loved you or that they haven't been happy in the marriage for years. This is the illness talking. Remind yourself not to take it personally and don't think that you've lost forever the loving person you once knew.

Keep in mind that a loss of sexual desire is a symptom of many mental disorders, not a rejection of you. These illnesses are physical as well as mental and, like heart disease or cancer, they dampen sexual interest. It's not that an individual who is depressed or anxious *won't* make love but that he or she *can't*.

Don't deny your own negative feelings. People with mental disorders can be decidedly less than lovable: They are often indifferent, irritable, self-absorbed, rejecting. However hard you try, you will not be able to hide the frustration you'll inevitably feel at times. Be honest about what you are feeling at the moment. If you say, "Of course I love you" with an edge to your voice, the person will ignore what you've said and pick up on how you said it. It is better to admit, "I love you but right now I could wring your neck" than to wait until you explode and let truly hurtful things out.

When you tell the truth, be tactful. Focus on your concerns, saying, "It scares me to see you this way" instead of "I can't stand you like this." Because many troubled individuals are exquisitely sensitive to criticism, try to limit negative comments to a few particularly irksome problems rather than attacking every shortcoming. The goal is to ease some of the pressure you are feeling without making your spouse feel even worse.

Protect yourself from catching a mental illness. This is literally possible. Some problems, such as depression, are so psychologically infectious that as many as a third of spouses eventually develop the same problem. Above all, resist the temptation to blame yourself. Talk to friends to help keep the problem in perspective. Get away for a few hours: See a movie, make a lunch date, browse through stores, take a walk. A growing number of mental health centers offer support groups for the families of individuals with psychiatric illnesses. Find out if there's one in your area and join. If you feel that you can't cope, get professional help yourself. You cannot help others get out of quicksand by jumping in with them.

Don't expect an overnight transformation. Recovery does not occur quickly. Sexual intimacy may take a particularly long time to restore. As a partner recovers, sexual desire does return, but it may take a while for a couple to rebuild a good sex life. Forms of affection other than sexual intercourse, such as kisses, hugs, and cuddling, can be comforting during this time.

When a parent of young children has a problem

When a parent develops a mental disorder, there are often concerns related to the children. Because of his or her own acute suffering, a father or mother may not be able to take care of or respond to youngsters' physical or psychological needs. A depressed mother may be so withdrawn that she doesn't talk or show affection. A manic father may frighten his children with his sudden mood changes or unexpected rages. The sheer unpredictability of daily life when a parent has a mental illness can make children feel abandoned, angry, confused, or hurt.

It is best to be straightforward in explaining a parent's condition to children. It is common for young children to assume they're to blame for Mommy's sadness or Daddy's anger. Let them know that their parent has an illness that makes him or her feel bad but that he or she will get better and is not unhappy or angry with *them*. You also can point out that talking about their feelings with you or with a close friend, relative, teacher, or pastor may help them to feel less alone.

Here are some other recommendations for talking to a child whose parent has a mental disorder:

Be careful not to put down or criticize the person. It can be tempting to let bad feelings out, but you'll only end up making the children feel angry, hurt, or afraid. If an upsetting episode occurs, try to avoid letting the children go off by themselves or go to sleep that night without first talking it over.

Encourage children to express their feelings, including the negative ones, as honestly as possible. But be careful not to use your children's reactions to a parent's behavior to try to get him or her to change or to seek help. This puts youngsters in an untenable position, and they may not want to share feelings with you in the future.

While dealing with a spouse's mental illness, be careful not to put your oldest child in the position of becoming a confidant or a surrogate parent. It is possible for this to happen without your being aware of it, yet it places far too much strain on a youngster and may anger your mate. Children usually want their parents to behave in ways that do not force them to take sides. If they are made to do so, they may face further problems in the future.

To the greatest extent possible, encourage youngsters to keep up their usual routines and to get involved in pleasurable activities at school or in the neighborhood. This can help them to forget about the problems at home for a while and to feel better about themselves. Let your children know that there is no need for them to feel guilty or ashamed about their parent's condition. Mental disorders are illnesses, and illnesses are nobody's fault.

When a young child has a problem

As noted in Chapter 26, mental health problems in children can create different and often difficult issues for their parents. When a child suffers in any way—whether the problem is mental or physical, temporary or chronic, the result of an accident or a hereditary disease—parents feel pain, guilt, and self-blame.

Obviously, the issues for families vary according to the age of the child and the nature of the problem. Severe behavioral or developmental disorders can shatter home routines, create an atmosphere of heightened tension and conflict, lead to spoken or unspoken resentments, and result in a breakdown in communication. Parents may feel torn between love for their youngster and frustration with the disruptions his or her behavior causes. They may also worry about the impact of their disturbed child on their other children. As discussed in Chapter 26 and later in this chapter, at every age siblings feel the impact of a brother's or sister's mental illness. In childhood they may resent the attention their troubled sibling receives or the embarrassment he or she may cause. In adulthood they may worry about the burden of assuming responsibility for a brother's or sister's care.

A marriage can undergo intense strain when a child has a mental disorder. Their nerves frayed, their emotional reserves drained, partners may lash out at each other. They may hold each other responsible, criticize the other's handling of the situation, or disagree about treatment. If they let themselves grow distant or distrustful, the relationship can be jeopardized. Counseling can be of great help in keeping a marriage on track. Often couples need permission from a therapist to acknowledge and respond to their own needs, including taking time to nurture their relationship. For the sake both of the marriage and their own mental health, it is so very important for couples to get much-needed time to themselves that it is worth the effort and cost of arranging for an occasional respite. Getting away, even if briefly, enables a couple to renew their relationship and bolsters their coping ability.

Parents also derive a great deal of benefit from participating in the education and support groups that have been set up by groups such as Children with Attention Deficit Disorders (CHADD), the Learning Disabilities Association of America, and the Autism Society of America. (See the Resource Directory at the back of the book for listings of these and similar organizations.)

When a teenager or young adult has a problem

For years, parents may nurture healthy children who blossom under their care and grow into bright, energetic, fun-loving teenagers. Then, just as they are on the verge of reaching their potential, something happens. The suntanned boy with the easy laugh becomes sullen and withdrawn. The loving daughter who had always been so responsible turns defiant and reckless, saying things that make no sense. As if out of the blue, parents feel they have strangers in their midst.

At first, they may suspect drugs. In some cases the problem is indeed substance abuse, and this must be confronted and treated. (See Chapter 9 on drugs and Chapter 26 on mental health in children and adolescents.) In others the difficulties stem from serious mental illnesses, such as schizophrenia or bipolar illness (manic depression), disorders most likely to develop in adolescence and early adulthood. Family members tend to respond in different ways, depending on the nature of the problem. Substance abuse often provokes anger and blaming; with schizophrenia or other severe mental disorders there is a greater sense of loss and of fear for the future. Because suicide can be a very real danger in these disorders (see Chapters 22 and 26), parents must face this terrifying possibility and learn as much as possible about recognizing the warning signals and getting prompt treatment.

The recovery process, whether it follows drug treatment or psychiatric hospitalization, presents challenges of its own. High school or college-age children are too old to be treated as babies, yet they may be too disabled, fragile, or unprepared to assume much responsibility. Those with residual symptoms of schizophrenia may not be capable of following through on a course of action. Parents may feel that they are back where they were many years before, when they were coping with the nonstop needs of very small youngsters.

"I've had to learn to live with her uncertain future, abandon my dreams, scale down my expectations," writes a mother of a schizophrenic daughter. "Vulture-like, fear of another episode always hovers." Counseling and support from groups such as NAMI can help enabling families come to terms with such feelings and develop realistic expectations for their loved ones.

When a sibling
has a problem

Brothers and sisters are sometimes called the hidden victims of mental illness. When one child develops a mental disorder, the parents may be forced by circumstances to devote most, if not all, of their energy, attention, and time to the child with the problem. As a result, the "healthy" youngsters in the family often feel pushed to the sidelines. Younger siblings may feel neglected; older siblings may pull away from the family or resent the shift in focus to their brother's or sister's needs. Even when parents try to keep daily family life as normal as possible, siblings may feel left out or resist the inevitable changes in their home. Their reactions depend on many factors, including the ages and number of children in the family, the nature and severity of the ill child's problem, and the parents' ability to cope (which may depend, in turn, on their financial resources and the support they receive from other family members). Although they may keep it to themselves, some siblings may be mortified by their brother's or sister's behavior on the school bus or around the neighborhood, and not bring friends home. Children can be cruel, and taunts about a "weird" brother or sister are painful.

Even young children need to understand that their sibling has an illness and that he or she may unintentionally do things that seem hurtful or embarrassing. If they respond inappropriately—by becoming disruptive, withdrawing from others, or showing other troubling changes in behavior—family therapy can be enormously beneficial. Meeting with a family therapist brings about better understanding about what is wrong with their brother or sister, helps them to accept the realities of the changes in their lives, and enhances their ability to communicate their own feelings and needs.

The issues involved in having a sibling with a serious mental disorder do not disappear as youngsters reach adulthood. "Even years later, siblings have lots of feelings about what has *not* happened to them, what they lost because of the other person's illness," says NAMI's Flynn. She also notes that many harbor a secret fear that they too may be vulnerable. "They wonder, 'Could I be next? Is it in the genes? What if I have children? Could I pass it on to them?'" Genetic counseling can provide answers, and in most cases reassurance.

As their parents age, adults who have a sibling with a severe mental disorder can develop new worries. "They look at what the mental illness has cost their parents—literally and figuratively," says Flynn. "They feel, 'I lost part of my childhood and now I may be asked to take on responsibility for my brother or sister as part of my adult life.'"

One woman, who recalls her little brother as her best childhood friend, has nightmares about people hurting the man he has become, a man diagnosed as having paranoid schizophrenia. His "appearance changes depending upon where he's living and what medication he's taking," she notes. "I never know if I will find him bearded or clean-shaven, with long hair or a buzz cut, a bit overweight or extremely thin. I never know what he will say or do. During one visit he asked me matter-of-factly if I ever heard voices coming out of the radio when it's off. 'I do,' he said." When he writes her, he always ends his letters with an "I love you." "He captures my heart," she says, "and breaks it."

Although the pain of a sibling's intractable mental illness never vanishes, learning about the disorder and understanding the nature of its prognosis can be a great help. Brothers and sisters often know surprisingly little about this, even though they have seen firsthand its effects on their entire family. NAMI has set up special programs and support groups for siblings and publishes a quarterly newsletter called *The Bond*. Among the common feelings that participants in such activities have voiced are:

- Grief and sadness over the emotional loss of a sibling

- Guilt because they have been spared while their sibling suffers

- Worry about developing the same problem or passing it on to their children

- Loss of esteem related to self and family

- Doubt and worry about what their responsibility is or should be

- Jealousy or resentment of the attention given to an ill sibling

- Shame and concern about what others will think

- Emotional numbness as a way of avoiding painful feelings

- Loss of faith because of God's cruelty or lack of mercy

- Hopelessness because the situation doesn't seem to get better

- A desire to escape and move on with their own life.

Nevertheless, however difficult their childhood years may have been, adult siblings, particularly those who become informed and understand the needs of the mentally ill, may be able to forge a new bond with their brothers and sisters. Mature enough to accept what happened in the past and what is possible in the present and future, some may be able to reach out and form a connection that enriches their lives as well as that of their ill sibling.

When an aging parent has a problem

Once your father may have seemed the strongest man alive and your mother's smile may have brightened even the gloomiest days. It can be hard to admit that the parents who once seemed so powerful and capable have become frail and vulnerable. If an older parent seems depressed, anxious, suspicious, or disoriented, adult children may be tempted to dismiss such behaviors as normal and understandable responses to the losses of late life and to physical aging. But this assumption is incorrect. Severe mental illnesses, including delusions and paranoia, affect 1 million elderly Americans. Many more suffer milder forms or significant symptoms. (Chapter 25 deals with mental health in the elderly and lists warning signals of possible disorders.)

Although occasional feelings of depression or anxiety, sleep disturbances, forgetfulness, or memory lapses are common among people of every age, adult children should be aware that persistent and significant changes in an elder are not normal. Sometimes they are caused by medications or by physical problems or ailments, and a comprehensive physical examination is essential to rule out medical causes, such as undiagnosed illness, drug interactions, or poor nutrition. If there appears to be the possibility of a mental disorder, it is best to consult a therapist with specialized training in geriatrics.

If your elderly parent resists the idea of therapy, you may want to consider more gradual approaches, such as having an initial meeting take place in a familiar place like the office of your parent's doctor or a senior center. You may want to accompany him or her on the early visits. (It is also important to make sure the therapist is aware of any medical problems or of medications your parent is taking.) If a psychiatric drug is prescribed, be sure that you and your parent completely understand when and how it is to be taken; you may need to monitor this if you feel that compliance is a potential problem.

One of the most beneficial things you can do is to provide frequent reassurance that the medication, psychotherapy, or other options proposed by the therapist will indeed help your parent feel better. With the exception of certain progressive conditions such as Alzheimer's disease, common problems such as depression and anxiety are just as likely to improve with treatment in older individuals as in younger ones. This is true whether the treatment consists of psychotherapy, medication, or a combination of both. Older adults are just as likely to benefit from the same strategies that enhance psychological well-being at younger ages, such as exercise and relaxation.

Special issues

Two of the most difficult and complex issues confronting the families of the mentally ill are the threat of aggression or violence and the high costs of mental health services.

AGGRESSIVE OR VIOLENT BEHAVIOR

Aggression and violence, which can range from mild verbal threats to the destruction of property and physical assaults, are major issues for families. In a survey of NAMI members by researchers from Johns Hopkins University, 11 percent reported that a family member with a mental disorder had physically harmed a relative or another individual during the preceding year. Almost twice as many reported that a family member had threatened to harm them or others; and 40 percent of those surveyed said that they had changed their behavior—for example, choosing not to give their relative a medication that had been refused or thrown away—in order to avoid a violent confrontation.

"A typical situation involves a sixty-year-old mother, alone because of divorce or her husband's death, trying to cope with a thirty-year-old son who may be physically aggressive," says NAMI's Flynn. "All sorts of families may have great fear of physical harm, yet they feel it's not their son or daughter who's responsible for such incidents, but the mental illness. It's only when weapons are involved that they call the police. Even then, they're ashamed. They try to forgive and forget, but the cycle tends to repeat itself. They fear that if they tell the psychiatrists, they'll just increase the medications and then their child won't take them. Ultimately there is just one too many violent or fearful experience or the family feels they just can't take it any more. That's when individuals are put into institutions."

It doesn't have to turn out this way. Agnes Hatfield, Ph.D., family education specialist for NAMI, says that in most cases "volatile behavior can be significantly reduced and/or families can protect themselves from personal attack." According to Hatfield, family members can lessen the likelihood of aggressive behavior by providing a supportive, nonstressful environment, characterized by:

- A predictable routine, which supplies structure so that individuals plagued by internal chaos can orient themselves to reality

- Reduced stimulation, which eliminates the anxiety and confusion caused by too many people and too many demands

- Realistic expectations, which relieve the pressure to perform at a level higher than the individual's capability

- Sensitivity to the individual's susceptibility to any slight or criticism. However, it is important for family members to understand the reasons for the violence and to take steps to prevent it. As Hatfield notes, "People with mental illnesses who have poor impulse control may direct hostility toward other family members for a variety of reasons, such as hypersensitivity to criticism, jealousy, or real or perceived obstruction to their needs and desires. Violence or the threat of violence may be an expression of the individual's psychotic thinking." People who are not in touch with reality may feel they are in danger and attack to protect themselves, or they may "hear" a command to hit someone or destroy something. In such cases the family should call the individual's psychiatrist to determine whether medication or hospitalization is necessary.

When a mental illness is accompanied by poor impulse control, episodes of aggression may occur even in a low-key, supportive environment. As a general precaution, guns should be removed from the home; knives and other dangerous objects should be locked away. Family members should train themselves to tune in to early warning signals of trouble, such as increasing fearfulness, confusion, suspiciousness, agitation, and disorganized behavior. Their reaction to these signs should be calm and reassuring, reflecting their expectation that their loved one will indeed stay in control. At the same time, they should give the individual physical and psychological space and avoid patronizing or talking down to him or her. If the person becomes increasingly agitated, it will be necessary to take steps to protect themselves and other family members. This may mean leaving the house, locking the person in a room, or calling neighbors or the police.

Once an upsetting incident is over, family members should discuss it with the individual so they can work together toward ways of avoiding such confrontations in the future. For example, a person may become so upset when a favorite television program is canceled that he throws a dinner tray at the TV, shattering his glass and plate. After calm has been restored, family members should make it clear that such actions will not be tolerated and that he will not be allowed to watch any television shows for a week if he ever behaves like this again.

If the violence is more extreme, such as pushing a family member down the stairs, some advocates urge families to file a police report. A history of verbal threats is not sufficient if a family decides it is necessary to seek involuntary commitment; evidence of physical dangerousness must be well-documented. A police report of all such incidents can provide needed evidence if the violence continues or escalates.

FINANCIAL ISSUES

Mental illness can create enormous financial difficulties. Treatment costs are high, and many insurance plans provide limited coverage, if any. Wanting to do everything they can for their loved one, families may drain their savings, mortgage and remortgage their homes, and incur huge debts.

Family members should find out exactly what their insurance policies cover and should check into such provisions as deductibles, copayments, and caps on lifetime coverage. Local chapters of NAMI and other advocacy groups may be able to provide information on other sources of reimbursement and income, such as Social Security Disability Insurance, for individuals who cannot work because of a mental disorder.

A great concern for parents is providing for the care of a mentally ill loved one when they become old or ill. Siblings also face this worry after the death of their parents. Planned Lifetime Assistance Networks (PLAN), a relatively new approach available in a growing number of states, offers long-term monitoring by social workers in nonprofit agencies. These professionals visit individuals with chronic mental disorders, coordinate needed services, and cut through bureaucratic obstacles. Families pay an initial membership fee and pledge a larger amount, usually payable at the death of both parents, to help fund the continuing care of their loved one.

Many parents provide for mentally ill children through a will or trust, but there can be complicating factors to doing this, such as entrusting money to a relative who may not be able to handle the responsibility. Local advocacy groups can usually provide the names of lawyers who specialize in trusts and wills involving a mentally ill person. There also are lawyers and agencies who specialize in handling the finances of aging parents.

What you can do

Just as individuals with mental disorders have been speaking and reaching out, family members are doing the same. One of the major contributions of the advocacy movement in mental health has been winning greater recognition and involvement for partners, parents, adult children, and siblings.

"For years, family members have been blamed, excluded, or given incomplete information," says NAMI's Flynn. "Mental health professionals have always said that they are protecting the confidentiality of what their patients tell them. Yet families don't want the secrets of therapy. We need to know what medications have been prescribed, what we should expect, what are their side effects, what should we watch for. We have to know enough to cope, especially now when people are being discharged more and more rapidly in a less and less stable state." As Flynn notes, because severe mental illnesses are chronic and the health care system is fragmented, families are often the linchpin of support. "Excluding them may pull away the only consistent support the person has. This sets up a disabling and often unnecessary cycle of crisis and relapse."

Like all families, each family of a mentally ill person is unique. Values, priorities, and goals differ. Each has developed its own ways of responding to crises and showing its commitment and love, but when a mental disorder strikes, these usual ways of responding may not be adequate or appropriate. Based on years of working with families affected by mental illness, the American and Canadian Mental Health Associations offer the following general recommendations:

Foster the will to be well. Talk in positive terms (about recovery, a new life, a new job), though not at the expense of honesty about feelings and fears. Give, and expect, respect and responsibility. Assign all family members household duties and a place in family discussions. Don't overprotect the sick one, provide special treatment, or let him or her hide behind "being different."

Seek out information. Though there are few cut-and-dried answers to the many questions that arise when mental illness confronts a family, there are broad guidelines that will help. Questions about financial assistance, education, employment opportunities, and other practical concerns do have definite answers. Check with therapists, read books and articles, and write to experts. Be prepared *before* a crisis.

Broaden the helping network. If this is done, less of the burden falls on the immediate family, especially the children. Friends, neighbors, and colleagues may be willing to give practical assistance if asked. Self-help groups, for both ex-patients and/or their friends and family, have been lifesavers for many.

Live your own life. Though it is difficult to do when confronted with a mentally ill family member, each person must continue to pursue his or her own interests and keep in touch with personal friends. Outlets like these relax us, help counterbalance the strained atmosphere at home, and keep us in touch with "ordinary" behavior.

Learn warning signals. Try to assess the words, actions, or attitudes that precede problems, and figure out their timetable. If in doubt, check with a helping professional.

Don't expect too much of yourself. You are likely to be tired, angry, or resentful now and then. Accept that your job and other personal relationships may suffer from time to time. Remember that few people can always be patient and giving.

Don't blame yourself. Mental illness can be caused by environmental stresses, biochemical imbalances, and many other factors, known and unknown. Family disruption or events in family history may not have helped, but they are rarely the cause of the illness.

Talk about your situation. It may be that, like many people, you will find it very difficult to discuss your circumstances with close friends because they have little or no sense of what you are going through and do not know how to respond. If you have trouble obtaining the understanding and support you need, contact a self-help group. People who have "been there" can listen objectively to your problems and give valid and useful advice.

Seek out counseling. If family members find it very difficult to cope, counseling for the entire family may be a wise alternative. There are many kinds of counseling available; check your community information sources.

Don't give up too soon. Recovery from a mental illness takes time. Like a wound, its healing is gradual and cannot be rushed. Don't be discouraged by temporary setbacks; don't lay blame when things go wrong. The family is in this together, for better or worse.*

---

*Reprinted from *Coping with Mental Illness in the Family*, Number 8 in a series published by the National Mental Health Association and the Canadian Mental Health Association.

Glossary

abreaction Release of previously repressed emotions after recall of a painful experience.

acetylcholine A **neurotransmitter** in the brain that helps to regulate memory. (*See also* **anticholinergic; cholinergic.**)

acquaintance rape Rape by a person known to the victim.

acquired immunodeficiency syndrome (AIDS) An incurable illness in which the **human immunodeficiency virus (HIV)** suppresses the body's immune system, resulting in vulnerability to a variety of "opportunistic" infections and diseases. AIDS is transmitted by direct exposure to the virus in blood, semen, or vaginal secretions; by an infected pregnant woman to her child before or during birth; or to an infant through breast milk.

acting out Expressing feelings through maladaptive actions rather than words.

addiction A behavioral pattern characterized by compulsion, loss of control, and continued repetition of a behavior or activity in spite of adverse consequences.

adjustment disorder The abnormal persistence of otherwise normal emotional or behavioral symptoms after a stressful event or trauma.

adrenaline *See* **epinephrine.**

adrenergic Pertaining to the neurotransmitter **epinephrine** (adrenaline).

aerobic exercise Physical activity in which oxygen is continually supplied to the body to meet increased demands.

affect External expression of emotion, feeling, or mood that accompanies a thought.

aftercare Rehabilitation and other therapies after hospitalization to help an individual adjust to a new environment and to prevent relapse.

aggression Forceful behavior with intent to dominate; physical or verbal force directed toward the environment, another person, or oneself.

agitation Excessive physical activity, usually associated with tension, such as an inability to sit still, fidgeting, pacing, or wringing of hands.

agoraphobia Fear of open spaces, leaving a familiar place (e.g., one's home), or being in places or situations in which escape may be difficult or embarrassing or where help may not be available.

AIDS   *See* **acquired immuno-deficiency syndrome.**

AIDS dementia   A rapidly progressive **dementia** in individuals with **acquired immuno-defiency syndrome (AIDS).**

akathisia   Uncontrollable motor restlessness and movement, commonly a side effect of certain medications.

akinesia   A state of reduced movement.

Al-Anon   An organization utilizing a **twelve-step program** for relatives of alcoholics.

Alateen   An organization utilizing a **twelve-step program** for teen-age children of alcoholic parents.

alcohol dependence   Alcohol use characterized by **tolerance** or development of **withdrawal** symptoms when alcohol intake is reduced or eliminated. (*Also called* **alcoholism.**)

alcoholic   An individual who loses control over use of alcohol and develops the characteristic symptoms of **alcoholism.** (*See also* **Type I alcoholic** and **Type 2 alcoholic.**)

Alcoholics Anonymous (AA)   A worldwide organization that developed the first **twelve-step program** for alcoholic persons based on group support.

alcoholism   A chronic, progressive, potentially fatal disease characterized by **physical dependence** on alcohol, **tolerance** to its effects, and **withdrawal**

symptoms when consumption is reduced or stopped.

Alzheimer's disease   An age-related, irreversible **dementia** in which gradual deterioration of mental capacity is caused by progressive degenerative changes in the brain, especially in the cortex and basal fore-brain; characterized by memory loss, personality changes, and increasing inability to function.

amenorrhea   Absence or abnormal cessation of menstruation.

amnesia   Permanent or temporary loss of memory.

amnestic disorder   A **cognitive** disorder characterized by impaired memory and the inability to learn new information or recall previous knowledge.

amphetamines   A group of stimulant chemicals often misused in order to overcome fatigue, induce **euphoria,** reduce appetite, or increase energy.

analgesics   Medications that relieve pain without inducing a loss of consciousness.

analysis   A common synonym for **psychoanalysis.**

anhedonia   The inability to experience pleasure; a loss of interest in once-pleasurable activities.

anorexia nervosa   An **eating disorder** in which refusal or inability to maintain normal food intake leads to malnutrition, severe weight loss, medical complications, and possibly death.

anorgasmia   The inability to achieve **orgasm.**

Antabuse (disulfiram)   An aversive drug used in the treatment of **alcohol dependence** that induces unpleasant symptoms (e.g., skin flushing, pounding heart, shortness of breath, nausea, and vomiting) when alcohol is consumed.

antagonists   Agents that limit or prevent the action of another substance.

anticholinergic   Impeding the action of the neurotransmitter **acetylcholine.** Anticholinergic side effects of certain antipsychotic, tricyclic antidepressant, and antiparkinson drugs include dry mouth, constipation, and blurred vision.

antidepressants   Drugs developed primarily to treat and relieve symptoms of **depression.**

antihistamines   Drugs used to treat allergic reactions and some cold symptoms; sometimes used as sleep aids because they may cause drowsiness. They work by inactivating histamine, a substance found in body tissues that plays a role in allergic reactions.

antipsychotics   Drugs used to treat the severe distortions in thought, perception, and emotion that characterize **psychosis.** (Also called *neuroleptics.*)

antisocial behavior   Actions performed without regard for another's rights, person, property, or for societal norms.

anxiety   Apprehension or uneasiness about an anticipated danger. Anxiety may be a normal reaction to danger or threat, or occur when no such such danger exists and cause troubling symptoms.

anxiety disorders   A group of conditions characterized by **anxiety,** affecting an individual's personal or work life, relationships, or emotional well-being. According to the **DSM-IV,** these disorders include **agoraphobia,** specific (simple) **phobia, social phobia, obsessive-compulsive disorder, posttraumatic stress disorder, acute stress disorder, generalized anxiety disorder,** mixed anxiety-depressive disorder, secondary anxiety disorder due to a general medical condition, and substance-induced anxiety disorder.

anxiolytics   Drugs that reduce **anxiety.**

apathy   Indifference, or lack of feeling, emotion, or interest.

aphasia   Impairment of the ability to use or to understand words, usually due to organic brain disease or trauma.

apnea   *See* **sleep apnea**.

assertiveness   The ability to be open and direct in expressing needs, feelings, and rights.

assertiveness training   A form of **behavioral therapy** that teaches individuals to express feelings and thoughts honestly and directly.

attention-deficit/hyperactivity disorder (AD/HD)   A mental disorder that usually develops before the age of seven, and is characterized by limited attention span, overactivity, restlessness, distractibility, and impulsiveness.

atypical depression   A form of major depression characterized by symptoms other than those usually associated with **depression** (e.g., increased appetite, weight gain, and sleeping more than usual).

autistic disorder   A developmental disorder that manifests itself in infancy or early childhood, and consists of severe impairment of social interaction and communication, behavior, and normal activity; thought to be neurophysiologic in origin.

aversion therapy   Treatment to overcome **substance dependence** or a bad habit by making the affected person feel disgusted or repelled by the behavior.

avolition   Lack of will, initiative, or motivation; one of the **negative symptoms** of **schizophrenia**.

barbiturates   A class of sedating drugs that depress the central nervous system.

behavioral modification   A method of changing behavior or eliminating a symptom by rewarding desired behavior and punishing unwanted behavior.

behavioral therapy   A form of treatment that aims to change behavior by means of **systematic desensitization, behavior modification,** or **aversion therapy.**

benzodiazepines   A group of drugs used as anti-anxiety agents or **sedatives.**

beta blocker   An agent that halts or inhibits the action of the beta-adrenergic receptors in the nervous system, which affect the blood vessels, heart, and lungs; in psychiatry, used most often in the treatment of performance anxiety.

binge eating   Uncontrollable eating of an amount of food significantly larger than most people would consume during a given period of time.

biofeedback   A technique, initially with the aid of an external monitoring device, of becoming aware of internal physiological activities so as to develop the capability of controlling them.

bipolar disorder   According to the *DSM-IV*, a **mood disorder** characterized by recurrent, alternating episodes of **depression** and either **mania** or **hypomania**. (Formerly called *manic depression; see also* **cyclothymic disorder**.)

bisexuality   Sexual attraction to, and relationships with, people of both sexes.

blood alcohol concentration (BAC)   The amount of alcohol in the blood, expressed in terms of a percentage and used as an indicator of intoxication. The U.S. Department of Transportation considers that a person with a BAC of 0.08 percent can be cited for drunken driving; a BAC of 0.05 percent is a level usually reached after one or two drinks.

body dysmorphic disorder   A **somatoform disorder** characterized by a preoccupation with an imagined defect in appearance.

brain imaging   Techniques used to visualize the structures and/or the functioning of the brain, including computed tomography (CT), positron emission tomography (PET), and magnetic resonance imaging (MRI).

breathing-related sleep disorder   A respiratory difficulty, such as **sleep apnea**, that interferes with sleep.

brief psychotherapy Any form of psychotherapy that is limited to a set number of sessions (usually not more than twenty-five) and to specific objectives or goals.

bulimia nervosa An **eating disorder** characterized by recurrent episodes of binge eating followed by vomiting, purging with diuretics and laxatives, or other methods to control weight such as fasting or extreme exercise regimens.

burn-out A state of physical, emotional, and mental exhaustion resulting from constant emotional pressure.

cataplexy Sudden loss of muscular strength without loss of consciousness, typically triggered by an emotion such as anger or excitement.

catatonia A motionless state, characterized by muscle rigidity or inflexibility, seen in states of extreme fear and in some types of **psychosis.**

catharsis The therapeutic release of emotions through talking and expressing feelings.

cerebral hemorrhage Bleeding in the brain caused by rupture of a blood vessel.

cholinergic Pertaining to the neurotransmitter **acetylcholine.**

chromosomes Microscopic structures within the cell nucleus that carry the **genes.** The normal human cell contains forty-six chromosomes, twenty-two of them paired and two, the X and Y chromosomes, dependent on the individual's sex. A female has two X chromosomes and a male has one X and one Y.

chronic Persisting over a long period of time or recurring frequently.

codependence An emotional and psychological behavioral pattern by the spouses, partners, parents, or friends of individuals with addictive behaviors that "enables" these individuals to continue their destructive habits.

cognitive Pertaining to the mental processes of thinking, understanding, perceiving, judging, remembering, and reasoning, in contrast to emotional processes.

cognitive-behavioral psychotherapy A short-term form of psychotherapy whose goal is to enable the individual to recognize and change specific conditions or symptoms, based on the complex interrelation of thoughts and behavior.

commitment A legal process for the admission of a mentally ill person to a psychiatric treatment program. Commitment may be voluntary or involuntary; the procedure varies from state to state.

comorbidity The coexistence of two or more illnesses in an individual.

compulsion A repetitive behavior (e.g., hand washing) or repetitive mental process (e.g., counting) that serves no rational purpose.

conduct disorder A persistent disruptive behavior disorder in children marked by repeated violations of the rights of others or of societal rules and norms.

confidentiality The ethical principle that forbids a therapist to reveal information disclosed by a patient during the course of treatment.

consciousness The aspects of mental functioning of which we are aware.

contract An explicit agreement between an individual and a therapist to follow a certain course of action.

conversion disorder A **somato-form disorder** in which a person develops a symptom suggestive of a neurologic disorder that cannot be fully explained by any medical condition, and is severe enough to impair functioning or require medical attention.

coping mechanisms Ways of dealing with **stress.**

counseling A general term for any interaction in which a person, who may or may not be a mental health professional, offers guidance or advice to another.

countertransference The **projection** of a therapist's emotions, wishes, and thoughts onto a client. (*See also* **transference.**)

couples therapy *See* **marital therapy.**

crisis intervention Emergency action to address a threat of suicide, violence, or similar urgency; also, a form of **brief psychotherapy** that focuses on a specific emotional trauma.

cross-addiction A state of **physical dependence** in which the physiologic need for one **psychoactive** substance leads to dependence on similar substances.

cross-tolerance The capacity to tolerate the effects of a **psychoactive** substance similar to another substance for which a **tolerance** has already developed.

cyclothymic disorder As described in the *DSM-IV*, a **bipolar disorder** characterized by **hypomanic** episodes and frequent periods of depressed mood or loss of interest or pleasure.

defense mechanism Any of several mental processes that work unconsciously to enable a person to cope with a difficult situation or problem, such as a major loss or trauma.

delirium A **cognitive** disorder characterized by impaired consciousness and attention, and by changes in thinking or other mental processes.

delirium tremens (DTs) The **delusions, hallucinations,** and agitated behavior that can follow **withdrawal** from long-term, chronic alcohol abuse.

delusion A false belief regarding the self or the world that a person persistently holds despite clear evidence to the contrary.

delusional disorder A psychotic disorder characterized by persistent false beliefs that involve the self, other persons, or situations in real life. (*See also* **paranoia.**)

dementia A **cognitive** disorder characterized by impaired memory, language, thinking, and perception.

denial A **defense mechanism** that enables a person to disclaim the existence of a behavior, thought, need, feeling, or desire that would be unendurable to acknowledge.

deoxyribonucleic acid (DNA) The "double helix" molecule found in all living cells that carries the organism's genetic information.

dependence, substance *See* **substance dependence.**

dependent personality disorder A condition characterized by an extreme lack of self-confidence, a continuing need to have others assume responsibility for one's life, and fear of separation.

depersonalization A strong sense of detachment from and unreality about the self, as if observing one's body or mental processes from the outside.

depersonalization disorder A dissociative disorder characterized by persistent or recurrent feelings of unreality and being detached from one's self. Occasional experiences of **depersonalization** are common; the diagnosis of depersonalization disorder is considered only when such episodes occur repeatedly and cause significant distress or impaired functioning.

depression A term that describes feelings of sadness, discouragement, and despair. It can be a normal and transitory reaction to events in a person's life, a symptom occurring in various physical and mental conditions, or a mental disorder in itself. The mental disorder involves slowed thinking, decreased pleasure, feelings of guilt, hopelessness, despair, and helplessness, and problems in eating and sleeping.

depressive disorders A group of mood disorders that includes **major depressive disorder** and **dysthymic disorder**.

derealization A feeling of detachment from one's environment, causing a person's perceptions of objects, other people, or time to be distorted.

detoxification A process that eliminates dependence-producing substances such as alcohol or addictive drugs from the body, usually combined with medication and supportive care.

Diagnostic and Statistical Manual of Mental Disorders The book that lists diagnostic criteria for all formally recognized mental disorders; used by mental health professionals in diagnosing mental disorders. It is regularly revised and updated, and is currently in its fourth edition. (Also called *DSM-IV.*)

disorientation Loss of awareness of one's relation to space, time, or other persons.

displacement A **defense mechanism** by which feelings are redirected from their true object to a more acceptable substitute.

dissociation The separation of some mental processes from conscious awareness; any altered form of consciousness that changes the sense of self or the ability to integrate memories and perceptions.

dissociative identity disorder A condition in which two or more distinct personalities coexist in a single individual. (Formerly called *multiple personality disorder;* renamed in the *DSM-IV.*)

distractibility The inability to sustain attention or the tendency to shift focus from one activity or topic to another.

dopamine A **neurotransmitter** found in the brain; elevated or decreased levels are associated with certain mental disorders, such as **schizophrenia**.

Down syndrome A form of congenital mental retardation of varying degrees of severity, sometimes accompanied by physical malformations, caused by a chromosome abnormality. (Also called *trisomy 21*; formerly called *mongolism*.)

drive A basic instinct or urge.

drug abuse *See* **substance abuse.**

drug dependence Habituation to, abuse of, and/or **addiction** to a chemical substance.

drug interaction A change in the way the body reacts to a drug when two or more drugs are taken simultaneously.

drug misuse The use of a drug for a purpose other than its original intent.

DSM-IV *See Diagnostic and Statistical Manual of Mental Disorders.*

dual diagnosis The simultaneous occurrence of a psychiatric disorder and a substance use disorder in the same individual at the time of diagnosis.

dysfunctional family A family characterized by negative and destructive patterns of behavior between the parents or among parents and their children.

dyskinesia Any disturbance of movement.

dyssomnias A major subgroup of **sleep disorders** distinguished by problems in the amount, quality, or timing of sleep.

dysthymic disorder A **depressive disorder** characterized by a chronically depressed mood.

Symptoms include feelings of inadequacy, hopelessness, and guilt; low self-esteem; low energy; fatigue; indecisiveness; and an inability to enjoy pleasurable activities.

eating disorders Unusual and often dangerous patterns of food consumption, including **anorexia nervosa** and **bulimia nervosa.**

ECT *See* **electroconvulsive therapy.**

ego In Freudian theory, one of the three divisions of the **psyche**; a person's consciousness or awareness of self.

ejaculation The expulsion of semen from the penis.

electroconvulsive therapy (ECT) The administration of a controlled electrical current into the brain, through electrodes placed on the scalp, that induces a convulsive seizure which can be effective in relieving certain mental disorders, such as an episode of major **depression**. Not to be confused with older, less effective forms of such treatment (*see* **shock treatment**).

emotional health The state of being able to express and acknowledge one's feelings and moods. (*See also* **mental health.**)

encopresis An elimination disorder in which a child of at least four years of age repeatedly passes feces in inappropriate places (e.g., clothing, floor).

endocrine disorder A disturbance in the function of any of the hormone-producing glands and tissues of the body.

endocrine system The network of glands and tissues that produce **hormones** and secrete them directly into the blood for transport to target organs.

endorphins Chemical substances produced by the brain that have mood-elevating and painkilling properties.

epinephrine A substance produced by the adrenal gland; it is responsible for many of the physical manifestations of fear and **anxiety**. (Also called *adrenaline; see also* **adrenergic**.)

erogenous Sexually sensitive.

estrogen The sex **hormone** that plays a major role in the development and maintenance of female secondary sex characteristics.

etiology Cause, particularly of a disease.

ethyl alcohol The intoxicating agent in alcoholic beverages. (Also called *ethanol*.)

euphoria An exaggerated feeling of physical and emotional well-being.

exhibitionism A **paraphilia** characterized by the urge to expose one's genitals to a stranger.

extrapyramidal syndrome Involuntary signs and symptoms, resulting from malfunction in the part of the central nervous system responsible for coordinating body movements, which include muscle rigidity, **tremors,** drooling, shuffling gait (parkinsonism); restlessness **(akathisia)**; peculiar involuntary postures (dystonia); and inertia **(akinesia)**. May be a side effect of **antipsychotic** or neuroleptic drugs.

factitious disorder A condition characterized by intentional production or feigning of physical or psychological symptoms in order to assume the sick role.

fetal alcohol syndrome (FAS) A group of irreversible, congenital abnormalities caused by maternal alcohol consumption during pregnancy. Characteristics include small head, small size, and mental retardation due to impaired brain development; other malformations may also be present. In milder forms of FAS, called fetal alcohol effects (FAE), the newborn may have low birth weight, irritability, and mental impairment.

fetishism A **paraphilia** characterized by urges involving the use of objects (fetishes), such as underclothing or shoes, to obtain sexual gratification.

flashback Reexperiencing of a traumatic event.

flooding (implosion) A **behavioral therapy** in which triggers of extreme **anxiety** (e.g., taking an elevator or flying on an airplane) are confronted directly, either in imagination or in actuality.

fragile X syndrome A common form of inherited mental retardation, caused by an abnormality in the X chromosome.

free association In psychoanalytic therapy, the spontaneous, uncensored expression of whatever comes to mind. (*See also* **psychoanalysis**.)

frotteurism A **paraphilia** consisting of recurrent, intense sexual urges to touch or rub against a nonconsenting person.

fugue A **dissociative identity disorder** marked by sudden, unplanned travel away from one's environment, together with an inability to recall the past and often the assumption of a new identity.

gender Maleness or femaleness, as determined by a combination of anatomical, physiological, and psychological factors and learned behaviors.

generalized anxiety disorder (GAD) An **anxiety disorder** characterized by unrealistic or excessive apprehensiveness and worry about life circumstances, which persists for a period of at least six months and interferes with normal functioning.

genes The biologic units of heredity, located on the **chromosomes,** that are the transmitters of genetic information.

geriatric psychiatry (geropsychiatry) A subspecialty of psychiatry concerned with the psychological aspects of aging and mental disorders of the elderly.

geriatrics The branch of medicine that focuses on the aging process, and problems and diseases of the elderly.

group psychotherapy The use of psychotherapeutic techniques by a therapist in a group setting. (*See also* **psychotherapy.**)

hair pulling *See* **trichotillomania.**

halfway house A specialized residence for individuals who do not require hospitalization but are not yet ready to return to independent living; usually operated under the supervision of trained staff.

hallucination A perception of sound, sights, physical sensations, or smells that do not exist.

hallucinogen A chemical substance that produces **hallucinations** in the user.

health A state of well-being, including physical, psychological, spiritual, social, intellectual, and environmental elements.

heterosexuality Sexual attraction to, and relationships with, people of the opposite sex.

history In a medical context, an individual's past and current health-related information collected during an interview by a health care professional.

HIV *See* **human immunodeficiency virus.**

homophobia Fear or dislike of homosexuals.

homosexuality Sexual attraction to, and relationships with, people of the same sex.

hormones Substances secreted by the **endocrine system** that are released into the bloodstream and regulate a wide variety of crucial body functions.

human immunodeficiency virus (HIV) A retrovirus transmitted via body fluids—including blood, semen, vaginal fluids, and breast milk—that gradually destroys cells of the immune system so that it cannot effectively defend the body against other infections; HIV is the cause of **AIDS.**

hyperactivity Excessive physical activity that may be purposeful or aimless.

hypersomnia A **dyssomnia** characterized by prolonged sleep or excessive daytime drowsiness.

hypertension High blood pressure.

hypnagogia The semiconscious state that immediately precedes sleep.

hypnosis A state of intense concentration that alters the way the brain processes perceptions and that makes an individual suggestible and accepting of instructions; of therapeutic value in breaking undesirable habits (e.g., smoking, overeating), in the treatment of certain disorders, and in alleviating pain.

hypnotic A drug used to induce relaxation or sleep.

hypochondriasis A **somatoform disorder** characterized by persistent worry about health or fear of having a disease, despite medical reassurance to the contrary.

hypomania A state of abnormal mood that falls between **euphoria** and **mania** and is characterized by unrealistic optimism, rapid speech and activity, and a decreased need for sleep.

id In Freudian theory, one of the three divisions of the **psyche;** the primitive part of the **unconscious,** composed of the unrestrained instincts for pleasure and survival.

illusion Misperception of a real occurrence.

impotence The inability to achieve or maintain a penile erection and to engage in successful sexual intercourse. (Also called *male erectile disorder.*)

impulse A sudden desire to act in a certain way to ease tension or feel pleasure.

impulse control disorders Disorders marked by the inability to resist an **impulse** or the temptation to perform an act that is harmful to self or to others. Problems of impulse control may occur as aspects of other mental disorders or as distinct conditions; among the latter are **kleptomania, pyromania, pathological gambling, trichotillomania,** and **intermittent explosive disorder.**

incest Sexual relations, with or without intercourse, between two individuals who are related by blood too closely to contract a legal marriage.

informed consent Permission for a procedure or treatment given voluntarily by a person after he or she has been fully briefed about it and understands its nature and consequences; must always be obtained in writing.

inhalants Substances that produce vapors having **psychoactive** effects when inhaled.

insanity An obsolete term for **psychosis**, used now in strictly legal contexts, such as the insanity defense.

insomnia A **dyssomnia** that consists of difficulty in falling or staying asleep.

instinct An innate drive.

institutionalization Long-term placement of an individual in a hospital, nursing home, residential center, or other care facility.

intermittent explosive disorder An **impulse control disorder** marked by discrete episodes of aggressive impulses that the individual is unable to resist, often resulting in serious assaults or the destruction of property.

interpersonal psychotherapy A form of **brief psychotherapy,** originally developed for the treatment of **depression,** which focuses on relationship issues in order to help individuals improve their interpersonal and communication skills.

interpretation The process by which a therapist encourages an individual to understand a particular problem.

intimacy A state of closeness between two people, characterized by the desire and ability to share their innermost feelings with each other in verbal and nonverbal ways.

intoxication The acute physiological effects of overdosage with a chemical substance.

intrapsychic Taking place within the **psyche,** or mind.

kleptomania An **impulse control disorder** characterized by theft of objects that are not needed for personal use or monetary value.

labile Rapidly changing, as applied to emotions; unstable.

libido In a psychoanalytic context, the psychic drive usually associated with the sexual instinct.

lifestyle An individual's way of life, as indicated and expressed by daily practices, interests, habits, and relationships.

lithium carbonate A naturally occurring mineral salt used to treat manic and depressive episodes and **bipolar illness.**

living will A written statement signed by a mentally competent individual that provides instructions for the use or withdrawal of life-sustaining procedures in the event of terminal illness or injury.

love addiction **Obsession** with a romantic partner.

magical thinking A conviction that thinking about something can make it happen.

maintenance therapy The continuation of a treatment, whether **psychotherapy** or medication or both, to prevent relapse or recurrence of a mental disorder.

major depressive disorder A **depressive disorder** characterized by depressed mood, loss of interest in pleasurable activities (**anhedonia**), changes in sleep or appetite patterns, fatigue, difficulty in concentrating, feelings of worthlessness, and thoughts of death or suicide.

malingering The deliberate production of false or exaggerated physical or psychological symptoms for the purpose of achieving a specific external objective, such as evading work or receiving insurance compensation.

mania A mood disturbance characterized by excessive elation, inflated self-esteem, **hyperactivity,** agitation, and rapid and often confused thinking and speaking; may occur in **bipolar disorder.**

manic depression *See* **bipolar disorder.**

marital therapy A treatment intended to improve or work out problems that are impairing or threatening a primary relationship between two people.

masochism, sexual A **paraphilia** characterized by the urge to suffer at the hands of a sexual partner.

masturbation Manual self-stimulation of the genitals, often leading to **orgasm.**

meditation Any of a variety of thought-focusing approaches that use breathing and other techniques to achieve relaxation, to improve concentration, and to become attuned to one's inner self.

memory The process of remembering or recalling.

menopause The period of time over which menstruation diminishes and eventually stops; when cessation is complete, a woman can no longer conceive.

mental disorder A behavioral or psychological condition or syndrome that causes significant distress, disability, disturbed functioning, or increased risk of harm or pain to one's self or others.

mental health A state of psychological and emotional well-being that enables an individual to work, love, relate to others effectively, and resolve conflicts.

mental status The level and style of a person's intellectual and psychological functioning, emotions, and personality.

mental status examination A process that evaluates psychological and behavioral functioning.

modeling A technique used in **behavioral therapy** in which a therapist performs a desired behavior that is then imitated by the patient; learning by imitation.

monoamine oxidase (MAO) An enzyme that breaks down certain **neurotransmitters** called biogenic amines and deactivates them.

monoamine oxidase inhibitors (MAOIs) A group of chemically related **antidepressant** drugs that act by inhibiting **monoamine oxidase (MAO)** in the brain, thereby raising the level of certain **neurotransmitters.**

mood disorders A group of disorders characterized by disturbances in mood; they include **depressive disorders, bipolar disorder**, and certain disorders caused by a general medical condition or substance use.

multiple personality disorder *See* **dissociative identity disorder**.

Munchausen syndrome A chronic form of **factitious disorder** characterized by physical symptoms that may be totally fabricated or self-inflicted for the purpose of gaining admission to, or staying in, hospitals.

narcissism Self-admiration or self-love; a tendency to overestimate one's abilities and importance.

narcolepsy A **sleep disorder** consisting of: irresistible attacks of sleep during the day; **cataplexy** (loss of muscle tone) typically associated with intense emotion; and recurrent intrusions of **REM sleep** into the transitional period between sleep and wakefulness.

narcotic Any drug, natural or synthetic, that is derived from or has a chemical structure related to that of an **opiate**; relieves pain and alters mood; addictive.

negative symptoms In the residual phase of **schizophrenia**, indications of a deficiency in certain mental functions and of an absence of normal behaviors; these include flattened or inappropriate emotions, lack of will, loss of spontaneous verbal expression, or lack of logic. (*See also* **positive symptoms**.)

neuroleptics *See* **antipsychotics**.

neuron Nerve cell; the basic unit of the nervous system.

neuroscience The study of brain and nervous system function and behavior.

neurosis In common usage, psychological distress beyond what might be considered appropriate for the circumstances of a person's life. (Once also used to refer to psychiatric problems in which individuals remained in touch with reality, the term has been replaced by the terms for specific mental disorders as defined in the *DSM-IV*.)

neurotransmitters Chemicals found in the nervous system that function as messenger molecules by facilitating the transmission of impulses across the **synapses** between **neurons**.

nicotine The addictive substance in tobacco.

nightmare disorder Dream anxiety disorder; a **parasomnia** consisting of repeated awakenings from sleep because of extremely frightening dreams.

non-REM sleep (NREM sleep) Regularly occurring periods of quiet sleep, comprising about 75 percent of a night's sleep, during which body functions slow down. (*See also* **rapid eye movement [REM] sleep**.)

norepinephrine A **neurotransmitter** that is chemically related to **epinephrine**; when in excess, may play a part in manic states, and when deficient, in certain depressive states. (Also called *noradrenaline*.)

nystagmus Abnormal eye movements.

obesity The excessive accumulation of fat in the body; a condition of being 20 percent or more above ideal weight.

obsession A recurrent, persistent, and senseless idea, thought, **impulse,** or image.

obsessive-compulsive disorder (OCD) An **anxiety disorder** characterized by recurrent, time-consuming **obsessions** and/or **compulsions** that impair the ability to function and to form relationships and are a source of significant distress.

opiate Any chemical derived from opium; relieves pain and produces a sense of well-being; addictive.

opioids Synthetic **narcotics** that are similar to **opiates** in their chemical structure and their effects; addictive.

oppositional defiant disorder A condition characterized by a pattern of negative, defiant, and hostile behavior that develops in childhood or early adolescence, lasts for at least six months, and causes significant impairments in everyday functioning.

organic disease An illness that impairs function in an organ or tissue.

orgasm Sexual climax.

orgasmic dysfunction The inability to achieve **orgasm** through physical stimulation.

orientation Awareness of self in relation to time, place, and person. (*See also* **disorientation**.)

outpatient A person who is receiving ambulatory care or treatment at a hospital or other health facility without being admitted to the facility.

over-the-counter (OTC) drugs Medications that can be legally obtained without a prescription.

pain disorder A **somatoform disorder** characterized by persistent pain that causes marked distress or impairs functioning.

panic attacks Sudden, unprovoked, emotionally intense experiences of impending doom, fear of dying, "going crazy," or losing control, marked by physical symptoms such as palpitations, dizziness, trembling, nausea, or shortness of breath.

panic disorder Recurrent **panic attacks**, at least one of which is followed by a month or more of persisting concern about having further attacks.

paranoia A tendency to view the actions of others as deliberately threatening or demeaning; suspicious thinking based on misinterpretation of an actual event.

paranoid ideation Suspiciousness about being harassed, persecuted, or unfairly treated.

paraphilias A major group of sexual disorders that involve recurrent, sexually arousing fantasies of various kinds; includes **exhibitionism, fetishism,** **transvestic fetishism, frotteurism, pedophilia, sexual masochism, sexual sadism,** and **voyeurism**.

parasomnias A group of **sleep disorders** occurring during sleep or in the period between wakefulness and sleep, and more prevalent in children than adults; includes **nightmare disorder, sleep terror disorder**, and **sleepwalking disorder**.

partial hospitalization A psychiatric treatment program for individuals who require hospitalization only during the day, overnight, or on weekends.

pastoral counseling The application of psychological principles by members of the clergy to assist persons in their congregations who have emotional problems.

pathological gambling An **impulse control disorder** characterized by an intense preoccupation with gambling and often-destructive behaviors to support the compulsion to gamble, which adversely affect the individual's personal, financial, occupational, and family life.

pedophilia A **paraphilia** characterized by urges to engage in sexual activity with a child.

personality The characteristic way in which a person thinks, feels, and behaves.

personality disorders A group of disorders marked by persistent, inflexible, maladaptive patterns of thought and behavior that develop in adolescence or early adulthood and significantly impair an individual's ability to function. The ten disorders in this group included in the *DSM-IV* are *paranoid, schizoid,* *schizotypal, antisocial, borderline, histrionic, narcissistic, avoidant, dependent,* and *obsessive-compulsive.*

personality trait A specific, characteristic way in which an individual thinks, feels, or acts in relation to his or her environment and self.

pharmacokinetics The study of drug metabolism.

phase of life problem Difficulty in adapting to a particular developmental period in an individual's life.

phobia Fear of a particular object or situation. Phobias may be specific, such as fear of animals, insects, storms, water, blood, injury, cars, airplane flights, heights, tunnels, elevators, etc.

physical dependence The physiological attachment to, and need for, a drug, characterized by **tolerance** and **withdrawal symptoms** if the drug is stopped. (*See also* **addiction; substance dependence; substance use disorders**.)

pica An **eating disorder** characterized by the repeated eating of non-nutritive substances (e.g., paint, dirt, clay); more common in children, and occasionally seen in pregnant women.

play therapy A technique in the treatment of children in which the child's play is a medium for expression and communication between patient and therapist.

polysomnography The all-night recording of brain waves, eye movements, muscle tone, respiration, heart rate, and penile tumescence (swelling) in order to diagnose sleep-related disorders.

positive symptoms In the acute or active phase of **schizophrenia**, signs that reflect abnormal mental activity and cause grossly abnormal behavior, including **delusions, hallucinations**, disorders in thought processes, disorganized speaking, and disorganized behavior. (*See also* **negative symptoms**.)

postconcussional disorder Physical symptoms and **cognitive** changes following head trauma and loss of consciousness.

postpartum depression A depressive episode in women who have recently borne a child; disinguishable by its symptoms, duration, and intensity from the normal downswing in mood that often follows childbirth.

posttraumatic stress disorder (PTSD) An **anxiety disorder** occurring after exposure to an extreme mental or physical stress—usually involving actual or threatened death or serious injury to self or others— and characterized by symptoms that persist for one month or more and include reexperiencing of the event, avoidance of stimuli associated with it, numbing of general responsiveness, and signs of increased arousal (e.g., sleeplessness, irritability, hypervigilance).

potentiating Making more effective or powerful.

preconscious thoughts Thoughts that are not in immediate awareness but that can be called up by conscious effort.

premature ejaculation Undesired ejaculation occurring immediately before or very early during sexual intercourse.

premenstrual dysphoric disorder An uncommon **depressive disorder**—more severe than **premenstrual syndrome (PMS)**—that occurs prior to the onset of menstruation and abates soon thereafter; symptoms are both psychological (e.g., emotional volatility, anxiety, depressed mood) and physical (e.g., sleep problems, breast tenderness or swelling, headaches, overeating or food cravings).

premenstrual syndrome (PMS) A common condition characterized by physical discomfort and psychological distress that occurs prior to the onset of a woman's menstrual period and abates soon thereafter.

prognosis The prediction of the outcome of an illness.

progressive relaxation A method of reducing muscle tension by contracting and then relaxing muscles in specific areas of the body in systematic order.

projection A **defense mechanism** by which unacceptable feelings or **impulses** are attributed to someone else.

proof A measure of the strength of an alcoholic beverage, expressed as twice the percentage by volume of alcohol present; thus a 70-proof beverage contains 35 percent alcohol.

psyche The mind; the sum of mental activity, including conscious and unconscious functions.

psychedelic A term applied to any of several drugs capable of inducing **hallucinations** and altered mental states.

psychiatric illness *See* **mental disorder**.

psychiatric nurse Any nurse with training and experience in psychiatric treatments; sometimes used to designate only those nurses who have a master's degree in psychiatric nursing and have passed a state examination.

psychiatric social worker A person trained in the specialty of social work that is concerned with prevention and treatment of **mental disorders**. (Also called *certified social worker [C.S.W.]* or *licensed clinical social worker [L.C.S.W.].*) Most states certify or license social workers as an independent profession and require two years of postgraduate clinical work and a qualifying examination.

psychiatrist A licensed medical doctor (M.D.) who has had specialized postgraduate training in the diagnosis, treatment, and prevention of mental and emotional disorders; the only mental health professional licensed to prescribe medication. Board-certified psychiatrists have passed national oral and written examinations ("boards") after completing a residency program in psychiatry.

psychiatry The medical science that deals with the **etiology** (origin), diagnosis, prevention, and treatment of mental disorders.

psychoactive Mood-altering; often used to describe both medications and illicit drugs that act on the brain to change feelings or emotions.

psychoanalysis A form of **psychotherapy,** originally developed by Sigmund Freud, that is intended to help patients become aware of long-repressed feelings and issues by using such techniques as **free association** and the interpretation of dreams. The process usually involves frequent sessions over a long period of time.

psychoanalyst A person, usually a **psychiatrist** or **psychologist,** who has had specialized training in **psychoanalysis** and who employs the techniques of psychoanalytic theory in the treatment of patients.

psychoanalytically oriented psychotherapy A form of **psychotherapy** that employs a variety of techniques, some of which are close to the practice of **psychoanalysis** (e.g., the use of **interpretation**), and others of which are quite different (e.g., the use of suggestion, reassurance, and advice-giving).

psychodynamic psychotherapy Treatments based on an understanding of an individual that takes into account the role of early experiences and unconscious influences in *actively* shaping his or her behavior.

psychodynamics The knowledge and theory of human behavior and its motivations.

psychologist A licensed professional who has completed a graduate program in **psychology** that includes clinical training and internships, and who provides care for individuals with mental and emotional problems. An increasing number of psychologists have a doctorate and have undergone postdoctoral training; however, they are not physicians and cannot prescribe medication.

psychology The study of mental processes and behaviors.

psychomotor A term referring to combined physical and mental activity.

psychomotor agitation Excessive motor activity associated with a feeling of inner tension.

psychomotor retardation Slowing of physical and emotional reactions.

psychopathology The study of the development and nature of **mental disorders.**

psychopharmacology The study of the actions and effects of **psychoactive** drugs on behavior in both animals and people.

psychosis A major **mental disorder** characterized by gross impairment of a person's perception of reality and ability to communicate and relate to others. A psychosis can be biological or emotional in origin.

psychosomatic A term describing an inseparable interaction of the mind (psyche) and the body (soma); often used to designate physical symptoms or conditions that have a mental or emotional component.

psychotherapist A person trained to practice **psychotherapy**.

psychotherapy Any type of counseling based on the exchange of words in the context of the special relationship that develops between a mental health professional and a person seeking help.

psychotic *See* **psychosis**.

psychotropic A term used to describe drugs that act in a particular way on the brain and affect the mind.

pyromania An **impulse control disorder** consisting of deliberate and purposeful firesetting.

rape Sexual assault; forced sexual relations without the other person's consent.

rape, statutory Unlawful sexual intercourse between a male over sixteen years of age and a female under the age of consent (which varies from state to state).

rapid cycling In **bipolar disorder**, the occurrence of four or more episodes of mood disturbance (**mania, depression**, or both) within one year.

rapid eye movement (REM) sleep A regularly occurring phase of the sleep cycle, during which the most active dreaming takes place; comprises about 25 percent of a night's sleep. (*See also* **non-REM sleep**.)

rationalization A **defense mechanism** in which "good," acceptable reasons for a behavior replace a person's real motivations.

reaction formation A **defense mechanism** in which an individual adopts attitudes and behaviors that are the opposite of what he or she really feels.

recall The process of bringing a memory into consciousness.

receptors Specialized molecules on the surface of **neurons** to which particular **neurotransmitters** bind after their release from another neuron; receptors receive the chemical "message" to activate or inhibit a nerve, blood vessel, or muscle.

rehabilitation In **psychiatry**, the methods and techniques used to achieve maximal functioning and adjustment.

reinforcement A **behavioral therapy** technique that involves the encouragement of a desired response through a system of rewards and/or punishments.

REM latency The time lag between sleep onset and the first **rapid eye movement (REM) sleep**.

REM sleep *See* **rapid eye movement sleep**.

repression A **defense mechanism** by which impulses, fantasies, memories, feelings, or wishes that the individual perceives as painful or threatening are kept from conscious awareness.

residual A term describing the phase of an illness that occurs after remission of active disease.

resistance A person's conscious or unconscious psychological defense against bringing repressed (unconscious) thoughts to light.

response A behavior or an action compelled by a stimulus.

retardation, mental Intellectual functioning and capacity that is significantly below average; may occur as a result of a genetic defect, a prenatal developmental impairment, or a mental or physical disorder.

ritual A repetitive activity, usually a distorted routine of daily life, that is employed to relieve anxiety.

sadism, sexual A **paraphilia** characterized by the urge to inflict physical or psychological suffering (including humiliation) on another person for the purpose of sexual gratification.

sadomasochistic relationship An interactive relationship between two people, characterized by sexual enjoyment of suffering in one person and a complementary sexual enjoyment, derived from inflicting pain, in the other person.

satiety A feeling of fullness after eating.

schizoaffective disorder A psychotic disorder in which either a major depressive or a manic episode develops concurrently with the symptoms of **schizophrenia**.

schizophrenia A major **mental disorder** with characteristic psychotic or **positive symptoms** (such as **delusions, hallucinations**, and disordered thought patterns) during the active phase of the illness, and **negative symptoms** (such as lack of logic or will) evident following psychotic episodes. The onset is generally between late adolescence and the mid-thirties. The prognosis varies, although complete remission is uncommon.

seasonal affective disorder (SAD) A recurrent **mood disorder** characterized by depressive episodes and related symptoms that develop at particular times of the year, most often in fall or winter, and remit when the season ends.

secondary gain The external benefit derived from any illness, such as additional attention or special nurturing.

sedative A general term applied to any quieting or sleep-producing agent.

selective serotonin reuptake inhibitor (SSRI) A medication that inhibits recapture of the neurotransmitter **serotonin** by the nerve cells.

self-actualization A state of wellness and fulfillment that can be achieved once certain human needs are satisfied; living to one's full potential.

self-esteem A sense of self-worth; the valuing of oneself as a person.

self-help group An assemblage of individuals with a common problem who collectively aid one another through personal and group support.

separation anxiety The fear and apprehension that occurs as a normal developmental phase in babies when removed from the mother (or surrogate mother) or when approached by strangers.

separation anxiety disorder A condition developing before the age of eighteen that is marked by inappropriate anxiety concerning separation from home or from persons to whom the child or young person is emotionally attached.

serotonin A **neurotransmitter** found both in the brain and elsewhere in the body that may play a role in several mental disorders, including **depression**.

sex Maleness or femaleness, resulting from genetic, structural, and functional factors.

sexual addiction A preoccupation with sex so intense and chronic that an individual cannot have a normal sexual relationship with a spouse or lover.

sexual arousal disorders A category of **sexual dysfunctions** that include female sexual arousal disorder and male erectile disorder.

sexual desire disorders A category of **sexual dysfunctions** that include hypoactive sexual desire disorder and sexual aversion disorder.

sexual dysfunctions A group of disorders characterized by disturbances in sexual desire and by psychophysiological changes in the sexual response cycle, which cause marked distress and interpersonal difficulty.

sexual orientation The focus of a person's sexual attractions, whether to individuals of the opposite sex, the same sex, or both.

sexuality The instincts, feelings, attitudes, and behaviors associated with being sexual.

shock treatment An obsolete and inaccurate term that was often used to refer to older, crude forms of electroconvulsive treatment; a more refined treatment, known as **electroconvulsive therapy (ECT)**, is used today in treating certain mental disorders.

short-term memory Technically, the recognition, recall, and reproduction of perceived material ten seconds or longer after initial presentation. The term is popularly used to refer to memory for recent events, as contrasted with events in the past.

side effect A drug response that accompanies the principal therapeutic response that is the purpose of a medication.

sleep apnea A **breathing-related sleep disorder** marked by repeated episodes in which a sleeping individual stops breathing for a short period of time.

sleep disorders A group of conditions involving sleep that include: primary sleep disorders (**dyssomnias** and **parasomnias**); sleep disorders related to another mental disorder (including **insomnia**); secondary sleep disorder due to a general medical condition; and substance-induced sleep disorder resulting from **intoxication** or **withdrawal**.

sleep terror disorder A **parasomnia** characterized by a pattern of abrupt awakening from sleep that is accompanied by a sense of panic and confusion.

sleepwalking disorder A **parasomnia** characterized by recurrent episodes of arising from the bed during sleep and walking about.

social phobia A persistent fear of finding oneself in situations that might lead to scrutiny by others and humiliation or embarrassment.

social work A profession whose primary concern is how human needs, both of individuals and of groups, can be met within society. (*See also* **psychiatric social worker**.)

somatic therapy In **psychiatry**, the biological treatment of mental disorders; examples are **electroconvulsive therapy** and psychopharmacological treatment.

somatization disorder A **somatoform disorder** characterized by multiple physical complaints occurring over several years that cannot be not fully explained by any known medical condition, yet are severe enough to require medical treatment or to cause alterations in lifestyle.

somatoform disorders A group of disorders with symptoms suggesting physical disorders but without demonstrable medical findings to explain the symptoms; included in this category are **somatization disorder, conversion disorder, pain disorder, hypochondriasis,** and **body dysmorphic disorder.**

splitting A **defense mechanism** by which an individual who cannot cope with ambivalent feelings about other people deals with these conflicting emotions by compartmentalizing such people as all good or all bad.

SSRI *See* **selective serotonin reuptake inhibitor.**

statutory rape *See* **rape, statutory.**

stimulus An environmental factor that evokes a response in an organism.

stress The nonspecific response of the body to any demands made upon it.

stress disorder, acute An **anxiety disorder** that develops when or immediately after a person experiences a highly traumatic stressor that induces feelings of intense fear, helplessness, or horror.

stress disorder/reaction, posttraumatic See **posttraumatic stress disorder.**

stressor A specific or nonspecific agent, event, or situation that causes the body to experience a **stress** response.

stupor A marked decrease in response to and awareness of the environment, with reduced spontaneous movements and activity; semiconsciousness.

sublimation A **defense mechanism** by which the energy originating from a sexual urge or other urge that a person perceives as unacceptable is redirected into socially acceptable channels.

substance In a **psychopharmacological** context, a chemical agent that is used to alter mood or behavior. (*See also* **psychoactive.**)

substance abuse The compulsive use of a substance, such as alcohol or a drug, despite evidence that it is impairing an individual's social and occupational functioning.

substance dependence Chemical dependence, usually defined in terms of **tolerance** or **withdrawal.**

substance use disorders Dependence, abuse, intoxication, and withdrawal syndromes associated with episodic or regular use of chemical substances. Use disorders are recognized for amphetamines; caffeine; cannabis; cocaine; hallucinogens; inhalants; nicotine; opioids; phencyclidine (PCP); alcohol and sedative/hypnotic/anxiolytic drugs; and combinations of drugs (*polysubstance use*).

suicide Taking of one's own life.

superego   In Freudian theory, one of the three divisions of the **psyche;** the internal voice bearing messages from parents and society regarding morals, behavior, and goals.

supportive psychotherapy   A type of therapy, which may be brief or long-term, that uses the therapist-patient relationship to help a person cope with specific crises or difficulties that he or she is currently facing. Its goal is to help individuals adapt and attain the best possible level of functioning given **personality**, life circumstances, ability, or illness.

suppression   The conscious inhibition of certain thoughts or impulses.

synapse   The gap or space between the surface of one nerve cell (**neuron**) and another.

syndrome   A group of signs and symptoms that appear together, suggesting a particular cause.

systematic desensitization   A **behavioral therapy** technique that teaches individuals how to reduce or control fears triggered by specific **stimuli.** (Also called *desensitization.*)

Tarasoff decision   A California court decision that in essence imposes a duty on the therapist to warn the appropriate person or persons when the therapist becomes aware that a patient may present a risk of harm to them.

tardive dyskinesia   A medication-induced movement disorder consisting of involuntary movements of the tongue, jaw, or extremities, that develops with long-term use (usually a period of months or more) of **antipsy-** chotic (neuroleptic) medication; sometimes irreversible.

therapeutic alliance   The relationship between an individual and a therapist that allows them to work together cooperatively and productively; based on trust on the individual's part, and on care and respect on the therapist's part.

tic   An involuntary, abrupt, rapid, and recurrent motor movement or vocalization.

tolerance   A characteristic of **substance dependence** marked by the need for increasing amounts of the substance to achieve the desired effect.

trance   A state of intensely focused attention in which an individual becomes detached from the physical environment. (*See also* **hypnosis**.)

tranquilizer   A drug that decreases anxiety and agitation.

transference   The unconscious assignment to others of feelings and attitudes originally associated with important figures in one's early life, such as parents or siblings; seen in the patient-analyst relationship in **psychoanalysis**. (*See also* **countertransference**.)

transsexual   A person whose psychological gender identity is the opposite of his or her biological sex.

transvestic fetishism   A **paraphilia** characterized by sexual urges that involve cross-dressing (wearing clothing associated with the opposite sex); found most frequently in heterosexual males.

transvestism   Sexual pleasure derived from dressing or masquerading in the clothing of the opposite sex.

tremor A trembling or shaking of the body or any of its parts.

trichotillomania An **impulse-control disorder** characterized by pathological hair pulling that results in noticeable hair loss.

twelve-step programs Self-help group programs based on the principles of **Alcoholics Anonymous.**

Type I alcoholic An **alcoholic** who becomes a heavy drinker usually after the age of twenty-five; drinks when external circumstances (such as stress) increase; abstains for long periods of time; and often experiences loss of control, guilt, and fear about the **physical dependence.** (Also called *milieu-limited alchoholic.*)

Type 2 alcoholic An **alcoholic** man who becomes a heavy drinker before the age of twenty-five; drinks regardless of external circumstances; has frequent fights and arrests; and experiences loss of control, guilt, or fear only infrequently. (Also called *male-limited alcoholic.*)

tyramine A chemical found in many foods and beverages that ordinarily has no effect on normal body functioning, but which can cause a dangerous rise in blood pressure when a type of drug called a **monoamine oxidase inhibitor (MAOI)** is taken. Persons using MAOIs must not consume foods and drinks containing tyramine.

unconscious In Freudian theory, that part of the mind or mental functioning of which a person is only rarely aware.

values The criteria by which individuals assess themselves, others, and the events in their life, and on which they base their choices and actions.

visualization An approach to stress management, self-healing, or motivating life changes that uses a technique of guided or directed imagery.

voyeurism A **paraphilia** characterized by the urge to observe unsuspecting people, usually strangers, who are naked, disrobing, or engaging in sexual activity. (Also called *peeping.*)

withdrawal The symptoms and signs that develop within a short period of time (usually hours) after cessation or reduced use of an addictive substance; may include sweating, rapid pulse, hand **tremor,** nausea or vomiting, agitation, **anxiety,** or temporary **hallucinations** or **illusions.**

Resource Directory

GENERAL MEDICAL INFORMATION RESOURCES

American Medical Association
AMA Publications

515 N. State Street
Chicago, IL 60610
(312) 464-5000

National Institutes of Health (NIH)

9000 Rockville Pike
Bethesda, MD 20892
(301) 496-4000

Public Health Service

2000 Independence
Avenue, S.W.
Washington, DC 20201
(202) 690-6867

Tel-Med Health Information Service provides taped messages on health concerns.

AIDS

National AIDS Hotline
(800) 342-AIDS

National STD Hotline
(800) 227-8922

San Francisco AIDS Foundation

P.O. Box 426182
San Francisco, CA 94142-6182
(415) 864-5855
(800) 367-2437 (FOR-AIDS)

Shanti Project

1546 Market Street
San Francisco, CA 94102
(415) 864-2273

Provides counseling and assistance to persons with AIDS.

ALCOHOL, DRUG, AND SUBSTANCE ABUSE

Al-Anon, Alateen, and Adult
Children of Alcoholics
Al-Anon Family Group
Headquarters, Inc.

P.O. Box 862
Midtown Station
New York, NY 10018
(212) 302-7240
(800) 344-2666

A fellowship of relatives and friends of alcoholics.

Alcohol, Drug Abuse and Mental
Health Association (ADAMHA)

5600 Fishers Lane
Rockville, MD 20852
(301) 443-2403

Alcohol Hotline
Adcare Hospital

107 Lincoln Street
Worcester, MA 01605
(800) ALCOHOL

Alcoholics Anonymous, Inc.

P.O. Box 459
Grand Central Station
New York, NY 10163

Voluntary, nonprofessional, twelve-step organization of recovering alcoholics.

American Council for Drug
Education

204 Monroe Street
Rockville, MD 20850
(301) 294-0600

Children of Alcoholics Foundation

555 Madison Avenue, 4th Floor
New York, NY 10022
(212) 754-0656

Cocaine Anonymous World Services

3740 Overland Avenue Suite G
Los Angeles, CA 90034
(800) 347-8998
(310) 559-5833

Self-help, nonprofessional, twelve-step fellowship program for men and women in recovery from cocaine addiction.

Co-Dependents Anonymous (CoDA)

P.O. Box 33577
Phoenix, AZ 85067-3577
(602) 277-7991

800-COCAINE

P.O. Box 100
Summit, NJ 07901

Referrals to local hotlines only.

Families Anonymous

World Service Office
P.O. Box 528
Van Nuys, CA 91408
(818) 989-7841
(800) 736-9805

Narcotics Anonymous

P.O. Box 9999
16155 Wyandotte
Van Nuys, CA 91409
(818) 780-3951

Support group for recovering narcotics addicts.

National Clearinghouse for Alcohol and Drug Information

P.O. Box 2345
Rockville, MD 20847–2345
(301) 468-2600
(800) 729-6686

National Drug Abuse Information and Treatment Referral Hotline *and* National Institute on Drug Abuse Helpline

12280 Wilkins Avenue
Rockville, MD 20852
(800) 662-HELP
(800) 66-AYUDA
(Spanish-speaking callers)

National Drug Information Center of Families in Action

2296 Henderson Mill Road,
Suite 204
Atlanta, GA 30345
(404) 934-6346

National Federation of Parents for a Drug Free Youth

1423 N. Jefferson
Springfield, MO 65802
(417) 836-3709

National Institute on Alcohol Abuse and Alcoholism

5600 Fishers Lane
Parklawn Building
Room 16C-14
Rockville, MD 20857
(301) 443-3860

Office for Substance Abuse Prevention
Alcohol, Drug Abuse and Mental Health Association (ADAMHA)

5600 Fishers Lane
Rockwall II Building
Rockville, MD 20852
(301) 443-0365

PRIDE (Parents' Resource Institute for Drug Education)

50 Hurt Plaza, Suite 210
Atlanta, GA 30303
(404) 577-4500

Women for Sobriety, Inc.

109 W. Broad Street
P.O. Box 618
Quakertown, PA 18951
(215) 536-8026
(800) 333-1606

Support group for women with drinking problems. A self-help program "whose purpose is to help all women recover from problem drinking."

ALZHEIMER'S DISEASE

Alzheimer's Disease and Related Disorders Association

919 No. Michigan Avenue,
Suite 1000
Chicago, IL 60611-1676
(312) 335-8700
(800) 272-3900
(800) 572-6037 (in Illinois)

ANXIETY DISORDERS AND PHOBIAS

Anxiety Disorders Association of America
(an expansion of the Phobia Society of America)

6000 Executive Boulevard,
Suite 513
Rockville, MD 20852
(301) 231-8368

PASS Group, Inc.

6 Mahogany Drive
Williamsville, NY 14221
(716) 689-4399

Support group to help treat agoraphobia.

TERRAP
(TERRitorial APprehensiveness)

648 Menlo Avenue, Suite 5
Menlo Park, CA 94025
(415) 327-1312

Headquarters for national network of treatment clinics for agoraphobia.

ATTENTION DEFICIT DISORDERS

Attention Deficit Disorder Association (ADDA)

8091 S. Ireland Way
Aurora, CO 80016
(508) 462-0495
(800) 487-2282

Information on support groups.

Children with Attention Deficit Disorders (CHADD)

1859 N. Pine Island Road,
Suite 185
Plantation, FL 33322
(305) 587-3700

Learning Disabilities Association of America (LDA)

4156 Library Road
Pittsburgh, PA 15234
(412) 341-1515

AUTISM

Autism Society of America

7910 Woodmont Avenue,
Suite 655
Bethesda, MD 20814
(301) 657-0881

Support and advocacy organization for people with autism and their families.

The New Jersey Center for Outreach and Services for the Autism Community, Inc.

123 Franklin Corner Road,
Suite 215
Lawrenceville, NJ 08648
(609) 895-0190

CANCER

American Cancer Society

1599 Clifton Road
Atlanta, GA 30329
(404) 320-3333
(800) 227-2345

Cancer Information Service
National Cancer Institute

9000 Rockville Pike
Building 31, Room 10A16
Bethesda, MD 20892-0001
(301) 496-4000
(800) 4-CANCER

National Coalition for Cancer Survivorship

1010 Wayne Avenue, 5th Floor
Silver Springs, MD 20910
(301) 650-8868

National Council of Independent Living

2111 Wilson Boulevard,
Suite 405
Arlington, VA 22201
(703) 525-3406

CAREGIVING

American Nurses Association

2420 Pershing Road
Kansas City, MO 64108
(800) 284-2378

Family Survival Project for Brain-Impaired Adults

425 Bush Street, Suite 500
San Francisco, CA 94108
(415) 434-3388

CHILD ABUSE

American Association for Protecting Children
The American Humane Association

63 Inverness Drive East
Englewood, CO 80112
(303) 792-9900

C. Henry Kempe National Center for the Prevention and Treatment of Child Abuse and Neglect

Department of Pediatrics
1205 Oneida Street
Denver, CO 80220
(303) 321-3963

Child Assault Prevention (CAP) Project
National Assault Prevention Center

P.O. Box 02005
Columbus, OH 43202
(614) 291-2540

Provides services to children, adoles-cents, mentally retarded adults, and the elderly.

National Child Abuse Hotline
Childhelp USA

1345 El Centro Avenue
P.O. Box 630
Los Angeles, CA 90028
(800) 422-4453

Focuses on crisis counseling and re-ferrals to professional organizations.

National Committee for the Prevention of Child Abuse (NCPCA)

332 S. Michigan Avenue,
Suite 1600
Chicago, IL 60604
(312) 663-3520

Provides literature on child abuse prevention programs.

National Domestic Violence Hotline

P.O. Box 7032
Huntington Woods, MI 48070
(800) 333-SAFE
(800) 873-6363 (for the hearing impaired)

Supportive listening, information and referral, and crisis intervention.

Parents Anonymous

6733 S. Sepulveda Blvd.
Los Angeles, CA 90045
(213) 388-6685

Self-help group for parents who feel "isolated, overwhelmed, or are afraid of their anger toward their children."

VOICES in Action, Inc.
(Victims of Incest Can Emerge Survivors in Action, Inc.)

P.O. Box 148309
Chicago, IL 60614
(312) 327-1500

Help for incest and child sexual abuse victims.

CRISIS INTERVENTION SERVICES

National Crisis Prevention Institute

3315K N. 124th Street
Brookfield, WI 53005
(414) 783-5787
(800) 558-8976

Offers programs on nonviolent physical crisis intervention.

DEATH AND GRIEVING

The Compassionate Friends, Inc.

900 Jorie Blvd.
P.O. Box 3696
Oak Brook, IL 60522
(708) 990-0010

Self-help organization for parents who have lost a child at any age, due to any cause.

Pregnancy and Infant Loss Center

1421 E. Wayzata Boulevard
Wayzata, MN 55391
(612) 473-9372

Provides "support, resources, and education on miscarriage, stillbirth, and newborn death."

SHARE

c/o St. John's Hospital
800 E. Carpenter Street
Springfield, IL 62769
(217) 544-6464

Support group for parents who have suffered the loss of a newborn baby.

DEPRESSIVE DISORDERS

Depression After Delivery

P.O. Box 1282
Morrisville, PA 19067
(215) 295-3994
(800) 944-4773

Support for women suffering from postpartum depression and psychosis.

Depression Awareness, Recognition and Treatment Program

National Institute of Mental Health
5600 Fishers Lane
Rockville, MD 20857

Depressives Anonymous

329 East 62nd Street, Suite 50
New York, NY 10021
(212) 689-2600

Self-help organization for people suffering from depression.

Lithium Information Center

c/o Department of Psychiatry
University of Wisconsin
600 Highland Avenue
Madison, WI 53792
(608) 263-6171

National Alliance for the Mentally Ill

2101 Wilson Boulevard,
Suite 302
Arlington, VA 22201
(703) 524-7600

Self-help and advocacy organiza-tion for persons with schizophrenia and depressive disorders and their families.

National Alliance for Research on Schizophrenia and Depression (NARSAD)

60 Cutter Mill Road, Suite 200
Great Neck, NY 11021
(516) 829-0091

National Depressive and Manic-Depressive Association (National DMDA)

730 N. Franklin Street
Chicago, IL 60610
(312) 939-2442

National Foundation for Depressive Illness

P.O. Box 2257
New York, NY 10116
(800) 248-4344

Assists in finding professional help.

DOMESTIC VIOLENCE

Batterers Anonymous

8485 Tamarinal Avenue, Suite D
Fontana, CA 92335
(714) 355-1100

Self-help group designed to rehabili-tate men who abuse women.

Batterers Anonymous

1269 N. "E" Street
San Bernardino, CA 92405
(714) 884-6809

*Self-help counseling program for men
who batter women.*

National Coalition Against
Domestic Violence

P.O. Box 34103
Washington, DC 20043
(202) 638-6388

National Domestic Violence Hotline

P.O. Box 7032
Huntington Woods, MI 48070
(800) 333-SAFE
(800) 873-6363 (for the hearing
impaired)

*Supportive listening, information and
referral, and crisis intervention.*

DOWN SYNDROME

National Association for Down
Syndrome

1800 Dempster
Park Ridge, IL 60068-1146
(708) 823-7550

*Provides information about Down
syndrome.*

National Down Syndrome Society
Hotline

666 Broadway
New York, NY 10012
(212) 460-9330
(800) 221-4602

EATING DISORDERS

American Anorexia/Bulimia
Association, Inc.

418 E. 76th Street
New York, NY 10021
(212) 734-1114

*Self-help group that provides informa-
tion and referrals to physicians and
therapists.*

Anorexia Nervosa and Related
Eating Disorders, Inc.

P.O. Box 5102
Eugene, OR 97405
(503) 344-1144

*Provides information and referrals for
people with eating disorders.*

Bulimia, Anorexia & Self-Help, Inc.

6125 Clayton Avenue, Suite 215
P.O. Box 39903
St. Louis, MO 63139
(314) 567-4080
(800) 762-3334

National Association of Anorexia
Nervosa and Associated Disorders

Box 7
Highland Park, IL 60035
(708) 831-3438

*Counseling and information for
anorexics, bulimics, their families,
and professionals.*

National Anorexic Aid Society

5796 Karl Road
Columbus, OH 43229
(614) 846-2833

Overeaters Anonymous

4025 Spencer Street, Suite 203
Torrance, CA 90503
(310) 618-8835

*Self-help fellowship of men and
women who wish to stop eating
compulsively.*

EPILEPSY

Epilepsy Foundation of America

4351 Garden City Drive
Landover, MD 20785-2267
(301) 459-3700
(800) 332-1000

GAMBLING AND COMPULSIVE SPENDING

Debtors Anonymous General
Service Board

P.O. Box 20322
New York, NY 10025-9992
(Enclose SASE)

Gam-Anon
International Service Office, Inc.

P.O. Box 157
Whitestone, NY 11357
(718) 352-1671

*Self-help fellowship for the families
of compulsive gamblers.*

Gamblers Anonymous

P.O. Box 17173
Los Angeles, CA 90017
(213) 386-8789
(213) 386-0300 FAX

*Self-help, nonprofessional organization
that follows the twelve-step program
of recovery used by AA.*

National Council on Compulsive
Gambling, Inc.

445 W. 59th Street
New York, NY 10019
(212) 765-3833
(800) 522-4700

Spender-Menders

P.O. Box 15000-156 (MC)
San Francisco, CA 94115
(Enclose $1 for
mailing/handling)

GENETIC DISEASES

National Clearinghouse for Human
Genetic Disease
National Center for Education in
Maternal and Child Health

2000 15th Street N., Suite 701
Arlington, VA 22201-2617
(703) 524-7802

*Provides information about inherited
diseases; publishes directory of genetic counseling services.*

IMPULSE-CONTROL DISORDERS

Trichotillomania Learning Center

1215 Mission Street, Suite 2
Santa Cruz, CA 95060
(408) 457-1004
(408) 426-4383 FAX

LEARNING DISORDERS

Association for Children and Adults
with Learning Disabilities

4156 Library Road
Pittsburgh, PA 15234
(412) 341-1515

National Center for Learning
Disabilities

99 Park Avenue, 6th Floor
New York, NY 10016
(212) 687-7211

The Orton Dyslexia Society
Chester Building
8600 LaSalle Road, Suite 382
Baltimore, MD 21204-6020
(410) 296-0232

MARRIAGE AND FAMILY

American Association for Marriage
and Family Therapy
1717 K Street N.W., Suite 407
Washington, DC 20006
(202) 452-0109
(800) 374-2638

American Family Therapy
Association
2020 Pennsylvania Avenue,
N.W., Suite 273
Washington, DC 20006
(202) 994-2776

Co-Dependents Anonymous (CoDA)
P.O. Box 33577
Phoenix, AZ 85067-3577
(602) 277-7991

Displaced Homemakers Network
1625 K Street, N.W., Suite 300
Washington, DC 20006
(202) 467-6346

*National advocacy group for women
over 35 who have lost their primary
means of support through death,
divorce, or disability of spouse.*

MENTAL HEALTH RESOURCES

American Mental Health Fund
2735 Harland Road
Falls Church, VA 22043
(703) 573-2200

American Psychiatric Press Inc.
1400 K Street, N.W.
Washington, DC 20005
(800) 368-5777

National Alliance for the Mentally Ill
2101 Wilson Boulevard,
Suite 302
Arlington, VA 22201
(703) 524-7600

*Self-help and advocacy organization
for persons with mental disorders and
their families.*

National Alliance for Research on
Schizophrenia and Depression
60 Cutter Mill Road, Suite 200
Great Neck, NY 11021
(516) 829-0091

National Association of Social
Workers
750 First Street, N.E., Suite 700
Washington, DC 20002
(202) 408-8600

National Mental Health Association
1021 Prince Street
Alexandria, VA 22314-2971
(703) 684-7722

National Mental Health Consumer
Self-Help Clearinghouse
311 S. Juniper Street, Room 902
Philadelphia, PA 19107
(215) 735-6367

Recovery, Inc.
Association of Nervous and Former
Mental Patients
802 N. Dearborn Street
Chicago, IL 60610
(312) 337-5661

*Self-help group for former mental
patients.*

MENTAL RETARDATION

National Association for Retarded
Citizens
500 E. Border Street, Suite 300
Arlington, TX 76010
(817) 261-6003

NEUROLOGICAL DISORDERS

National Institute of Neurological
and Communicative Disorders and
Stroke
National Institutes of Health
9000 Rockville Pike
Bethesda, MD 20892
(301) 496-4000

Tardive Dyskinesia/Tardive
Dystonia National Association
4244 University Way, N.E.
P.O. Box 45732
Seattle, WA 98145
(206) 522-3166

OBSESSIVE-COMPULSIVE DISORDERS

Obsessive Compulsive Disorder
Foundation, Inc.
P.O. Box 9573
New Haven, CT 06535
(203) 772-0565

*A voluntary organization "dedicated
to early intervention in controlling
and finding cures for OCD, and for
improving the welfare of people with
this disorder."*

PARENT SUPPORT GROUPS

Emotions Anonymous—Children
ages 5–13
Emotions Anonymous—Children
ages 13–19
P.O. Box 4245
St. Paul, MN 55104
(612) 647-9712

*Self-help, nonprofessional organization
for help with either short-term or chronic
emotional problems.*

Families Anonymous
World Service Office
P.O. Box 528
Van Nuys, CA 91408
(818) 989-7841
(800) 736-9805

*Self-help, volunteer organization of
parents, friends, and relatives of children and adults with drug and alcohol
and associated behavioral problems.*

Parents Anonymous
6733 S. Sepulveda Boulevard
Los Angeles, CA 90045
(213) 388-6685

Self-help group for abusive parents.

Toughlove
P.O. Box 1069
Doylestown, PA 18901
(215) 348-7090
(800) 333-1069

Support group for parents of problem
teenagers.

PROFESSIONAL ORGANIZATIONS

American Academy of Child and
Adolescent Psychiatry
3615 Wisconsin Avenue, N.W.
Washington, DC 20016
(202) 966-7300

American Group Psychotherapy Association

25 E. 21st Street, 6th Floor
New York, NY 10010
(212) 477-2677

American Mental Health Counselors Association (a division of the American Association for Counseling and Development)

5999 Stevenson Avenue
Alexandria, VA 22304
(703) 823-9800

American Psychiatric Association

1400 K Street N.W.
Washington, DC 20005
(202) 682-6000

American Psychological Association

1200 17th Street, N.W.
Washington, DC 20002
(202) 336-5500

Association for the Advancement of Behavioral Therapy

15 W. 36th Street
New York, NY 10018
(212) 279-7970

Center for Cognitive Therapy University of Pennsylvania

133 S. 36th Street, Room 602
Pennsylvania, PA 19104
(215) 898-4100

National Association for the Advancement of Psychoanalysis and the American Board for Accreditation and Certification, Inc.

80 Eighth Avenue, Suite 1210
New York, NY 10011
(212) 741-0515

National Association of Private Psychiatric Hospitals

1319 F Street, N.W., #1000
Washington, DC 20004
(202) 393-6700

National Association of Social Workers

750 First Street, N.E., Suite 700
Washington, DC 20002
(202) 408-8600

National Council of Community Mental Health Centers

12300 Twinbrook Parkway,
Suite 320
Rockville, MD 20852
(301) 984-6200

National Institute of Mental Health

Information Resources and Inquiries Branch
5600 Fishers Lane,
Room 15-C-105
Rockville, MD 20857
(301) 443-4515

RAPE

National Clearinghouse on Marital and Date Rape

2325 Oak Street
Berkeley, CA 94708
(510) 524-1582

National Coalition Against Sexual Assault

P.O. Box 21378
Washington, DC 20009
(202) 483-7165

SCHIZOPHRENIA

National Alliance for the Mentally Ill

2101 Wilson Boulevard,
Suite 302
Arlington, VA 22201
(703) 524-7600

Self-help and advocacy organization for persons with mental disorders and their families.

National Alliance for Research on Schizophrenia and Depression

60 Cutter Mill Road, Suite 200
Great Neck, NY 11021
(516) 829-0091

SELF-CARE/SELF-HELP

National Self-Help Clearinghouse

25 W. 43rd Street
New York, NY 10036
(212) 642-2944

Provides information about self-help groups.

SEXUAL ABUSE AND ASSAULT

National Assault Prevention Center

P.O. Box 02005
Columbus, OH 43202
(614) 291-2540

Parents United

P.O. Box 952
San Jose, CA 95108
(408) 453-7616

Support group for individuals and families who have experienced sexual molestation as children.

SEXUAL DIFFICULTIES

American Association of Sex Educators, Counselors, and Therapists

11 Dupont Circle, N.W., Suite 220
Washington, DC 20036

Impotence Information Center

P.O. Box 9
Minneapolis, MN 55440
(800) 843-4315
(612) 933-4666 (in Minnesota)

Provides information on causes and treatment of impotence.

Impotents Anonymous
I-Anon (for partners)
Impotence World Service

P.O. Box 5299
Maryville, TN 37802
(615) 983-6064

Support group network of community self-help chapters for impotent men; I-Anon is for their partners.

Sexaholics Anonymous

P.O. Box 300
Simi Valley, CA 93062
(818) 704-9854

Self-help group for sexual addicts.

SLEEP AND SLEEP DISORDERS

American Narcolepsy Association

425 California Street, Suite 201
San Francisco, CA 94104
(415) 788-4793

American Sleep Disorders Association

1610 14th Street, N.W., Suite 300
Rochester, MN 55901
(507) 287-6006

Better Sleep Council (of the
International Sleep Products
Association)
> 333 Commerce Street
> Alexandria, VA 22314
> (703) 683-8371

STRESS REDUCTION

Association for Applied
Psychophysiology and Biofeedback
> 10200 W. 44th Avenue,
> Suite 304
> Wheat Ridge, CO 80033
> (303) 422-8436

STROKE

Council on Stroke
> American Heart Association
> 7320 Greenville Avenue
> Dallas, TX 75231
> (214) 373-6300

National Institute of Neurological
and Communicative Disorders
and Stroke
National Institutes of Health
> 9000 Rockville Pike
> Bethesda, MD 20892
> (301) 496-4000

SUICIDE PREVENTION

Directory of Suicide Prevention
and Crisis Intervention Agencies
in the U.S.
> 2459 Ash Street
> Denver, CO 80222
> (303) 692-0985

Youth Suicide National Center
> 1824 I Street, N.W., Suite 400
> Washington, DC 20006

TERMINAL ILLNESS

Make Today Count, Inc.
> P.O. Box 6063
> Kansas City, KS 66106
> (913) 362-2866

CLEARINGHOUSES FOR LOCAL SELF-HELP LISTED BY STATE

*The quickest way to find a self-help group is through clearinghouses that have been
set up in many states. This list can help you find one in or near your community.*

ARIZONA

The Rainy Day People
> P.O. Box 472
> Scottsdale, AZ 85252
> (602) 840-1029

CALIFORNIA

Fresno County Information Referral
Network
> 2420 Mariposa Street
> Fresno, CA 93721
> (209) 488-3857

California Self-Help Center
U.C.L.A.
> 405 Hildgard Avenue
> Los Angeles, CA 90024
> (800) 222-LINK
> (213) 825-1799

Mental Health Association of
Contra Costa County
> 604 Ferry Street
> Martinez, CA 94553
> (510) 603-1212

Sacramento Self-Help
Clearinghouse
Mental Health Association of
Sacramento
> 5370 Elvos Avenue, Suite B
> Sacramento, CA 95819
> (916) 368-3100

San Francisco Self-Help
Clearinghouse
Mental Health Association
> 2398 Pine Street
> San Francisco, CA 94115
> (415) 921-4401

CONNECTICUT

Self-Help Mutual Support Network
Consultation Center
> 19 Howe Street
> New Haven, CT 06511
> (203) 789-7645

FLORIDA

Hotline Information Referral
> P.O. Box 13087
> St. Petersburg, FL 33733
> (813) 531-4664

ILLINOIS

Self-Help Center
> 405 State Street
> Champaign, IL 61820
> (217) 352-0099

Illinois Self-Help Center
> 1600 Dodge Avenue,
> Suite S-122
> Evanston, IL 60201
> (708) 328-0470(800)
> 322-MASH (in Illinois)

INDIANA

Indianapolis Hotline
> (317) 926-HELP

Information and Referral Network
> 1828 N. Meridian Street
> Indianapolis, IN 46202
> (317) 921-1305

IOWA

Iowa Self-Help Clearinghouse
> 33 N. 12th Street
> P.O. Box 1151
> Fort Dodge, IA 50501
> (515) 576-5870

KANSAS

Kansas Self-Help Network
Campus Box 34
Wichita State University
Wichita, KS 67208-1595
(316) 689-3170

MASSACHUSETTS

Clearinghouse of Mutual
Self-Help Groups
Massachusetts Cooperative
Extension

113 Skinner Hall
University of Massachusetts
Amherst, MA 01003
(413) 545-2313

MICHIGAN

Center for Self-Help
Riverwood Center

1485 Highway M-139
Benton Harbor, MI 49022
(616) 925-0585

Michigan Self-Help Clearinghouse
Michigan Protection & Advocacy
Service

109 W. Michigan Avenue,
Suite 900
Lansing, MI 48933
(517) 484-7373
(800) 752-5858 (in Michigan)

MINNESOTA

Minnesota Mutual Help
Resource Center
Wilder Foundation Community
Care Unit

919 LaFond Avenue
St. Paul, MN 55104
(612) 242-4060

MISSOURI

Kansas City Association for
Mental Health

706 W. 42 Street
Kansas City, MO 64111
(816) 472-5000

Mental Health Association of
St. Louis

3617 Shaw Boulevard
St. Louis, MO 63110
(314) 773-1399

NEBRASKA

Self-Help Information Services

1601 Euclid Avenue
Lincoln, NE 68502
(402) 476-9668

NEW HAMPSHIRE

New Hampshire Self-Help
Clearinghouse
Office of Public Education
Division of Mental Health &
Developmental Services

105 Pleasant Street
State Office Park South
Concord, NH 03301
(603) 271-5060

NEW JERSEY

New Jersey Self-Help
Clearinghouse
St. Clare's Riverside Medical Center

Pocono Road
Denville, NJ 07834
(201) 625-9565
(800) 367-6274 (in New Jersey)

NEW YORK

New York State Self-Help
Clearinghouse
N.Y. Council on Children &
Families

Empire State Plaza Tower 2
Albany, NY 12224
(518) 474-6293

New York City Self-Help
Clearinghouse

P.O. Box 022812
Brooklyn, NY 11202

Erie County Self-Help
Clearinghouse
Mental Health Association of
Erie County

1237 Delaware Avenue
Buffalo, NY 14209
(716) 886-1242

Long Island Self-Help
Clearinghouse
New York Institute of Technology

Central Islip Campus
Central Islip, NY 11722
(516) 348-3030

Monroe County Self-Help
Clearinghouse
Mental Health Chapter of
Rochester/Monroe

One Mount Hope Avenue
Rochester, NY 14620
(716) 423-9490

Onondaga County Self-Help
Clearinghouse
The Volunteer Center, Inc.

115 Jefferson Street, Suite 300
Syracuse, NY 13202
(315) 474-7011

Westchester Self-Help
Clearinghouse
Westchester Community College

75 Grasslands Road
Valhalla, NY 10595
(914) 949-6301

NORTH CAROLINA

Supportworks

1012 Kings Drive, Suite 923
Charlotte, NC 28283
(704) 331-9500

OHIO

Ohio Self-Help Clearinghouse
Family Service Association

184 Salem Avenue
Dayton, OH 45406
(513) 222-9481

OREGON

Northwest Regional Self-Help
Clearinghouse

718 W. Burnside Avenue
Portland, OR 97209
(503) 222-5555

PENNSYLVANIA

Self-Help Information & Networking
Exchange
Voluntary Action Center of
Northeast Pennsylvania

225 N. Washington Avenue
Park Plaza, Lower Level
Scranton, PA 18503
(717) 961-1234

Self-Help Group Network of the Pittsburgh Area

710 South Avenue
Wilkinsburg, PA 15221
(412) 261-5363

RHODE ISLAND

Support Group Helpline
Rhode Island Department of Health

Cannon Building, Davis Street
Providence, RI 09208
(401) 277-2223

SOUTH CAROLINA

The Support Group Network
Lexington Medical Center

2720 Sunset Boulevard
West Columbia, SC 29169
(803) 791-9227

TENNESSEE

Support Group Clearinghouse
Mental Health Association of
Knox County

6712 Kingston Pike, Suite 203
Knoxville, TN 37919
(615) 584-6736

TEXAS

Dallas Self-Help Clearinghouse
Mental Health Association of
Dallas County

2500 Maple Avenue
Dallas, TX 75201-1998
(214) 871-2420

Tarrant County Self-Help
Clearinghouse
Tarrant County Mental Health
Association

3136 W. 4th Street
Fort Worth, TX 76109
(817) 335-5405

Houston Self-Help Clearinghouse
Mental Health Association in
Houston and Harris County

2211 Norfolk, Suite 810
Houston, TX 77098
(713) 523-8963

Greater San Antonio Self-Help
Clearinghouse
Mental Health Association

1407 N. Main
San Antonio TX 78212
(512) 222-1571

VERMONT

Vermont Self-Help Clearinghouse

P.O. Box 829
Montpelier, VT 05602
(802) 229-5724

VIRGINIA

Greater Virginia Self-Help Coalition
Mental Health Association of
Northern Virginia

100 N. Washington Street,
Suite 232
Falls Church, VA 22046
(703) 642-0800

WASHINGTON

Crisis Clinic/Thurston & Mason
Counties

P.O. Box 2463
Olympia, WA 98507
(800) 627-2211

WASHINGTON, D.C.

Greater Washington Self-Help
Coalition

100 N. Washington Street,
Suite 232
Falls Church, VA 22046
(703) 642-0800

Family Stress Services of D.C.

2001 O Street, N.W., Suite 6
Washington, DC 20036
(202) 628-FACT

WISCONSIN

Health and Human Services
Outreach
University of Wisconsin–Madison

414 Lowell Hall
610 Langdon Street
Madison, WI 53706
(608) 263-4432

Readings and Selected References

CONSUMER BOOKS

Andreasen, Nancy. *The Broken Brain: The Biologic Revolution in Psychiatry.* New York: Harper & Row, 1984.

Beck, Aaron. *Love Is Never Enough.* New York: Harper & Row, 1988.

Bruckner-Gordon, Fredda, Barbara Gangi and Geraldine Wallman. *Making Therapy Work.* New York: Harper & Row, 1988.

Burns, David. *Feeling Good.* New York: William Morrow & Company, 1980.

Copeland, Mary Ellen. *The Depression Workbook.* Oakland, Ca.: New Harbinger Publications, 1992.

Cronkite, Kathy. *On the Edge of Darkness.* New York: Doubleday, 1994.

Duke, Patty, and Gloria Hochman. *A Brilliant Madness.* New York: Bantam Books, 1992.

Engler, Jack, and Daniel Goleman. *The Consumer's Guide to Psychotherapy.* New York: Fireside, 1992.

Fishman, Katharine Davis. *Behind the One-Way Mirror: Psychotherapy and Children.* New York: Bantam Books, 1995.

Garber, Steven, Marianne Garber and Robyn Spizman. *If Your Child Is Hyperactive, Inattentive, Impulsive, Distractible: A Practical Program for Changing Your Child's Behavior with and without Medication.* New York: Villard Books, 1990.

Gorman, Jack. *The Essential Guide to Psychiatric Drugs.* New York: St. Martin's Press, 1990.

Griest, John, and James Jefferson. *Depression and Its Treatment.* Washington, D.C.: American Psychiatric Press, 1992.

Griest, John, and James Jefferson. *Panic Disorder and Agoraphobia: A Guide.* Madison, Wis.: Anxiety Disorders Center and Information Centers, University of Wisconsin, 1992.

Hales, Dianne. *Depression.* New York: Chelsea House, 1989.

———. *How to Sleep like a Baby.* New York: Ballantine, 1987.

———. *Invitation to Health,* 6th ed. Redwood City: Benjamin-Cummings, 1994.

Hallowell, Edward, and John Ratey. *Driven to Distraction.* New York: Pantheon Books, 1994.

Jamison, Kay Redfield. *An Unquiet Mind: A Memoir of Moods and Madness.* New York: Alfred A. Knopf, 1995.

Kaysen, Susanna. *Girl, Interrupted.* New York: Random House, 1993.

Kernodle, William. *Panic Disorder,* 2nd ed. Richmond, Va.: William Byrd Press, 1993.

Klein, Donald, and Paul Wender. *Understanding Depression.* London: Oxford University Press, 1993.

Kramer, Peter. *Listening to Prozac.* New York: Viking, 1993.

Kutner, Lawrence. *Parent and Child.* New York: William Morrow & Company, 1991.

Marks, Jane. *We Have a Problem: A Parent's Sourcebook.* Washington, D.C.: American Psychiatric Press, 1992.

Oldham, John, and Lois Morris. *The Personality Self-Portrait.* New York: Bantam Books, 1990.

Quinnett, Paul. *Suicide: The Forever Decision.* New York: Continuum Books, 1987.

Rapoport, Judith. *The Boy Who Couldn't Stop Washing: The Experience and Treatment of Obsessive-Compulsive Disorder.* New York: Penguin, 1990.

Reinisch, June, and Ruth Beasley. *The Kinsey Institute New Report on Sex.* New York: St. Martin's Press, 1990.

Restak, Richard. *The Mind.* New York: Bantam Books, 1988.

———. *Receptors.* New York: Bantam Books, 1994.

Ross, Jerilyn. *Triumph over Fear.* New York: Bantam Books, 1994.

Seligman, Martin. *Learned Optimism: The Skill to Conquer Life's Obstacles, Large and Small.* New York: Alfred A. Knopf, 1991.

Selye, Hans. *Stress Without Distress.* Philadelphia: J.B. Lippincott, 1974.

Silver, Larry. *Dr. Larry Silver's Advice to Parents on Attention Deficit Hyperactivity Disorder.* Washington, D.C.: American Psychiatric Press, 1993.

Turecki, Stanley. *The Emotional Problems of Normal Children.* New York: Bantam Books, 1994.

Yudofsky, Stuart, Robert E. Hales and Tom Ferguson. *What You Need to Know about Psychiatric Drugs.* New York: Grove, 1991.

PROFESSIONAL BOOKS

Alonso, A., and H.I. Swiller, eds. *Group Therapy in Clinical Practice.* Washington, D.C.: American Psychiatric Press, 1993.

American Psychiatric Association. *Diagnostic and Statistical Manual of Mental Disorders*, 4th ed. Washington, D.C.: American Psychiatric Association, 1994.

Andreasen, Nancy, ed. *Schizophrenia: From Mind to Molecule.* Washington, D.C.: American Psychiatric Press, 1994.

Andreasen, Nancy, and Donald Black. *Introductory Textbook of Psychiatry.* Washington, D.C.: American Psychiatric Press, 1990.

Austin, Linda. *Responding to Disaster.* Washington, D.C.: American Psychiatric Press, 1992.

Beck, Aaron, et al. *Cognitive Therapy of Depression.* New York: Guilford Press, 1979.

Ciraulo, Domenic, and Richard Shader. *Clinical Manual of Chemical Dependence.* Washington, D.C.: American Psychiatric Press, 1991.

Dubovsky, Steven. *Concise Guide to Clinical Psychiatry.* Washington, D.C.: American Psychiatric Press, 1988.

Dulcan, Mina, and Charles Popper. *Concise Guide to Child and Adolescent Psychiatry.* Washington, D.C.: American Psychiatric Press, 1991.

Favazza, Armando. *Bodies Under Siege.* Baltimore: Johns Hopkins University Press, 1987.

Frances, Richard, and John Franklin. *Concise Guide to Treatment of Alcoholism and Addictions.* Washington, D.C.: American Psychiatric Press, 1989.

Glick, Ira, et al. *Marital and Family Therapy*, 3rd ed. Washington, D.C.: American Psychiatric Press, 1987.

Goodwin, Frederick, and Kay Jamison. *Manic-Depressive Illness.* New York: Oxford University Press, 1990.

Hales, Robert E., and Allen Frances, eds. *Psychiatric Update: American Psychiatric Association Annual Review*, Vols. 4-8. Washington, D.C.: American Psychiatric Press, 1985-1989.

Hales, Robert E., Stuart Yudofsky and John Talbott, eds. *American Psychiatric Press Textbook of Psychiatry*, 2nd ed. Washington, D.C.: American Psychiatric Press, 1994.

Harper-Guiffre, Heather, and K. Roy MacKenzie, eds. *Group Therapy for Eating Disorders.* Washington, D.C.: American Psychiatric Press, 1992.

Hollander, Eric. *Obsessive-Compulsive Related Disorders.* Washington, D.C.: American Psychiatric Press, 1993.

Husain, Syed, and Dennis Cantwell. *Fundamentals of Child and Adolescent Psychopathology.* Washington, D.C.: American Psychiatric Press, 1991.

Institute of Medicine. *Sleeping Pills, Insomnia and Medical Practice.* Washington, D.C.: U.S. National Academy of Medical Sciences, 1979.

Jamison, Kay Redfield. *Touched with Fire: Manic-Depressive Illness and the Artistic Temperament.* New York: The Free Press/Macmillan, 1992.

Kane, John (Task Force Chair). *Tardive Dyskinesia.* Washington, D.C.: American Psychiatric Press, 1992.

Karasu, T. Byram (Task Force Chair). *Treatments of Psychiatric Disorders.* Washington, D.C.: American Psychiatric Press, 1989.

Kellner, Robert. *Psychosomatic Syndromes and Somatic Symptoms.* Washington, D.C.: American Psychiatric Press, 1991.

Oldham, John, et al., eds. *American Psychiatric Press Review of Psychiatry,* Vols. 12, 13. Washington, D.C.: American Psychiatric Press, 1993, 1994.

Pato, Michele, and Joseph Zohar. *Current Treatments of Obsessive-Compulsive Disorder.* Washington, D.C.: American Psychiatric Press, 1991.

Reite, Martin, et al. *Concise Guide to the Evaluation and Management of Sleep Disorders.* Washington, D.C.: American Psychiatric Press, 1990.

Ross, Colin. *Multiple Personality Disorder.* New York: John Wiley & Sons, 1989.

Silver, Larry. *Attention-Deficit Hyperactivity Disorder.* Washington, D.C.: American Psychiatric Press, 1992.

Stoudemire, Alan, ed. *Clinical Psychiatry for Medical Students.* Philadelphia: J.B. Lippincott, 1990.

Tardiff, Kenneth. *Concise Guide to Assessment and Management of Violent Patients.* Washington, D.C.: American Psychiatric Press, 1989.

Ursano, Robert. *Concise Guide to Psychodynamic Psychotherapy.* Washington, D.C.: American Psychiatric Press, 1991.

Waldinger, Robert. *Psychiatry for Medical Students,* 2nd ed. Washington, D.C.: American Psychiatric Press, 1990.

Wiener, Jerry, ed. *Textbook of Child and Adolescent Psychiatry.* Washington, D.C.: American Psychiatric Press, 1994.

Wise, Michael, and J.R. Rundell. *The Concise Guide to Consultation Psychiatry*, 2nd ed. Washington, D.C.: American Psychiatric Press, 1994.

Yager, Joel, et al. *Special Problems in Managing Eating Disorders.* Washington, D.C.: American Psychiatric Press, 1992.

Yudofsky, Stuart, and Robert E. Hales. *American Psychiatric Press Textbook of Neuropsychiatry*, 2nd ed. Washington, D.C.: American Psychiatric Press, 1992.

Zerbe, Kathryn. *The Body Betrayed: Women, Eating Disorders, and Treatment.* Washington, D.C.: American Psychiatric Press, 1993.

ARTICLES, CHAPTERS, AND REPORTS

AACAP Work Group on Quality Issues. "Practice Parameters for the Assessment and Treatment of Attention Deficit Hyperactivity Disorder." *Journal of the American Academy of Child and Adolescent Psychiatry*, Vol. 30, i-iii (1991).

AACAP Work Group on Quality Issues. "Practice Parameters for the Assessment and Treatment of Conduct Disorders," *Journal of the American Academy of Child and Adolescent Psychiatry*, Vol. 31, iv-vii (1992).

American Psychiatric Association. *Legal Sanctions for Mental Health Professional-Patient Sex.* June 1993.

Blazer, Dan. "Depression in the Elderly." *New England Journal of Medicine*, 320 (1989).

Cross-National Collaborative Group. "The Changing Rate of Major Depression." *Journal of the American Medical Association*, Vol. 268, No. 21 (December 2, 1992).

Depression Guideline Panel. *Depression in Primary Care.* Rockville, Md.: U.S. Department of Health and Human Services, 1993.

"Drugs That Cause Psychiatric Symptoms." *The Medical Letter*, Vol. 35 (July 23, 1993).

Dulcan, Mina. "Brief Psychotherapy with Children and Their Families: The State of the Art." *Journal of the American Academy of Child and Adolescent Psychiatry*, 23 (1984).

Elkin, E., et al. "National Institute of Mental Health Treatment of Depression Collaborative Research Program: General Effectiveness of Treatment." *Archives of General Psychiatry*, 46 (1989).

Frank, Ellen, et al. "Three-Year Outcomes for Maintenance Therapies in Recurrent Depression." *Archives of General Psychiatry*, Vol. 47 (December 1990).

Gelenberg, Alan, ed.-in-chief. "Anxiety: Special Problems and New Approaches." *The Journal of Clinical Psychiatry*, Vol. 54 (supplement; May 1993).

———. "Recent Advances in Bulimia Nervosa." *The Journal of Clinical Psychiatry*, Vol. 52 (supplement; October 1992).

———. "Treatment Strategies for Complicated Anxiety." *The Journal of Clinical Psychiatry*, Vol. 54 (supplement; May 1993).

Jensen, M.P., et al. "Coping with Chronic Pain: A Critical Review." *Pain*, Vol. 47 (1991).

Kandel, Eric. "Psychotherapy and the Single Synapse: The Impact of Psychiatric Thought on Neurobiologic Research." *New England Journal of Medicine*, 301 (1979).

Katon, Wayne. "Somatization Disorder, Hypochondriasis, and Conversion Disorder." In: *Current Psychotherapy*. Philadelphia: W.B. Saunders, 1993.

Katzman, R., and J.E. Jackson. "Alzheimer's Disease: Basic and Clinical Advances." *Journal of Geriatric Psychiatry*, 39 (1991).

Kessler, Ronald, et al. "Lifetime and 12-Month Prevalence of DSM-IIIR Psychiatric Disorders in the United States: Results from the National Comorbidity Study." *Archives of General Psychiatry*, Vol. 51, No. 1 (January 1994).

Kiecolt-Glaser, Janice, and Ronald Glaser. "Stress and the Immune System: Human Studies." In: *American Psychiatric Press Review of Psychiatry*, Vol. 11. Washington, D.C.: American Psychiatric Press, 1992.

Kluft, Richard. "Multiple Personality Disorder." In: *American Psychiatric Press Review of Psychiatry*, Vol. 10. Washington, D.C.: American Psychiatric Press, 1991.

Kupfer, David, et al. "Five-Year Outcome for Maintenance Therapies in Recurrent Depression." *Archives of General Psychiatry*, 49 (October 1992).

Levenson, Hanna, and Robert E. Hales. "Brief Psychodynamically Informed Therapy: Relevance for the Medically Ill." In: *Medical Psychiatric Practice*, Vol. 2. Washington, D.C.: American Psychiatric Press (in press).

MacKenzie, K.R. "Principles of Brief Intensive Psychotherapy." *Psychiatric Annals*, 21 (1991).

McGrath, Ellen, et al. *Women and Depression: Risk Factors and Treatment Issues.* Washington, D.C.: American Psychological Association, 1990.

National Commission on Sleep Disorders Research. *Wake Up, America: A National Sleep Alert.* 1993.

National Institutes of Health. NIH Consensus Development Conference Statement. *The Treatment of Sleep Disorders in Older Persons.* Washington, D.C.: U.S. Government Printing Office, 1990.

National Institutes of Health. NIH Consensus Development Conference Statement. *Treatment of Panic Disorder.* Bethesda, Md.: NIH, September 1991.

Nierenberg, Andrew. "A Systematic Approach to Treatment-Resistant Depression." *Journal of Clinical Psychiatry Monograph,* Vol. 10, No. 1 (May 1992).

Nolen-Hoeksma, Susan, et al. "Predictors and Consequences of Childhood Depressive Symptoms: A 5-Year Longitudinal Study." *Journal of Abnormal Psychology,* Vol. 101, No. 3 (1992).

Phillips, Kathleen. "Body Dysmorphic Disorder: The Distress of Imagined Ugliness." *American Journal of Psychiatry,* 148 (1991).

Regier, Darrel, et al. "The De Facto U.S. Mental and Addictive Disorders Service System." *Archives of General Psychiatry,* 50 (1993).

Regier, Darrel, et al. "The NIMH Depression Awareness, Recognition, and Treatment Program: Structure, Aims and Scientific Basis." *American Journal of Psychiatry,* Vol. 145, No. 11 (November 1988).

Robins, L.N., et al. "Lifetime Prevalence of Specific Psychiatric Disorders in Three Sites." *Archives of General Psychiatry,* 41 (1984).

Ryan, N.D. "The Pharmacologic Treatment of Children and Adolescents." *Psychiatric Clinics of North America,* 15 (1992).

Solomon, Susan, et al. "Efficacy of Treatments for Posttraumatic Stress Disorder." *Journal of the American Medical Association* (August 5, 1992).

Spiegel, David. "Dissociative Disorders." In: *American Psychiatric Press Review of Psychiatry,* Vol. 10. Washington, D.C.: American Psychiatric Press, 1991.

———. "Hypnosis in the Treatment of Victims of Sexual Abuse." *Psychiatric Clinics of North America,* Vol. 12, No. 2 (June 1989).

Terr, Lenore. "Childhood Traumas: An Outline and Overview." *American Journal of Psychiatry,* Vol. 148 (1991).

Weiss, Kenneth, et al. "The Functioning and Well-being of Depressed Patients." *Journal of American Medical Association,* Vol. 262, No. 7 (August 18, 1989).

Weissman, Myrna, and John Markowitz. "Interpersonal Psychotherapy: Current Status." *Archives of General Psychiatry,* Vol. 51 (August 1994).

Wise, Michael, and Sally Taylor. "Anxiety and Mood Disorders in Medically Ill Patients." *Journal of Clinical Psychiatry,* Vol. 51, No. 1 (supplement; January 1990).

Index

*In the United States, aspirin is a generic term; in Canada, Aspirin is a registered trademark.